T0181590

Register Now for Online Access to Your Book!

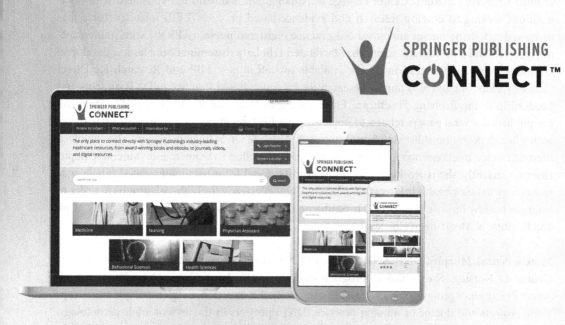

Your print purchase of *Research for Advanced Practice Nurses, Fourth Edition*, **includes online access to the contents of your book**—increasing accessibility, portability, and searchability!

Access today at:
http://connect.springerpub.com/content/book/978-0-8261-5133-9
or scan the QR code at the right with your smartphone
and enter the access code below.

1VNM8CPX

Scan here for quick access.

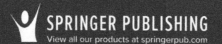
SPRINGER PUBLISHING
View all our products at springerpub.com

Beth A. Staffileno, PhD, FAHA, is a professor in the department of Adult Health and Gerontological Nursing and co-director of the Center for Clinical Research and Scholarship at Rush University Medical Center College of Nursing. Dr. Staffileno has consulted with organizations seeking to develop research and evidence-based practice (EBP) infrastructures, has mentored practicing nurses and advanced practice registered nurses (APRNs) with implementing research and EBP initiatives, and has facilitated scholarly dissemination. She has developed an online continuing education course available to staff nurses, EBP and Research for Direct Care Providers. She has also taught Research for Evidence-Based Practice to DNP students and Leadership in the Evolving Healthcare Environment to DNP and PhD students. Dr. Staffileno has published several papers related to implementing EBP initiatives, and is an active researcher with a health promotion/disease prevention focus. Much of Dr. Staffileno's research has involved lifestyle change interventions for cardiovascular risk reduction in women and vulnerable populations. Currently, she is working with an interprofessional team using augmented intelligence technology to tailor health information efficiently and effectively for high-risk groups in order to promote healthy lifestyle behaviors. Dr. Staffileno is a Fellow of the American Heart Association and Institute of Medicine of Chicago.

Marcia Pencak Murphy, DNP, ANP, FAHA, FPCNA, is a professor emeritus at Rush University College of Nursing. She served as program director of the Adult-Gerontology Primary Care Nurse Practitioner program for 15 years. She has extensive experience supervising master's capstone projects and doctor of nursing practice (DNP) projects in the area of adult-gerontology. Dr. Murphy has over 30 years of experience as an advanced practice registered nurse (APRN) in both acute care and community settings. She has published and presented several papers on the topic of clinical scholarship for APRNs. Dr. Murphy has received several distinguished awards including Fellow of the American Heart Association, Fellow of the Preventive Cardiovascular Nurses Association, and Fellow of the Institute of Medicine of Chicago, and is active in several organizations, including the Preventive Cardiovascular Nurses Association, the American Heart Association, and the Institute of Medicine of Chicago.

Susan Weber Buchholz, PhD, RN, FAANP, FAAN, is a professor, Associate Dean for Research, and Director of the PhD Program at Michigan State University College of Nursing. Dr. Buchholz is funded by the National Institutes of Health's (NIH's) National Institute of Nursing Research. The long-term goal of her research program is to develop cost-effective strategies to increase physical activity among low physically active adults. Within her research, she uses innovative mHealth strategies to promote physical activity. Globally, she is one of the first researchers to use a Sequential Multiple Assignment Randomized Trial design to explore how to optimize adaptive interventions to improve physical activity. She has conducted and published on her quantitative and qualitative research, including integrative and systematic reviews. As an adult nurse practitioner faculty member, she is committed to high-quality nurse practitioner education and is currently serving as President-Elect on the National Organization of Nurse Practitioner Faculties Board. She is a Fellow in the American Academy of Nursing. She is also a Fellow in the American Association of Nurse Practitioners and served as the Chair of the inaugural American Association of Nurse Practitioners Nursing Research Committee.

RESEARCH FOR ADVANCED PRACTICE NURSES

FROM EVIDENCE TO PRACTICE

FOURTH EDITION

Beth A. Staffileno, PhD, FAHA

Marcia Pencak Murphy, DNP, ANP, FAHA, FPCNA

Susan Weber Buchholz, PhD, RN, FAANP, FAAN

Editors

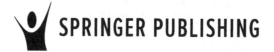 SPRINGER PUBLISHING

Springer Publishing Company, LLC
11 West 42nd Street, New York, NY 10036
www.springerpub.com
connect.springerpub.com/

Acquisitions Editor: Joseph Morita
Compositor: Exeter Premedia Services Private Ltd.

ISBN: 978-0-8261-5132-2
ebook ISBN: 978-0-8261-5133-9
DOI: 10.1891/9780826151339

Qualified instructors may request supplements by emailing textbook@springerpub.com

Instructor's PowerPoints ISBN: 978-0-8261-5134-6

21 22 23 24 25 / 5 4 3 2 1

The author and the publisher of this Work have made every effort to use sources believed to be reliable to provide information that is accurate and compatible with the standards generally accepted at the time of publication. Because medical science is continually advancing, our knowledge base continues to expand. Therefore, as new information becomes available, changes in procedures become necessary. We recommend that the reader always consult current research and specific institutional policies before performing any clinical procedure or delivering any medication. The author and publisher shall not be liable for any special, consequential, or exemplary damages resulting, in whole or in part, from the readers' use of, or reliance on, the information contained in this book. The publisher has no responsibility for the persistence or accuracy of URLs for external or third-party Internet websites referred to in this publication and does not guarantee that any content on such websites is, or will remain, accurate or appropriate.

Library of Congress Control Number: 2020952107

Contact us to receive discount rates on bulk purchases.
We can also customize our books to meet your needs.
For more information please contact: sales@springerpub.com

Publisher's Note: **New and used products purchased from third-party sellers are not guaranteed for quality, authenticity, or access to any included digital components.**

Beth A. Staffileno: https://orcid.org/0000-0003-3712-2207
Susan Weber Buchholz: https://orcid.org/0000-0002-6311-9709

CONTENTS

CONTRIBUTORS

Anne W. Alexandrov, PhD, AGACNP-BC, ANVP-BC, NVRN-BC, CCRN, FAAN, Professor of Nursing and Neurology, University of Tennessee Health Science Center (UTHSC), Memphis, Tennessee

Mary D. Bondmass, PhD, RN, CNE, Associate Professor in Residence, School of Nursing, University of Nevada, Las Vegas, Nevada

Susan Weber Buchholz, PhD, RN, FAANP, FAAN, Professor, Associate Dean for Research, Director of the PhD Program, Michigan State University, College of Nursing, East Lansing, Michigan

Elizabeth A. Carlson, RN, PhD, Professor Emerita, Adult Health and Gerontological Nursing, Rush University, College of Nursing, Chicago, Illinois

Leslie A. Christensen, MLIS, Health Sciences Librarian, Ebling Library, University of Wisconsin School of Medicine and Public Health, Madison, Wisconsin

Claire Cunningham, DNP, NP-C, Neurology Advanced Practice Nurse, Loyola University Medical Center, Maywood, Illinois

Uchita A. Dave, MS, Manager, Institutional Research, Rush University, Chicago, Illinois

Susan K. Frazier, PhD, RN, FAHA, Associate Professor, Co-Director, RICH Heart Program, College of Nursing, University of Kentucky, Lexington, Kentucky

Carol Glod, RN, PhD, FAAN, Professor and Chair, Department of Public Health and Nutrition School of Health Sciences, Merrimack College, North Andover, Massachusetts

Lindsey Gradone, DNP, APRN-CNP, Division of Pulmonary and Critical Care, Northwestern Memorial Hospital, Chicago, Illinois

Mary Heitschmidt, RN, PhD, APRN, CCRN-K, Assistant Professor, Women, Children and Family Nursing, Rush College of Nursing; Co-Director, Center for Clinical Research and Scholarship, Rush College of Nursing; Director of Clinical Research, Rush University Medical Center and Rush Oak Park Hospital, Chicago, Illinois

Mary E. Hitchcock, MA, MLIS, Health Sciences Librarian, Ebling Library, University of Wisconsin School of Medicine and Public Health, Madison, Wisconsin

Lisa J. Hopp, PhD, RN, FAAN, Dean and Professor, College of Nursing, Purdue University Northwest, Hammond, Indiana

Briana J. Jegier, PhD, Associate Professor and Chair, Health Administration, Baptist Health Sciences University, Memphis, Tennessee; Adjunct Assistant Professor, College of Health Sciences, Rush University, Chicago, Illinois

Mary E. Johnson, PhD, RN, PMHCNS (retired), CNE, FAAN, Professor Emerita, Community Systems and Mental Health Nursing, Rush University College of Nursing, Chicago, Illinois

Tricia J. Johnson, PhD, Professor, Department of Health Systems Management, Rush University, Chicago, Illinois

Izabela Kazana, DNP, APRN, AGPCNP-BC, CPHQ, CHCQM, Director of Quality, University of Illinois Health Oncology Service Line, University of Illinois Cancer Center, Chicago, Illinois

Tracy Klein, PhD, FNP, ARNP, FAANP, FRE, FAAN, Associate Professor, College of Nursing, Washington State University Vancouver, Vancouver, Washington

Katherine A. Maki, PhD, APRN, AGPCNP-BC, Laboratory for Sleep Neurobiology, College of Nursing, University of Illinois at Chicago, Chicago, Illinois

Lea Ann Matura, PhD, RN, FAAN, Associate Professor, University of Pennsylvania, School of Nursing, Philadelphia, Pennsylvania

Jessica Mauleon, DNP, AGPCNP-C, Internal Medicine Nurse Practitioner, Senior Care Physicians of Illinois, Lincolnshire, Illinois

Kerry A. Milner, DNSc, RN, EBP-C, Associate Professor, Sacred Heart University, Davis & Henley College of Nursing, Fairfield, Connecticut

Marcia Pencak Murphy, DNP, ANP, FAHA, FPCNA, Professor Emerita, Adult Health and Gerontological Nursing, Rush University, College of Nursing, Chicago, Illinois

Patricia F. Pearce, PhD, FNP-BC, FAANP, FNAP, Professor and Interim Chair, Department of Nursing, Clarke University, Dubuque, Iowa

Vivian Nowazek, PhD, MSN, APRN, FNP-BC, CNS-CC, Clinical Associate Professor, School of Nursing, College of Health Sciences, Sam Houston State University, The Woodlands, Texas

Marcia Phillips, PhD, RN, Assistant Professor, Adult Health and Gerontological Nursing College of Nursing, Assistant Professor, Department of Internal Medicine, Rush Medical College, Chicago, Illinois

Lisa A. Rauch, DNP, APHA-BC, RN, Assistant Director and Curriculum Coordinator, The Valley Foundation School of Nursing at San Jose State University, San Jose, California

Beth Rodgers, PhD, RN, FAAN, Professor Emerita, University of Wisconsin–Milwaukee, College of Nursing, Milwaukee, Wisconsin

Karen J. Saewert, PhD, RN, CPHQ, ANEF, Clinical Professor, Edson College of Nursing and Health Innovation, Arizona State University, Phoenix, Arizona

Beth A. Staffileno, PhD, FAHA, Professor, Adult Health and Gerontological Nursing, Co-Director, Center for Clinical Research and Scholarship, Rush University, College of Nursing, Chicago, Illinois

Kathleen R. Stevens, RN, EdD, ANEF, FAAN, Castella Endowed Distinguished Professor, University of Texas Health Science Center San Antonio, San Antonio, Texas

Rosemarie Suhayda, PhD, RN, Assistant Dean Emerita, Rush University, Chicago, Illinois

Karen M. Vuckovic, PhD, APRN ACNS-BC, FAHA, Clinical Associate Professor, College of Nursing, University of Illinois, Chicago, Illinois

Mary C. Zonsius, PhD, RN, Associate Professor, Adult Health and Gerontological Nursing Department, Assistant Dean—Evaluation, Rush University, College of Nursing, Chicago, Illinois

PREFACE

The increasing focus on evidence needed for practice decisions propels us to re-envision how we teach graduate students about research and evidence-based practice (EBP). This book serves as a resource for graduate students and practicing advanced practice registered nurses (APRNs) who contribute to the scholarly output in the discipline, particularly in the area of clinical practice. Similar to the previous editions, this book is unique because it is designed specifically for APRNs. Increasing numbers of APRNs are prepared with a doctorate in nursing practice (DNP) degree. DNP graduates are expert clinicians who have the knowledge and skills to address problems and improve outcomes in real-world health settings. APRNs prepared with a PhD degree are also engaged in practice scholarship. Collaborative teams, comprising APRNs prepared with master's and doctoral degrees, can accelerate the translation of evidence into practice to improve health outcomes. Therefore, this book teaches APRNs prepared at the master's and doctoral levels how to (a) find relevant and current evidence, (b) appraise the evidence, (c) translate evidence into practice to improve patient care and outcomes, and (d) disseminate findings. This book expands on the previous edition by:

- Providing a chapter on quality improvement (QI) models, processes, and tools
- Expanding Chapter 14 (systematic reviews) to include integrative and literature reviews
- Adding a chapter with exemplars of APRN-led initiatives that showcase improved processes and health outcomes

Part I: Evidence-Based Practice. The chapters in Part I focus on an overview of EBP: the definitions of EBP that have evolved over time, types of evidence, and models of EBP. Strategies for finding evidence are presented to guide the reader to respond to the mandate for EBP. Additionally, a brief history of QI is presented along with various models, processes, and tools. This information on EBP and QI is vital to graduate students who are developing skills that will prepare them to assume their advanced practice role in health care.

Part II: Building Blocks for Evidence. The section starts with appraising a single research article, a building block for evidence. Components of the research process are presented from a reviewer's perspective of using the article as supporting evidence for practice in subsequent chapters. One of the documented barriers to EBP is that practitioners feel inadequate reading and interpreting research findings. Gaining knowledge about the research process is crucial for practitioners who must read, interpret, and determine the relevance of research findings (evidence) to practice.

Part III: Using Available Evidence. Meta-analyses, systematic reviews, integrative reviews, and practice guidelines from various sources, such as professional organizations and government websites, are other types of evidence that may be used in establishing EBP. Appraising information from these sources is suggested in this section. Program evaluation provides an opportunity for use of evidence. Considerations when planning and implementing EBP activities are also included in this section—that is, identifying the focus of EBP activities (unit or organizational) and developing an EBP protocol.

Part IV: Evaluating the Impact of Evidence-Based Practice, Ethical Aspects of a Study, and Communicating Results. Cost, outcomes, and ethical aspects are essential components of EBP and QI. Communicating ideas through oral and written avenues is valuable in making EBP and QI a reality. Techniques for acquiring oral and written methods for presenting ideas are included; such techniques are helpful in writing protocols and reporting outcomes of EBP and QI activities. This section concludes with exemplars of APRN-led initiatives that highlight improved healthcare processes, outcomes, and resultant dissemination.

Although graduate students are the primary audience for this book—a textbook for a graduate course in nursing research or an interdisciplinary health care course—nurses in clinical settings will also find the book helpful in fulfilling their research role toward achieving hospital Magnet® status. Our hope is that the information presented in this book will be used to provide optimal cost-efficient care to patients, which will increase their quality of life.

We acknowledge the work of Marquis D. Foreman, PhD, RN, FAAN, for his contributions to previous editions of this book.

Beth A. Staffileno
Marcia Pencak Murphy
Susan Weber Buchholz

EVIDENCE-BASED PRACTICE

OVERVIEW OF EVIDENCE-BASED PRACTICE

MARY D. BONDMASS

▨ INTRODUCTION

This chapter begins with an overview of evidence-based practice (EBP) including generally accepted definitions, central tenets, barriers and facilitators, and trends over time. Additionally, an overview of the necessary underlying components of EBP are explored, these being the actual providers of EBP and the competencies required of EBP providers, specifically advanced practice registered nurses (APRNs).

▨ EBP DEFINITIONS

Multiple definitions of EBP have been proposed and have evolved over the years. One of the most common definitions of EBP in use today was derived from an initial proposal for evidence-based medicine by Sackett et al. (2000). Over time the Sackett et al.'s definition evolved, such that many contemporary texts and publications agree on the definition of EBP to be "the integration of best research evidence with clinical expertise and patient values and circumstances" (Straus et al., 2005, p. 1). While many other excellent definitions are used in the literature, most would agree that Straus et al.'s definition is inclusive enough for universal use.

Regardless of the exact definition, or which discipline supports which nomenclature, there exists today much discussion and debate about implementation, barriers, facilitators, evaluation, and perhaps more importantly, the health outcomes for patients in an EBP environment. Positive health outcomes should logically result from knowledge generated from research and be reflec-tive of an effective EBP environment; however, positive health outcomes in the United States lag far behind what we know about safe and effective healthcare, especially considering the high cost of U.S. healthcare. The knowledge-to-practice gap is even more apparent when health status outcomes are compared with those of other countries. Current data from the Organisation for Economic Cooperation and Development (OECD, 2019), indicate that the worldwide spending on health is about $4,000 per person (adjusted for purchasing power) on average across OECD countries (Figure 1.1), but the United States spends more than all other countries by a consid-erable margin, at over $10,000 per resident (Institute of Medicine [IOM], 2015b; OECD, 2019). Indeed the United States spends more than twice as much on healthcare than other developed countries, yet according to multiple indicators of health status, the United States is ranked con-siderably lower (OECD, 2019). Unsurprisingly, studies continue to indicate that the U.S. health system is inefficient. In 2013, the IOM estimated that upward of $750 billion of healthcare spend-ing could be attributed to excess costs. Moreover, despite an increased knowledge base and a

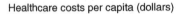

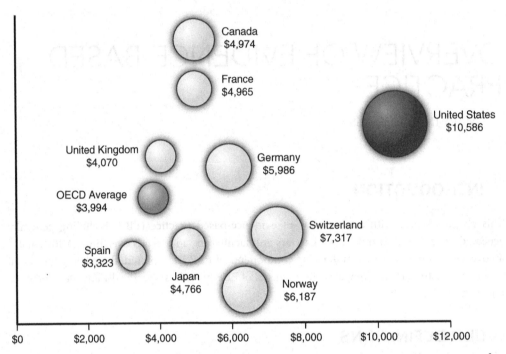

FIGURE 1.1 United States per capita healthcare spending is more than twice the average of other developed countries.

Source: Data from Organisation for Economic Co-operation and Development, OECD Health Statistics, 2019, November 2019.

Notes: Data are from 2018. Chart uses purchasing power parities to convert data into U.S. dollars.

considerable monetary investment, there is no corresponding improvement in U.S. health outcomes; in fact, the United States falls measurably behind our international peers across essential measures of access, equity, and efficiency (IOM, 2015b).

Extending back two decades, this concerning trend in the knowledge-to-practice gap has been acknowledged and written about (IOM, 2000, 2001, 2003, 2010, 2015a; OECD, 2019). While strategic direction from policymakers needs to continually address quality and safety issues at the system or macro level, nurses (academic educators, advanced practitioners, and hospital administrators) have a role in ensuring competent practice, to the end of improving various health-related outcomes. While some may be discouraged by the slow pace of EBP implementation, progress has been made regarding the competence and the competencies expected of the nursing healthcare workforce. Insistence on EBP competence and competencies are strategies that nurses may consider within our collective scope of practice.

Providers from many health-related professions believe the implementation of EBP promotes safety, quality of care, and consistency, and improves patient outcomes while decreasing healthcare costs (Aste et al., 2020; Copeland et al., 2020; Jin & Yi, 2019; Lewis et al., 2019; Melnyk, 2016; Taxman, 2018). The IOM further recommended that 90% of clinical decisions be evidence-based by 2020 (IOM, 2010). Despite this recommendation, a persistent gap remains between what care providers do and what care providers should do based on the best available evidence (IOM, 2010; Melnyk et al., 2018), yet barriers to EBP implementation persist.

▩ BARRIERS AND FACILITATORS

Regardless of profession or country of practice, much has been written over the past 20-plus years about the barriers and facilitators to implementing EBP. Data relating to EBP barriers and facilitators were found in the literature even before the first of the IOMs sentinel reports and extend through today. Primarily, lack of general EBP knowledge and skills (e.g., searching and critically appraising the literature) lead the list of barriers and overcoming these barriers is believed to be the most effective way to facilitate an EBP environment (Al-Jamei et al., 2019; Alqahtani et al., 2020; Baig et al., 2016; Bhor et al., 2019; Bianchi et al., 2018; Garcia et al., 2019; Hallum-Montes et al., 2016; Haynes & Haines, 1998; Hong et al., 2019; Labrague et al., 2019; Newman et al., 1998; Nolan et al., 1998; Oliver & Lang, 2018; Renolen et al., 2020; Rojjanasrirat & Rice, 2017; Rossi et al., 2020; Shayan et al., 2019; Skela-Savič et al., 2017; Youssef et al., 2018). Other barriers include difficulty with time constraints, limited support from organizations (Connor et al., 2016; Melnyk et al., 2012), and perhaps the most disheartening of all, resistance from colleagues (Melnyk et al., 2012).

However, despite the barriers, when nurses specifically are surveyed about their beliefs and attitudes toward EBP, they continue to indicate that they value EBP and that critical appraisal of the literature is essential to translate current knowledge into practice to produce positive patient outcomes (Alqahtani et al., 2020; Azmoude et al., 2018; Bhor et al., 2019; Li et al., 2019; Stokke et al., 2014; van Der Goot et al., 2018).

▩ EVIDENCE-BASED PRACTICE COMPETENCE AND COMPETENCIES FOR EDUCATION AND PRACTICE

Core practice needs were identified in 2001, indicating that healthcare should be safe, effective, patient-centered, timely, efficient, and equitable. Subsequently, in 2003, five core competencies were recommended by the IOM for the healthcare education curriculum with a focus on EBP. Today, as the latest edition of this text is prepared for publication, EBP, and the need for an effective EBP curriculum in healthcare education, still exist. Data are clear and compelling that healthcare education must produce competent practitioners to meet the needs of EBP (IOM, 2010, 2015a; Melnyk et al. 2018; QSEN Institute, 2012; Stevens, 2009). Following the implementation of the 2010 legislation of the Health Care and Education Reconciliation Act and the Affordable Care Act, nursing is at the forefront of leading this change in both education and practice. *The Future of Nursing: Leading Change, Advancing Health* report from the IOM (2010), and the *Quality and Safety Education for Nurses* (QSEN) initiative from the University of North Carolina and the American Association of Colleges of Nursing (AACN, 2012), are two examples of exciting initiatives available to advise and guide nursing on leading change in education and on EBP (IOM, 2010, 2015a; QSEN Institute, 2012).

▩ COMPETENCY/COMPETENCE DEFINITIONS

Most might agree that the general definition of competency or competence is the ability or capability to accomplish something. Merriam-Webster defines competence as ". . . possession of sufficient knowledge or skill . . ." and competency ". . . as a specific area of competence . . ." (Merriam-Webster, 2020). More specifically, for our profession, the American Nurses

Association (ANA, 2014, p. 64) define competency as "an expected and measurable level of nursing performance that integrates knowledge, skills, abilities, and judgment, based on established scientific knowledge and expectations for nursing practice." Moreover, in the past two decades, multiple authors, from various disciples, have published similar definitions of competence or competencies when teaching or evaluating EBP (Claus et al., 2020; Kim et al., 2015; Jin & Yi, 2019; Lee & Seomun, 2016; Melnyk, 2016, 2017; Odhwani et al., 2019; Saunders & Vehvilainen-Julkunen, 2018; Stevens, 2005, 2009; Stiffler & Cullen, 2010; Ruzafa-Martinez et al., 2013).

■ EXISTING EBP COMPETENCIES

While *The Future of Nursing* report (IOM, 2010, 2015a) plotted a course to position nurses for advanced practice, the QSEN competencies provide specific knowledge, skills, and attitudes that are quite similar to, and no doubt developed from, the original five core competencies proposed by the IOM in 2003 to ensure quality in patient care. Comparisons of the core competencies recommended by the IOM in 2003 and the 2012 QSEN competency categories are displayed in Table 1.1. The graduate-level QSEN competencies for EBP are listed in Table 1.2.

Of note, *The Baccalaureate Essentials for Professional Nursing Practice* (AACN, 2008), *The Essentials of Master's Education in Nursing* (AACN, 2011), and *The Essentials of Doctoral Education for Advanced Nursing Practice* (AACN, 2006, 2015) were also developed using data and recommendations from the IOM (2003) report; however, all the AACN Essentials are currently in the process of revision; therefore, this chapter will briefly discuss some of the proposed conceptual, forward-focused changes to the AACN Essentials related to competencies and their role in evidence-based nursing education (AACN, 2019).

■ ADDITIONAL EVIDENCE-BASED PRACTICE COMPETENCIES FOR EDUCATION AND PRACTICE

Competency-based education, as preparation for practice, is emerging within the health professions to address training deficits (Claus et al., 2020; Englander et al., 2013; Jin & Yi, 2019;

TABLE 1.1 Comparisons of the Core Competencies Proposed by the Institute of Medicine (IOM) in 2003 and the 2012 Quality and Safety Education for Nurses (QSEN) Competency Categories

IOM (2003)	QSEN: SKILL, KNOWLEDGE, AND ATTITUDE (2012)
• Patient-centered care	• Patient-centered care
• Interdisciplinary skills	• Teamwork and collaboration
• Quality improvement skills	• Quality improvement
• Information technology	• Informatics
• Evidence-based practice	• Evidence-based practice
	• Safety

TABLE 1.2 Graduate-Level Quality and Safety Education for Nurses (QSEN) Competencies for Evidence-Based Practice (EBP)

KNOWLEDGE	SKILLS	ATTITUDES
Demonstrate knowledge of health research methods and processes	Use health research methods and processes, alone or in partnership with scientists, to generate new knowledge for practice	Appreciate the strengths and weaknesses of scientific bases for practice
Describe evidence-based practice to include the components of research evidence, clinical expertise, and patient/family/community values	Role model clinical decision-making based on evidence, clinical expertise, and patient/family/community preferences	Value all components of evidence-based practice
Identify efficient and effective search strategies to locate reliable sources of evidence	Employ efficient and effective search strategies to answer focused clinical or health system practices	Value development of search skills for locating evidence for best practice
Identify principles that comprise the critical appraisal of research evidence	Critically appraise original research and evidence summaries related to the area of practice	Value knowing the evidence base for one's practice specialty area
Summarize current evidence regarding major diagnostic and treatment actions within the practice specialty and healthcare delivery system	Exhibit contemporary knowledge of best evidence related to practice and healthcare systems	Value cutting-edge knowledge of the current practice
Determine evidence gaps within the practice specialty and healthcare delivery system	Promote a research agenda for evidence that is needed in the practice specialty and healthcare system	Value working in an interactive manner with the institutional review board
Identify strategies to address gaps in evidence-based guidelines	Use quality improvement methods to address gaps in evidence-based guidelines	Appreciate the gaps in evidence related to practice
Develop knowledge that can lead the translation of research into evidence-based practice	Build consensus among key stakeholders through the use of change theory to create evidence-based care	Champion the changes required that support evidence-based practice
Analyze how the strength of available evidence influences care (assessment, diagnosis, treatment, and evaluation)	Implement care practices based on strength of available evidence	Appreciate the strength of evidence on provision of care
Evaluate organizational cultures and structures that promote evidence-based practice	Participate in designing organizational systems that support evidence-based practice	Appreciate that organizational systems can significantly influence nursing's efforts in evidence-based practice
Understand the need to define critical questions related to practice and healthcare system delivery	Use coaching skills to engage nurses in evidence-based practice and research	Appreciate that all nurses can participate in creating evidence-based practice

Source: From Cronenwett, L., Sherwood, G., Pohl, J., Barnsteiner, J., Moore, S., Sullivan, D. T., Ward, D., & Warren, J. (2009). Quality and safety education for advanced nursing practice. Nursing Outlook, 57(6), 338–348. https://doi.org/10.1016/j.outlook.2009.07.009; data were retrieved from http://www.qsen.org.

Nodine, 2016). Moreover, at the national level, consensus is growing related to competency-based education to prepare health professionals (Englander et al., 2013; Jin & Yi, 2019; Josiah Macy Jr. Foundation, 2017; Kavanagh & Szweda, 2017; Litwack & Brower, 2018; Tharp-Barrie et al., 2020; Wagner et al., 2018).

There remains, however, a continued challenge to translate research results into evidence-based clinical nursing practice. Many educators and researchers suggest that nurses who are educated in the EBP methodology believe their most effective clinical decisions are based on scientific knowledge, practice expertise, and client preference in the context of the healthcare delivery setting (Stevens, 2009; Stokke et al., 2014). The IOM (2010, 2015a) wrote that professionals should be educated to deliver patient-centered care, as members of an interprofessional team emphasizing EBP and quality improvement. Moreover, in the seminal report *The Future of Nursing*, the IOM recommended that faculty partner with healthcare organizations to develop and prioritize competencies, regularly updating curricula to ensure graduates meet future healthcare needs (IOM, 2010). Education-based competencies can translate into clinical practice, whereas continuing education of nurses within healthcare organizations or through professional development may sustain competency (Kesten et al., 2019).

Stevens (2005, 2009) developed and published the first national consensus-based essential EBP competencies in nursing based on, and corresponding to, the Stevens Star Model of Knowledge Transformation (Stevens, 2004). The five star points of the Stevens Star Model of Knowledge Transformation include *Primary Research* (new knowledge discovered through traditional research methodologies), *Evidence Summary* (the body of research synthesized into the state of the knowledge), *Translation* (evidence translated into clinical practice guidelines), *Integration* (implementation of changes in individual, organizational, and environmental practices), and *Evaluation* (outcome evaluation of efficacy, efficiency, and satisfaction for both providers and patients). The EBP competency development project used a survey and content analysis approach and a consensus-forming expert panel to identify and gain consensus on EBP competency statements. These EBP competencies were leveled across nursing education, including associate, baccalaureate, master, and doctoral knowledge. Steven's 2005 and 2009 national consensus editions for essential EBP competencies are inclusive of the EBP skills and content for nursing education, and provide a basis for professional competencies in clinical practice (Kesten et al., 2019). Stevens's EBP competencies have additionally served as an assessment strategy for undergraduate and graduate research and EBP courses (Bondmass, 2009; Bondmass, 2011; Kesten et al., 2013; Kesten et al. 2019; Whorley et al., 2018).

In a comprehensive text, Melnyk and Fineout-Overholt (2018) describe the two-step process of research and consensus-building, which began in 2014, and resulted in the publication of 24 EBP competencies; 11 of which are for generalist RNs and all 24 applicable for APRNs (Gallagher-Ford et al., 2020; Melnyk et al., 2014; Melnyk, 2016; Melnyk et al., 2018). While the core EBP competencies may be similar to previously discussed competencies (IOM, 2003; QSEN Institute, 2012; Stevens, 2005, 2009), Melnyk et al. incorporate the formulation of clinical questions using the PICOT format, which represents patient population, intervention or area of interest, comparison intervention or group, outcome, and time. The use of PICOT questions, widely used in many current EBP courses, differentiates Melnyk et al.'s EBP competencies from others. However, whichever set of competencies you may choose in your classroom or practice setting, the achievement of the essential knowledge and skills associated with EBP should be the goal to ensure the best outcome for our patients and their families.

▦ PROPOSED AMERICAN ASSOCIATION OF COLLEGES OF NURSING *ESSENTIALS* REVISIONS

The AACN and the IOM (2010) have identified EBP as a fundamental competency for nursing. The AACN specifically addresses EBP in *The Essentials of Master's Education in Nursing* (2011) as Essential IV: Translating and Integrating Scholarship into Practice: "Program graduates must possess the skills necessary to bring evidence-based practice to both individual patients for whom they directly care and to those patients for whom they are indirectly responsible" (AACN, 2011, p. 16).

Currently, and consistent with the current literature, the AACN formed an *Essentials* Task Force to begin revisions of the existing Baccalaureate, Masters, and DNP Essentials. In the *Executive Summary of AACN's Vision for Academic Nursing*, the *Essentials* Task Force addresses overarching academic nursing considerations and future goals. One of the primary suggested actions for moving toward this AACN vision includes the transition to competency-based education and assessment (AACN, 2019).

The AACN's vision for the revision of all the *Essentials* is based on a competency-based framework, adapting the work of Englander et al. (2013), to include a set of core domains and essential skills within each respective domain. The *Essentials* Task Force is in the process of building awareness and consensus around developing the new *Essentials* via national faculty meetings, webinars, and conference presentations. A date for the final version of the revised *Essentials* to be published is not yet set, but given the enormity and the thoughtful depth needed for this project, it is not expected in the immediate future.

▦ SUMMARY

"Knowing is not enough; we must apply. Willing is not enough; we must do."

—*Goethe*

This chapter provided a brief overview of EBP definitions, barriers, facilitators, and academic and clinical EBP competencies as a snapshot of the future challenges and expectations for APRNs in an interprofessional EBP environment. Additionally, the expectations and responsibilities of the DNP, APRNs, and other advanced nursing practice specialties are included in the EBP competencies with leading initiatives to improve health outcomes. In the following chapters of this text, in-depth and specific material will be presented with the intent to prepare APRNs for their leadership role in healthcare related to research and EBP.

SUGGESTED LEARNING ACTIVITIES

1. Search the literature or look within your healthcare organization for an example of how a nurse, educated to the level of advanced nursing practice (preferably an MSN or DNP), implemented an evidence-based change initiative or quality improvement project that measurably improved health outcomes, thus demonstrating an EBP competency.

2. Gather a group of colleagues, either in your clinical or classroom setting, and conduct a self-assessment using the QSEN's graduate-level EBP competencies related to your knowledge, skills, and attitudes; then compare your results.

3. With colleagues at your institution, discuss which of the EBP competencies or combination of the competencies referenced in this chapter would fit best within your institution's culture.

REFERENCES

Aste, R., Hjalmhult, E., Hoye, S., Danbolt, L. J., & Kirkevold, M. (2020). Creating room for evidence-based practice: Leader behavior in hospital wards. *Research in Nursing & Health, 43*(1), 90–102. https://doi.org/10.1002/nur.21981

Al-Jamei, S., Abu Farha, R., Zawiah, M., Kadi, T., & Al-Sonidar, A. (2019). Perceptions, knowledge, and perceived barriers of Yemeni pharmacists and pharmacy technicians towards evidence-based practice. *Journal of Evaluation in Clinical Practice, 25*(4), 585–590. https://doi.org/10.1111/jep.12988

Alqahtani, N., Oh, K. M., Kitsantas, P., & Rodan, M. (2020) Nurses' evidence-based practice knowledge, attitudes and implementation: A cross-sectional study. *Journal of Clinical Nursing, 29*(1–2), 274–283. https://doi.org/10.1111/jocn.15097

American Association of Colleges of Nursing. (2006). *The essentials of doctoral education for advanced nursing practice.* http://www.aacn.nche.edu/publications/position/DNPEssentials.pdf

American Association of Colleges of Nursing. (2008). *The essentials of baccalaureate education for professional Nursing Practice.* https://www.aacnnursing.org/Portals/42/Publications/BaccEssentials08.pdf

American Association of Colleges of Nursing. (2011). *The essentials of master's education in nursing.* https://www.aacnnursing.org/Portals/42/Publications/MastersEssentials11.pdf

American Association of Colleges of Nursing. (2012). *Graduate-level QSEN competencies knowledge, skills, and attitudes.* National Academies Press. http://www.aacn.nche.edu/faculty/qsen/competencies.pdf

American Association of Colleges of Nursing. (2015). *Report from the Task Force on the Implementation of the DNP; Current Issues and Clarifying Recommendations.* http://www.aacn.nche.edu/news/articles/2015/dnp-white-paper

American Association of Colleges of Nursing. (2019). *AACN's vision for academic nursing: Executive Summary.* https://www.aacnnursing.org/Portals/42/News/White-Papers/Vision-Academic-Nursing.pdf

American Nurses Association. (Reaffirmed November 12, 2014). ANA Position Statement: Professional Role Competence. https://www.nursingworld.org/practice-policy/nursing-excellence/official-position-statements/id/professional-role-competence/

Azmoude, E., Aradmehr, M., & Dehghani, F. (2018). Midwives' attitude and barriers of evidence based practice in maternity care. *The Malaysian Journal of Medical Sciences, 25*(3), 120–128. https://doi.org/10.21315/mjms2018.25.3.12

Baig, M., Sayedalamin, Z., Almouteri, O., Algarni, M., & Allam, H. (2016). Perceptions, perceived barriers and practices of physicians' towards evidence-based medicine. *Pakistan Journal of Medical Sciences, 32*(1), 49–54. https://doi.org/10.12669/pjms.321.8841

Bhor, K. Shetty, V., Garcha, V., Vinay, V., & Nimbulkar, G. (2019). Knowledge, attitude, and perceived barriers toward evidence-based practice among dental and medical academicians and private practitioners in Pune: A comparative cross-sectional study. *Journal of Indian Association of Public Health Dentistry, 17*(1), 48–53. https://doi.org/10.4103/jiaphd.jiaphd_93_18

Bianchi, M., Bagnasco, A., Bressan, V., Barisone, M., Timmins, F., Rossi, S., Pellegrini, R., Aleo, G., & Sasso, L (2018). A review of the role of nurse leadership in promoting and sustaining evidence-based practice. *Journal of Nursing Management, 26*(8), 918–932. https://doi.org/10.1111/jonm.12638

Bondmass, M. (2009, July 8). Using the ACE STAR Model for teaching/learning evidence-based practice [Poster presentation]. Summer Institute of the Academic Center of Excellence for Evidence Based Practice.

Bondmass, M. (2011, July 29). Application of the ACE Star Model and Essential Competencies in a DNP Program [Conference session]. Summer Institute of the Academic Center of Excellence for Evidence Based Practice.

Claus, N., Watts, P., & Moss, J. (2020). Medical-surgical nurse self-perceived competency in posttraumatic stress disorder/substance use disorder veteran care in a non-Veterans Health Administration setting. *Journal of Nursing Administration, 50*(4), 203–208. https://journals.lww.com/jonajournal/Fulltext/2020/04000/Medical_Surgical_Nurse_Self_perceived_Competency.7.aspx

Connor, L., Dwyer, P., & Oliveira, J. (2016). Nurses' use of evidence-based practice in clinical practice after attending a formal evidence-based practice course: A quality improvement evaluation. *Journal for Nurses in Professional Development, 32*(1), E1–E7. https://doi.org/10.1097/NND.0000000000000229

Copeland, W. E., Gaydosh, L. M., Hill, S. N., Godwin, J., Harris, K. M., Costello, E. J., & Shanahan, L. (2020). Associations of despair with suicidality and substance misuse among young adults. *JAMA Network Open, 3*(6), e208627. https://doi.org/10.5167/uzh-191374

Cronenwett, L., Sherwood, G., Pohl, J., Barnsteiner, J., Moore, S., Sullivan, D. T., Ward, D., & Warren, J. (2009). Quality and safety education for advanced nursing practice. *Nursing Outlook, 57*(6), 338–348. https://doi.org/10.1016/j.outlook.2009.07.009

Englander, R., Cameron, T., Ballard, A. J., Dodge, J., Bull, J., & Aschenbrener, C. A. (2013). Toward a common taxonomy of competency domains for the health professions and competencies for physicians. *Academic Medicine, 88*(8), 1088–1094. https://doi.org/10.1097/ACM.0b013e31829a3b2b

Gallagher-Ford, L. Thomas, B. K., Connor, L., & Sinnott, L, & Melnyk. (2020). The effects of an intensive evidence-based practice educational and skills building program on EBP competency and attributes. *Worldviews on Evidence-based Nursing, 17*(1), 71–81. https://doi.org/10.1111/wvn.12397

Garcia, A. R., Denard, C., Morones, S. M., & Eldeeb, N. (2019). Mitigating barriers to implementing evidence-based interventions in child welfare: Lessons learned from scholars and agency directors. *Children and Youth Services Review, 100*, 313–331. https://doi.org/10.1016/j.childyouth.2019.03.005

Hallum-Montes, R., Middleton, D., Schlanger, K., & Romero, L. (2016). Barriers and facilitators to health center implementation of evidence-based clinical practices in adolescent reproductive health services. *Journal of Adolescent Health, 58*(3), 276–283. https://doi.org/10.1016/j.jadohealth.2015.11.002

Haynes, B., & Haines, A. (1998). Barriers and bridges to evidence based clinical practice. *British Medical Journal, 317*(7153), 273–276. https://doi.org/10.1136/bmj.317.7153

Hong, B., O'Sullivan, E. D., Henein, C., & Jones, C. M. (2019). Motivators and barriers to engagement with evidence-based practice among medical and dental trainees from the U.K. and Republic of Ireland: A national survey. *British Medical Journal Publishing Group BMJ Open, 9*(10), 1–10. https://bmjopen.bmj.com/content/bmjopen/9/10/e031809

Institute of Medicine. (2000). *To err is human: Building a safer health system.* National Academies Press. https://www.nap.edu/9728

Institute of Medicine. (2001). *Crossing the quality chasm: A new health system for the 21st century. Committee on Quality of Health Care in America, Institute of Medicine.* National Academies Press. https://www.nap.edu/download/10027

Institute of Medicine. (2003). *Health professions education: A bridge to quality.* National Academies Press. https://www.nap.edu/download/10681

Institute of Medicine. (2010). *The future of nursing: Leading change, advancing health.* National Academies Press. https://www.nap.edu/download/12956

Institute of Medicine: National Academies of Sciences, Engineering, and Medicine. (2015a). *Assessing progress on the Institute of Medicine report "The Future of Nursing."* National Academies Press. https://www.nap.edu/download/21838

Institute of Medicine. (2015b). *Vital signs: Core metrics for health and health care progress.* The National Academies Press. https://doi.org/10.17226/19402

Jin, J., & Yi, Y. J. (2019). Patient safety competency and the new nursing care delivery model. *Journal of Nursing Management, 27*(6), 1167–1175. https://doi.org/10.1111/jonm.12788

Josiah Macy Jr. Foundation. (2017, June). *Achieving competency-based, time-variable health professions education recommendations from the Macy Foundation Conference.* https://macyfoundation.org/publications/achieving-competency-based-time-variable-health-professions-education

Kavanagh, J. M., & Szweda, C. (2017). A crisis in competency: The strategic and ethical imperative to assessing new graduate nurses' clinical reasoning. *Nursing Education Perspectives, 38*(2), 57–62. https://doi.org/10.1097/01.NEP.0000000000000112

Kesten, K., Bondmass, M., & Dennison, R. (2013, April 12). Application of the ACE Star Model and essential competencies in a MSN program [Poster presentation]. NONPF 39th Annual Meeting. https://nonpf.confex.com/nonpf/2013pa/webprogram/Paper5756.html

Kesten, K., White, K. A., Heitzler, E. T., Chaplin, L. T., & Bondmass, M. D. (2019). Perceived Evidence-based practice competency acquisition in graduate nursing students: Impact of intentional course design. *Journal of Continuing Education in Nursing, 50*(2), 79–86. https://doi.org/10.3928/00220124-20190115-07

Kim, K., Han, Y., Kwak, Y., & Kim, J. (2015). Professional quality of life and clinical competencies among Korean nurses. *Asian Nursing Research, 9*(3), 200–206. https://doi.org/10.1016/j.anr.2015.03.002

Labrague, L. J., Mcenroe-Petitte, D., D'Souza, M. S., Cecily, H., Fronda, D. C., Edet, O. B., Ibebuike, J. E., Venkatesan, L., Almazan, J. U., Al Amri, M., Mirafuentes, E. C., Cayaban, A. R. R., . . . Bin Jumah, J. A. (2019). A multicountry study on nursing students' self-perceived competence and barriers to evidence-based practice. *Worldviews on Evidence-Based Nursing, 16*(3), 236–246. https://doi.org/10.1111/wvn.12364

Lee, Y., & Seomun, G. (2016). Role of compassion competence among clinical nurses in professional quality of life. *International Nursing Review, 63*(3), 381–387. https://doi.org/10.1111/inr.12295

Lewis, C. C., Boyd, M., Puspitasari, A., Navarro, E., Howard, J., Kassab, H., Hoffman, M., Scott, K., Lyon, A., Douglas, S., Simon, G., & Kroenke, K. (2019). Implementing measurement-based care in behavioral health: A review. *JAMA Psychiatry, 76*(3), 324–335. http://doi.org/10.1001/jamapsychiatry.2018.3329

Li, S., Cao, M., & Zhu, X. (2019). Evidence-based practice: Knowledge, attitudes, implementation, facilitators, and barriers among community nurses-systematic review. *Medicine, 98*(39), e17209. https://doi.org/10.1097/MD.0000000000017209

Litwack, K., & Brower, A. M. (2018). The University of Wisconsin-Milwaukee flexible option for bachelor of science in nursing degree completion. *Academic Medicine, 93*. S37–S41. https://doi.org/10.1097/ACM.0000000000002076

Merriam-Webster. (2020). Competency. In *Merriam-Webster.com dictionary*. Retrieved August 26, 2020, from https://www.merriam-webster.com/dictionary/competency

Melnyk, B. M. (2016). Development of and evidence to support the evidence-based practice competencies. In B. M. Melnyk, L. Gallagher-Ford, & E. Fineout-Overholt (Eds.), *Implementing Evidence-Based Practice (EBP) Competencies in Healthcare*. Sigma Theta Tau International.

Melnyk, B. M. (2017). The difference between what is known and what is done is lethal: Evidence-based practice is a key solution urgently needed. *Worldviews on Evidence-Based Nursing, 14*(1), 3–4. https://doi.org/10.1111/wvn.12194

Melnyk, B. M., & Fineout-Overholt, E. (2015). Making the case for evidence-based practice and cultivating a spirit of inquiry. In B. M. Melnyk & E. Fineout-Overholt (Eds.), *Evidence-based practice in nursing & healthcare: A guide to best practice* (pp. 3–23). Wolters Kluwer.

Melnyk, B. M., & Fineout-Overholt, E. (2018). *Evidence-based practice in nursing & healthcare: A guide to best practice* (4th ed.). Wolters Kluwer Health, Inc.

Melnyk, B. M., Fineout-Overholt, E., Gallagher-Ford, L., & Kaplan, L. (2012). The state of evidence-based practice in U.S. nurses: Critical implications for nurse leaders and educators. *Journal of Nursing Administration, 42*(9), 410–417. https://doi.org/10.1097/NNA.0b013e3182664e0a

Melnyk, B. M., Gallagher-Ford, L., Long, L., & Fineout-Overholt, E. (2014). The establishment of evidence-based practice competencies for practicing registered nurses and advanced practice nurses in real-world clinical settings: Proficiencies to improve healthcare quality, reliability, patient outcomes, and costs. *Worldviews on Evidence-Based Nursing, 11*(1), 5–15. https://doi.org/10.1111/wvn.12021

Melnyk, B. M., Gallagher-Ford, L., Zellefrow, C., Tucker, S., Van Dromme, L., & Thomas, B. K. (2018). Outcomes from the first Helene Fuld Health Trust National Institute for Evidence-based Practice in Nursing and healthcare invitational expert forum. *Worldviews on Evidence-Based Nursing, 15*(1), 5–15. https://doi.org/10.1111/wvn.12272

Newman, M., Papadopoulos, I., & Sigsworth, J. (1998). Barriers to evidence-based practice. *Intensive and Critical Care Nursing, 14*(5), 231–238. https://doi.org/10.1016/S0964-3397(98)80634-4

Nodine, T. R. (2016). How did we get here? A brief history of competency-based higher education in the United States. *The Journal of Competency-Based Education, 1*(1), 5–11. https://doi.org/10.1002/cbe2.1004

Nolan, M., Morgan, L., Curran, M., Clayton, J., Gerrish, K., & Parker, K. (1998). Evidence-based care: Can we overcome the barriers? *British Journal of Nursing, 7*(20), 1273–1278. https://doi.org/10.12968/bjon.1998.7.20.5567

Odhwani, A. S., Sarkar, P. K., Giggleman, G. F., Holmes, M. M., & Pohlman, K. A. (2019). Self-perceived evidence-based practice competencies: A survey of faculty and students at a chiropractic institution. *The Journal of Chiropractic Education in Press, November*, 1–6. https://doi.org/10.7899/JCE-18-24

OECD. (2019). *Health at a Glance 2019: OECD Indicators*. OECD Publishing. https://doi.org/10.1787/4dd50c09-en

Oliver, J. A., & Lang, J. M. (2018). Barriers and consultation needs regarding implementation of evidence-based treatment in community agencies. *Children and Youth Services Review, 94*, 368–377. https://doi.org/10.1016/j.childyouth.2018.10.004

QSEN Institute. (2012). *Quality and Safety Education for Nurses project*. https://www.uclahealth.org/nursing/competency-assessment-criteria#Evidence-Based%20Practice

Renolen, A., Hjälmhult, E., Høye, S., Danbolt, L. J., & Kirkevold, M. (2020). Creating room for evidence-based practice: Leader behavior in hospital wards. *Research in Nursing & Health, 43*(1), 90–102. https://doi.org/10.1002/nur.21981

Rojjanasrirat, W., & Rice, J. (2017). Evidence-based practice knowledge, attitudes, and practice of online graduate nursing students. *Nurse Education Today, 53*, 48–53. https://doi.org/10.1016/j.nedt.2017.04.005

Rossi, S., Bagnasco, A., Barisone, M., Bianchi, M., Bressan, V., Timmins, F., Pellegrini, R., Aleo, G., Sasso, L., & Rossi, S. (2020) Research awareness among children's nurses: An integrative review. *Journal of Clinical Nursing, 29*(3–4), 290–304. https://doi.org/10.1111/jocn.15068

Ruzafa-Martinez, M., Lopez-Iborra, L., Moreno-Casbas, T., & Madrigal-Torres, M. (2013). Development and validation of the competence in evidence based practice questionnaire (EBP-COQ) among nursing students. *BMC Medical Education, 13*(1), 19. https://doi.org/10.1186/1472-6920-13-19

Sackett, D. L., Straus, S. E., Richardson, W. S., Rosenberg, W., & Haynes, R. B. (Eds.). (2000). *Evidence-based medicine: How to practice and teach EBM*. Churchill Livingstone.

Saunders, H., & Vehvilainen-Julkunen, K. (2018). Key considerations for selecting instruments when evaluating healthcare professionals' evidence-based practice competencies: A discussion paper. *Journal of Advanced Nursing, 74*(10), 2301–2311. https://doi.org/10.1111/jan.13802

Shayan, S. J., Kiwanuka, F., & Nakaye, Z. (2019). Barriers associated with evidence-based practice among nurses in low-and middle-income countries: A systematic review. *Worldviews on Evidence-Based Nursing, 16*(1), 12–20. https://doi.org/10.1111/wvn.12337

Skela-Savič, B., Hvalič-Touzery, S., & Pesjak, K. (2017). Professional values and competencies as explanatory factors for the use of evidence-based practice in nursing. *Journal of Advanced Nursing, 73*, 1910–1923. https://doi.org/10.1111/jan.13280

Stevens, K. R. (2004). *ACE star model of knowledge transformation*. Academic Center for Evidence-based Practice. University of Texas Health Science Center San Antonio. https://www.uthscsa.edu/academics/nursing/star-model

Stevens, K. R. (2005). *Essential competencies for evidence-based practice in nursing* (1st ed.). Academic Center for Evidence-Based Practice: The University of Texas Health Science Center at San Antonio. https://www.uthscsa.edu/academics/nursing/star-model

Stevens, K. R. (2009). *Essential competencies for evidence-based practice in nursing* (2nd ed.). Academic Center for Evidence-Based Practice: The University of Texas Health Science Center at San Antonio. https://www.uthscsa.edu/academics/nursing/star-model

Stevens, K. R. (2013). The impact of evidence-based practice in nursing and the next big ideas. *Online Journal of Issues in Nursing, 18*(2). https://doi.org/10.3912/OJIN.Vol18No02Man04

Stiffler, D., & Cullen, D. (2010). Evidence-based practice for nurse practitioner students: A competency-based teaching framework. *Journal of Professional Nursing, 26*(5), 272–277. https://doi.org/10.1016/j.profnurs.2010.02.004

Stokke, K., Olsen, N. R., Espehaug, B., & Nortvedt, M. W. (2014). Evidence based practice beliefs and implementation among nurses: A cross-sectional study. *BMC Nursing, 13*, 1–10. https://bmcnurs.biomedcentral.com/articles/10.1186/1472-6955-13-8

Straus, S. E., Richardson, W. S., Glasziou, P., & Haynes, R. B. (2005). *Evidence-based medicine* (3rd ed.). Churchill Livingstone.

Taxman, F. S. (2018). The partially clothed emperor: Evidence-based practices. *Journal of Contemporary Criminal Justice, 34*(1), 97–114. https://doi.org/10.1177/1043986217750444

Tharp-Barrie, K., Williams, T. E., Howard, P. B., El-Mallakh, P., & MacCallum, T. (2020). DNP practice improvement initiative: Staff nurse competency evaluation. *The Journal of Nursing Administration, 50*(1), 22–27. https://www.ncbi.nlm.nih.gov/pubmed/31809453

van Der Goot, W. E., Keers, J. C., Kuipers, R., Nieweg, R. M. B., & de Groot, M. (2018). The effect of a multifaceted evidence-based practice programme for nurses on knowledge, skills, attitudes, and perceived barriers: A cohort study. *Nurse Education Today, 63*, 6–11. https://doi.org/10.1016/j.nedt.2018.01.008

Wagner, L. M., Dolansky, M. A., & Englander, R. (2018) Entrustable professional activities for quality and patient safety. *Nursing Outlook, 66*(3), 237–243. https://doi.org/10.1016/j.outlook.2017.11.001

Whorley, E., Aucoin, J., Edmonds, A., Ortelli, T., & Stevens, K. (2018). The implementation of the essential competencies for evidence-based practice in baccalaureate nursing education. (Publication No. 10839539)[Doctoral dissertation, Nova Southeastern University]. ProQuest Dissertations Publishing.

Youssef, N., Alshraifeen, A., Alnuaimi, K., & Upton, P. (2018). Egyptian and Jordanian nurse educators' perception of barriers preventing the implementation of evidence-based practice: A cross-sectional study. *Nurse Education Today, 64*, 33–41. https://doi.org/10.1016/j.nedt.2018.01.035

SEARCHING FOR EVIDENCE

MARY E. HITCHCOCK AND LESLIE A. CHRISTENSEN

■ INTRODUCTION

The changing shape of information and how it is retrieved and evaluated has profound effects at every level of the research process. The emphasis on evidence-based decision-making in healthcare, coupled with the exponential increase in the volume of scientific literature, have resulted in a more complicated research environment. Although the core concepts of research have remained relatively consistent, new tools and technologies continue to evolve and multiply. This chapter discusses the search for evidence as a systematic process consisting of four distinct phases including preparation and planning, searching the literature, going beyond the literature, and pulling it all together.

One of the most dramatic changes over the past 10 years affecting all types of information gathering has been the sheer increase of available information. In 2014, Larosa estimated that PubMed, a health sciences literature database, adds approximately 500,000 new records every year and its collection doubles every 13 years (Larosa, 2014). More recent statistics show that the pace of new records is increasing, with an average 1.2 million additional new records every year since 2014 (National Library of Medicine, 2019). While the explosion of information continues, the skills to navigate through denser and more crowded information landscapes seldom keep pace (Christenbery et al., 2016). Advanced practice registered nurses (APRNs) may be overwhelmed with available evidence and find it difficult to maintain searching skills and to keep up-to-date in their fields. Barriers such as time, lack of resources, or appropriate skill sets remain an issue in translating research into clinical practice (Fencl & Matthews, 2017). The heightened focus in recent years on improving clinical outcomes through support of scientific knowledge has resulted in a greater emphasis on the integration of evidence-based practice (EBP) at all levels of healthcare (Fencl & Matthews, 2017; Taylor et al., 2016). As nursing students and healthcare professionals learn to incorporate EBPs into their clinical workflow, they must learn to identify evidence-based information resources and construct related information-seeking strategies. Effective EBPs will be increasingly important in saving clinician's time and energy and, ultimately, in achieving improved clinical outcomes (Polit & Beck, 2020).

■ PHASE I—PREPARATION AND PLANNING

Since 2001 when the Institute of Medicine (IOM, now known as the National Academy of Medicine) called for all healthcare professionals to incorporate the concept of EBP into practice, the need to search for evidence has become paramount (Cypress, 2019). The concept of literature searching encompasses far more than merely entering words into a search box. The process includes formulating search statements, selecting appropriate search terminology, and locating databases and strategies; a literature review, in actuality, is a robust project waiting to be organized. Contemplating and identifying its various parts before approaching a database is time well spent. Not only will this prep work benefit the searcher in time saved, it will instill order in what may seem to be a frustrating string of chaotic activities. The preliminary literature review preparation phase will be discussed in this section.

To use an analogy, anyone who has been challenged by the prospect of cooking using a new recipe can find the task either daunting or unnerving. In order to make sense of the process, we find ourselves first reading the entire recipe from beginning to end before assembling the ingredients for the dish. Once we understand what the finished product should be, we gather appropriate ingredients and the necessary utensils. As the cook gains more confidence in their skills, there is more certainty in the procedure and a pattern begins to develop. As patterns develop, variations are incorporated with ease and confidence increases over time.

Research is much the same. If searching a database is a rare occurrence, it will seem to be a slow, laborious, and unwelcomed process. As the practice of research is integrated into clinical cultures and professional workflows, the familiarity of the process will become second nature as well.

Ask Yourself Some Questions

Before diving head-first into database searching, it is important to ask a few questions to guide subsequent actions (Exhibit 2.1). Pre-search preparation will tease out existing strengths and weaknesses, define the skills needed, and pinpoint knowledge gaps. Questioning the purpose of the literature review will determine the intent and the appropriate intensity, depth, and scope of the search(es).

An inclusive search for all relevant literature, such as demanded by systematic reviews and meta-analyses, requires more time and involves more databases than a selective review of limited scope. Which resources are best for the research question? It is advisable to identify the best information resources for the topic before constructing search strategies. Good preparation prevents

---

EXHIBIT 2.1

QUESTIONS TO ASK DURING PHASE I

- What is the purpose of the literature search?
- Which resources are best for the research question?
- How are the resources best searched?
- Where can help be obtained?
- What resources are available?
- Is time a limiting factor?
- Which citation manager will be used?
- How is the information to be evaluated?

distracting detours and lost time, resolves confusion, and serves to sequence the order in which databases are searched. In Phase I, exploratory searches are important for discovery and to determine the viability of the research topic.

Define the Search Goal

Defining the scope of the planned research is an important element in moving forward. Assessing the intended outcome of the search will provide a clarity of purpose and direction. Is the impending literature review a class assignment with specific guidelines, requirements, and deadlines? Is it generated by unanswered healthcare questions that need immediate attention? Is it part of a team project leading to the creation of evidence-based guidelines in the clinical setting? Answers to these questions may drive the momentum of the literature review down slightly different search paths. Decisions made at this juncture will also impact the choice of databases and resources consulted. One size does not fit all. A small-sized research goal does not warrant an extensive research approach. Each literature review is a sum of its smaller parts.

Gather Background Information

One important preliminary step is to understand how the research topic fits into its related field of knowledge. The APRN must attain some degree of comfort with the nomenclature and the topic-at-large before moving into serious search phases. A good background builds an information foundation that will support increased awareness of vocabulary (important when searching) and related issues. Background information can be found in many places, including textbooks, trusted websites, reference resources, clinical summary databases (CSDs; discussed later in this chapter), and review articles. If the topic is interdisciplinary, as many nursing topics are, the information destinations will be broader in scope, more numerous, and often less familiar. Reaching across disciplines can be a stretch, especially for the less experienced searcher. During the background gathering, it is advisable to clearly list and expand related terminology to aid in search strategy construction later.

Construct a Searchable Question

First, formulating a searchable or answerable question is a technique that focuses on the most basic elements of the research topic. A poorly constructed research question makes searching frustrating by wasting time or returning too many or off target results. Spending time to create a "searchable question" will allow the researcher to focus search terms, database limiters, and find appropriate and useful literature (Bramer et al., 2018).

By focusing on only the core elements of a complex healthcare scenario, the central question gains clarity and more precise definition. Precision and focus are also enhanced by the use of the PICO method developed by proponents of EBP. The PICO mnemonic (P = patient, population, problem; I = intervention; C = comparison; O = outcome) provides a useful instrument for peeling away the outer layers of the research question and directs the focus to only the most essential components. PICO is widely used for quantitative research questions.

Alternatively, the PEO mnemonic (P = populations and their problems; E = exposure; O = outcomes or themes) provides a useful instrument for peeling away the outer layers of qualitative research questions. Either structure can be used to create a clinical question; however, not every clinical question will fit neatly into both frameworks, but the approach of deconstructing the parts to their meaningful essence will clarify the purpose, help develop more effective search

---

EXHIBIT 2.2

CHECKLIST: PHASE I

- Research topic
- Due date
- Background information
- Searchable question/PICO
- Knowledge gaps
- Core and peripheral databases/resources
- Citation manager

---

strategies, and remove other "noisy" narratives that may prove distracting when constructing search strategies (Bettany-Saltikov, 2012; Gerberi & Marienau, 2017).

Eliminate Search Barriers

Nursing literature is replete with documentation of potential barriers to the integration of evidence-based methods into practice. The most commonly identified barriers include the perceived lack of value of EBP to practice, time constraints, lack of access to computers and databases at the point of need, limited database searching skills, and continued underutilization of evidence-based information in healthcare environments. Even trusted online resources are not as accessible or viewed as useful as consultation with a colleague as each hospital or university may have different resources available to staff (Brown et al., 2009; Pravikoff et al., 2005).

Uncertainties surrounding the research process can inhibit forward momentum. It is important to identify and manage research uncertainties early and throughout the process. Johnston et al. (2016) identified basic themes of the barriers nurses may face when conducting research. These themes, with additional "subthemes" noted, are: keeping up-to-date with the evidence, using a clinical tool, education/training, and implementation. Practicing nurses may not face approval, encouragement, or support for their research, which also leads to hesitancy to continue in the research field after their formal education.

Researchers are advised to follow a basic prescription when contemplating literature reviews: (a) spend pre-search time on discovery, planning, reflection; then (b) choose the appropriate information destinations and execute well-formulated searches; (c) critically evaluate and expand search parameters; and (d) sort, store, and organize gathered information throughout the process. Using a checklist, such as the one in Exhibit 2.2, will promote effective search habits.

▪ PHASE II—MINING THE LITERATURE DATABASES

Choose the Best Resources

Once a well-formulated question is created, researchers must look for the best evidence to answer the question. An understanding of the EBP hierarchy, adequate searching skills, and access to appropriate resources are all required to succeed. There is a remarkable amount of health research now published. With 75 trials and 11 systematic reviews published each day and an estimated 2 million-plus research papers on biomedical topics published annually, it is essential for a researcher to have a solid grasp of the resources to find the proper evidence to answer clinical questions (Bastian et al., 2010).

Start With Reviews

From an evidence-based perspective, the best bet is to start by using resources containing the secondary literature—articles that review or summarize peer-reviewed research on a topic. Keep in mind there are several types of reviews. Reviews published in the literature can be divided into two broad types: narrative and systematic. A *narrative review* (often referred to as simply a literature review) tends to be an article that states the current knowledge on a topic from a wide variety of sources, often by an expert in the field. This type of review is designed to be informative and can consist of nonsystematic methods of obtaining and appraising the information. A *systematic review*, conversely, focuses on a specific clinical topic or question, includes a thorough and explicit literature search, appraises all individual studies on a topic, and offers a conclusion to answer the clinical question. A *meta-analysis* is a type of systematic review that applies statistical methods to combine or pool the evidence from individual trials. *Practice guidelines* are commonly placed into the evidence category of "review," but this is proper only if their statements are developed using rigorous scientific evidence (i.e., systematic reviews and randomized controlled trials).

Search the Primary Literature

Although the amount (and value) of the review literature has seen phenomenal growth in the last decade, much of the evidence, particularly in the nursing and allied health fields, still resides within the *primary literature*—individual reports of findings. These single studies are the building blocks from which the systematic reviews, meta-analyses, and evidence-based guidelines are built. Studies, however, are not created equal and there is a great range of publication types found in the journal literature. All levels of the evidence hierarchy from randomized controlled trials, cohort and case–control studies, to qualitative and descriptive studies are found in journals. Researchers should initiate a search in the review literature and turn to primary literature to fill in the gaps both in content and currency.

Select the Resources to Search

There are thousands of resources that cover the scholarly output of the health sciences. Some are freely available on the internet through government agencies, health organizations, or even commercial enterprises; others are restricted to individuals and/or institutions with, at times costly, subscriptions. The highest quality health research is normally found in the scholarly, peer-reviewed, journals and literature databases that cover them. Literature databases are indices of journal articles. The majority of these databases contain citations and abstracts of articles from journals covering specific topics. Some also provide either the full articles or links to providers of the articles.

It is in the best interest of the health researcher to commence with searches in the core health databases. Three literature databases considered essential for APRNs are MEDLINE (via PubMed), CINAHL (Cumulative Index to Nursing and Allied Health Literature), and the Cochrane Database of Systematic Reviews. These databases are the best starting point for both clinical and research topics in the health sciences. For a list of core database descriptions and features see Table 2.1.

TABLE 2.1 Selected Core Literature Databases

	COVERAGE	PUBLICATION TYPES	FEATURES	FINDING REVIEWS
CINAHL (Cumulative Index to Nursing and Allied Health Literature)	Comprehensive source for nursing and allied health journals, providing coverage of 5,300 journals along with 80 other document types.	Systematic reviews Guidelines Primary literature Dissertations Books Book chapters Audiovisual Pamphlets etc.	Controlled vocabulary Advanced search EBM filters Explode Major concept Allows Boolean limits Excludes MEDLINE option	Use the systematic review publication type limit or Evidence-based practice special interest filter
Cochrane Database of Systematic Reviews	Includes approximately 7,500 full reviews and approximately 2,500 protocols (detailed plan to create a Cochrane review) involving therapy and prevention in all areas of healthcare. Recently added reviews of diagnostic tools.	Systematic reviews Protocols	Offers MeSH search Allows Boolean limits (systematic review or protocol)	If available, use reviews limit
MEDLINE (PubMed)	PubMed offers free searching of MEDLINE, a biomedical database covering more than 5,600 journals, and some other publication types in all areas of the health sciences.	Systematic reviews Guidelines Primary literature	Controlled vocabulary Explode (automatic) Major topic Allows Boolean limits Filters (clinical queries)	Use clinical queries: systematic review filter or Systematic reviews article type filter or Review article type filter

There are, of course, other databases with unique content that might be useful, if not integral, to the searcher. For instance, EMBASE, a large international health database, contains unique global literature with particularly strong coverage in topics related to drugs/pharmaceuticals; ERIC can be tapped for articles, reports, and other publications concerning education; PsycINFO, as its name implies, covers the mental health literature; and SocINDEX can be a useful resource to find evidence in sociology and related areas. Table 2.2 lists peripheral databases of interest to researchers and clinicians in nursing.

TABLE 2.2 Selected Peripheral Literature Databases

DATABASES	COVERAGE
Allied and Complementary Medicine Database (AMED)	AMED covers references to articles from approximately 600 journals in three separate subject areas: professions allied to medicine; complementary medicine; and palliative care. The scope of coverage is mainly European.
British Nursing Index (BNI)	BNI is a UK nursing and midwifery database, covering more than 270 UK journals and other English-language titles, including international nursing and midwifery journals, and selected content from medical, allied health, and management titles.
Cochrane Central Register of Controlled Trials (CENTRAL)	CENTRAL includes citations and summaries of more than 1.6 million controlled trials culled from literature databases and other published and unpublished sources used to create Cochrane reviews. Subscription required.
EMBASE	EMBASE is a large international biomedical and pharmacological database containing more than 32 million records from 8,500 biomedical journals including more than 2,900 titles not covered in MEDLINE. EMBASE has a broad biomedical scope, with in-depth coverage of pharmacology, pharmaceutical science, and clinical research. EMBASE also includes approximately 2.4 million conference abstracts from more than 7,000 conferences.
ERIC	Sponsored by the U.S. Department of Education, ERIC provides free access to more than 1.6 million records of journal articles from 1,000 journals and other education-related materials (books, research syntheses, conference papers, tech reports, policy papers, etc.) and, if available, includes links to full text.
HealthSource: Nursing/Academic Edition	This EBSCO database provides coverage of nursing and allied health and includes citation/abstracts from 840 journals and the full text of more than 320 scholarly journals.
PsycINFO	Produced by the American Psychological Association, PsycINFO is a large behavioral science and mental health database with more than 4.7 million records from 2,500 journals, books, book chapters, and dissertations.
Scopus	This large multidisciplinary database from Elsevier has over 75 million records, including citation/abstracts from 24,600 journals, 9 million conference papers, and 194,000 books. Coverage includes records from both MEDLINE and EMBASE databases.
SocINDEX	SocINDEX is a sociology database with coverage of all subdisciplines and other related topics. It includes indexing/abstracting of 1800 core journals, as well as 320 priority coverage and 2300 selective coverage journals. There are more than 2.6 million records, going back to 1895.

Speak the Database Language

Nurses have identified a lack of searching skills as a barrier to EBP (Fencl & Matthews, 2017). It is therefore essential for database users to develop a skill set to gain confidence and to search efficiently. This chapter proceeds with a discussion of some of the basic search concepts and tools that all researchers should understand and employ when utilizing health databases. Keep in mind that attending a continuing education (CE) session provided by a health library or institution, a consultation with a librarian, or even a few moments viewing a resource-specific tutorial will often pay great dividends.

The search terms (keywords or phrases) entered into a literature database search box will have a significant bearing on the quality of the results. Terminology in the health literature is replete with synonyms (different words, same definition) and homonyms (same word, different definition). For example, the concept *cancer* can be entered in a database as: *cancer, tumor, malignancy, neoplasm, carcinoma*, and so forth. Therefore, challenging decisions need to be made regarding the selection of appropriate terms.

In some cases, using common or everyday language is effective and appropriate. This is called *free-text* or *keyword* searching. However, searching with terms offered from a database-specific thesaurus, often referred to as a *controlled vocabulary*, will often prove the best way to improve the breadth and accuracy of the retrieval set.

Search Using Keywords

Keyword (free-text, natural language, common language) searches are commonly used in search boxes on the internet (e.g., Google), and all literature databases allow searchers to create search queries with keywords. Keyword searches are by nature fairly restrictive, as records retrieved by the database must have the exact term(s) entered in the search box. For example, if an author of an article uses the term *ascorbic acid* and the searcher enters *vitamin C*, the searcher would not necessarily retrieve that specific potentially relevant article.

Keyword searches can be used to find good information on a topic and are appropriate in certain circumstances. Expert searchers will often begin the process of searching a database by entering a few important keywords to obtain a quick initial retrieval set. This set is then scrutinized to uncover any appropriate additional search terms to refine the query.

Although the use of natural language may not be the best way to search a given resource (see Search Using a Controlled Vocabulary), there are techniques to improve the results of your search query:

- *Truncation*, also called stemming, allows searching for various word endings and spellings of a keyword term simultaneously. Databases that allow truncation will designate database-specific characters, or wildcards, to initiate the truncation feature. The asterisk (*), question mark (?), and dollar sign ($) are commonly used wildcards. For example, entering *communit** in the PubMed search box will retrieve records with the terms: *community, communities, communitarian, communitarians*, and so forth. Some resources also allow for internal (wom?n) or beginning truncation ($natal).

- *Phrase searching* is a good way to search for specific phrases or words that are unusually formed. Many resources will allow a searcher to surround a phrase with brackets, parentheses, or quotes (depending on the resource) to retrieve only results with the exact specific phrase within the database record. This modification can reduce irrelevant results by requiring the resource to locate the component words in that specific order. For example, entering "community acquired pneumonia" in the PubMed search box will retrieve only the results containing that particular string of words.

Search Using a Controlled Vocabulary

A *controlled vocabulary* is a carefully selected standardized list of terms, or thesaurus, that indexers (individuals who review articles before inclusion into a database) use to determine the main and minor topics discussed in the article. These standardized terms may or may not be the same words the author uses in their writings, but are embedded within the database record. Consequently, a searcher using a standardized or controlled term will retrieve articles on a topic, regardless of the ambiguity of terms. Many studies have shown that utilizing a controlled term will improve searches in both size and accuracy. Be aware that not all health databases use a controlled vocabulary system, and even in databases that do, many concepts do not have precise matches within the system. Also, it takes a database time to incorporate new concepts/terms into its thesaurus. For example, the term AIDS was coined in 1981, but it took more than 2 years before it was introduced into MEDLINE's Medical Subject Heading (MeSH) thesaurus. In these cases, a searcher must resort to a keyword search.

There are several examples of a controlled vocabulary in the health literature and many are database specific:

■ MeSH is the National Library of Medicine's controlled vocabulary for MEDLINE. The 2020 MeSH list contains a hierarchy of more than 27,000 descriptive terms covering virtually all medical concepts.

■ CINAHL uses a different set of controlled vocabulary, named CINAHL Headings. Although CINAHL Headings follow the structure of MeSH, they were developed to reflect the terminology used by nursing and allied health professionals. This controlled vocabulary thesaurus should be used when searching the CINAHL database.

Some databases have addressed the ease, and also the problems, associated with keyword searches by developing a built-in term mapping system where free-text terms are matched (mapped) against a controlled vocabulary translation table. For example, MEDLINE's MeSH list includes over 27,000 terms, yet another 200,000 synonyms are included in the translation table. A search query with term *vitamin C* will be matched (and searched) with the proper MeSH term *ascorbic acid*. Although this is reliable for many common health terms, not all have such straightforward and successful mapping. It is very important to look for additional headings that may be synonymous with your terms because every database has numerous choices of appropriate terms.

Explode and Focus Terms

The subject headings of a controlled vocabulary are often presented in a hierarchical structure. This type of structure in MEDLINE's MeSH thesaurus is called the "MeSH tree," which presents broad to narrower terms. Here is the MeSH tree for the term *depressive disorder*:

Mood Disorders
  Cyclothymic Disorder
  Depressive Disorder
    Depression, Postpartum
    Depressive Disorder, Major
    Depressive Disorder, Treatment-Resistant
    Dysthymic Disorder
    Premenstrual Dysphoric Disorder
    Seasonal Affective Disorder

Many databases allow searchers to *explode* a subject heading, which instructs the database to retrieve records with the requested subject heading as well as any more specific/narrower terms that are related to the topic. In MEDLINE, a search query with the exploded MeSH term *Depressive Disorder* will search not only the MeSH term *Depressive Disorder*, but also the terms *Depression, Postpartum; Depressive Disorder, Major; Depressive Disorder, Treatment-Resistant; Dysthymic Disorder; Premenstrual Dysphoric Disorder,* and *Seasonal Affective Disorder*. Be aware that when searching using MeSH terms, PubMed automatically explodes the MeSH term(s). It is possible to prevent that by selecting the box titled *Do not include MeSH terms found below this term in the MeSH hierarchy*.

The *major* command instructs the database to retrieve only those articles in which the subject term selected is considered to be a primary focus of the article. This command narrows your search by eliminating articles that peripherally discuss the topic of the subject heading. In PubMed's MeSH one can apply the focus command by checking the *Restrict to MeSH Major Topics* box and in CINAHL by checking the *Major Concepts* box within CINAHL Headings.

Combine Concepts (Boolean Operators)

Boolean logic defines the relationship between terms in a search. There are three Boolean operators: AND, OR, NOT. Database searchers can apply these operators to create broader or narrower searches:

- AND combines search terms so that the retrieval set contains all of the terms. The AND operator is generally placed between different concepts. For example, the search *St John's Wort* AND *Depression* will retrieve results containing *both* terms.

- OR combines search terms so that the retrieval set contains at least one of the terms. The OR operator is generally placed between synonyms of the same concept. For example, *St John's Wort* OR *Hypericum* will retrieve results containing *either* term.

- NOT excludes search terms so that the retrieval set will not contain any of the terms that follow the operator NOT. For example, *St John's Wort* NOT *Adolescent* will retrieve results containing the term *St John's Wort* without the term *Adolescent*. Searchers should apply the NOT operator with caution, since it often excludes relevant results with only a passing mention of the term *NOTed* out.

For more efficient searching using Boolean operators, parentheses (brackets) should be used to nest search terms within other search terms. By nesting terms, searchers can specify the order in which the database interprets the search. It is recommended that synonyms (i.e., terms *ORed* together) should be nested. For example, *(St John's Wort* OR *Hypericum)* AND *(Depression* OR *Depressive Disorder)*.

Advanced Versus Basic Search Modes

Several resources offer the searcher an option of using a *basic* search interface with limited and rudimentary options for conducting and refining a search, or a more *advanced* mode that will provide more sophisticated search features and allow searchers to employ many of the techniques discussed in this section. The advanced search mode is the only choice for earnest researchers.

Utilize Filters and Limits

To aid in retrieval relevancy and precision, databases may offer options to filter and/or limit searches by certain parameters. Several databases have devised valuable and effective filters for researchers and clinicians specifically for finding the evidence to answer clinical questions. One example is PubMed's *Clinical Queries*, which offers essential built-in evidence-based medicine search filters to retrieve systematic reviews (and meta analyses, evidence-based guidelines, etc.) and individual studies at the highest tier of the evidence hierarchy (e.g., randomized controlled trials for therapy scenarios). Other examples include the *Evidence-Based Practice* or the *Systematic Review* publication type limit within CINAHL. These filters can be particularly helpful in finding the best evidence on a topic.

Literature databases also offer several ways to limit the retrieval set. Common limits include:

- **Date:** Allows searchers to restrict the publication dates of the articles retrieved. Keep in mind that newer literature is not always better.

- **Language:** Databases include articles from many different countries and languages, so it may be helpful to limit the results of a search to a specific language.

- **Publication Type:** Journal articles are not created equal. Case reports, cohort studies, controlled trials, editorials, systematic reviews, comments, practice guidelines, audiovisuals, book chapters, dissertations, and so on, are found in the journal literature.

- **Age:** Some databases offer limits by specific age groups. For example, by selecting the *Infant* limit in CINAHL or MEDLINE, the majority of articles concerning infancy will be retrieved. However, articles that include additional age groups will also be retrieved.

- **Full Text:** Several databases include a small selection of free full-text (entire) articles. Use of the full-text limit will restrict the results to only items that include, or provide links to, the full text. Selecting this option will often greatly reduce the retrieval set and give no guarantee in the quality of items retrieved. Many health organizations, centers, academic institutions, and so on, have the ability to embed a much larger set of full-text content into a database that would not be picked up by the generic full-text option. If the purpose of a literature search is to produce a comprehensive set of relevant articles, this limit should not be applied. However, if the purpose is simply to get a quick grasp of a clinical topic, this option might prove useful since whole articles could be obtained.

PHASE III—BEYOND THE LITERATURE DATABASES: SEARCHING THE INTERNET

Target Health Websites for Guidelines, Reviews, and Reports

There are plenty of health-related websites that provide quality information for both researchers and clinicians. It is often necessary to venture beyond the literature databases to find guidelines, reports, consensus statements, and other documents not published in the commercial literature. Table 2.3 presents a selective list of valuable sites for EBP.

Some look and act much like commercial literature databases and provide access to information created by others (meta-sites). TRIP database, for example, is a sophisticated tool that searches dozens of evidence-based resources in addition to the millions of articles in MEDLINE. SUMSearch 2 also searches the internet for evidence-based medical information by scanning literature databases and high-impact medical journals, and employs a unique method of searching and filtering for the best results.

Whereas large meta-sites include citations from a wide variety of documents, others are designated as repositories for specific publication types. Practice guidelines are valuable components in

TABLE 2.3 Select Examples of Websites

WEBSITE	NOTES
ACP Clinical Guidelines http://www.acponline.org/clinical_information/guidelines	ACP Clinical Guidelines cover many areas of internal medicine, including screening for cancer or other major diseases, diagnoses, treatment, and medical technology. Included are Clinical Practice Guidelines, Clinical Guidance Statements, and Best Practice Advice.
Agency for Healthcare Research and Quality Evidence-Based Practice Centers https://www.ahrq.gov/research/findings/evidence-based-reports/overview/index.html	A collection of high-quality reports, reviews, and technology assessments based on rigorous, comprehensive syntheses and analyses of the scientific literature on topics relevant to clinical, social science/behavioral, economic, and other healthcare organization and delivery issues.
Agency for Healthcare Research and Quality U.S. Preventive Services Task Force http://www.uspreventiveservicestaskforce.org	The U.S. Preventive Services Task Force is an independent panel of experts in primary care and prevention that systematically review the evidence for effectiveness and develop recommendations for clinical preventive services.
American Heart Association Scientific Statements and Guidelines http://professional.heart.org/professional/index.jsp	A collection of AHA's scientific statements and practice guidelines that are published in *Circulation; Stroke; Arteriosclerosis, Thrombosis, and Vascular Biology; Hypertension; Circulation Research*; or other journals.
CDC Infection Prevention & Control Guidelines & Recommendations https://www.cdc.gov/infectioncontrol/guidelines/index.html	This site includes an overview of how infections spread, ways to prevent the spread of infections, and more detailed recommendations by type of healthcare setting.
The Community Guide http://www.thecommunityguide.org	Developed by the nonfederal Task Force on Community Preventive Services, whose members are appointed by the Director of the Centers for Disease Control and Prevention (CDC), The Community Guide summarizes what is known about the effectiveness, economic efficiency, and feasibility of interventions to promote community health and prevent disease.
ECRI Guidelines Trust™ https://www.ecri.org/library/general-topics/	ECRI Institute, an independent, nonprofit patient safety organization, developed this new resource in response to urgent pleas from healthcare professionals after substantial federal funding cuts forced the Agency for Healthcare Research and Quality (AHRQ) to shut down the National Guideline Clearinghouse™ (NGC). ECRI had developed and maintained the NGC website for 20 years.
Guideline Central https://www.guidelinecentral.com	Guideline Central is dedicated to providing healthcare professionals with evidence-based clinical decision-support tools that are current, practical, and easily accessible. It partners with over 35 medical societies and government agencies to provide quick-reference tools that physicians can rely on for credible guidance in the management of a medical condition.
Healthy People 2020 https://www.healthypeople.gov/	Healthy People 2020 is the product of an extensive stakeholder feedback process that is unparalleled in government and health. It integrates input from public health and prevention experts, a wide range of federal, state and local government officials, a consortium of more than 2,000 organizations, and perhaps most importantly, the public.

(continued)

TABLE 2.3 Select Examples of Websites (*continued*)

WEBSITE	NOTES
Infectious Diseases Society of America Practice Guidelines https://www.idsociety.org/practice guidelines#/name_na_str/ASC/0/+/	Includes standards, practice guidelines, and statements developed and/or endorsed by the IDSA.
The Joanna Briggs Institute https://joannabriggs.org	JBI is an initiative of the Royal Adelaide Hospital and the University of Adelaide. The Institute provides "a collaborative approach to the evaluation of evidence derived from a diverse range of sources, including experience, expertise and all forms of rigorous research and the translation, transfer and utilization of the 'best available' evidence into healthcare practice." Many resources are available only to member institutions, although selected systematic reviews and best practices information sheets are available to nonmembers.
National Cancer Institute Clinical Trials https://www.cancer.gov/clinicaltrials	Allows users to search and browse recent clinical trial results by type of cancer or topic or search NCI's list of thousands of clinical trials now accepting participants. Also included are educational materials about clinical trials, a list of noteworthy clinical trials, and more information for research teams interested in conducting clinical trials.
Nursing Best Practice Guidelines http://rnao.ca/bpg	Presents best practice guidelines for client care developed for Ontario Nurses. Includes almost 50 published guidelines as well as a Toolkit and an Educator's Resource to support implementation.
SUMSearch 2 http://sumsearch.org	A free meta-search engine for evidence-based medical information, scanning databases (MEDLINE, DARE, and National Guidelines Clearinghouse) as well as various high-impact medical journals. To automate searching, SUMSearch 2 combines meta- and contingency searching. Meta-searching is designed to scan multiple databases and sites simultaneously, and returns one single retrieval document to the user. If a high number of results are obtained, more restrictive searches (called contingency searches) are conducted by activating additional filters. Conversely, if the result is small, more databases are added to the search.
TRIP Medical Database https://www.tripdatabase.com	A free meta-search engine providing quick access to evidence-based and other high-quality medical information resources via a single interface. TRIP identifies/searches numerous internet resources that allow access to their content such as MEDLINE, Cochrane, National Guidelines Clearinghouse, ACP Journal Club, and top peer-reviewed journals. These resources are then categorized by type: Evidence-Based Synopses, Clinical Questions, Systematic Reviews, Guidelines, Core Primary Research, E textbooks, and Calculators.
Virginia Henderson Global Nursing e-Repository (Sigma Repository) https://www.sigmarepository.org/vhlonrnl/	This repository is an online digital service that collects, preserves, and disseminates digital materials in both abstract and full-text format without charge. Submissions may be made by individual nurses, nursing students, and nursing organizations and may include preprints, working papers, theses, dissertations, conference papers, presentations, faculty-created learning objects, data sets, etc.

ACP, The American College of Physicians; AHA, American Heart Association; IDSA, Infectious Diseases Society of America; JBI, The Joanna Briggs Institute; NCI, National Cancer Institute.

the delivery of evidence-based healthcare practice. Consequently, researchers should have some familiarity with sites specifically focusing on guidelines, such as the ECRI Guidelines Trust™.

Government agencies and professional associations that have developed clinical guidelines and practice statements may include them on their websites. Examples of this include standards, practice guidelines, statements, and clinical updates available online from the Infectious Diseases Society of America and the American Heart Association.

Websites of health agencies and associations organized around specific diseases or conditions also frequently post valuable reviews, reports, and studies that may or may not be included in the pages of journals. The website for the Agency for Healthcare Research and Quality delivers agency-funded, evidence-based research reports on clinical topics, healthcare services, and research methodologies. The website of the National Cancer Institute provides summaries of recently released results from clinical trials.

Search the Whole Internet

There is never one perfect location to find information on a health topic. Some people quickly turn to the ease of the internet as a starting place, which can be quite useful if you know where to look or how to search for pertinent and reliable information. The capability for "publishers"—whether they are healthcare institutions, corporate entities, government agencies, even individuals—to quickly and inexpensively publish permits immediate information transfer to the internet user. This also allows groups to distribute potentially important relevant information that may go unpublished through commercial channels. This type of literature is often referred to as the *grey literature* and can include scientific and technical reports, guidelines, care plans, patent documents, conference papers, internal reports, government documents, newsletters, factsheets, and theses.

Third-party informational sites such as Wikipedia are quickly becoming the initial stopping point for information on diagnoses, treatments, and prognoses of conditions. The use of these sites has tended to be negative in nature due to their open editing and lack of verification of research and/or resources. Wikipedia, for example, continues to be both a positive and negative resource to use during a research project. Aibar et al. (2015) conducted a large study looking at the use of Wikipedia and what faculty thought about it as a teaching tool. Aibar et al.'s study found that "academic disciplines [were] a key factor in explaining attitudes towards Wikipedia. This study also showed that age correlates with having a more negative view and that faculty who frequently use other online resources are more sceptical [sic] of Wikipedia" (p. 670). As with any online resource, the researcher should use critical analysis to determine the validity and reliability of the information contained within and not automatically assume the information is correct (London et al., 2019).

The information available via the internet is neither entirely trustworthy nor well organized. There are numerous popular search engines that scour the internet to retrieve materials that match keywords entered in the search box. Search engines use specific algorithms to sort retrieved results and in many cases retrieval order depends on a mixture of keyword matches, currency, and other factors (not necessarily quality of content). To eliminate some of the vagaries of internet searching, there are techniques to improve the quality and reliability of the retrieval set. The first is to try a selective search engine. A good example of a selective multidisciplinary search engine is Google Scholar (scholar.google.com), which restricts an internet search to "scholarly" publications such as journal articles, technical reports, preprints, theses, books, and vetted web pages from academic publishers, professional societies, preprint repositories, universities, and other scholarly organizations. Another good technique is to seek and employ search tools or an *advanced search* option, which may offer numerous options for making searches more precise and getting more

---

EXHIBIT 2.3

STRATEGIES TO DETERMINE WEBSITE QUALITY

1. Identify the website sponsor and author and credentials of the author.
2. Identify the date when the page was produced or revised.
3. View the HTML or page source of web pages to look for author/organization identification and/or publication date.
4. If you are not already knowledgeable about the topic, ask an expert to review the information.
5. Find reviews of internet resources by reviewers in reputable print and online sources, or use selective subject directory/electronic library collections you trust to identify resources.
6. Peruse related trustworthy websites to see whether there is a link to the site you are questioning.
7. Email the author or responsible organization/sponsor and ask about credentials.

Source: From Al-Jefri, M., Evans, R., Uchyigit, G., & Ghezzi, P. (2018).What is health information quality? Ethical dimension and perception by users. *Frontiers in Medicine, 5*, 260. https://doi.org/10.3389/fmed.2018.00260

---

reliable results. Do keep in mind, however, that much of the internet is not peer-reviewed or vetted in any way, so the searcher carries the burden of evaluating the quality and accuracy of the information presented. Strategies to assess website quality are presented in Exhibit 2.3.

Be Aware of Emerging Resources

Searching for, perusing, and validating either the review or the primary literature take skill and precious time. New practical resources to support evidence-based decisions are becoming readily available to healthcare practitioners. CSDs are designed to act as quick, single-stop, point of care tools that quickly connect users to evidence-based information on treatment and diagnostic options for common conditions. Examples of CSDs are listed in Box 2.1.

BOX 2.1 Clinical Summary Database Examples

Clinical Evidence (BMJ)
http://clinicalevidence.bmj.com

ClinicalKey or ClinicalKey for Nurses
https://www.elsevier.com/solutions/clinicalkey

DynaMed
https://www.dynamed.com

Essential Evidence Plus
http://www.essentialevidenceplus.com

UpToDate
http://www.uptodate.com

BOX 2.2 Surveillance Tool Examples

Evidence-Based Nursing
http://ebn.bmj.com

ACP Journal Club
http://www.acpjc.org

EvidenceAlerts
http://evidencealerts.com

Essential Evidence Plus: Daily POEMs
http://www.essentialevidenceplus.com/content/poems

The best CSDs summarize and synthesize current, high-quality research for answers to specific clinical questions, often adding practice implications specifically supported by a rationale and pertinent, current evidence. The centerpiece of these products includes a database of hundreds of entries on the treatment and prevention of medical conditions, which are developed from synthesized information obtained by searching quality evidence-based medicine resources and health-related literature databases. Creation of these entries is generally overseen by recognized experts and clinical specialists. Most CSDs tend to be updated monthly, although some are updated quarterly and/or will insert news items and urgent updates as needed. Although there is great variation in searchability, most interfaces offer browsable tables of contents and rudimentary search boxes; some include means to target or narrow search results.

Most researchers and practitioners commonly scan a fairly narrow set of journals to find articles of interest. To broaden their radar, readers should consider utilizing specialty resources that survey large sets of journals in selected disciplines. These *surveillance tools* summarize important articles that warrant the attention of their readership. In general, editors associated with these resources scan the health literature (often hundreds of journals) and highlight published topic reviews and individual studies from prominent journals. With few exceptions, reviews or studies that appear in these sources are sound and have met established quality criteria. Much like the CSDs, these resources boil down lengthy systematic reviews and detailed studies to a consumable package of value-added information. Selected examples of sources that provide this service are listed in Box 2.2.

■ PHASE IV—PULLING IT ALL TOGETHER

The search for evidence does not end with successful retrieval from a database or website. The relevant information needs to be retained and organized for further analysis, and full-text copies of articles, reports, and guidelines, and similar documents need to be obtained and stored. In addition, any search queries used should be retained and available for future searches on the topic.

Save Your Search Query

Experienced searchers are well aware of the benefits of saving database search queries at the conclusion of a search. One good motivation to do so is to prevent that sting of frustration when a literature search gets interrupted or misplaced and the entire search progression needs to be retraced. Another is to simply be in a position to quickly rerun a search at designated intervals to keep abreast of the literature on the particular topic. As a valuable convenience, databases now allow users to create individual accounts that will retain user information, search queries, and search results. My NCBI (PubMed) and My EBSCOhost are examples of user-created personal accounts within databases.

Invest in a Citation Manager

Databases allow searchers to output their retrieval sets in a variety of displays and a range of output formats. The most common display options are citation only, citation with abstract, or full record, which would include descriptors, accession numbers, and other useful data. Databases also offer different output options such as a text file, Microsoft Word file, preserved in an email, or sent to printer. Websites, on the other hand, give virtually no output choice other than the browser-supported PRINT and SAVE AS options.

The most efficient researcher, however, will enlist the help of commercial software called a *citation manager* to transfer, store, and manage the bibliographic references/citations retrieved from databases or websites. These products consist of a database in which full bibliographic citations (abstracts, subject headings, etc.) can be imported, as well acting as a conduit for generating selective lists or reference lists in the different formats required by publishers.

Citation managers can integrate themselves within word processing software and format citations automatically in any chosen style such those from the American Medical Association, American Psychological Association, and so on. These products also give researchers the ability to switch between citation styles based on the specific style the selected journal wishes manuscripts be formatted. Commonly used citation managers in the health sciences include:

- EndNote—www.*endnote.com*
- Mendeley—*www.mendeley.com*
- RefWorks—*www.refworks.com/refworks2/*
- Zotero—www.*zotero.org*

There are many citation managers available on the market and the best of them allow:

- Direct export from online databases such as PubMed, CINAHL, PsycINFO, etc. into the citation manager.
- Ability to create multiple folders and subfolders for the organization of citations.
- Output to format bibliographies in all major styles (AMA, APA, etc.).
- Automatic integration with word processor formats (Microsoft Word, RTF [rich text format], HTML, etc.).
- Attachments such as image files, Adobe PDFs, Microsoft Word docs to be embedded into a record to a citation within the database for opening at a later time.
- Group accounts that allow several researches to access the citation database.

Find the Full Article (Full Text)

One of the barriers to conducting a successful literature search is simply obtaining the entire (full-text) articles of the retrieved results. Access to full-text articles has improved dramatically with the growth of electronic publishing, yet this usually remains a multistep process. The majority of databases and websites tend to only provide citations and abstracts to items of interest, but entire articles are not always immediately available online. Certain databases are making an effort to assist the user by allowing publishers and academic institutions to insert a link within item records to lead users to the full article. Keep in mind that commercial and academic publishers rarely give anything away for free and often charge fees, some exorbitant, to grant access to articles. A searcher may want to first contact a local clinic, hospital, academic, or even turn to a public library. Libraries often have established access to journal collections or offer interlibrary loan services.

Keep Current

Current awareness of the published information on any given topic is no longer difficult. Several options are available for practitioners to stay current with the new information or update information on a given topic (Ross & Cross, 2019). Mobile apps, RSS feeds and readers, podcasts, blogs, or databases now offer *alert* or *current awareness* services that allow users automatically to receive new results (via email) from saved search queries at prescribed intervals. Search queries can involve topics of interest, or can pertain to specific authors or a set of relevant journals. Blogs and podcasts are varied and can be selected on personal interest; these can be found by running general searches on the interest or from publishers, journals, or professional organizations.

Really simple syndication (RSS) is a technology that automatically retrieves information from favorite sources. RSS is more or less an electronic table of contents service where one can quickly scan the contents (called feeds) of any number of the latest journals, headlines from favorite news sources, news from relevant organizations, entries from blogs and websites, and even updates from literature searches, at one location, a feed reader. There are many free feed readers available. Here are some selected examples, but the final choice will be yours depending on the features you are interested in:

- Feedly—*feedly.com*
- FlowReader—*www.flowreader.com*
- NewsBlur—*www.newsblur.com*

Getting started with RSS is relatively easy and is likely to become an indispensable tool for keeping a researcher or clinician current and saving time.

Mobile apps are the hottest avenues to follow the rapidly changing health science field. While not exactly RSS readers, there are several dedicated apps on the market to help you stay on top of the journal literature and other scholarly information. In addition to the raw tables of contents, they offer other services and/or functionality. Here are a few examples:

- Read by QxMD is "a single place to discover new research, read outstanding topic reviews and search PubMed." It is available for a variety of devices and covers about a dozen medical specialties.
- docphin is a free app for all smartphones and tablets, and the web billed as "the best way to keep up with medical research." It has an integrated institutional login function to allow access to full-text PDFs, the Medstream news service, and powerful search features to find the articles you need quickly and efficiently.
- BrowZine is a current awareness service to help you keep up with the latest research in your field. You can use it on the web, through a mobile app, or both as it syncs your account across all devices. Users need be affiliated with an origination that subscribes to this service. No personal subscriptions are available.

Social Media

Social media sites have become a tremendous access point for staying current with research or trends in the health sciences. Twitter, Facebook and YouTube all offer continuous professional development, lectures, access to professional content or up-to-the-minute conversations regarding health-related research or scholars. Researchers in 2010 estimated Twitter contained over 19,100 accounts created by nurses (Moorley & Chinn, 2015). Coupled with today's Facebook, YouTube, LinkedIn, podcast, or blog accounts created by professional organizations or nurses, the amount of emerging research promoted outside of traditional venues is impressive (Reinbeck & Antonacci, 2019). However, being able to evaluate any information from the social media realm still requires the user to approach these tweets or posts with a critical eye as one would a traditional research article.

If you have any questions about current awareness topics in your area of interest, look to the literature, discuss possible items of interest with colleagues, or speak with a health science librarian close to you.

■ SUMMARY

Literature reviews are not mysterious manifestations of scholarly pursuits. Nor should they be merely academic exercises. They are, and are increasingly being required to be, vital components of quality healthcare. Literature reviews are the sum of many definable parts and the application of systematic procedures as illustrated in this chapter in four phases: (a) pre-search preparations and planning, (b) mining core and peripheral literature databases for evidence-based information, (c) mining additional resources across the internet, and (d) using new technologies to organize, store, and update found information. This systematic process builds a researcher's toolkit and can be adapted to meet the demands of EBP.

SUGGESTED LEARNING ACTIVITIES

1. You are planning a research study to determine adherence to diet by diabetic patients. Perform a literature search to locate articles published in the past 3 to 5 years that describe how diabetics conform to their prescribed diets. Use at least two appropriate databases (e.g., CINAHL and MEDLINE [PubMed]) to find pertinent articles. Compare and contrast articles you retrieve for levels of evidence, strength of evidence presented, and their usefulness for defined needs.

2. Locate practice guidelines on the treatment of foot ulcers in diabetics. Use at least two appropriate resources (e.g., ECRI Guidelines Trust™ and MEDLINE [PubMed]). How do the search results compare?

REFERENCES

Aibar, E., Lladós-Masllorens, J., Meseguer-Artola, A., Minguillón, J., & Lerga, M. (2015). Wikipedia at university: What faculty think and do about it. *Electronic Library, 33*(4), 668–683. https://doi.org/10.1108/EL-12-2013-0217

Al-Jefri, M., Evans, R., Uchyigit, G., & Ghezzi, P. (2018). What is health information quality? Ethical dimension and perception by users. *Frontiers in Medicine, 5*, 260. https://doi.org/10.3389/fmed.2018.00260

Bastian, H., Glasziou, P., & Chalmers, I. (2010). Seventy-five trials and eleven systematic reviews a day: How will we ever keep up? *PLOS Medicine, 7*(9), e1000326. https://doi.org/10.1371/journal.pmed.1000326

Bettany-Saltikov, J. (2012) *How to do a systematic literature review in nursing: A step-by-step guide.* McGraw-Hill/Open University Press.

Bramer, W. M., de Jonge, G. B., Rethlefsen, M., Mast, F., & Kleijnen, J. (2018). A systematic approach to searching: An efficient and complete method to develop literature searches. *Journal of the Medical Library Association, 106*(4), 531–541. https://doi.org/10.5195/JMLA.2018.283

Brown, C. E., Wickline, M. A., Ecoff, L., & Glaser, D. (2009). Nursing practice, knowledge, attitudes and perceived barriers to evidence-based practice at an academic medical center. *Journal of Advanced Nursing, 65*(2), 371–381. https://doi.org/10.1111/j.1365-2648.2008.04878.x

Christenbery, T., Williamson, A., Sandlin, V., & Wells, N. (2016). Immersion in evidence-based practice fellowship program: A transforming experience for staff nurses. *Journal for Nurses in Professional Development, 32*(1), 15–20. https://doi.org/10.1097/NND.0000000000000197

Cypress, B. S. (2019). Qualitative research: Challenges and dilemmas. *Dimensions of Critical Care Nursing: DCCN, 38*(5), 264–270. https://doi.org/10.1097/DCC.0000000000000374

Fencl, J. L., & Matthews, C. (2017). Translating evidence into practice: How advanced practice RNs can guide nurses in challenging established practice to arrive at best practice. *AORN Journal, 106*(5), 378–392. https://doi.org/10.1016/j.aorn.2017.09.002

Gerberi, D., & Marienau, M. S. (2017). Literature searching for practice research. *AANA Journal, 85*(3), 195–204.

Johnston, B., Coole, C., Narayanasamy, M., Feakes, R., Whitworth, G., Tyrell, T., & Hardy, B. (2016). Exploring the barriers to and facilitators of implementing research into practice. *British Journal of Community Nursing, 21*(8), 392–398. https://doi.org/10.12968/bjcn.2016.21.8.392

Larosa, S. S. (2014). The science of caring. *Discoveries Magazine, Cedars-Sinai, 2014*(Fall), 20–25.

London, D. A., Andelman, S. M., Christiano, A. V., Kim, J, H., Hausman, M. R., & Kim, J. M. (2019). Is Wikipedia a complete and accurate source for musculoskeletal anatomy? *Surgical and Radiologic Anatomy, 41*(10), 1187–1192. https://doi.org/10.1007/s00276-019-02280-1

Moorley, C., & Chinn, T. (2015). Using social media for continuous professional development. *Journal of Advanced Nursing, 71*(4), 713–717. https://doi.org/10.1111/jan.12504

National Library of Medicine. (2019). *MEDLINE PubMed production statistics.* https://www.nlm.nih.gov/bsd/medline_pubmed_production_stats.html

Polit, D. F., & Beck, C. T. (2020). *Nursing research: Generating and assessing evidence for nursing practice* (11th ed.). Wolters Kluwer Health/Lippincott Williams & Wilkins.

Pravikoff, D. S., Tanner, A. B., & Pierce, S. T. (2005). Readiness of U.S. nurses for evidence-based practice. *The American Journal of Nursing, 105*(9), 40–51; quiz 52. https://doi.org/10.1097/00000446-200509000-00025

Reinbeck, D., & Antonacci, J. (2019). How nurses can use social media to their advantage. *Nursing, 49*(5), 61–63. https://doi.org/10.1097/01.NURSE.0000554624.05347.6e

Ross, P., & Cross, R. (2019). Rise of the e-Nurse: The power of social media in nursing. *Contemporary Nurse: A Journal for the Australian Nursing Profession, 55*(2/3), 211–220. https://doi.org/10.1080/10376178.2019.1641419

Taylor, M. V., Priefer, B. A., & Alt-White, A. C. (2016). Evidence-based practice: Embracing integration. *Nursing Outlook, 64*(6), 575–582. https://doi.org/10.1016/j.outlook.2016.04.004

RESEARCH AND THE MANDATE FOR EVIDENCE-BASED PRACTICE, QUALITY, AND PATIENT SAFETY

KATHLEEN R. STEVENS

■ INTRODUCTION

The development of science to guide nursing practice and healthcare is a response to the need for knowledge to improve care and advance the health of the public. Nursing science has the ultimate aim of discovering effective interventions to resolve actual and potential health problems and to point to interventions that reliably produce intended health-related outcomes. Nursing research has been well institutionalized since 1984, with the establishment of the National Institute of Nursing Research (NINR; originally, the National Center for Nursing Research). As a result, nursing science has greatly expanded, providing research results and a foundation for evidence-based practice (EBP); however, it is widely recognized that many years pass before even a small percentage of EBPs are adopted into routine care. The gap between what is known to work and what is practiced is responsible for less-than-possible care quality and patient safety.

There is increased public demand for moving new knowledge into practice to increase care quality and safety and increase the likelihood that our nursing interventions will produce intended health outcomes. The recent past has seen growing emphasis on *how* to move research findings into everyday practice. Research across all health disciplines is investigating strategies to move evidence into practice through the new field of implementation science. The focus of implementation science is to evaluate strategies that overcome organizational, individual, and policy barriers in adoption of EBP.

During the past 25 years, research has grown the science of quality and safety, providing a foundation for (a) knowing what works in healthcare, as well as (b) how to implement changes in practice. This chapter presents events and findings that influence this scientific interest in healthcare quality and safety. Included are descriptions of the underlying reasons for the emphasis on quality improvement and safety, frameworks for conceptualizing and studying improvement and safety, methods used for such investigations, and new resources and future trends in improvement and safety research. In addition, this chapter explores how EBP achieves quality and safety in healthcare by reflecting nursing theory, research, science, and practice to meet the mandate for improved population health.

To provide a broad context, our discussion first presents an overview of the relationship among research, EBP, quality, and safety, providing a framework through which to view these aspects of healthcare. Sections of the chapter define the relationship among EBP, implementation science, and quality. Additional sections of the chapter are devoted specifically to quality and to safety, highlighting dominant thinking and research advances. Exemplars led by advanced practice nurses illustrate their central role in transforming healthcare. The chapter concludes with a look to the future of quality and safety, examining recent advances and suggesting directions in theory, research, and science.

■ SHIFTS IN NURSING RESEARCH FOCUS

Because of the emphasis on quality improvement in regard to patient safety, the relationship between research and clinical care has changed. In the past, primary research was conducted to test the efficacy of interventions; now, researchers investigate ways to render healthcare systems and processes effective and safe. A number of these approaches involve integrating research into practice—so nurses are called on to be part of the team that transforms research knowledge into clinical practice. Clients demand that healthcare be based on *best scientific evidence* in combination with *client preferences* and the *clinician's expertise* (the definition of EBP).

This paradigm of EBP has required a shift in thinking about EBP competencies that are needed in clinical care. This is particularly true of competencies at intermediate and advanced levels to promote uptake of evidence into daily care. Prior to the new knowledge forms offered by EBP, educational programs prepared nurses to "conduct" research to discover new knowledge. Although an important function, conducting research is insufficient to achieve evidence-based quality improvement. Increasingly, advance practice nurses assume roles that emphasize evidence-based quality improvement—competencies not widely included in basic and professional development education. These competencies involve managing both the research-based evidence and the organizational activities necessary to translate research into practice (Stevens, 2009). Research has led to identification of these EBP competencies which make clear the distinction between conducting research and translating research into practice. National consensus on 83 EBP competencies (Stevens, 2009) has galvanized changes in nursing practice and in nursing education programs. EBP competencies are being integrated throughout undergraduate, graduate, and professional development education and clinical practice. Additional work identified learning outcomes for quality and safety education (Dolansky & Moore, 2013), which contributed to this growing effort toward a workforce that is prepared to translate research into practice. However, nurses still face significant barriers in employing EBP (Yoder et al., 2014) and it is imperative to continue efforts to embed these competencies into the core of our profession.

■ CHANGES IN NURSING RESEARCH

Now, over 20 years into the pioneering EBP work in nursing, nurses, managers, and healthcare system leaders are still making the paradigm shift to a system that rapidly adopts best practices; this is owing to the challenge of complex healthcare systems and entire industries. Gains made in the transformation of healthcare to be safe, effective, efficient, equitable, and patient-centered can be accelerated as emphasis on discovery through nursing research is joined by expanding horizons noted in nursing science.

The focus of nursing research has recently expanded to include the study of healthcare delivery systems, quality, and patient safety. In the past, nursing research produced knowledge about individual clients through primary research studies. Research was largely based on designs used to investigate individual client interventions (such as experimental psychology and anthropology). The resulting research reports were found to be difficult to translate into practice. Single research studies were presented in terms of inferential statistics and multiple studies and often produced varying results on the efficacy of a given intervention.

Today's healthcare redesign and evidence-based quality initiatives call on nurse scientists and clinicians to embrace what is known about best (effective) practices and system change to support quality healthcare. Prior methods, such as true experiments, and theory are important to our scientific fundamentals. Research designs such as systematic reviews (SR) and new models such as complex adaptive systems (CASs) are being added to place nurses at the cutting edge of advancing the science of improvement. New competencies in translational science have been added to prior investigative competencies to conduct primary research studies. Nurse researchers are realigning previous research approaches and adopting new research designs as members of translational science teams that produce knowledge about effective healthcare and systems.

New fields of study have set about to investigate improvement strategies and to understand factors that facilitate or hinder implementation and adoption of EBP. The aim of implementation and improvement science is to determine which strategies work as we strive to ensure safe and effective care. Improvement and implementation competencies are primarily focused on evolving the healthcare delivery system and microsystem (Berwick, 2008). Implementation science is important to improvement in that it assesses ways to link evidence into practice; it adds to our understanding of the usefulness of strategies to "adopt and integrate evidence-based health interventions and change practice patterns within specific settings" (National Institutes of Health [NIH], 2019). Together, improvement and implementation sciences add to an increased understanding of the *system* aspects of the care we deliver.

▨ OVERVIEW: RESEARCH, EVIDENCE-BASED PRACTICE, QUALITY, AND SAFETY

Quality, safety, and efficiency are top priorities in contemporary healthcare. The responsibility and accountability for ensuring effective and safe care are inescapable for all health professionals and are a social obligation of every healthcare agency. Delivering the right care at the right time in the right setting is the goal of efforts to advance safety and quality. This challenge requires that well-prepared nurses play key roles in moving research into action to evolve today's healthcare system. Progress requires competencies at the individual clinician level; in addition, operational leaders and organizational climate must be open to continued learning and change. For nurses to effectively guide the movement for quality and safety, skills and competencies in evidence-based practice (e.g., Stevens, 2013), change management, and organizational development are required. In tandem, organizational leaders must adopt system approaches that reflect improvement principles and principles of high-reliability industries.

The morbidity and mortality toll of both ineffective care and unsafe care requires that all health professionals take a serious look at what must be done to address lapses in quality and to avoid the loss of hundreds of thousands of lives. To meet this challenge, it is vital to ensure that healthcare is error free, that all existing best (research-based) practices are used, and that individual clinicians and organizations implement the highest quality and most reliable processes for every patient. The narrow notion of safety as the absence of medication errors or falls has been broadened. This is the challenge of quality and patient safety in healthcare. The foundation of success is translation of research results into clinical care; the infrastructure of success is conducting research to elucidate change interventions that improve clinical care processes at the individual clinician, organization, system, environment, and policy levels. Thus, translational research is the key to determining clinical effectiveness of care and redesigning healthcare systems that are safe, effective, and efficient.

■ PROBLEMS IN HEALTHCARE QUALITY

Research has built a large body of science about "what works" in healthcare, yet actual care lags behind what has been reported to be effective (Institute of Medicine [IOM], 2008). The end result is healthcare that is ineffective in producing intended patient health outcomes and care that is unsafe. These circumstances are prevalent in nursing and across all health professions, even though massive numbers of research reports provide "best evidence" for care. Healthcare processes and outcomes will be greatly improved when research results are adopted into routine care.

■ QUALITY AND EVIDENCE-BASED PRACTICE

The quality of healthcare is based on the degree to which decisions about patient care are guided by "conscientious, explicit, and judicious use of current best evidence" (IOM, 2008, p. 3). The following definition of healthcare quality emphasizes this point.

Definition: Quality of Healthcare

Degree to which health services for individuals and populations increase the likelihood of desired health outcomes and are consistent with current professional knowledge.

(IOM, 1990)

This definition makes clear that research evidence is a core element in predictably producing intended health outcomes. Unless patient care is based on the most current and best evidence, it falls short of quality.

The aim of EBP is to standardize healthcare practices using the best scientific base (best evidence) and to reduce illogical variations in care, which lead to uncertainty that clinical interventions will lead to better health outcomes. Development of EBP is fueled by public and professional demand for accountability in safety and quality improvement in healthcare. It is imperative that healthcare is based on current professional knowledge in order to produce the quality necessary for intended patient outcomes.

Leaders in the field have classically defined EBP as the "integration of best research evidence with clinical expertise and patient values" (Sackett et al., 2000, p. ii). Therefore, EBP melds research evidence with clinical expertise and encourages individualization of care through incorporation of patient preferences and the circumstances of the setting.

Just as evidence and quality are linked, so are safety and quality. The ties across safety, errors, quality, and care are explained as concentric circles or subsets of a common flaw (Woolf, 2004). The innermost concentric circle is safety, followed by errors, then quality, and, finally, caring as the outermost circle. The model suggests that safety is a subcategory of healthcare errors. Such errors include mistakes in health promotion and chronic disease management that cost lives but do not affect safety—these are errors of omission. Following this model, errors are a subset of quality lapses, which result from both errors and systemic problems. Systemic problems that reduce quality in healthcare may stem from lack of access, inequity, and flawed system designs. Finally, this model suggests that lapses in quality are a subset of deficient caring; such deficiencies can be seen in lack of access, inequity, and faulty system designs (Woolf, 2004). In nursing research, such a model can serve to frame investigations of healthcare safety and quality.

Healthcare quality and safety have emerged as a principal concern. Multiple reports were produced since 2000 that still guide our national thinking about how to improve our healthcare system to impact better population health. In 1990, interprofessional opinion leaders began an intensive initiative to improve the quality of healthcare (IOM, 1990). These leaders proclaimed that there is a chasm between what we *know* (through research) to be the best healthcare and what we *do*. In a series of influential reports, these national advisers called for one of our nation's most far-reaching health reforms, called the IOM Quality Initiative. A series of reports known as the *Quality Chasm Series*, dissected healthcare problems and recommended fundamental and sweeping changes in healthcare (IOM, 2001). The directions set by the *Quality Chasm Series* continue to have marked impact on every aspect of healthcare and health professionals, with the "IOM Principles" deeply integrated into requirements in nursing education and practice. Each of the trendsetting IOM reports (2001, 2003a, 2003b, 2004, 2008, 2011a, 2011b) identify EBP as *crucial* in closing the quality chasm. This movement is likely to continue beyond the next decade. Because of their enduring impact on the transformation of healthcare, we offer the following summary of some of the IOM *Chasm* reports.

In 2000, the IOM reviewed studies and trends and concluded that 48,000 to 98,000 Americans die annually in hospitals due to medical errors caused by defective systems rather than caregivers themselves. *To Err Is Human: Building a Safer Health System* (IOM, 2000) offered impressive documentation regarding the severity and pervasive nature of the nation's overall quality problem. In fact, using statistical approaches, the report showed that more people die from medical mistakes each year than from highway accidents, breast cancer, or AIDS. In addition to deaths, it was noted that medical errors cause permanent disabilities and unnecessary suffering. This report raised the issue of patient safety to a high priority for every healthcare provider, scientist, agency leader, and policy maker.

The next report in this series further unfolded the story of quality in American healthcare. In *Crossing the Quality Chasm: A New Health System for the 21st Century* (IOM, 2001), healthcare leaders reviewed research that highlighted other widespread defects in our healthcare system. Defects included overuse, misuse, and underuse of healthcare services and described a wide gulf between ideal care (as supported by research) and the reality of the care that many Americans experience. The 2001 *Quality Chasm* report presented research evidence documenting a lack of quality in healthcare, cost concerns, poor use of information technology, absence of progress in restructuring the healthcare system, and underutilization of resources. Throughout these analyses of healthcare safety and quality, a deep-rooted problem was highlighted: Although health science and technology were advancing at a rapid pace, the healthcare delivery system was failing to deliver high-quality healthcare services (IOM, 2001). The report emphasized that a major part of the problem is that research results are not translated into practice and that practice lags behind research-generated knowledge.

The profession of nursing is central to many of the interprofessional and discipline-specific changes that must be accomplished to provide safe and effective care. The Interdisciplinary Nursing Quality Research Initiative (INQRI, 2013) supported by the Robert Wood Johnson Foundation (RWJF, 2008) funded studies to discover how nurses contribute to and can improve the quality of patient care.

After a series of public input meetings, the IOM issued the 2011 report, *The Future of Nursing: Leading Change, Advancing Health.* The report identified the 3 million (now 4 million) nurses in the profession as the largest segment of the nation's healthcare workforce. Among the eight recommendations was urging nurses to lead and manage collaborative efforts within an interdisciplinary team to redesign and improve practice and healthcare systems (IOM, 2011c). Since this publication, a nationwide campaign for action emerged to address the recommendations. Recent assessment of the campaign highlights progress made through nurses' addressing the areas of healthcare delivery, scope of practice, education, collaboration, leadership, diversity in the nursing profession, and workforce data (Altman et al., 2016). Efforts are underway to update the recommendations and set the course for the Future of Nursing 2020–2030, specifying how nurses might continue to contribute to healthcare quality and safety.

■ NURSING PROGRESSION: RESEARCH UTILIZATION AND EVIDENCE-BASED PRACTICE

Because the purpose of research ultimately is to uncover causal relationships, the primary goal is to determine which interventions are most effective in assisting patients and clients to resolve actual and potential health problems. In other words, research shows us "what works best" to produce the intended health outcome for a given health problem. Knowledge discovered through research is then translated into practice guidelines and ultimately affects health policy through commonly accepted healthcare practices.

In health professions, research is conducted to build a case for specific practices and interventions. The reason for conducting research is to illuminate effective practices, so it follows that the end goal is that research findings be translated into clinical decision-making at the point of care. Although this goal is clear, health professionals have struggled to achieve research utilization since the 1970s.

Nurses, along with other health professionals, have sought ways to move research results into practice; however, early attempts were not fully successful. Barriers to knowledge translation became a crucial topic of investigation in nursing in the early 1990s. A number of research utilization models were developed to explain the barriers and challenges in applying research results in practice. An early program of study established a dissemination model (Funk et al., 1989) and developed a scale with which to quantify nurses' perceptions of barriers to applying research in practice (Funk et al., 1990). The BARRIERS scale is framed in the old paradigm of research utilization, in which results of a single study were examined for direct application, and clinical nurses were expected to read, critique, and translate primary research reports into point-of-care practice, and to devote time to these activities.

This early work in research utilization resulted in a clearer focus on clinical investigations. Nurse scientists who conducted research, largely in academic settings, were criticized for their shortcomings in making research results clinically meaningful. Such criticism included claims that research did not address pressing clinical problems, results were not expressed in terms understood by clinicians, and clinicians were not in positions to apply the results in care. In tandem, nurse scientists gathered momentum to establish what is today the NINR, dedicated to funding clinical research.

Initial research utilization models were developed prior to the emergence of EBP. The Stetler Model (Stetler, 1994) mapped a step-by-step approach that could be used by individual clinicians to critique research, restate findings, and consider the findings in their own decision-making. The model focuses on a bottom-up approach to change in clinical practice. The Iowa Model outlined a process to guide implementation of research results into clinical practice in the context of provider, patient, and infrastructure (Titler et al., 2001). The Iowa Model gives heavy emphasis to nurse managers as key instruments of change. Both models have moved from their original roots in research utilization to reflect a broader approach used in EBP. These early efforts underscored the importance of moving research into direct patient care.

■ SHIFT FROM RESEARCH UTILIZATION TO EVIDENCE-BASED PRACTICE

Frequently, research results are either inadequately translated into clinical practice recommendations or applied inconsistently in the delivery of healthcare. Additionally, poor healthcare system design contributes to the chasm; healthcare design inadequacies include a lack of interprofessional teams to provide comprehensive and coordinated care and a complex system that is a maze to patients and that fails to provide patients the services from which they would likely benefit (IOM, 2001).

As the EBP movement grew, it became apparent that the hurdles to translating research to practice required complex answers not yet formulated. The EBP movement has provided new scientific means with which to overcome these hurdles (Stevens, 2013).

Until recently, emphasis was placed on designing and conducting research studies to fill knowledge gaps about efficacy of clinical care. While generating this new knowledge is critically important, it falls short of the goal of adopting new knowledge into routine care to improve health and healthcare. The evidence-based practice paradigm and particularly the newer field of implementation science provide foundations for clinicians to spur adoption and sustainment of evidence-based practices. In the EBP approach, emphasis is placed on applying this new knowledge and the steps needed to increase clinical utility and usefulness of the research results. It became clear that knowledge transformation must occur in order for research results to be readily accessible to clinicians and transformed into practice (Stevens, 2015).

As the healthcare quality paradigm expanded to EBP, challenges in transforming research results into common practice became apparent. EBP approaches, derived from clinical epidemiology, provided new insights and changed the approach to moving research into routine care. With the paradigm shift, these two hurdles became apparent: (a) the large volume and complexity of health research literature and (b) the low clinical utility of the form of knowledge that is available to the clinician (Stevens, 2015).

Advancements in the EBP movement produced a number of models and techniques to meet the challenges of adopting research into care to improve care and patient safety (Nilsen, 2020). Nurse scientists contributed a number of models to understand the various aspects of EBP. These models guide implementation approaches intended to strengthen evidence-based decision-making. Forty-seven prominent EBP models identified in the literature were grouped into four thematic areas: "(a) EBP, Research Utilization, and Knowledge Transformation Processes. . ., (b) Strategic/ Organizational Change Theory to Promote Uptake and Adoption of New Knowledge..., (c) Knowledge Exchange and Synthesis for Application and Inquiry. . ., and (d) Designing and Interpreting Dissemination Research" (Mitchell et al., 2010, pp. 288–289). Listed among models is the widely-adopted Stevens Star Model of Knowledge Transformation (Stevens, 2015). The following discussion expands on the Star Model to frame important aspects of the advance practice nurse's role in evidence-based quality improvement.

The Star Model addresses two key challenges in moving evidence into action, First, research results from multiple studies must be combined and repackaged to maximize utility for clinical decision-making. Second, systematic facilitation is requisite for successful implementation of the EBP. As depicted in Figure 3.1, the stages represented in the Stevens Star Model are arranged around a 5-point star representing (a) discovery research, (b) evidence summary, (c) translation into clinical guidelines, (d) integration into practice, and (e) evaluation of impact on outcomes (Stevens, 2015).

POINT 1: Discovery Research

As described, the NINR provided great stimulus, resources, and focus for primary nursing research studies. The upshot was that the number of nursing research studies rapidly expanded. However, a large collection of single research studies is not manageable to inform clinical choices at the point of care. Moreover, various studies may show different conclusions about the efficacy of a clinical intervention (e.g., skin-to-skin neonatal care).

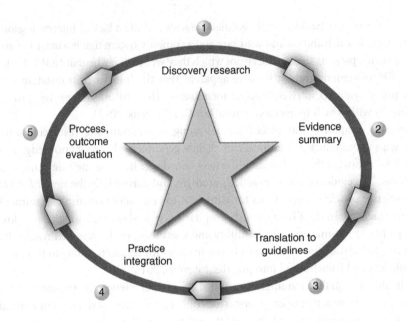

FIGURE 3.1 Stevens Star Model of Knowledge Transformation.
Source: Copyright 2015, Kathleen Stevens, EdD, FAAN, RN, ANEF. Used with permission.

POINT 2: Evidence Summary

To overcome the hurdle to clinical application posed by the growing volume of single research studies, a new approach to knowledge management was developed in the mid-1990s. The new approach systematically combined research results from multiple studies and evidence summaries became a key to bridging knowledge to practice. The most rigorous scientific method for synthesizing all research into a single summary is called a *systematic review* (SR). A SR is defined as a scientific investigation that focuses on a specific question and uses explicitly preplanned scientific methods to identify, select, assess, and summarize similar but separate studies (IOM, 2008).

A SR produces a concise, comprehensive, comprehensible statement about the state of the science regarding clinical effectiveness. It is identified as the cornerstone to understanding whether a clinical intervention works (IOM, 2008, 2011b). Indeed, it is recognized that an evidence summary is requisite to "getting the evidence [about intervention efficacy] straight" (Glasziou & Haynes, 2005). The sobering flip side of this logic is that *not* conducting an rigorous evidence summary or conducting a non-SR will likely result in *not* getting the evidence straight, leading to a misinformed clinical decision and poor patient outcomes. Nursing care must be driven by research evidence—not knowing the state of the science about clinical effectiveness results in ineffective, unnecessary, or harmful care. From EBP, we now realize that basing care on results of a single primary research study can lead to the selection of a wrong intervention and produce poor outcomes. With this new realization, we have moved away from using single research studies to change practice to a much more rigorous knowledge form—the evidence summary.

SRs serve two important knowledge functions in selecting high-quality clinical interventions. First, a SR provides evidence about the clinical efficacy of a particular intervention in relation to specified outcomes. Second, a SR provides a view of gaps in the scientific field and points to further research needed to fill these voids. A prime advantage of an evidence summary, such as a SR,

BOX 3.1 Advantages of a Systematic Review

1. Reduces information into a manageable form

2. Increases power in cause and effect

3. Assesses consistencies across studies

4. Integrates information for decisions

5. Establishes generalizability—participants, settings, treatment variations, and study designs

6. Reduces bias and improves true reflection of reality

7. Reduces time between research and implementation

8. Offers a basis for continuous update as new knowledge is discovered

9. Points to further research to address gaps

Source: From Mulrow, C. D. (1994). Rationale for systematic reviews. *British Medical Journal (Clinical Research Edition), 309*(6954), 597–599. https://doi.org/10.1136/bmj.309.6954.597

is that all research results on a given topic are transformed into a single, harmonious statement (Mulrow, 1994).

With a SR, the state of the science on a given topic is placed at the fingertips of the clinician in terms of what is known and what remains to be discovered. SRs are deemed one of the two key ways of *knowing what works* in healthcare (IOM, 2008, 2011b). With regard to providing evidence-based direction for clinical care, a SR offers other advantages (Mulrow, 1994) as outlined in Box 3.1.

Box 3.2 illustrates a systematic review of a topic of high interest to individual clinicians, healthcare organizations, and patients: falls prevention.

BOX 3.2 Example of a Systematic Review

A recent systematic review identified 62 randomized clinical trials ($N = 35{,}058$) which investigated 7 types of fall prevention interventions. The conclusions were:

- Multifactorial and exercise interventions were associated with fall-related benefit.

- Evidence was most consistent across multiple fall-related outcomes for exercise.

- Vitamin D supplementation interventions had mixed results, with a high dose being associated with higher rates of fall-related outcomes.

Source: From Guirguis-Blake, J. M., Michael, Y. L., Perdue, L. A., Coppola, E. L., & Beil, T. L. (2018). Interventions to prevent falls in older adults: Updated evidence report and systematic review for the U.S. Preventive Services Task Force. *JAMA, 319*(16), 1705–1716. https://doi.org/10.1001/jama.2017.21962

POINT 3: Translation to Guidelines

The next stage of knowledge transformation is producing evidence-based clinical practice guidelines (CPGs). In the Star Model, CPGs represent the "translation" of the evidence summary into recommendations for clinical practice. Evidence-based CPGs have the potential to reduce illogical variations in practice by encouraging use of clinically effective practices (IOM, 2008, 2011a, 2011b). CPGs articulate the likelihood that a chosen intervention will produce the intended patient outcome, or more succinctly, "what works in healthcare" (IOM, 2008). Importantly, CPGs enhance the uptake of EBP by presenting trustworthy recommendations that are directly related to clinical care. CPGs are "systematically defined statements that are designed to help clinicians and patients make decisions about appropriate healthcare for specific clinical circumstances" (IOM, 1990, p. 38). The current definition is: "CPGs are statements that include recommendations intended to optimize patient care that are informed by a systematic review of evidence and an assessment of the benefits and harms of alternative care options" (IOM, 2011a, p. 4). Guidelines can be considered a convenient way of packaging evidence and presenting recommendations to healthcare decision-makers.

The trustworthiness of a CPG is enhanced when it is firmly based on the best evidence relating to clinical effectiveness and cost-effectiveness. Standards for trustworthy CPGs include transparent processes for developing the recommendations and criteria for appraising reliability. Well-developed guidelines include specification and rating of supporting evidence. Defining characteristics of trustworthy guidelines are included in Box 3.3.

An example of nurses engaged in development of guidelines is noted in the U.S. Preventive Services Task Force. This entity is an independent, volunteer panel of national experts in prevention and evidence-based medicine. The Task Force works to improve the health of all Americans by making evidence-based recommendations (CPGs) about clinical preventive services such as screenings, counseling services, and preventive medications. Table 3.1 presents two examples of "Grade A or B" guidelines (U.S. Preventive Services Task Force, 2020).

When developed in a systematic and transparent way, CPGs are a critical form of knowledge, making evidence far more accessible during clinical decision-making.

BOX 3.3 Characteristics of Trustworthy Clinical Practice Guideline

- Based on a systematic review of the existing evidence.
- Developed by a knowledgeable, multidisciplinary panel of experts and representatives from key affected groups.
- Considers important patient subgroups and patient preferences.
- Based on an explicit and transparent process that minimizes distortions, biases, and conflicts of interest.
- Provides a clear explanation of the logical relationships between various care options and health outcomes.
- Provides ratings of the quality of evidence and the strength of the recommendations.
- Reflects revisions when important new evidence warrants modifications of recommendations.

Table 3.1 Two Examples of "Grade A or B" Guidelines

POPULATION	RECOMMENDATION
Pregnant Women	Grade A "The USPSTF recommends screening for HBV infection in pregnant women at their first prenatal visit." https://www.uspreventiveservicestaskforce.org/uspstf/recommendation/hepatitis-b-virus-infection-in-pregnant-women-screening
School-aged children and adolescents who have not started to use tobacco	Grade B "The USPSTF recommends that primary care clinicians provide interventions, including education or brief counseling, to prevent initiation of tobacco use among school-aged children and adolescents." https://www.uspreventiveservicestaskforce.org/uspstf/recommendation/tobacco-and-nicotine-use-prevention-in-children-and-adolescents-primary-care-interventions

HBV, hepatitis B virus; USPSTF, U.S. Preventive Services Task Force.

POINT 4: Integration

Once high quality evidence-based guidelines have been developed, routine practice and clinical decisions must be realigned to these new standards to improve healthcare processes and outcomes. Introduction of EBP into ongoing care is accomplished through change management to promote uptake and sustainment at the individual clinician, organizational, and policy levels. The challenges of changing provider practices within an organizational context are many and complex. New approaches to studying organizational change, CASs, and culture shifts are adding to our understanding of the challenge of integration. Research will fill the gap in what we know about "getting the straight evidence used" (Glasziou & Haynes, 2005) in practice.

Rapid advancement in the new field of implementation science contributes greatly to our growing understanding of changing practice and promoting uptake of EBP. Similar to the development of the field of EBP, this new field has quickly expanded to invent new models, frameworks, methodologies, and metrics. As in most new sciences, the terms, models, and frameworks proliferate. Reviews of the broad scientific field identified more than 100 theories, models, and frameworks (TMFs) (Nilsen, 2020; Tabak et al., 2012). Many grew out of Rogers's seminal Diffusion of Innovations Theory (Rogers, 2003), describing the ways that innovations diffuse and the elements that speed innovation adoption from scientific research to end users (Nilsen, 2020; Rogers, 2003). Given the advance practice nurse role in improvement, theories are especially useful as practice models for implementing EBP and can lead to successful incorporation of evidence into clinical care.

Other models and frameworks are useful in planning the process of integration in the Star Model Point 4, defining domains that are associated with the adoption, implementation, and maintenance of evidence-based interventions. The Consolidated Framework for Implementation Research (CFIR; Damschroder et al., 2009) and the i-PARIHS model (Harvey & Kitson, 2015) take into account the importance of "context" or organizational setting of the proposed practice change to explain or predict adoption of evidence into practice. The widely used CFIR model provides a comprehensive framework to systematically identify factors in multi-level contexts that may influence implementation of EBP. In particular, the CFIR model identifies the following characteristics that can help or hinder adoption of the EBP improvement: intervention characteristics; outer setting; inner setting; characteristics of individuals; and process of implementation

(Damschroder et al., 2009). Similarly, core constructs of the i-PARIHS model are facilitation, innovation, recipients, and context; facilitation is a process that assesses, aligns, and integrates the other three constructs (Harvey & Kitson, 2015). As implementation research provides principles to direct integration into practice, reliable tools are also developed, such as those that assess organizational readiness for change (Weiner et al., 2020).

Applying these theories and tools in practice is useful for maximizing influences of implementation strategies to promote adoption and improve care and patient outcomes and for planning and evaluating implementation efforts. Advanced practice nurses are well-positioned in the healthcare system to outline effective system strategies that promote the integration of EBP into care.

The focus on implementation has grown what is known about successful implementation strategies. Implementation strategies target multiple outcomes, including outcomes related to implementation (e.g., feasibility, fidelity, sustainment); service outcomes (the IOM standards of care—safe, timely, effective, efficient, equitable, and patient centered), and client outcomes (health status and satisfaction; Proctor et al., 2011). To be successful in a complex system, implementation strategies must target a range of stakeholders and multilevel contextual factors across different phases of implementation. For example, strategies may include factors related to patients, providers, organizations, communities, and policy and financing levels.

Implementation strategies are described as those methods and techniques used to enhance the adoption, implementation, and sustainability of a clinical program or practice (Proctor et al., 2013). These strategies assist in overcoming barriers to adoption of evidence-based quality improvement changes. Examples of implementation strategies include audit-feedback loops, reminders, decision support, communication technology, incentives, and disincentives. Commonly used strategies include pay-for-performance, professional education, facilitation and championing, opinion leaders, and policy mandates. To date, meta-analyses performed through the Cochrane Collaboration have been performed on seven categories of implementation strategies, showing small effect sizes. The categories are as follows: printed educational materials, educational meetings, educational outreach, local opinion leaders, audit and feedback, computerized reminders, and tailored implementation strategies. A full discussion of effectiveness of implementation strategies is offered by Grimshaw et al. (2012). Strategies vary by their impact and studies continue to evaluate the strategies.

Implementation strategy nomenclature is under development, with a total of 73 implementation strategies identified through expert panels (Powell et al., 2015). This common nomenclature is recommended to guide implementation practice and research. Clinicians can use this foundation to systematically match implementation strategies to the barriers and facilitators for a specific EBP (Powell et al., 2017) in order to maximize success in the practice change and improvement.

An example of an evidence-based program that is packaged for implementation is the program called "Team Training for Enhancement of Performance and Patient Safety" (TeamSTEPPS®). TeamSTEPPS® is a comprehensive evidence-based program aimed at optimizing communication performance in healthcare professionals engaged in team care, reducing adverse events. Although the program is well-developed and includes a full curriculum, implementation guidance, and tools such as posters and flip cards, integrating the program into practice has proven challenging. A recent project used the CFIR model to plan implementation of the TeamSTEPPS® program for school mental health. Implementation challenges were those that are common in implementation projects, including leader and staff turnover, agency policies, and logistical barriers (e.g., securing private space for interviews in schools). This example underscores the importance of considering stakeholder and organizational features within a complex organization to support change management (Wolk et al., 2019).

Given the neophyte field of implementation science, efforts toward research (e.g., Brownson et al., 2017) have overshadowed the *practice* of implementation. One resource stands out as a definitive reference for advanced practice nurses who are leading initiatives to implement EBP, rather than studying it. Greenhalgh (2018) offers a clear and comprehensive capture of the scientific principles discovered to date. In her book, she explains *how to successfully apply* evidence-based healthcare to practice in order to ensure safe and effective practice. Doing so requires mastery of a breadth of skill across a number of factors, including evidence, people, groups and teams, organizations, citizens, patients, technology, policy, networks, and systems (Greenhalgh, 2018). This definitive practice resource includes tools and techniques across each of these factors.

Nurses were significantly involved in "packaging" and creating plans to spread the practices recommended in the Million Hearts Campaign® (Centers for Disease Control and Prevention [CDC], 2018). An all-inclusive tool kit reflects the many elements of successful implementation planning, including multi-level stakeholder engagement, policy impact, and metrics to evaluate success of the national program.

POINT 5: Evaluation

Evaluation is a critical step in the change process as evidence-based practices are implemented. The new quality improvement investigation movement includes estimating costs and savings over time, for the customer and other stakeholders. Once integrated, the practice change is evaluated for its impact on multiple outcomes, including care processes, healthcare services, and patient and population health outcomes. An unresolved issue in implementation science is how to conceptualize and evaluate successful implementation; to that end, conceptual distinctions are made between implementation effectiveness and treatment effectiveness (Proctor et al., 2011). In their seminal discussion, Proctor and her associates list the types of outcomes in implementation research as shown in Table 3.2.

Evaluation of implementation success quantifies the feasibility, fidelity, cost, and sustainment of the evidence-based practice as it moves into care. Improvement in healthcare service can be assessed in terms of safety, timeliness, effectiveness, efficiency, equitability, and patient-centeredness resulting from the change. Client, patient, family, and population outcomes can be evaluated in terms of health status, symptomology, and satisfaction. (Proctor et al., 2011). Building on this conceptual map, implementation scientists have extended the work to develop implementation outcome measures, considered essential for monitoring and evaluating the success of implementation efforts. Consensus and psychometric testing resulted in three noteworthy measures to evaluating three implementation outcomes: Acceptability of Intervention, Intervention Appropriateness, and Feasibility of intervention (Weiner et al., 2017). Table 3.3 further defines each construct.

TABLE 3.2 Types of Implementation Outcomes

Implementation Outcomes	Service Outcomes	Client Outcomes
Acceptability	IOM "STEEEP" Standards of Care	Satisfaction
Adoption	Safety	Function
Appropriateness	Timeliness	Symptomatology
Costs	Effectiveness	
Feasibility	Efficiency	
Fidelity	Equity	
Penetration Sustainability	Patient-centeredness	

TABLE 3.3 Three Concepts of Fit and Match of an EBP Intervention

CONCEPT DEFINITION	4 LIKERT-TYPE QUESTIONS FOR EACH CONCEPT
Acceptability—Personal views of stakeholder (e.g., clinicians, administrators) perception that a given treatment, service, practice, or evidence-based innovation is agreeable, palatable, or satisfactory	Approval Appeal Preference Openness
Appropriateness—Technical or social views on perceived fit, relevance, or compatibility of the innovation for a given practice setting, provider, consumer for a given problem	Fitting Suitable Applicable Good match
Feasibility—Practical views on the extent to which a new treatment or evidence-based innovation can be successfully used or carried out in a given setting	Implementable Possible Doable Easy to use

Source: Adapted from Proctor, E., Silmere, H., Raghavan, R., Hovmand, P., Aarons, G., Bunger, A., Griffey, R., & Hensley, M. (2011). Outcomes for implementation research: conceptual distinctions, measurement challenges, and research agenda. *Administration and Policy in Mental Health and Mental Health Services Research, 38*(2), 65–76. https://doi.org/10.1007/s10488-010-0319-7; Weiner, B. J., Lewis, C. C., Stanick, C., Powell, B. J., Dorsey, C. N., Clary, A. S., Boynton, M. H., & Halko, H. (2017). Psychometric assessment of three newly developed implementation outcome measures. *Implementation Science, 12*(1), 108. https://doi.org/10.1186/s13012-017-0635-3

One of the most frequently applied implementation evaluation frameworks, the Research-Effectiveness-Adoption-Implementation-Maintenance (RE-AIM) framework is useful not only in public health behavior change, but also in clinical settings (Glasgow et al., 2019). RE-AIM identifies metrics for evaluating implementation success: that is, high reach and effectiveness resulting in practice change.

The field of implementation science has greatly advanced and a number of priorities have been identified for continuation. Among these is a call for economic evaluations of implementation strategies (Ovretveit, 2017; Powell et al., 2019). The goal of EBP is to improve healthcare and the cost of the change and maintenance is central in the value equation (Kilbourne et al., 2019). Every practice change requires an up-front investment of time and resources, with the intent of improving patient and service outcomes. Process costs (e.g., clinician orientation to the new practice, supplies) are examined in light of outcomes. Examples of outcomes are shortened length of hospital stay, reduced injurious falls, and avoidance of unplanned re-admissions. Cost analysis is an approach to examine the return on investment of EBP, including implementation. Such analysis often includes determining the costs avoided and cost of implementing the change to estimate the return on investment. Organizational and individual endorsement of the change is enhanced when the benefits of the investment are demonstrated.

■ NATIONAL COMPETENCIES IN EVIDENCE-BASED QUALITY IMPROVEMENT

Evidence-based quality improvement remains a relatively new field; for the advanced practice nurse, the field brings with it the need for new competencies and skills. Healthcare leaders and organizations have responded to the quality and safety healthcare agenda with unprecedented speed. Few other movements in healthcare have gained such widespread and rapid momentum.

Nurses have risen to the occasion to lead and join evidence-based quality efforts through improvement activities, development of explanatory models and science of EBP, and educational programs to embed EBP into the profession.

Early in the movement, nurses responded to national urging to integrate EBP into practice and education. Pivotal to building this nursing EBP capacity is the specification of EBP competencies and skills deemed necessary. Along with national experts, Stevens (2009) developed consensus on EBP competencies. This consensus established these competencies to guide the practice of EBP as well as the professional development and preparation of nurses. Because of the breadth of the Stevens Star Model across the knowledge transformation process, the Star Model was used as the framework for organizing the EBP competencies, providing a theory-based, stable foundation as EBP moved forward. The work resulted in consensus on skills that are requisite to employing EBP in a clinical role (Stevens, 2009). Using a systematic process, expert panels generated, validated, endorsed, and disseminated competency statements that guide nursing practice in basic (associate and undergraduate), intermediate (masters), and advanced (doctoral) roles. Between 10 and 32 specific competencies are enumerated for each of four levels of nursing roles/education. This consensus document categorizes requisite skills, including knowledge management, accountability for scientific basis of nursing practice, organizational and policy change, and development of scientific underpinnings for EBP (Stevens, 2013); they are published in *Essential Competencies for EBP in Nursing* (Stevens, 2009) and are reviewed annually. Table 3.4 displays examples of competencies in each level.

Although EBP competencies are established, health professionals are still in the early adoption stage of fully integrating these into their roles and into healthcare delivery. Individual clinicians face barriers in EBP improvement that include any knowledge deficits including lack of preparation in EBP competencies, lack of experience, and lack of confidence (Saunders et al., 2016). New programs

TABLE 3.4 Examples of National Consensus Competency Statements for Evidence-Based Quality Improvement

STAR POINT	INTERMEDIATE (5 OF 32 COMPETENCIES)	ADVANCED (5 OF 31 COMPETENCIES)
1	Critically appraise original research reports for practice implications in context of EBP using existing standards.	Design primary research to address factors within the system, the microsystem, and the individual that are associated with uptake of evidence-based CPG and quality improvement processes.
2	Interpret statistical analyses commonly used in evidence summaries.	Critically appraise evidence summaries for practice implications in context of EBP and as the basis for proposing primary research studies.
3	Critically appraise CPG in the context of EBP using valid instruments.	As part of planned organizational change, outline systematic approaches to develop evidence-based CPG.
4	Provide leadership for integrating EBP in clinical practice.	Represent nursing in developing interdisciplinary national initiatives to redesign healthcare to infuse quality and safety into healthcare.
5	Interpret analysis of indicators/ outcomes in terms of quality of care.	Design processes to determine impact of EBP on multiple outcomes.

CPG, clinical practice guidelines; EBP, evidence-based practice.

Source: From Stevens, K. R. (2009). *Essential competencies for evidence-based practice in nursing* (2nd ed.). Academic Center for Evidence-Based Practice (ACE), University of Texas Health Science Center.

have successfully boosted nursing scholarship in clinical settings through EBP internships and fellowship opportunities (e.g., Black et al, 2015; Saunders et al., 2016). These programs increase nurses' EBP confidence and knowledge, strengthening their EBP readiness at least in the short term.

In tandem, while individual clinicians may possess EBP competencies, they often face organizational obstacles for implementing EBP in the clinical setting. These obstacles include lack of time, lack of facilities or resources, and lack of institutional leadership support (Yoder et al., 2014). One exemplar program housed in a major hospital established dedicated human resources to promote clinical nursing inquiry in evidence-based quality improvement. Key elements of the ongoing program include opportunities to contribute to the science of nursing, culture change for nursing inquiry, institutionalized professional development and mentoring, and bridging between practice and academic sectors (Whalen et al., 2020).

To enable nurses to achieve EBP competencies, leaders have developed, tested, and made available in-depth online learning programs. The web-based Evidence-Based Research (EBR) program incorporates sound instructional design, theoretical basis, including the Stevens Star Model of Knowledge Transformation (Stevens, 2015), and broad EBP skills. The EBR program is usable on multiple devices and is effective in helping interprofessional clinicians acquire skills and tap into important EBP resources. The e-learning strategy places evidence-based resources at the fingertips of users by addressing some of the most commonly cited barriers to research utilization while exposing users to information and online literacy standards of practice, meeting a growing need (Long et al., 2016).

Advancing evidence-based quality improvement, requires that providers, organizational leaders, and the environment continue to support individual clinician and organizational capacity building and infrastructure evolution so that EBP is fully implemented.

Identifying and De-Implementing Low-Value Care: Choosing Wisely® Campaign

In tandem with the nation's focus on safe, high-quality care, there is grave concern about the overuse of healthcare resources. As much as 30% ($760 billion to $935 billion) of healthcare delivered annually is wasteful and more than half of this is spent on ineffective, inefficient, harmful, duplicative, and unnecessary care; these experts call for wise care decisions (American Board of Internal Medicine [ABIM] Foundation, 2016; Berwick & Hackbarth, 2012; Shrank et al., 2019).

Initially, efforts to improve quality focused on underuse (i.e., not doing the right thing) and misuse (i.e., preventable complications). In 2012, attention was drawn to overuse (i.e., doing too much) amid a growing emphasis on optimizing care value (Schpero, 2014). Value reflects a balance between net clinical benefit and cost. The term *low-value care* refers to healthcare services with little potential benefit and harm, or for which less expensive alternatives are available. Low-value care includes overtesting and overdiagnosis, leading to overtreatment.

Nurses and nurse leaders have aligned with the NQS to achieve better care for individuals, better health for populations, and greater value (lower per capita costs). Elimination of low-value healthcare services as a cost control strategy has economic appeal because it improves quality while reducing costs (ABIM Foundation, 2016). Unnecessary and ineffective procedures and interventions add to cost while desired health outcomes are not reached, eroding the value of care.

An important strategy is to choose care for which evidence indicates it is nonduplicative, truly necessary, and will cause no harm. In response to cost and overtreatment concerns, the national Choosing Wisely® (CW) campaign was launched by the ABIM Foundation in 2012 with the objective of assisting providers and patients to make informed decisions, to choose wisely among diagnostic and treatment options to avoid overuse, and to avoid "low-value" care (Wolfson et al., 2014). Over 70 health professional organizations in the nation and multiple countries are currently part of the effort, representing a wide array of disciplines including medicine, nursing, dentistry, and other health professions. Each participating organization has contributed lists of "Things to Question" that providers and patients can use to make wise decisions as they select best care in the individual situation (ABIM Foundation, 2016).

Definition: Overtreatment

The waste that comes from subjecting patients to care that, according to sound science and the patients' own preferences, cannot possibly help them—care rooted in outmoded habits, supply-driven behaviors, and ignoring science. Examples include excessive use of antibiotics, use of surgery when watchful waiting is better and unwanted intensive care at the end of life for patients who prefer hospice and home care.

(Berwick & Hackbarth, 2012, p. 1514)

The CW initiative represents what could be called the "flip side" of EBP, that is, *removing* from practice those approaches for which there is evidence of ineffectiveness, inefficiency, or harm (Stevens, 2019; Woodward et al., 2015). Organizations in the CW campaign generate evidence-based recommendations to help clinicians and consumers engage in conversations to make informed decisions and avoid unnecessary and ineffective care and cost. Such decisions are enacted by the healthcare team, with nurses playing a vital role.

Nurses are represented in the campaign by the nursing organizations convened by the American Academy of Nursing, which was among the first nonphysician organizations to release a CW list in 2014 (Sullivan, 2015). Recommendations are presented as "avoid" or "don't" statements and are accompanied by background information and reference citations on the website. Two of the 25 recommendations are presented in Exhibit 3.1 (American Academy of Nursing, 2018).

Additional nursing implications for CW recommendations cross over from medicine. For example, the recommendation to avoid elective labor induction or cesarean birth before 39 weeks from the American College of Obstetricians and Gynecologists is often a highly charged decision for the mother; in this situation, the nurse's role in wise choices is to support both physician and patient decisions. Whether the nurse is supporting a decision for medical treatment or advocating for a nursing care decision, the trusted voice of the nurse in making wise decisions will help patients navigate the complex health system with evidence-based information.

The removal of wasteful or ineffective practices from our collective thinking and healthcare system is challenging. Many times ineffective clinical approaches are embedded in common practices and held there by multiple factors in the complexity of healthcare and public literacy. While no parallel studies are yet available in nursing, a study in medicine substantiates widespread overuse and variation in overuse in the Medicare population by measure and by geography (Colla et al., 2015). Eleven CW recommendations were tracked to determine the prevalence of the delivery of low-value services (e.g., don't perform preoperative cardiac tests for cataract surgeries and don't use antipsychotics as first choice to treat behavioral and psychological symptoms of dementia). The prevalence of low-value services was significant. For example, the prevalence of use of nonrecommended preoperative cardiac testing for low-risk, noncardiac procedures was 46.5% (Colla et al., 2015).

Just as nurse leaders employ principles to promote adoption of best practices, they may also draw on principles to *remove* useless and harmful practices from daily care. This effort to "de-adopt" low-value interventions requires change management for individual care providers,

EXHIBIT 3.1

EXAMPLES* OF NURSING RECOMMENDATIONS IN THE *CHOOSING WISELY* CAMPAIGN

Don't automatically initiate continuous electronic fetal heart rate (FHR) monitoring during labor for women without risk factors; consider intermittent auscultation (IA) first. As a routine procedure in many hospitals, continuous FHR is associated with increased cesarean or instrument assisted (e.g., forceps) births and do not improve Apgar scores, NICU admission rates, or intrapartum fetal death rates. Advantages of IA is freedom of movement during labor, pain management, shorter first stage of labor and less epidural medication use.
Don't let older adults lie in bed or only get up to a chair during their hospital stay. During hospitalization, around 65% of older adults lose their ability to walk. Mobilization during hospital stays maintains functional ability. This in turn reduces length of stay, avoids need for rehabilitation services, reduces risk for falls, and reduces burden on caregivers. Older adults who walk during hospitalization can walk farther at discharge, are discharged sooner, and are able to perform basic activities of daily living.

*Two of 25 recommendations on nursing care

Source: From American Academy of Nursing. (2018). *Twenty-five things nurses and patients should question.* https://higherlogicdownload.s3.amazonaws.com/AANNET/c8a8da9e-918c-4dae-b0c6-6d630c46007f/UploadedImages/AAN_Nursing-Choosing-Wisely-List__11_19_18_.pdf

the general public, and healthcare delivery systems. Practical principles can be derived from a number of sources commonly used in promoting adoption of best practices. These include principles of change, team leadership, creating a sense of urgency, and empowering through capacity building (Stevens, 2019). However, actions to remove low-value care are predicated on *awareness* of nationally-accepted recommendations. Surveys indicate that frontline clinicians were minimally aware of recommendations on low-value care: 21% of RNs and 26% of advanced practice nurses were aware of the AAN Choosing Wisely® recommendations (Stevens, 2019).

The CW campaign will be judged successful if there are changes in (a) provider behavior, (b) patient knowledge of overuse, and (c) utilization of low-value or negligible-value care while at the same time, avoiding underuse and dissatisfaction with healthcare.

A CULTURE OF SAFETY

A culture of safety has emerged as a crucial element in providing safe patient care. A culture shares norms, values, and practices associated with a nation, organization, or profession. The model of cultural maturity (Westrum, 2004) explains stages in the evolution of a safety culture. These stages progress from a pathological stage where safety is a problem of the worker; the business is the main driver and the goal is to avoid being caught by regulators. Reactive cultures take action only after an error occurs. In a calculative culture, safety is driven by management, which collects much data and imposes safety on the worker. In a proactive culture, workforce involvement begins to move away from the top-down approach, focusing instead on improving performance where the unexpected is a challenge. The final evolutionary stage of an organizational culture is the generative stage, where everyone participates in safety because all workers understand that safety is an inherent part of the business.

Patient Safety Research

Safety research has emerged as one of the nation's top priorities in healthcare research. Following the shocking report, *To Err Is Human: Building a Safer Health System* (IOM, 2000), further examination has shown medical errors to be the third leading cause of death in the nation, behind heart disease and cancer (Makary & Daniel, 2016). The science of safety has matured to directly connect these problems with patient harm and death: communication breakdowns, diagnostic errors, poor judgment, and inadequate skill. Although the epidemiology of errors receives much attention, investigating the prevalence of adverse events is hindered by the prevalent culture of blame. This culture squelches adequate reporting of adverse events and prevents healthcare providers from making adverse events visible for further analysis and correction of causes of unsafe care.

Enhancing patient safety in healthcare includes three complementary actions: (a) preventing adverse events, (b) making adverse events visible, and (c) mitigating the effects of adverse events when they occur (World Health Organization [WHO], 2005). These three actions have stimulated development of theories to guide safety and the testing of those theories to produce safety science.

Safety science in healthcare is relatively new. The IOM (2000) report raised awareness of the hazards associated with healthcare, identifying errors as the eighth leading cause of death in the United States. Safety science was well established in other industries, such as aviation and nuclear power. Such high-risk industries are inherently dangerous and have developed safety management systems that nurture a culture of safety, thereby reducing errors and risks for errors and maximizing lessons learned. Safety practices established in these high-risk industries are now being adapted and tested in healthcare.

As in any new field of science, key concepts must be defined, theories generated to guide investigations, and new methods employed to study the topic. Likewise, theories and models with which to frame the investigation must be developed and tested.

An *adverse event* is defined as an untoward and usually unanticipated outcome that occurs in association with healthcare. *Patient safety* has been defined by the Agency for Healthcare Research and Quality (AHRQ) as the freedom from accidental injuries during the course of medical care and encompasses actions taken to avoid, prevent, or correct adverse outcomes that may result from the delivery of healthcare.

In seeking to improve safety, one of the most frustrating aspects for both patients and professionals is the apparent failure of healthcare systems to learn from their mistakes. It is the management of errors and risks that becomes the priority of everyone in an organization. Organizations that have fewer accidents than normal as a result of a change in organizational culture are high-reliability organizations.

■ SAFETY MODELS IN NURSING

There are four safety models that are seen as an integral part of the culture of safety. These models are: (a) Reason's Swiss Cheese Model of System Accidents; (b) Helmreich's Threat and Error Management (TEM) Model for Medicine, which was developed from aviation's Crew Resource Management (CRM); (c) Marx's Just Culture; and (d) Complex Adaptive System (CAS) theory.

Reason (2000) advanced one of the most widely used theories on human error, one that has been used extensively in high-risk industries and cited in IOM reports. In Reason's model, human error is recognized as being inevitable. Reason identified two ways to view human error: the person approach and the system approach. The person approach has been the longstanding tradition in healthcare, which focuses on individual providers, blaming providers for forgetfulness, inattention, or moral weakness. The system approach holds as its basic premise that humans are fallible and errors are to be expected. The theory suggests that, to avert or mitigate errors, interventions must focus on conditions under which individuals work and must build defenses against error (Reason, 2000).

Reason's Swiss Cheese Model of System Accidents describes high-technology systems that have many defensive layers; when holes in these defenses momentarily line up, the opportunity for accidents occurs. A hole in any one defensive layer does not normally cause a bad outcome. There are two reasons that holes occur in the defensive layers: active failures and latent conditions. An active failure is an unsafe act committed by people who are in direct contact with the system. Latent conditions arise from decisions made by designers, builders, procedure writers, and management. Latent conditions may lie dormant in a system for years until they combine with active failures and local triggers to create an accident opportunity (Reason, 2000). Human-error research in nursing has been valuable in examining barriers to safety in a neonatal intensive care unit (Jirapaet et al., 2006).

The Threat and Error Management (TEM) Model was developed to analyze adverse events, define training needs for medical personnel, and define organizational strategies to recognize and manage threat and error (Helmreich, 2000). Threats are factors that can increase the likelihood of an error being committed. In this model, threats are either latent or overt and serve as settings or overarching variables that increase the potential for error to occur. Latent threats are aspects of the hospital or medical organization that are not always easily identifiable but that predispose it to the commission of errors or the emergence of overt threats; examples of latent threats are failure to maintain equipment and high nurse–patient staffing ratios. Overt threats include environmental factors such as poor lighting and excessive noise, individual factors such as fatigue, team- or staff-related factors such as poor communication, and patient-related factors such as high acuity level. For example, Pape (2003) significantly reduced nursing distractions during medication administration by having staff use protocols from high-risk industries (Pape, 2003).

David Marx's Just Culture describes four behavioral concepts (evils) that are necessary to the comprehension of the interrelationship between discipline and patient safety: human error, negligent conduct, knowing violation of rules, and reckless conduct (Marx, 2001). Human errors are the mistakes, slips, and lapses that occur in our everyday behaviors. *Negligence* is a legal term used when a person has been harmed by a failure to provide reasonable and safe care in a manner consistent with that of other prudent healthcare workers. Intentional rule violations occur when an individual knowingly works around policy and procedures while performing a task or skill. Reckless conduct is the conscious disregard of obvious and significant risk; it differs from negligence in that negligence involves a failure to recognize the risk. The purpose of a Just Culture is to promote nonpunitive reporting of all types of errors, either anonymously or confidentially, and at the same time, holding individual and organizational responsibility. Only when this information is gained can solutions be generated.

Healthcare systems have been described as complex adaptive systems. A prominent theory in complexity science is the CAS theory (Begun et al., 2003). CASs are collections of various agents, individuals, and groups that interact with other groups, and with their environment in a way that allows them to sometimes learn and act in nonlinear and unpredictable directions. These systems are dynamic and evolve over time. CASs encompass individual, interdisciplinary, and system facets of quality and safety. Characteristics of CASs are their ability to self-organize, the emergence of new patterns from nonlinear interactions, and their coevolution as the agent and the environment mutually transform in response to the interactions (Stroebel et al., 2005). The complexity of the healthcare system has been a challenge to those trying to adapt safety models of other high-risk industries. Usually, in other high-risk industries (such as aviation), the individuals involved in the error die themselves, unlike in healthcare, where the healthcare worker is seldom directly harmed by the actions or the error. A CAS framework helps researchers understand the complexity of the work of the clinician (Begun et al., 2003; Ebright et al., 2004).

The High-Reliability Organization (HRO) model is a new approach to framing the dynamic and numerous aspects of the organization. Heightened awareness of the functioning of health-care systems and subsystems is required throughout the organization in order to achieve safe and effective care. In addition to employing best clinical practices, organizations must address the processes of the delivery system, which can become more reliable by applying an HRO frame-work (Chassin & Loeb, 2013; Frankel et al., 2017). Continuous improvement requires heightened awareness of the functioning of systems and subsystems in order to achieve high reliability in the delivery of safe and effective care. HROs include an environment of "collective mindfulness," in which all workers engage in detecting and reporting operational problems before they result in safety risk.

Thought leaders suggest that organizations can become HROs when organizational mind-fulness is employed, observations gained from the study of high-risk industries such as nuclear power plants. This HRO mindfulness includes five principles: preoccupation with failure, reluc-tance to simplify interpretations of events, sensitivity to operations, commitment to resilience, and recognition of frontline expertise (Chassin & Loeb, 2013; Weick & Sutcliffe, 2015). While seemingly simple, these practices are often difficult to implement and/or sustain in hospitals due to system complexities in administration, discipline boundaries, and ingrained habits and culture. Chassin and Loeb describe the ongoing lack of sensitivity to operations as "one of the most per-vasive safety problems in hospitals" (2013, p. 463).

One national study framed nursing workflow problems in the HRO model, positing that heightened awareness of the functioning of healthcare systems is requisite to achieve safe and effective care (Stevens et al., 2017). High reliability organizations embrace an environment of "collective mindfulness," in which all workers detect and report operational problems before they result in workarounds and safety risk. To that end, participating acute care nurses systematically recorded data about operational failures (OF) in which essential care supplies, equipment, infor-mation, staff, and so forth, were not made available to the front line. Across 10 work shifts, 774 nurses in 67 adult and pediatric medical-surgical units in 23 hospitals reported 27,298 OFs over 4,497 shifts, a rate of 6.05 OFs per shift (Stevens et al., 2017).

Clearly, nurses' detection of OFs can provide the organization with rich, real-time information about system operations to improve organizational reliability and safety. Embedding HRO prin-ciples into the healthcare delivery system holds promise of promoting quality and patient safety.

■ RISK MANAGEMENT MODELS

Incident reports are a primary method for data collection on errors. Other high-risk industries have criticized healthcare for not having a standardized method of investigating, documenting, and disseminating information on medication errors. Studies have been conducted on failures within the incident reporting system. The current incident reporting system is voluntary. The present rate of medical errors underestimates the full scope of the problem because of incomplete reporting. Studies have shown that nurses use the incident report system more frequently than physicians and other healthcare workers, which results in nurses appearing to commit a dispro-portionate number of medication errors.

Root cause analysis (RCA) is a retrospective approach to error analysis that has been widely used in high-risk industries. The Joint Commission mandated the use of the multidisciplinary RCA in 1997 to investigate sentinel events in hospitals. RCAs are uncontrolled case studies (qualitative approach) that predominantly use Reason's taxonomy of error to uncover the latent errors that underlie a sentinel event. The majority of RCAs investigate serious adverse events that resulted in patient death. Limitations of the RCA are the hindsight bias of the investigators and the voluntary nature of reporting the incident and outcomes. The Joint Commission suggests that hospitals underreport incidents because they fear being put on probationary status and because of the legal implications of the disclosure of a sentinel event. Nursing researchers have used RCAs to change current nursing practice in the transport of sick newborns in an effort to improve patient outcomes (Mordue, 2005).

Most errors that affect patient safety occur at the microsystem level within a hospital macrosystem. For example, as part of an effort to increase error reporting and to capture Reason's active failures, *near miss* or *close call* (errors that do not reach the patient) incident reporting was improved with the Good Catch Pilot Program at MD Anderson Cancer Center (Mick et al., 2007). Three strategies were employed to improve reporting of close-call errors. First, the terminology for a potential error was changed to *good catch*. Second, an end-of-shift safety report was implemented that gave nurses an opportunity to identify and discuss patient safety concerns that had come up during the shift. Third, awards and other patient safety incentives were sponsored by executive leadership to recognize the efforts of individual nurses to improve patient safety. For example, in one hospital, scores based on the anonymous reporting by individual nurses on the various units were kept at the unit level. Buy-in by the upper level of nursing management was instrumental in promoting open discussions about patient safety and the distribution of "Good Catch" tokens to reward unit team members. At 9 weeks, more than 800 potential errors were reported, and at 6 months that number had increased to 2,744, which represents an increase of 1,468% in the reporting of potential errors. Changes that occurred as a result of the Good Catch program were highlighted in a weekly nursing newsletter as a source of feedback to employees (Mick et al., 2007).

The failure modes and effects analysis (FMEA) tool has been adapted from high-risk industries outside healthcare. Its purpose is to prospectively assess risks of failures and harm within a system and to identify the most important areas for improvement. This process is conducted with a multidisciplinary team approach that identifies any and all possible failure modes and causes, assigns risk priority numbers to these failures, and then plans, implements, and evaluates interventions to reduce potential failures (Reams, 2011).

■ PRACTICE SCHOLARSHIP

The definition of practice scholarship is still evolving. However, it can be considered in context of relatively new educational programs, such as the doctor of nursing practice (DNP) and clinical nurse leader (CNL). The commonality across these is the goal of systematic improvement of clinical practice and healthcare services, resulting in better population health. The level of improvement may be at the microsystem, facility, or policy level.

In an effort to improve patient outcomes, a number of aspects are examined, including structures and processes leading to outcomes. Data and information are examined for trends in terms of desired outcomes, such as national benchmarks. For example, if rate of "retained foreign objects" after surgery is above the national benchmark (a never event), then further problem identification is warranted. Often, performance improvement and alignment with evidence-based (best) practices are the targets.

Best practices are specified in credible evidence-based CPGs (IOM, 2011a). The practice scholar often conducts a gap analysis between local practice and evidence-based best practice. Because the gap analysis may point to solutions that cross practice, processes, infrastructure, and environment, multiple layers of the clinical system and multiple disciplines and stakeholders are engaged to accomplish successful change.

Framing the improvement initiative as a CAS intervention will assist the practice scholar in anticipating the many aspects and stakeholders that can be involved to support adoption of the proposed improvement change. EBP adoption can be supported by using the following change management strategies: embed change champions in care settings; garner buy-in from executive, frontline nurses, and multiple disciplines; manage organizational culture; promote public awareness and engagement of patients and families; engage policy agents; and track the practice change and its impact. This last strategy is crucial to building and sustaining; from the impact and outcome information, the business case can be made for continuing and spreading the new practice.

Further details on change champions have emerged from a review of how the role was operationalized (Miech et al., 2018). Recognizing that champions are crucial to effective healthcare implementation is broadly accepted; for example, the terms *hand hygiene champion, guideline champion, nurse champion, clinical champion* have been used. The review concluded that champions produced positive and significant associations with implementation outcomes. Characteristics of a successful champion include: communication and persuasion, proactivity, humility, horizontal and collective leadership style; sense of responsibility and accountability; action-oriented; empathetic; dedicated; ability to inspire and motivate others; steady eye on the vision (Demes et al., 2020).

With a focused definition of practice scholarship as the *adoption of best practices*, the practice scholar will gain from the emerging field of implementation science. Implementation science has enjoyed a rapid swell of uptake because it is seen as providing solutions to move EBP through successful adoption in clinical practice. The new concept of "implementation" is defined as "the use of strategies to adopt and integrate evidence-based health interventions into clinical and community settings to improve individual outcomes and benefit population health (NIH, 2019). Advancements in the field are rapid; for example, national infrastructure established by the NIH Clinical and Translational Science Award (CTSA) program provides clear focus on the entire range of activities necessary to move research to practice and then to population health.

In tandem, the annual NIH Dissemination and Implementation Conference highlights the rapidly moving field. Implementation science now is boosted by research methodologies, specific theories, tools and instruments, defined competencies, emphasis on interprofessional investigative teams, dedicated journal emphasis, and research training programs across the nation. In addition, an increased emphasis for dissemination and implementation research is evident in the NIH multi-institute announcement calling for research proposals in the field, paving the way for discovery of effective strategies to promote uptake of evidence-based best practices. While implementation scientists design rigorous studies to evaluate such strategies, the practice scholar will benefit from the results produced in the new field, pointing to key approaches to improving practice in clinical settings.

INSTRUMENTS, TOOLS, AND RESOURCES FOR MEASURING PATIENT SAFETY

There are various approaches to quantifying variables important in patient safety research. Through methodological research designs, scientists have developed and estimated psychometric qualities (reliability and validity) of a number of such instruments. The following describes several important instruments used in quality and safety research, including the Hospital Survey on Patient Safety Culture (HSOPS; AHRQ, 2016b). The Practice Environment Scale of the Nursing Work Index (PES-NWI) was developed specifically to address issues relevant to nursing in Magnet® hospitals (Lake, 2007).

A valuable instrument for assessing the system context for safety is the HSOPS. This widely used survey gathers data about staff perceptions and opinions regarding patient safety issues, medical error, and event reporting. It provides hospital staff, managers, and administrators with basic knowledge necessary to assess safety culture and to help them evaluate how well they have established a culture of safety in their institution. In addition, benchmarking based on data voluntarily provided by other, similar hospitals can be accomplished (AHRQ, 2016b). The highly reliable 42-item questionnaire measures 13 domains: openness of communication, feedback and communication of errors, frequency of events, handoffs and transitions, management support, nonpunitive response to error, organizational learning, overall perceptions of patient safety, staffing, manager expectations, actions that promote patient safety, teamwork across units, and teamwork within units.

The PES-NWI was developed to measure five subscale domains of the hospital nursing practice environment. Two of the subscales measure the hospital-wide environment: Nurse Participation Hospital Affairs and Nursing Foundations for Quality of Care. The other three subscales are more unit specific: Nurse Manager Ability, Leadership, and Support; Staffing and Resource Adequacy; and Collegial Nurse–Physician Relations (Lake, 2007).

From a microsystem level, the performance of the care team is critical in safeguarding patient safety. Communication failures have been shown to be the leading cause of sentinel events, including preventable patient deaths, accounting for up to 80% of adverse events (AHRQ, 2016a). The evidence-based program, Team Strategies and Tools to Enhance Performance and Patient Safety (TeamSTEPPS®) is rooted in more than 20 years of evidence from human factor research and is a powerful solution to improving patient safety through team performance (AHRQ, 2016a). Instruments have been developed to measure impact of the TeamSTEPPS® program on specific performance outcomes: the TeamSTEPPS® Team Attitude Questionnaire (AHRQ, 2014a) and the TeamSTEPPS® Teamwork Perception Questionnaire (AHRQ, 2014b).

THE FUTURE OF QUALITY IMPROVEMENT AND SAFETY RESEARCH

Research in healthcare quality improvement and safety is evolving at an unprecedented speed. As healthcare is redesigned, providers, administrators, and policy makers look to scientists to develop and evaluate sound approaches. In response, scientists are developing and evolving new research designs, theories, and measurement approaches. Top priorities for healthcare organizations include providing high-quality and safe patient care. The quality and patient safety movement is accelerating in healthcare organizations, and progress is evident (Buerhaus, 2007).

Key national quality reports have been a major impetus for healthcare improvements in quality and safety. The 2001 IOM report *Crossing the Quality Chasm: A New Health System for the 21st Century* (IOM, 2001) identified the need for fundamental change in the U.S. healthcare system; the recommendations in the report still resonate as a blueprint for today's healthcare transformation efforts. The redesign of the healthcare system involves providing healthcare that is safe, timely, effective, efficient, equitable, and patient centered. In addition, the IOM's *Health Professions Education: A Bridge to Quality* (2003b) was another key report that identified five core competencies needed by healthcare professions to provide quality care in the 21st century. The essential five core competencies identified were (a) providing patient-centered care, (b) working in multidisciplinary teams, (c) using EBP, (d) applying quality improvement, and (e) using informatics.

In subsequent IOM reports, experts then pointed to "what works" (IOM, 2008, 2011a; 2011b). These reports identified two key forms of knowledge that are helpful in supporting clinical decision-making and selecting best practices for quality improvement: (a) SRs and (b) evidence-based CPGs. "Systematic reviews identify, select, assess, and synthesize the findings of similar but separate studies, and can help clarify what is known and not known about the potential benefits and harms of drugs, devices, and other healthcare services" (IOM, 2011b). To be credible, CPGs are backed by strong scientific evidence from reviews and methodically fashioned into clinical recommendations through a systematic process with clinical experts. CPGs are often developed through professional clinical associations and are considered "best practice," and therefore a vital part of practice scholarship (IOM, 2011a).

National agencies such as the AHRQ, The Joint Commission, and the Institute for Healthcare Improvement (IHI) have been instrumental in setting initiatives designed to advance quality and safety in the healthcare arena. The AHRQ's nine Evidence-Based Practice Centers (EPCs) and the AHRQ's Translating Research Into Practice (TRIP) initiatives are important resources that assist in moving EBPs into clinical practice, promoting quality and patient safety in healthcare.

In a history-making initiative, the IHI's 100,000 Lives and 5 Million Lives campaigns were outstanding examples of how national initiatives could improve quality and safety and incorporate evidence-based knowledge into clinical practice. The 100,000 Lives campaign focused on six interventions to reduce morbidity and mortality. The six interventions were (a) deployment of rapid response teams, (b) improvement of care of patients with acute myocardial infarction by delivering reliable evidence-based care, (c) prevention of adverse drug events through medication reconciliation, (d) prevention of central line infections, (e) prevention of surgical site infections, and (f) prevention of ventilator-associated pneumonia. This initiative involved the participation of 3,100 hospitals and saved an estimated 122,000 lives in 18 months (IHI, 2008). The IHI expanded the quality and safety focus with the 5 Million Lives campaign to address the issue of protecting patients from 5 million incidents of medical harm between December 2006 and December 2008. The 5 Million Lives campaign continues with the six interventions in the 100,000 Lives campaign, in addition to six new interventions targeted on harm: (a) preventing harm from high-alert medications (i.e., anticoagulants, sedatives, narcotics, and insulin); (b) reducing surgical complications; (c) preventing pressure ulcers; (d) reducing methicillin-resistant *Staphylococcus aureus* (MRSA) infection; (e) delivering reliable, evidence-based care for congestive heart failure; and (f) defining the roles of hospital boards of directors in promoting and sustaining a culture of safety. Frequent new initiatives introduced by the IHI are adding greatly to the nation's quality movement. Similarly, the Million Hearts Campaign® was jointly launched by the Centers for Medicare & Medicaid Services (CMS) and the Centers for Disease Control and Prevention (CDC) in tandem with other parts of the U.S. Department of Health and Human Services (DHHS) and the U.S. Department of Veterans Affairs (VA). This excellent improvement exemplar offers well-developed tools, including the Cardiac

Rehabilitation Change Package useful for interprofessional teams implementing the evidence-based change (CDC, 2018).

The Joint Commission is another national agency that focuses on improving quality and safety of healthcare. The Joint Commission's annual National Patient Safety Goals are reviewed by healthcare organizations to ensure that their clinical practices are addressing these quality and safety areas. In addition, The Joint Commission's Patient Safety Practices is an online resource providing more than 800 links that healthcare professionals can use to address patient safety issues (The Joint Commission, 2020). These goals have stimulated many innovative interventions, the impact of which is evaluated using research approaches.

■ QUALITY INDICATORS, MEASURES, AND REPORTING

Performance measures are necessary to determine the impact of ongoing quality improvement efforts. Such efforts require that specific quality indicators be identified and measurement approaches validated through research. In the recent past, a number of healthcare entities have responded to the need for such indicators by developing consensus on indicators that should be tracked and by launching annual quality reports from national surveys. These efforts are reflected in the work of the AHRQ and the NQF. Other groups have undertaken efforts to create nursing-sensitive quality indicators reflected in the following sources: National Database of Nursing Quality Indicators (NDNQI), Veterans Affairs Nursing Sensitive Outcomes Database, Military Nursing Outcomes Database, and California Nursing Outcomes Coalition Database.

These groups note that many barriers to the widespread adoption of consensus standards exist and that overcoming them will require significant resources. Despite progress in quality improvement, challenges remain. These include inadequately developed measures, lack of standardization of performance measures and quality indicators, the need to refine measures, misalignment of measures of outcomes and baseline measures, and the burdens of data collection.

■ THE AGENCY FOR HEALTHCARE RESEARCH AND QUALITY'S NATIONAL HEALTHCARE QUALITY REPORTS

Since 2003, the AHRQ has reported on progress and opportunities for improving healthcare quality. One of the key functions of the AHRQ *National Healthcare Quality and Disparities Report* (NHQR) is to track the nation's progress in providing safe healthcare. For 16 years, the reports have presented a snapshot of the safety of healthcare provided to the American people. The NHQR surveys the healthcare system through quality indicators, such as the percentage of heart attack patients who receive recommended care when they reach the hospital or the percentage of children who receive recommended vaccinations. In all, 218 measures are used, categorized across four dimensions of quality—effectiveness, patient safety, timeliness, and patient centeredness (AHRQ, 2018).

As a result of such research efforts in improvement science, a clearer picture of healthcare quality and safety is beginning to emerge. The report assessed the state of healthcare quality using core report measures that represent the most important and scientifically credible measures of quality for the nation (AHRQ, 2018). The data reflected that clear progress has been made in improving the healthcare delivery system, focused on the three aims of better care, better value, and a healthier population, and pointed to areas for additional emphasis. As reported, the NQS has six priorities: patient safety, person-centered care, care coordination, effective treatment, healthy living, and care affordability. The trends are presented in Exhibit 3.2.

EXHIBIT 3.2

NATIONAL HEALTHCARE QUALITY AND DISPARITIES REPORT—TRENDS

- Half of the *patient safety* measures improved, led by a 17% reduction in rates of hospital-acquired conditions.
- *Person-centered care* improved steadily, especially for children.
- *Care coordination* improved as providers enhanced discharge processes and adopted health information technologies.
- *Effective treatment* in hospitals achieved high levels of performance, led by measures publicly reported by Centers for Medicare & Medicaid Services on Hospital Compare.
- *Healthy living* improved in about half of the measures followed, led by selected adolescent vaccines from 2008 to 2012.
- *Care affordability* worsened from 2002 to 2010 and then leveled off.

Source: From The Agency for Healthcare Research and Quality's National Healthcare Quality and Disparities Report.

QUALITY INDICATORS: THE NATIONAL QUALITY FORUM

The National Quality Forum (NQF) is a nonprofit organization with diverse stakeholder membership from the public and private health sectors, including consumers, healthcare professionals, providers, health plans, public and private purchasers, researchers, and quality improvement organizations. Established in 1999, the NQF seeks to implement a national strategy for healthcare quality measurement and reporting. The NQF's mission includes improving healthcare by "setting national goals for performance improvement, endorsing national consensus standards for measuring and publicly reporting on performance, and promoting the attainment of national goals through education and outreach programs" (NQF, 2020).

Since the formation of the NQF, healthcare quality has become a major public policy issue. The diverse NQF stakeholders agreed on standards by which the healthcare industry would be measured, and data on these measures are publicly reported. Together with the other forces in effect, the NQF has fostered public reporting of performance. Such reporting, once a rare event, is becoming the norm. NQF-endorsed voluntary consensus standards are widely viewed as the "gold standard" for the measurement of healthcare quality.

SELECTED NURSING PERFORMANCE QUALITY INDICATORS

Because of the sheer number of nurses and the frequency of contact with patients, nurses have a major impact on patient safety and healthcare outcomes (NQF, 2020). Research points to the influence of nursing on patient outcomes (e.g., IOM, 2004); however, only recently have advances in building a platform for public reporting reflecting nursing-sensitive performance measures been made.

National Quality Forum-15

NQF endorsed a set of 15 consensus-based nursing-sensitive standards. These uniform metrics will increase understanding of nurses' influence on inpatient hospital care and advance internal quality improvement. The measures were recommended to evaluate the impact that nurses in acute care settings have on patient safety, healthcare quality, and professional work environment. Of note, the NQF addressed improving care through nursing, pointing to initiatives and results that are part of the "national mosaic of ongoing nursing-led initiatives to improve the healing environment for patients and the nurses who care for them" (NQF, 2020).

Definition: Nursing-Sensitive Performance Measures

Nursing-sensitive performance measures are processes and outcomes—and structural proxies for these processes and outcomes (e.g., skill mix, nurse staffing hours)—that are affected, provided, and/or influenced by nursing personnel—but for which nursing is not exclusively responsible. Nursing-sensitive measures must be quantifiably influenced by nursing personnel, but the relationship is not necessarily causal.

(NQF, 2020)

The NQF undertook a 15-month study to better understand the adoption of NQF-15 and to identify the successes, challenges, and technical barriers experienced by those implementing the measure. In 2006 and 2007, interviews were conducted with critical leaders, hospital representatives, quality organization leaders, and representatives of implementation initiatives. Interview data were augmented with a web-based survey. Content and descriptive analyses led to recommendations to accelerate adoption of the NQF-15. The 10 recommendations focus on aligning the NQF-15 with priorities, advancing science, improving regulatory and reporting requirements, fostering adoption of the standard through education, holding nurses accountable for public reporting, and creating a business case for nursing quality measurement (NQF, 2020).

National Database of Nursing Quality Indicators

Another major quality and safety measurement effort is reflected in the National Database of Nursing Indicators (NDNQI). The American Nurses Association developed the NDNQI in 1998. The NDNQI is designed to assist healthcare organizations in patient safety and quality improvement initiatives by supplying research-based national comparative data on nursing care and its impact on patient outcomes. The NDNQI reflects nursing-sensitive indicators related to the structure, process, and outcomes of nursing care. Structure of nursing care is reflected by the supply, skill level, and education and certification of nursing staff. Process indicators reflect nursing care aspects such as assessment, intervention, and RN job satisfaction. Outcome indicators reflect patient outcomes that are nursing sensitive; these improve with both greater quantity and greater quality of nursing care (e.g., pressure ulcers, falls, and IV infiltrations; NQF, 2020).

▪ KEY INITIATIVES CONTRIBUTING TO NURSING QUALITY AND SAFETY

A number of initiatives are proving to be the key in the forefront of quality and safety. These include additional IOM/NAS reports, the Magnet Recognition Program®, and the INQRI, each of which is described here.

Institute of Medicine Reports

Keeping Patients Safe: Transforming the Work Environment of Nurses (2004) identified mandates for quality and safety specifically aimed at nurses' roles. The report emphasized a call for change for healthcare organizations, the federal government, state boards of nursing, educational institutions, professional organizations, labor organizations, and professional nurses and urged them to take an active role in improving quality and safety in healthcare. This report identified essential patient safeguards in the work environment of nurses, calling for (a) governing boards that focus on safety, (b) leadership and evidence-based management structures and processes, (c) effective nursing leadership, (d) adequate staffing, (e) organizational support for ongoing learning and decision support, (f) mechanisms promoting multidisciplinary collaboration, (g) work designs promoting safety, and (h) an organizational culture that enhances patient safety. Additional research addressing patient safety is necessary in the following areas: information on nurse's work including on how nurses divide their time among various activities; information on nursing-related errors; safer nursing work processes and workspace design; standardized measurements of patient acuity; and safe nursing staff levels on various nursing units (IOM, 2004).

The Future of Nursing Recommendations

A key initiative in the transformation of the profession of nursing was outlined by the IOM in 2011 in its report *The Future of Nursing: Leading Change, Advancing Health*, calling for nurses to advance the nursing profession and take a greater role in the transformation of the healthcare delivery system. This report triggered a nation-wide campaign with multiple initiatives embedded to address the recommendations and make significant contributions by addressing challenges in the areas of healthcare delivery and scope of practice, education, collaboration, leadership, diversity in the nursing profession, and workforce data. Recent examination led to an assessment on the progress on *The Future of Nursing* recommendations. The authors concluded that "No single profession, working alone, can meet the complex needs of patients and communities. Nurses should continue to develop skills and competencies in leadership and innovation and collaborate with other professionals in healthcare delivery and health system redesign" (Altman et al., 2016, p. 3). An update of the recommendations will set the course for *The Future of Nursing 2020–2030*, specifying how nurses might continue to contribute to healthcare quality and safety.

Magnet Recognition Program

The Magnet Recognition Program developed by the American Nurses Credentialing Center (ANCC) has been a driving factor urging nursing to develop a research agenda focused on EBP, quality, and safety. The Magnet Recognition Program was developed to recognize healthcare organizations that provide nursing excellence and to provide a channel for spreading successful nursing practices. Providing high-quality and safe patient care and integrating evidence-based knowledge into clinical practice are important components in achieving the esteemed Magnet recognition certification (ANCC, 2008). The program has had a significant impact on quality and safety in nursing and in increasing the amount of attention paid to employing EBP and conducting research.

Interdisciplinary Nursing Quality Research Initiative

The RWJF is a leading funder of research on nursing quality care. The primary goal of the INQRI was to "generate, disseminate and translate research to understand how nurses contribute to and can improve the quality of patient care" (RWJF, 2008). The program of research began to fill the gap in what is known about nurses' effects on quality and on keeping patients safer and healthier. Forty interdisciplinary research teams examined nurses' practices, processes, and work environments to determine the impact that nurses have on the quality of patient care. The ultimate goal is to support research to reduce healthcare errors and improve patient care. These studies comprised the first large-scale effort to identify the ways in which nurses can improve the quality of patient care and the contributions that nurses make to keep patients safer (RWJF, 2008). Lessons learned from this program have paved the way for future work in nursing quality research (e.g., Newhouse et al., 2013).

▮ SUMMARY

The national effort to ensure that healthcare systems provide quality and safe care will continue to be a major focus for healthcare professionals. Nurses are essential in creating and sustaining a culture of safety, translating evidence-based research into clinical practice in healthcare, and creating the science of safety and evidence-based quality to improve healthcare and maximize positive health outcomes.

SUGGESTED LEARNING ACTIVITIES

1. Review an example of an evidence-based quality improvement initiative in the literature.
    a. What implementation framework was used?
    b. What were the targeted patient outcomes?
    c. What were the targeted organization outcomes?
    d. Was cost analysis used to determine return on investment in the change?
2. Search a bibliographic database such as CINAHL. Locate a research study using "complex adaptive systems" or "high reliability organizations" as a framework. List the primary variables in the investigation. Relate the results to quality and/or safety in healthcare.

ACKNOWLEDGMENTS

The author is grateful for the contributions of Katherine McDuffie and Paula C. Clutter to the original chapter.

REFERENCES

Agency for Healthcare Research and Quality. (2014a). *TeamSTEPPS Team Attitudes Questionnaire (T-TAQ)*. http://www.ahrq.gov/teamstepps/instructor/tools.html

Agency for Healthcare Research and Quality. (2014b). *TeamSTEPPS Teamwork Perception Questionnaire.* http://www.ahrq.gov/teamstepps/instructor/tools.html

Agency for Healthcare Research and Quality. (2016a). *TeamSTEPPS 2.0.* http://teamstepps.ahrq.gov

Agency for Healthcare Research and Quality. (2016b). *Patient safety culture surveys.* http://www.ahrq.gov/professionals/quality-patient-safety/patientsafetyculture/hospital

Agency for Healthcare Research and Quality. (2018). *2018 National healthcare quality and disparities report.* https://www.ahrq.gov/research/findings/nhqrdr/nhqdr18/index.html

Altman, S. H., Butler, A. S., & Shern, L. (Eds.). (2016). *Assessing progress on the Institute of Medicine report: The future of nursing.* National Academies Press.

American Academy of Nursing. (2018). *Twenty-five things nurses and patients should question.* https://higherlogicdownload.s3.amazonaws.com/AANNET/c8a8da9e-918c-4dae-b0c6-6d630c46007f/UploadedImages/AAN_Nursing-Choosing-Wisely-List__11_19_18_.pdf

American Board of Internal Medicine Foundation. (2016). *Choosing Wisely®: About the campaign.* http://www.choosingwisely.org/wp-content/uploads/2015/04/About-Choosing-Wisely.pdf

American Nurses Credentialing Center. (2008). *Magnet recognition program.* https://www.nursingworld.org/organizational-programs/magnet/

Begun, J. W., Zimmerman, B., & Dooley, K. (2003). Healthcare organizations as complex adaptive systems. In S. M. Mick & M. Wyttenbach (Eds.), *Advances in healthcare organization theory* (pp. 253–288). Jossey-Bass.

Berwick, D. M. (2008). The science of improvement. *Journal of the American Medical Association, 299*(10), 1182–1184. https://doi.org/10.1001/jama.299.10.1182

Berwick, D. M., & Hackbarth, A. D. (2012). Eliminating waste in U.S. healthcare. *Journal of the American Medical Association, 307*(14), 1513–1516. https://doi.org/10.1001/jama.2012.362

Black, A. T., Balneaves, L. G., Garossino, C., Puyat, J. H., & Qian, H. (2015). Promoting evidence-based practice through a research training program for point-of-care clinicians. *The Journal of Nursing Administration, 45*(1), 14. https://doi.org/10.1097/NNA.0000000000000151

Brownson, R. C., Colditz, G. A., & Proctor, E. K. (Eds.). (2017). *Dissemination and implementation research in health: translating science to practice* (2nd ed.). Oxford University Press.

Buerhaus, P. (2007). Is hospital patient care becoming safer? A conversation with Lucian Leape. *Health Affairs, 26*(6), w687–w696. https://doi.org/10.1377/hlthaff.26.6.w687

Centers for Disease Control and Prevention. (2018). *Cardiac Rehabilitation Change Package.* Centers for Disease Control and Prevention, U.S. Department of Health and Human Services. https://millionhearts.hhs.gov/index.html

Chassin, M. R., & Loeb, J. M. (2013). High-reliability health care: Getting there from here. *The Milbank Quarterly, 91*(3), 459–490. https://doi.org/10.1111/1468-0009.12023

Colla, C. H., Morden, N. E., Sequist, T. D., Schpero, W. L., & Rosenthal, M. B. (2015). Choosing wisely: Prevalence and correlates of low-value health care services in the United States. *Journal of General Internal Medicine, 30*(2), 221–228. https://doi.org/10.1007/s11606-014-3070-z

Demes, J. A. E., Nickerson, N., Farand, L., Montekio, V. B., Torres, P., Dube, J. G., Coq, J. G., Pomey, M-P., Champagne, F., & Jasmin, E. R. (2020). What are the characteristics of the champion that influence the implementation of quality improvement programs?. *Evaluation and Program Planning, 80*, 101795. https://doi.org/10.1016/j.evalprogplan.2020.101795

Damschroder, L. J., Aron, D. C., Keith, R. E., Kirsh, S. R., Alexander, J. A., & Lowery, J. C. (2009). Fostering implementation of health services research findings into practice: a consolidated framework for advancing implementation science. *Implementation Science, 4*(1), 50. https://doi.org/10.1186/1748-5908-4-50

Dolansky, M. A., & Moore, S. M. (2013). Quality and safety education for nurses (QSEN): The key is systems thinking. *Online Journal of Issues in Nursing, 18*(3), 1.

Ebright, P. R., Urden, L., Patterson, E., & Chalko, B. (2004). Themes surrounding novice nurse near-miss and adverse-event situations. *Journal of Nursing Administration, 34*(11), 531–538. https://doi.org/10.1097/00005110-200411000-00010

Frankel, A., Haraden, C., Federico, F., & Lenoci-Edwards, J. (2017). A framework for safe, reliable, and effective care. *White paper. Institute for Healthcare Improvement and Safe & Reliable Healthcare.*

Funk, S. G., Champagne, M. T., Wiese, R. A., & Tornquist, E. M. (1990). BARRIERS: The barriers research utilization scale. *Applied Nursing Research, 4*(1), 39–45. https://doi.org/10.1016/S0897-1897(05)80052-7

Funk, S. G., Tornquist, E. M., & Champagne, M. T. (1989). Application and evaluation of dissemination model. *Western Journal of Nursing Research, 11*(4), 486–491. https://doi.org/10.1177/019394598901100411

Glasgow, R. E., Harden, S. M., Gaglio, B., Rabin, B. A., Smith, M. L., Porter, G. C., Ory, M. G., & Estabrooks, P. A. (2019). RE-AIM planning and evaluation framework: adapting to new science and practice with a twenty-year review. *Frontiers in Public Health, 7*, 64. https://doi.org/10.3389/fpubh.2019.00064

Glasziou, P., & Haynes, B. (2005). The paths from research to improved health outcomes. *ACP Journal Club, 142*(2), A8–A10. https://doi.org/10.1136/ebn.8.2.36

Greenhalgh, T. (2018). *How to implement evidence-based healthcare.* Wiley Blackwell.

Grimshaw, J. M., Eccles, M. P., Lavis, J. N., Hill, S. J., & Squires, J. E. (2012). Knowledge translation of research findings. *Implementation Science, 7*(1), 50. https://doi.org/10.1186/1748-5908-7-50

Guirguis-Blake, J. M., Michael, Y. L., Perdue, L. A., Coppola, E. L., & Beil, T. L. (2018). Interventions to prevent falls in older adults: updated evidence report and systematic review for the U.S. Preventive Services Task Force. *JAMA, 319*(16), 1705–1716. https://doi.org/10.1001/jama.2017.21962

Harvey, G., & Kitson, A. (2015). PARIHS revisited: From heuristic to integrated framework for the successful implementation of knowledge into practice. *Implementation Science, 11*(1), 33. https://doi.org/10.1186/s13012-016-0398-2

Helmreich, R. L. (2000). On error management: Lessons from aviation. *British Medical Journal (Clinical Research Edition), 320*(7237), 781–785. https://doi.org/10.1136/bmj.320.7237.781

Institute for Healthcare Improvement. (2008). *About us.* http://www.ihi.org/ihi/about

Institute of Medicine. (1990). *Clinical practice guidelines: Directions for a new program.* National Academies Press.

Institute of Medicine. (2000). *To err is human: Building a safer health system.* National Academies Press.

Institute of Medicine. (2001). *Crossing the quality chasm: A new health system for the 21st century.* National Academies Press.

Institute of Medicine. (2003a). *Priority areas for national action: Transforming health care quality.* National Academies Press.

Institute of Medicine. (2003b). *Health professions education: A bridge to quality.* National Academies Press.

Institute of Medicine. (2004). *Keeping patients safe: Transforming the work environment of nurses.* National Academies Press. https://www.nap.edu/read/10851/chapter/1

Institute of Medicine. (2008). *Knowing what works: A roadmap for the nation.* National Academies Press.

Institute of Medicine. (2011a). *Clinical guidelines we can trust.* National Academies Press. https://www.nap.edu/catalog/13058/clinical-practice-guidelines-we-can-trust

Institute of Medicine. (2011b). *Finding what works in healthcare: Standards for systematic reviews.* https://www.nap.edu/catalog/13059/finding-what-works-in-health-care-standards-for-systematic-reviews

Institute of Medicine. (2011c). *The future of nursing: Leading change, advancing health* (prepared by Robert Wood Johnson Foundation Committee Initiative on the Future of Nursing). National Academies Press.

Interdisciplinary Nursing Quality Research Initiative. (2013). *Program overview.* https://www.rwjf.org/en/library/research/2013/04/the-interdisciplinary-nursing-quality-research-initiative.html

Jirapaet, V., Jirapaet, K., & Sopajaree, C. (2006). The nurses' experience of barriers to safe practice in the neonatal intensive care unit in Thailand. *Journal of Obstetric, Gynecologic, and Neonatal Nursing, 35*(6), 746–754. https://doi.org/10.1111/j.1552-6909.2006.00100.x

The Joint Commission. (2020). *National patient safety goals.* https://www.jointcommission.org/standards_information/npsgs.aspx

Kilbourne, A. M., Goodrich, D. E., Miake-Lye, I., Braganza, M. Z., & Bowersox, N. W. (2019). Quality enhancement research initiative implementation roadmap: Toward sustainability of evidence-based practices in a learning health system. *Medical Care, 57*(10 Suppl 3), S286. https://doi.org/10.1097/MLR.0000000000001144

Lake, E. T. (2007). The nursing practice environment: Measurement and evidence. *Medical Care Research and Review, 64* (Suppl. 2), 104S–122S. https://doi.org/10.1177/1077558707299253

Long, J. D., Gannaway, P., Ford, C., Doumit, R., Zeeni, N., Sukkarieh-Haraty, O., Milane, A., Byers, B., Harrison, L., Hatch, D., Brown, J., Proper, S., . . . Brown, J. (2016). Effectiveness of a technology-based intervention to teach evidence-based practice: The EBR Tool. *Worldviews on Evidence-Based Nursing, 13*(1), 59–65. https://doi.org/10.1111/wvn.12132

Makary, M. A., & Daniel, M. (2016). Medical error—the third leading cause of death in the U.S. *BMJ, 353*, i2139. https://doi.org/10.1136/bmj.i2139

Marx, D. (Ed.). (2001). *Patient safety and the "Just Culture": A primer for health care executives.* Trustees of Columbia University.

Miech, E. J., Rattray, N. A., Flanagan, M. E., Damschroder, L., Schmid, A. A., & Damush, T. M. (2018). Inside help:An integrative review of champions in healthcare-related implementation. *SAGE Open Medicine, 6,* 2050312118773261. https://doi.org/10.1177/2050312118773261

Mitchell, S. A., Fisher, C. A., Hastings, C. E., Silverman, L. B., & Wallen, G. R. (2010). A thematic analysis of theoretical models for translational science in nursing: Mapping the field. *Nursing Outlook, 58*(6), 287–300. https://doi.org/10.1016/j.outlook.2010.07.001

Mick, J. M., Wood, G. L., & Massey, R. L. (2007). The good catch pilot program: Increasing potential error reporting. *Journal of Nursing Administration, 37*(11), 499–503. https://doi.org/10.1097/01.NNA.0000295611.40441.1b

Mordue, B. C. (2005). A case report of the transport of an infant with a tension pneumopericardium. *Advances in Neonatal Care, 5*(4), 190–200; quiz 201. https://doi.org/10.1016/j.adnc.2005.03.003

Mulrow, C. D. (1994). Rationale for systematic reviews. *British Medical Journal (Clinical Research Edition), 309*(6954), 597–599. https://doi.org/10.1136/bmj.309.6954.597

National Institutes of Health. (2019). *Dissemination and implementation research in health.* PAR 19-274. https://grants.nih.gov/grants/guide/pa-files/PAR-19-274.html

National Quality Forum. (2020). *Forum endorses National Consensus Standards promoting accountability and public reporting.* http://www.qualityforum.org/About_NQF

Newhouse, R., Bobay, K., Dykes, P. C., Stevens, K. R., & Titler, M. (2013). Methodology issues in implementation science. *Medical Care, 51*(4, Suppl. 2), S32–S40. https://doi.org/10.1097/MLR.0b013e31827feeca

Nilsen, P. (2020). Making sense of implementation theories, models, and frameworks. In B. Albers, A. Shlonsky, & R. Mildon (Eds.), *Implementation Science 3.0* (pp. 53–79). Springer International Publishing.

Ovretveit, J. (2017). Perspectives: Answering questions about quality improvement: Suggestions for investigators. *International Journal for Quality in Health Care, 29*(1), 137–142. https://doi.org/10.1093/intqhc/mzw136

Pape, T. M. (2003). Applying airline safety practices to medication administration. *Medsurg Nursing, 12*(2), 77–93; quiz 94.

Powell, B. J., Beidas, R. S., Lewis, C. C., Aarons, G. A., McMillen, J. C., Proctor, E. K., & Mandell, D. S. (2017). Methods to improve the selection and tailoring of implementation strategies. *The Journal of Behavioral Health Services & Research, 44*(2), 177–194. https://doi.org/10.1007/s11414-015-9475-6

Powell, B. J., Fernandez, M. E., Williams, N. J., Aarons, G. A., Beidas, R. S., Lewis, C. C., McHugh, S. M., & Weiner, B. J. (2019). Enhancing the impact of implementation strategies in healthcare: A research agenda. *Frontiers in Public Health, 7,* 3. https://doi.org/10.3389/fpubh.2019.00003

Powell, B. J., Waltz, T. J., Chinman, M. J., Damschroder, L. J., Smith, J. L., Matthieu, M. M., Proctor, E. K., & Kirchner, J. E. (2015). A refined compilation of implementation strategies: Results from the Expert Recommendations for Implementing Change (ERIC) project. *Implementation Science, 10*(1), 21. https://doi.org/10.1186/s13012-015-0209-1

Proctor, E. K., Powell, B. J., & McMillen, J. C. (2013). Implementation strategies: Recommendations for specifying and reporting. *Implementation Science, 8*(1), 139. https://doi.org/10.1186/1748-5908-8-139

Proctor, E., Silmere, H., Raghavan, R., Hovmand, P., Aarons, G., Bunger, A., Griffey, R., & Hensley, M. (2011). Outcomes for implementation research: Conceptual distinctions, measurement challenges, and research agenda. *Administration and Policy in Mental Health and Mental Health Services Research, 38*(2), 65–76. https://doi.org/10.1007/s10488-010-0319-7

Reams, J. (2011). Making FMEA work for you. *Nursing Management, 42*(5), 18–20. https://doi.org/10.1097/01.NUMA.0000396500.05462.6e

Reason, J. (2000). Human error: Models and management. *British Medical Journal (Clinical Research Edition), 320*(7237), 768–770. https://doi.org/10.1136/bmj.320.7237.768

Robert Wood Johnson Foundation. (2008). *Interprofessional nursing quality research initiative.* https://www.rwjf.org/en/library/research/2013/04/the-interdisciplinary-nursing-quality-research-initiative.html

Rogers, E. M. (2003). *Diffusion of innovations* (5th ed.). Free Press.

Sackett, D. L., Straus, S. E., Richardson, W. S., Rosenberg, W., & Haynes, R. B. (2000). *Evidence-based medicine: How to practice and teach EBM* (2nd ed.). Churchill Livingstone.

Saunders, H., Stevens, K. R., & Vehviläinen-Julkunen, K. (2016). Nurses' readiness for evidence-based practice at Finnish university hospitals: A national survey. *Journal of Advanced Nursing, 72*(8), 1863–1874. https://doi.org/10.1111/jan.12963

Schpero, W. L. (2014). Limiting low-value care by "choosing wisely." *AMA Journal of Ethics, 16*(2), 131–134. https://doi.org/10.1001/virtualmentor.2014.16.2.pfor2-1402

Shrank, W. H., Rogstad, T. L., & Parekh, N. (2019). Waste in the U.S. healthcare system: estimated costs and potential for savings. *JAMA, 322*(15), 1501–1509. https://doi.org/10.1001/jama.2019.13978

Stetler, C. B. (1994). Refinement of the Stetler/Marram model for application of research findings to practice. *Nursing Outlook, 42*(1), 15–25. https://doi.org/10.1016/0029-6554(94)90067-1

Stevens, K. R. (2009). *Essential competencies for evidence-based practice in nursing* (2nd ed.). Academic Center for Evidence-Based Practice (ACE), University of Texas Health Science Center.

Stevens, K. (May 31, 2013). The impact of evidence-based practice in nursing and the next big ideas. *The Online Journal of Issues in Nursing, 18*(2), Manuscript 4. https://doi.org/10.3912/OJIN.Vol18No02Man04. http://ojin.nursingworld.org/MainMenuCategories/ANAMarketplace/ANAPeriodicals/OJIN/TableofContents/Vol-18-2013/No2-May-2013/Impact-of-Evidence-Based-Practice.html

Stevens, K. R. (2015). *Stevens star model of knowledge transformation.* Academic Center for Evidence-based Practice. The University of Texas Health Science Center at San Antonio. https://www.uthscsa.edu/academics/nursing/star-model

Stevens, K. R. (2019). *Awareness of Low-Value Care as a Requisite for De-Implementation: Nurses' Choosing Wisely® Campaign.* Poster Presentation. NIH/Academy Health Dissemination & Implementation Conference. December 4-5, 2019. Washington, DC. https://academyhealth.confex.com/academyhealth/2019di/meetingapp.cgi/Session/23255

Stevens, K. R., Engh, E. P., Tubbs-Cooley, H., Conley, D. M., Cupit, T., D'Errico, E., DiNapoli, P., Fischer, J. L., Freed, R., Kotzer, A. M., Lindgren, C. L., Marino, M. A., . . . Lindgren, C. L. (2017). Operational failures detected by frontline acute care nurses. *Research in Nursing & Health, 40*(3), 197–205. https://doi.org/10.1002/nur.21791

Stroebel, C. K., McDaniel, R. R., Crabtree, B. F., Miller, W. L., Nutting, P. A., & Stange, K. C. (2005). How complexity science can inform a reflective process for improvement in primary care practices. *Joint Commission Journal on Quality and Patient Safety, 31*(8), 438–446. https://doi.org/10.1016/S1553-7250(05)31057-9

Sullivan, C. G. (2015). *American Academy of Nursing announced engagement in National Choosing Wisely® campaign.* http://www.choosingwisely.org/american-academy-of-nursing-announces-engagement-in-national-choosing-wisely-campaign

Tabak, R. G., Khoong, E. C., Chambers, D. A., & Brownson, R. C. (2012). Bridging research and practice: models for dissemination and implementation research. *American journal of preventive medicine, 43*(3), 337–350. https://doi.org/10.1016/j.amepre.2012.05.024

Titler, M. G., Kleiber, C., Steelman, V. J., Rakel, B. A., Budreau, G., Everett, L. Q., Buckwalter, K. C., Tripp-Reimer, T., & Goode, C. J. (2001). The Iowa model of evidence-based practice to promote quality care. *Critical Care Nursing Clinics of North America, 13*(4), 497–509. https://doi.org/10.1016/S0899-5885(18)30017-0

U.S. Preventive Services Task Force. (2020). *Home Page.* https://www.uspreventiveservicestaskforce.org/uspstf

Weick, K. E., & Sutcliffe, K. M. (2015). *Managing the unexpected: Sustained performance in a complex world.* John Wiley & Sons.

Weiner, B. J., Lewis, C. C., Stanick, C., Powell, B. J., Dorsey, C. N., Clary, A. S., Boynton, M. H., & Halko, H. (2017). Psychometric assessment of three newly developed implementation outcome measures. *Implementation Science, 12*(1), 108. https://doi.org/10.1186/s13012-017-0635-3

Weiner, B. J., Clary, A. S., Klaman, S. L., Turner, K., & Alishahi-Tabriz, A. (2020). Organizational readiness for change: What we know, what we think we know, and what we need to know. In B. Albers, A. Shlonsky, & R. Mildon (Eds.), *Implementation Science 3.0* (pp. 101–144). Springer International Publishing.

Westrum, R. (2004). A typology of organisational cultures. *Quality & Safety in Health Care, 13* (Suppl. 2), ii22–ii27. https://doi.org/10.1136/qshc.2003.009522

Whalen, M., Baptiste, D. L., & Maliszewski, B. (2020). Increasing nursing scholarship through dedicated human resources: Creating a culture of nursing inquiry. *JONA: The Journal of Nursing Administration, 50*(2), 90–94. https://doi.org/10.1097/NNA.0000000000000847

Wolfson, D., Santa, J., & Slass, L. (2014). Engaging physicians and consumers in conversations about treatment overuse and waste: A short history of the Choosing Wisely® campaign. *Academic Medicine, 89*(7), 990–995. https://doi.org/10.1097/ACM.0000000000000270

Wolk, C. B., Stewart, R. E., Eiraldi, R., Cronholm, P., Salas, E., & Mandell, D. S. (2019). The implementation of a team training intervention for school mental health: Lessons learned. *Psychotherapy, 56*(1), 83. https://doi.org/10.1037/pst0000179

Woodward, L. J., Bradshaw, P. J., & Stevens, K. R. (2015). *Curbing the use of ineffective and costly healthcare: Nursing evidence for Choosing Wisely®*. Symposium at the Sigma Theta Tau Biennial Convention, Las Vegas. https://stti.confex.com/stti/bc43/webprogram/Session20862.html

Woolf, S. H. (2004). Patient safety is not enough: Targeting quality improvements to optimize the health of the population. *Annals of Internal Medicine, 140*(1), 33–36. https://doi.org/10.7326/0003-4819-140 -1-200401060-00009

World Health Organization. (2005). *WHO draft guidelines for adverse event reporting and learning systems*. Author.

Yoder, L. H., Kirkley, D., McFall, D. C., Kirksey, K. M., StalBaum, A. L., & Sellers, D. (2014). Staff nurses' use of research to facilitate evidence-based practice. *American Journal of Nursing, 114*(9), 26–38. https://doi .org/10.1097/01.NAJ.0000453753.00894.29

CONTINUOUS QUALITY IMPROVEMENT

MARY C. ZONSIUS AND KERRY A. MILNER

◼ THE HISTORY OF QUALITY IMPROVEMENT IN HEALTHCARE

In the late 1980s, with the beginning transition from fee for service to a prospective payment plan, healthcare organizations were first challenged to evaluate their inefficiencies. With further changes in the financing of healthcare to rein in costs (e.g., capitation and contracting by large insurers and managed care organizations), hospitals began to recognize the competitive nature of healthcare and that inefficiency cut into profits. Healthcare organizations began to shift from quality assurance, a retrospective review of individual's compliance with policies and procedures, to proactive analysis of system's processes and outcomes called quality improvement (QI; Colton, 2000).

In addition to financial factors, several sentinel events accelerated the evolution of QI in healthcare organizations. The National Demonstration Project in QI in Health Care examined whether or not the industrial QI paradigm was transferable to healthcare organizations (Colton, 2000). The industrial QI paradigm was based on the founding work of Walter Shewhart, W. Edwards Deming, and Joseph Juran and results supported the use of this paradigm to drive patient safety and quality care in healthcare organizations (Burda, 1988). Bolstered by these results, co-author and physician Donald Berwick, made the case, in the *New England Journal of Medicine,* for using industrial-based QI methods to improve American healthcare (Berwick, 1989). Another sentinel event was The Joint Commission's Agenda for Change that included the use of QI in hospitals and included input from key stakeholders (e.g., patients, healthcare workers, and hospital administrators) to achieve its goal of rewriting its accreditation standards (Colton, 2000). The new standards focused on the QI process and included the use of run charts, Pareto charts and statistical process control to evaluate and improve systems to achieve better outcomes.

The Institute for Healthcare Improvement (IHI) emerged from the National Demonstration Project on QI in Health Care in 1991 in Cambridge, Massachusetts (IHI, n.d.). The creators of the IHI envisioned clinicians in healthcare systems using QI methods to fix unreliable common care practices (Berwick et al., 1990). The IHI recognized the need to build capacity for change in the U.S. healthcare system by creating an organization that would engage in knowledge sharing and training on performance improvement.

From 2005 to the present, the IHI has been establishing patient safety initiatives in the United States and abroad (IHI, n.d.). As part of this work, the IHI launched the Triple Aim in 2006 with a call to enhance the patient experience, improve population health, and reduce costs to optimize health system performance (Berwick et al., 2008). Clinicians in primary care practices across the United States have adopted the Triple Aim framework; however, stressful work life has interfered with their ability to achieve the three aims. In response to this, Bodenheimer and Sinsky (2014) proposed the Quadruple Aim that includes the tenets of the Triple Aim plus the aim of improving the work life of the healthcare workforce. The Quadruple Aim recognizes that a healthy workforce is needed to optimize health system performance.

■ DEFINING CHARACTERISTICS OF QUALITY IMPROVEMENT IN HEALTHCARE

The IHI, whose mission is to improve healthcare quality and safety for all, defines QI in terms of using a team of managers and staff that have the relevant expertise to analyze the current process (Scoville & Little, 2014). This team is supported by QI specialists who work behind the scenes to improve the overall quality of care of that health facility. The team identifies the symptoms and causes of poor quality and devises a theory of what is needed to improve the process. The team uses a variety of improvement methods and tools to develop, test, and implement changes and redesigns the process if needed. The redesigned process is then monitored to ensure it performs at a new level (with new upper and lower control limits), with new work specifications, improved results, and reduced variation.

The National Quality Forum (NQF) was established in 1999 to improve the quality of U.S. healthcare. The forum works to define national goals and priorities for healthcare QI and develops standard metrics for measuring performance in healthcare nationally (Marjoua & Bozic, 2012). They have metrics for processes (appropriate use), structures, outcomes, cost/resource use, and efficiency. The NQF stakeholders include hospitals, healthcare providers, consumer groups, purchasers, accrediting bodies, and research. Having national measures to assess healthcare performance is a critical component of ensuring appropriate and high-quality patient care.

The Health Resources and Services Administration (HRSA) is a federal agency whose mission is to improve access to healthcare and health outcomes of vulnerable populations. The HRSA defines QI as systematic and continuous actions that lead to measurable improvement in healthcare services and the health status of targeted patient groups (Department of Health and Human Services and HRSA, 2011). HRSA collaborates with other federal and state entities to improve care. For example, HRSA partners with the Centers for Medicare & Medicaid Services (CMS) to improve care for vulnerable populations. The CMS defines QI as standardized behavior that is made systematic so that the same inputs result in the same outputs (CMS, n.d.). In this definition, behavior is aligned with best evidence. Donabedian's structure, process, and outcome (Donabedian, 2005) are used to increased desired health outcomes and Deming's PDSA (plan-do-study-act) cycle (Moen & Norman, 2010) is used to standardize behavior.

The Quality and Safety Education for Nurses (QSEN) initiative began in 2005 with the mission of preparing competent nurses to improve the quality and safety of the healthcare system. The founding faculty members adapted the Institute of Medicine (IOM) competencies from the *Health Professionals Education: A Bridge to Quality* (Greiner & Knebel, 2003) report and defined essential knowledge, skills, and attitudes (e.g., competency) in the areas of patient-centered care, evidence-based practice (EBP), teamwork and collaboration, safety, QI, and informatics for undergraduate (Cronenwett et al., 2007) and graduate nursing levels (American Association of Colleges of Nursing QSEN Education Consortium, 2012). The QSEN faculty defined QI in terms of "use data to monitor the outcomes of care processes and use improvement methods to design and test changes to continuously improve the quality and safety of healthcare systems" (Cronenwett et al., 2007, p. 127). QSEN has helped to bridge the gap between what is and what should be in delivering healthcare.

ADVANCED PRACTICE REGISTERED NURSE ENGAGEMENT IN QUALITY IMPROVEMENT

The 2019 American Association of Nurse Practitioners (AANP) standards for practice include APRN engagement in QI. Standard VII: Quality Assurance and Continued Competence calls for "participation in quality assurance review, including the systematic, periodic review of records and plans of care that may result in quality improvement plan." Standard IX: Research as Basis for Practice calls for APRNs to "support research and dissemination of evidence-based practice by developing clinical research questions, conducting or participating in studies, implementing quality improvement, and incorporating system changes into practice" (AANP, n.d.).

Reimbursement is another key reason for APRNs to be engaged in QI activities. APRNs are eligible clinicians under the CMS value-based initiative called Merit-Based Incentive Payment System (MIPS; Curtin, 2019). In this new payment system, performance is measured using data that APRNs report in three areas: quality (50% of score), promoting interoperability requirements (25% of score) and improvement activities (15% of score) and cost makes up the last 10%. For quality, APRNs pick performance measures that best fit their practice from a provided list (e.g., appropriate use, patient safety, efficiency, patient experience or care coordination; AANP, n.d.). Promoting interoperability is fulfilled by hospitals and APRNs demonstrating compliance with information sharing. Improvement activities include how clinicians improve care processes, enhance patient engagement and access to care. It is assumed that these activities will promote ongoing improvement and innovation in healthcare.

Additionally, reimbursement under MIPS relies on performance measures. These performance measures should be based on metrics that assess the outcomes of APRN care on patient care and quality of care measures (Kapu & Kleinpell, 2013). APRN outcomes must also be included in the benchmarks for hospital performance. Thus, APRNs must engage in the development of APRN-associated metrics in order to generate relevant data to accurately assess their performance and contributions to patient safety and quality care nationally.

QUALITY IMPROVEMENT COMPETENCIES FOR ADVANCED PRACTICE REGISTERED NURSES

The National Organization for Nurse Practitioner Faculty (NONPF) developed core competencies for nurse practitioners that include a quality competency. NONPF defines quality as the degree to which health services increase the desired health outcomes consistent with professional knowledge and standards, the understanding of how to access and use information databases, and how to critically evaluate research findings. Other QI competencies for nurse practitioners include:

- Uses best available evidence to continuously improve quality of clinical practice.
- Evaluates the relationships among access, cost, quality, and safety and their influence on healthcare.
- Evaluates how organizational structure, care processes, financing, marketing, and policy decisions impact the quality of healthcare.
- Applies skills in peer review to promote a culture of excellence.
- Anticipates variations in practice and is proactive in implementing interventions to ensure quality.

TABLE 4.1 Comparison of Research, Evidence-Based Practice (EBP), Quality Improvement (QI)

	RESEARCH	EBP	QI
Definition	Use scientific method to investigate a gap in knowledge	A problem-solving process that integrates existing evidence (research, QI), nursing expertise and patient preferences to guide care decisions	Appraise the efficiency of clinical interventions and provide guidance for achieving quality outcomes, productivity, cost containment
Prompted by	Gap in knowledge	New evidence from research	Process breakdown or system failure
Purpose	Generate new knowledge	Integrate best evidence, clinician's expertise, and patient values and preferences to improve health outcomes	Improve system and process of healthcare delivery
Questions	What is the best thing to do?	Are we doing the best thing?	Are we doing the best thing right, all of the time?
Results	Generalizable to population	Recommendation for practice change, clinical research study, or no change	Applicable to the patients studied or local setting

◼ DIFFERENCES AMONG RESEARCH, EVIDENCE-BASED PRACTICE, AND QUALITY IMPROVEMENT

APRNs need to be knowledgeable about the differences among research, EBP, and QI, and how they form the basis for practice inquiry. Table 4.1 outlines the specific characteristics of each method of inquiry. Research is pursued when there is a lack of knowledge upon which to base practice. EBP is a problem-solving approach to practice and EBP projects are undertaken when new evidence from research needs to be translated into practice. QI inquiry is followed when the current practice is the best thing to do (e.g., based on best available evidence), however there is breakdown in the process or structures, or the outcomes are not meeting expectations.

◼ QUALITY IMPROVEMENT AS THE CENTRAL COMPONENT OF THE NURSING INQUIRY PROCESS

Figure 4.1 displays the Clinical Inquiry Process from Virginia Commonwealth University where performance improvement, also known as QI, is a central component of clinical inquiry. The EBP steps of problem identification, question development using the PICOT format, search for evidence, and appraisal of evidence appear across the top of Figure 4.1. If the Appraise Evidence step reveals adequate evidence but the current practice is not fully implemented, then the performance improvement (Process Enhancement/Improvement) inquiry should be followed. If the practice setting is not following the evidence-based recommendation for practice, then the EBP (Change in Practice) inquiry should be followed. If the current practice is fully implemented, then the APRN can stop or pursue new questions. If the Appraise Evidence step reveals a lack of evidence upon which to base practice, then the research inquiry (Creation of New Knowledge) should be followed.

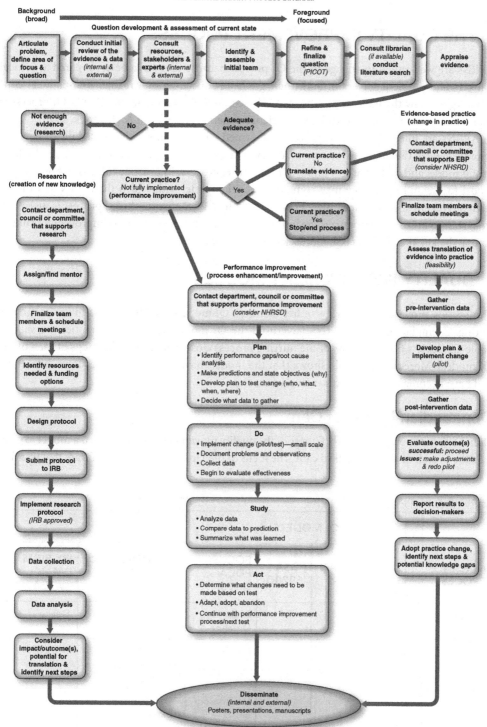

THE CLINICAL INQUIRY PROCESS DIAGRAM

FIGURE 4.1 Nursing inquiry process diagram.

EBP, evidence-based practice; IRB, institutional review board; NHSRD, Not Human Subjects Research Determination; PICOT, P=Patient population, I=Intervention, C=Comparison intervention, O=Outcome, T=Time.

Source: Used with permission from Roy, R. E. (2020). The Clinical Inquiry Process diagram. https://scholarscompass.vcu.edu/libraries_pubs

THE QUALITY IMPROVEMENT PROCESS

APRNs are well-suited to engage in the QI process because they have been prepared as critical thinkers and problem solvers in both their graduate education and in their foundational education (guided by the nursing process that is based on the scientific method). The QI process is considered an extension or rework of the scientific method (Cleghorn & Headrick, 1996).

APRNs are integral to the QI process and armed with the knowledge and skills to navigate improvement at the micro, meso, and macro system levels. As a QI team leader, the APRN selects the QI model and tools that will improve the existing process. In practice there is not one "right" model to use and the choice may come down to the model with which the APRN and the QI team has the most experience (Silver et al., 2016). The APRN ensures the QI process is successful from start to finish and recognizes the importance of instilling a continuous improvement culture among the key stakeholders (Chandrasekaran & Toussaint, 2019).

QUALITY IMPROVEMENT MODELS

This section provides an overview of five common QI models used by APRNs in the healthcare setting. Exemplars of how APRNS have used the QI models to improve practice are shared. Table 4.2 depicts how the steps of the nursing process closely align with the steps of each of the QI models. Moreover, the table shows that the models have more similarities than differences and have become more comprehensive across time.

Donabedian Model of Care

Donabedian was one of the early fathers of the quality movement who developed a model to evaluate the overall quality of medical care. The focus of the Donabedian Model of Care that was first

TABLE 4.2 Comparison of Common Quality Improvement Models

	COMMON QI MODELS				
NURSING PROCESS	DONABEDIAN (1960s)	PDSA (1920s)	FOCUS-PDCA (1993)	IHI MODEL FOR IMPROVEMENT (1990s)	SIX SIGMA/ DMAIC (LATE 1980s)
Assess			Find/ Organize	What are we trying to accomplish?	Define
			Clarify	How we know that a change is an improvement?	Measure
Diagnose			Understand/ Select	What change can we make that will result in an improvement?	Analyze
Plan	Structure	Plan	Plan	Plan	
Implement	Process	Do	Do	Do	Improve
Evaluate	Outcome	Study	Check	Study	Control
		Act	Act	Act	

presented in the 1960s is an evaluation of quality that includes the triad of structure, process, and outcome (Donabedian, 2005). The thought was that to fully evaluate quality one had to have the proper structures in place that would influence the given process and ultimately the outcomes of care. Structure refers to the inputs; characteristically the setting where the process occurs, the staff involved in the process, and the material and organizational resources. Process is as stated, the process to be implemented and/or evaluated: What are the technical and interpersonal activities involved in delivering care? The outcome is the output, the effect of whether care of patients or population groups was improved (Donabedian, 1988).

The Donabedian model can be used to implement a QI change as well as to evaluate an existing process. APRNs Compton and Carrico (2018) used Donabedian's model to develop and implement a chronic obstructive pulmonary disease (COPD) tool to improve the patient and provider communication process and thereby improve patient outcomes by decreasing emergency department visits, hospitalizations, and healthcare costs.

The Plan-Do-Study-Act (PDSA) Cycle

The PDSA cycle that is commonly used in healthcare settings today stems from the original work of Walter Shewhart that began in the 1920s at Bell Telephone Laboratories that was later modified by W. Edwards Deming (Re & Krousel-Wood, 1990). Together Shewhart and Deming are viewed as the founders of the industrial quality movement and fathers of the modern-day QI movement.

This four-step iterative model (PDSA) is best used to test interventions in a pilot setting using multiple cycles to refine the process prior to expanding system-wide. This model allows for rapid-cycle change (Taylor et al., 2014).

1. *Plan.* Assemble the team, understand current process, and identify possible solutions. Develop goals of the planned change and delineate who will do what and when to carry out the planned change.

2. *Do.* Implement the change and note any unexpected deviations from the plan.

3. *Study.* The analysis phase. Did the intervention go as planned? Was the plan successful? What was learned?

4. *Act.* If successful, sustain the change. If not, make modifications and retest.

The PDSA cycle is one of the most common QI models used by APRNs to improve the patient safety and quality care related to delirium (Fraire & Whitehead, 2019), falls (Cangany et al., 2018; Grillo et al., 2019; Kohari, 2018), 30-day readmission rates (House et al., 2016), heparin infusion protocols (Johnson et al., 2018), pediatric asthma care (Kennedy & Jolles, 2019), colon screening rates (Florea et al., 2016), sleep disturbances (Lopez et al., 2018), and medical management for older adults (Vejar et al., 2015).

▬ FOCUS-PDCA MODEL

In 1993, the Hospital Corporation of America created the Find, Organize, Clarify, Understand, Select (FOCUS) model from Deming's PDSA model (Taylor et al., 2014) to guide the QI efforts of their healthcare workers. The five steps in this model are:

1. *Find* a process to improve.

2. *Organize* a team that knows the process.

3. *Clarify* current knowledge of the process.

4. *Understand* causes of process variation.

5. *Select* the process improvement.

The five step FOCUS is followed by the Plan-Do-Check-Act (PDCA) cycle. However, small tests of change using PDCA are used in steps 3 and 4 to inform the improvement implemented in the PDCA cycle that begins following step 5 (Batalden & Stoltz, 1993).

Note that in the PDCA cycle "C" is used for "Check" rather than the "S" for "Study." Many organizations use the "S" and "C" interchangeably although Deming stressed that semantically "check" was not appropriate because it means "to hold back" (Moen & Norman, 2010).

The FOCUS-PDCA model provides additional structure and guidance to the planning of the QI process. An example of APRNs' use of this model in practice is the work by Watts and Nemes (2018) who used the FOCUS-PDCA model to guide the implementation of a hypoglycemic protocol to increase rechecks within 30 minutes of treatment.

Institute for Healthcare Improvement Model for Improvement

The IHI Model for improvement (MFI), an outgrowth of the more common PDSA cycle from Deming, was designed by Langley and colleagues concurrent to the FOCUS-PDCA model (Langley et al., 2009). The MFI, a comprehensive QI model, begins with three questions that inform the subsequent PDSA cycle. Note that the IHI MFI uses *study* for the third step of the cycle.

The three questions are (a) What are we trying to accomplish? — purpose or aim; (b) How do we know that a change is an improvement? — feedback/data are needed; and (c) What change can we make that will result in an improvement? — what specific change can be made that will address the purpose or aim? Next, rather than randomly implementing a change and hoping to get the expected result, the MFI supports a pilot test of the change using the PDSA model. The overall goal is to spread and sustain the change (Langley et al., 2009).

The IHI MFI provides additional structure and direction to guide the QI process. APRNs have used the model to improve suicide screening practices in an outpatient mental health clinic (Spear, 2018); implement a mobility plan in a long-term care facility (Kazana & Murphy, 2018); and implement scripted post-discharge phone calls to heart failure patients to improve outcomes (Ruggiri et al., 2019).

Six Sigma (DMAIC)

The development of Six Sigma quality methodology, in the late 1980s, is attributed to the Motorola Corporation with the goal of decreasing process variability but also improving financial performance and customer satisfaction. The use of data to establish pre-change baseline performance, and statistical analysis tools distinguish this data-driven methodology from previous QI models that have been discussed (Glasgow et al., 2010; Takao, 2017).

Sigma uses the 5-step DMAIC model (define, measure, analyze, improve, and control):

1. *Define.* Identify the problem, scope of the project, key customer needs, and current process.

2. *Measure.* Collect data to determine the performance of the current process.

3. *Analyze.* Identify and prioritize root causes of variation.

4. *Improve.* Address opportunities for improvement in the process. Develop and implement solutions to reduce/eliminate root causes and decrease variation.

5. *Control.* Did the process improve? If so, sustain the gains.

TABLE 4.3 DMAIC Tools

	SIX SIGMA ANALYSIS TOOLS	DESCRIPTION OF SIX SIGMA TOOL	COMMON QUALITY IMPROVEMENT TOOLS*
Define	Voice of the customer (VoC)	To gather customer feedback on needs/wants	Pareto diagram
Measure	Value stream map	Identify where in the process value is enabled/added or nonvalue added.	
Analyze	Failure Effects Mode Analysis (FMEA)	Proactive assessment of the process to identify where failure is occurring and consequences of the failures. Prioritize potential failures by severity/frequency. Eliminate failures, addressing highest priority first.	Root cause analysis Pareto diagram Histogram Brainstorming Cause and effect - Fishbone
Improve	Kaizen events	Rapid improvement event. Gathering of key stakeholders to review and improve process based on their knowledge of the work.	
Control	Statistical process control (SPC) e.g. control charts	Based on Shewhart's work – using a statistical process to determine if process variation is common cause or special cause variation.	

*Common QI tools are defined in the next section.

Additionally, Six Sigma analysis tools and common QI tools are used with each step of the DMAIC model. Extensive training is needed for effective use of the Six Sigma analysis tools described in Table 4.3. The common QI tools listed in the table are described later in the chapter (see Table 4.4).

The term Six Sigma is specific to manufacturing as it literally means to have less than 3.4 defects per 1 million opportunities. However, adaptations of Six Sigma have been used successfully to guide QI in the healthcare industry (Glasgow et al., 2010). APRNs have used the DMAIC model to successfully improve practice to decrease central line-associated bloodstream infection (CLABSI) rates below national benchmarks in a neurotrauma intensive care unit (Loftus et al., 2015).

TABLE 4.4 Common Quality Improvement Tools Categorized by Function

UNDERSTANDING THE CURRENT PROCESS	IDENTIFYING ROOT CAUSE	DATA DISPLAY/ANALYSIS
Process flowchart	Cause and effect/Fishbone	Histogram
Benchmarking	5 Whys	Pie chart
Focus group	Pareto chart	Pareto chart
	Focus groups	Run charts
		Control charts

Common QI models used by APRNs have been presented. It is interesting to note that Cleghorn and Headrick (1996) assert that the scientific method is (a) foundational to the education of health professionals and (b) that the QI process is an extension of or rework of the scientific method. This assertion supports why APRNs are well suited to engage in QI because both their foundational education (guided by the nursing process that is also based on the scientific method) and graduate education have prepared them as critical thinkers and problem solvers. Table 4.3 depicts how the steps of the nursing process closely align with the steps of each of the QI models. Moreover, the table shows that the models have more similarities than differences and have become more comprehensive across time.

Quality Improvement Tools

A graduate-level QSEN competency for QI is to "select and use quality improvement tools (e.g., run charts, control charts, root cause analysis, flow diagrams and GANTT charts) to achieve best possible outcomes" (American Association of Colleges of Nursing QSEN Education Consortium, 2012). Therefore, it is important that APRNs have a working knowledge of common QI tools. Common QI tools are used in tandem with the selected QI model to help achieve the desired result(s). As a rule, QI tools can be grouped by function: (a) understanding of the current process, (b) understanding of the root cause of the issue, and 3) data display/analysis (see Table 4.4).

Quality Improvement Tools for Understanding the Current Process

"If you do not ask the right questions, you do not get the right answers. A question asked in the right way often points to its own answer. Asking questions is the A-B-C of diagnosis. Only the inquiring mind solves problems."

—Edward Hodnett, poet (1841–1920)

One of the first steps in the QI process is to understand the current process, regardless of the QI model being followed. It is important to determine what is the baseline performance and what is working well before determining what can be improved. Commonly people rush to implement a solution before fully understanding the problem which leads to frustration and waste of resources. The process flowchart, benchmarking, and focus groups are three QI tools used to understand the current process.

Process Flowchart

The process flowchart or flow diagram is a graphic display of each step in a given process. Each step of the process is clarified and displayed from start to finish using a series of symbols connected by arrows to depict the chronological flow of the process. The rounded rectangle is used to depict the beginning and end of the process, rectangles denote steps in the process, and a diamond designates a decision (Heher & Chen, 2017). See Figure 4.2.

Once the flowchart has been designed, a thoughtful analysis of the process helps to identify specific steps in the process where improvement opportunities exist (waste, duplication, complexity, delay). This analysis is best done with a team of committed stakeholders who can provide insight into the nuances of the process.

Benchmarking

Benchmarking is a tool used to evaluate if a process is meeting "best practices." The current metrics of a process are compared against the internal and/or external organizational standards to

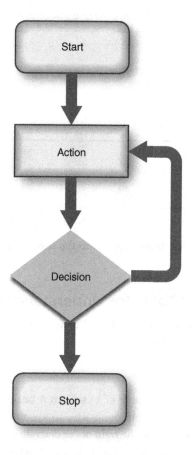

FIGURE 4.2 Example of a process flowchart.

provide baseline information on how well a process is currently performing (Wind & van Harten, 2017). Sources for benchmarking include internal metrics that may be collected by the quality department in a health system. Performance and quality measures from national practice organizations (e.g. American Heart Association, American Diabetes Association, American College of Cardiology or the National Database of Nursing Quality Indicators) are sources of external benchmarks to evaluate quality of care.

A bar graph is one way to display the data to get a snapshot of current practice in relation to the benchmark against one or more data points. In Figure 4.3 the benchmark is the national 80th percentile. In the first two time periods, the organization was below benchmark and above benchmark in the final three time periods.

Focus Group

A focus group is an effective strategy to gather baseline information from a group of stakeholders involved in a given process. This strategy can be used to identify stakeholder expectations as well as what they view as facilitators and barriers to the optimal performance of a process. Bringing small groups of stakeholders together face to face with a moderator allows for targeted and open conversation. Conducting a focus group takes careful planning and systematic delivery. Krueger and Casey (2015) support a step by step approach to conducting focus groups.

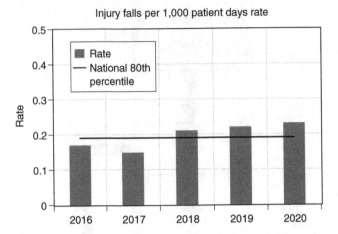

FIGURE 4.3 Benchmark with the use of a bar graph.

Quality Improvement Tools for Understanding the Root Cause

The cause-and-effect diagram (fishbone) and the 5 whys are two QI tools commonly used to help understand the root cause of a problem.

Cause-and-Effect Diagram

When attempting to establish the root cause of a problem A cause-and-effect diagram, also known as "Ishikawa" or "fishbone diagram, is commonly used to identify contributing factors impacting a problem. The problem (effect) is listed at the right of the diagram (the head) and the probably causes are placed on the diagonal lines (the bones). Typically, six categories are used to help sort the causes. As shown in Figure 4.4 these may include people (healthcare personnel), environment, process/methods, patient. These categories can be altered as needed to guide the process. The best results are attained from a group brainstorming session to elicit multiple probable causes (Tague, 2005). Next the diagram is analyzed to review the cause-and-effect relationships among the probable causes.

The 5 Whys

Asking the "5 whys" is a simple exercise to drill down to the ultimate root cause of a problem. To perform this exercise the learner repeatedly asks the question "why?" five times. The response to each "why" is one step closer to identifying the underlying cause of the problem. It is important that each "why" refocuses the user to keep digging deeper. The key to a successful "5 whys" outcome is that the analysis must not end too early before the ultimate cause of the problem is identified. The process may take only two or three "whys" or could take more than five "whys" depending on the complexity of the problem (Barsalou, 2017). The "5 whys" can also be used when performing a root cause analysis of a sentinel event or in combination with the fishbone as shown in Figure 4.4.

Quality Improvement Tools for Data Analysis/Display

"Data are not taken for museum purposes; they are taken as a basis for doing something. If nothing is to be done with the data, then there is no use in collecting any. The ultimate purpose of taking data is to provide a basis for action or a recommendation for action."

—*W. Edwards Deming, 1942*

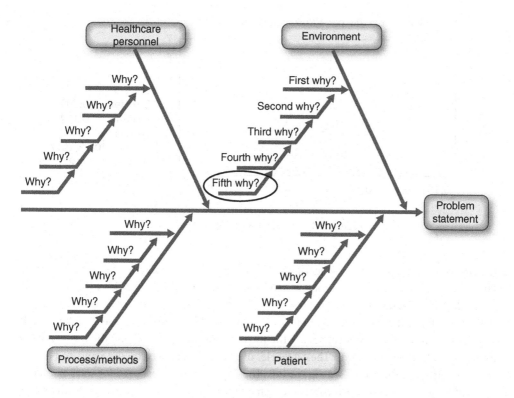

FIGURE 4.4 Fishbone diagram.

The histogram, bar chart, pie chart, and Pareto chart are common options to display frequency data (Dawson, 2019). First, consider whether the data are quantitative or categorical. The histogram is used for quantitative data whereas the bar, pie, and Pareto chart are used for categorical data. Displaying data by the frequency of occurrence provides a quick way to analyze visually the contributing factors to a problem.

Histogram

A histogram displays the frequency distribution of the values of a quantitative variable dataset (e.g., age, length of stay). This visual summary of the data can be used as an exploratory analysis tool to identify the range of the data, whether the data are normally distributed or skewed, and any outliers (Nuzzo, 2019). To construct a histogram, the horizontal or x axis displays the quantitative variable and the frequency or count is graphed on the left vertical or y axis and the percent on the right. Equally spaced adjacent columns are drawn to correspond with each of the quantitative variables and the height of each column aligns with the frequency. The highest column denotes the highest frequency. See Figure 4.5.

Pareto Chart

The Pareto chart is named for Vilfedo Pareto an Italian economist who in his study of income distribution identified the inequities of wealth distribution with a small percentage of the population holding the majority of the wealth (Pareto's law). Pareto's law is also known commonly as the 80/20 rule. Juran transferred this principle to quality improvement, noting that a small percent of factors contributed to the most causes of defects (Kelly et al., 2013). Focusing on the 20% of

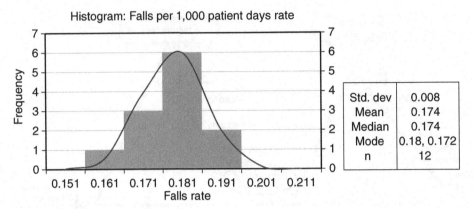

FIGURE 4.5 Example of a histogram.

causes that have the most direct impact on the effects or outcomes can improve process variation by 80%. Simply stated, 80% of the problem can be resolved by addressing 20% of the root causes (Kelly et al., 2013; Livesay et al., 2020).

After identifying the contributing causes of variation, the Pareto chart (vertical bar graph) is used to determine which root causes are the most significant by displaying the most frequent causes left to right across the x axis. The categories of causes are depicted on the *x* axis and the frequency is depicted by the *y* axis (see Figure 4.6). The Pareto chart is best used for categorical data and provides a quick look at which contributing factor is occurring most frequently by displaying the descending order of frequency.

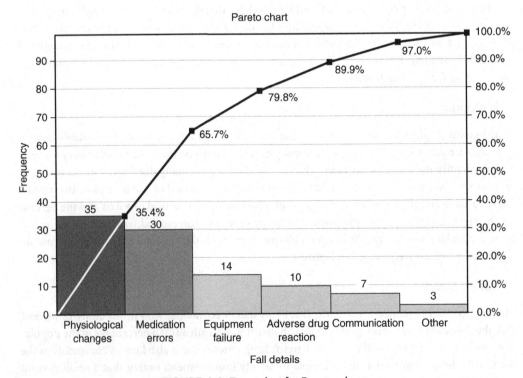

FIGURE 4.6 Example of a Pareto chart.

Bar Graph or Pie Chart

A bar graph or pie chart can be used for categorical data such as gender or race (Nuzzo, 2016). The bar graph is displayed like the histogram, however there are gaps between the bars as each bar is self-contained whereas the histogram adds to 100%. Relative frequency is displayed using a pie chart where each category is displayed as the percentage of the total (100%) and the highest percentage is shown as the "biggest piece of the pie."

Patterns/Trends in a Process

Monitoring the QI process to observe patterns or trends in data across time is an important step to determine whether an improvement has occurred. Generally, 15 or more data points are needed to strengthen the data interpretation (Lloyd, 2019). Two tools to display the data include a run chart and a control chart. The control chart, also known as the Shewhart chart or statistical process control chart (SPC), was developed by Shewhart during his work at Bell Laboratories in the 1920s (Connelly, 2018).

Run Chart

The run chart or timed-series chart displays data across time using the x axis as the time scale and the y axis as the frequency measure in number, percent, or rate (e.g., the fall rate per month). The distinctive feature of a run chart is a line drawn at the median where half of the data points fall above, and half the data points fall below. The run chart provides a visual and analytical display of the process performance and can be used to detect process variation after the implementation of a planned change (Perla et al., 2011). It allows for a quick display of the progress of a planned change to determine if the planned intervention is having the intended effect and whether that effect is sustained (Provost & Murray, 2011).

To interpret the data on a run chart, there are two basic rules that can be used "to identify non-random signals on a run chart" (Lloyd, 2019, p. 192). The first step is to review how the data points cluster either above or below the median. A *shift* occurs when there are six or more consecutive data points clustered either above or below the median. Data points directly on the median are not counted. A *trend* is considered when there are five or more consecutive points that are moving in the same direction – either all up or all down (Lloyd, 2019; Perla et al., 2011).

Control Chart (Also Known as the Shewhart Chart or Statistical Process Control Chart)

Like a run chart, a control chart provides a visual display of process variation and is one tool to monitor and evaluate the effect of the planned change/QI across time. However, the control chart provides a more detailed approach to determine whether the process variations is normal fluctuation, in control (within the control limits), or is out of control (special cause variation; Fretheim & Tomic, 2015). Ideally, adequate baseline data are also plotted so one can review the process variation pre-implementation of the planned change (Shaughnessy et al., 2018).

For a control chart the x and y axes are constructed similarly to the run chart, however a minimum of 20 data points is suggested for the control chart (Lloyd, 2019). Between the two charts, the key differences are that the mean is used for the central line, and upper control limits (UCL) and lower control limits (LCL) are calculated and inserted on the graph as an upper and lower line. Often the UCL and the LCL are described as three standard deviations from the mean, however the IHI and others stress that this is inaccurate and technically the upper and lower limits should reflect

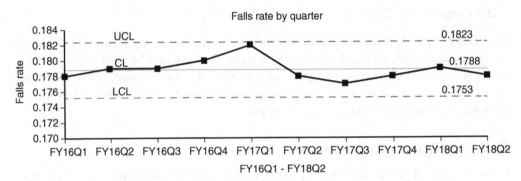

FIGURE 4.7 A control chart with common-cause variation.
CL, central line; LCL, lower control limit; UCL; upper control limit.

+/− 3 sigma limits from the mean (Lloyd, 2019). The limits can be determined readily using a software program such as Microsoft Excel. Remember to mark on the chart when the planned change or other contributing events occurred as this information strengthens the data interpretation.

Within the Control Limit

When reviewing the control chart, two types of process variation are considered, common-cause and special-cause variation. A common-cause variation (Figure 4.7) points to expected process variation. In this case, the process variation is attributed to expected fluctuations and the process is considered to be "in control" (Brady et al., 2018; Fretheim & Tomic, 2015). However, a special-cause variation (Figure 4.8) suggests that a change in the process has occurred due to a specific cause, most likely the planned intervention has affected a true change in the process.

The IHI outlines five control chart analysis rules that can be used to evaluate the data and detect special causes, three of which are outlined here (Lloyd, 2019). Rule 1 is one data point that is outside either the UCL or LCL and is named a 3-sigma violation. Given that this is an outlier, the first step to take is to verify the origin of the data point. Rule 2 refers to a shift, visualized by eight consecutive points either above or below the mean. This differs from the

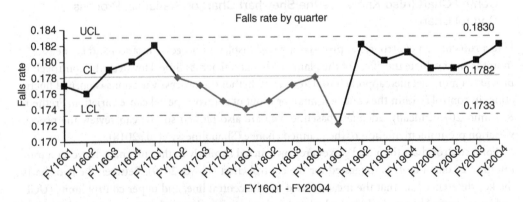

FIGURE 4.8 Special-cause variation, Rule 2 – a shift, eight consecutive points below the mean, one data point outside the lower control limits.

CL, central line; LCL, lower control limit; UCL; upper control limit.

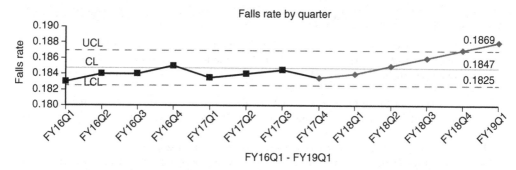

FIGURE 4.9 Special-cause variation, Rule 3 – a trend, six data points moving consecutively upward, one data point outside the upper control limits.
CL, central line; LCL, lower control limit; UCL; upper control limit.

shift on a run chart where only six consecutive points are needed. A shift—provided it is in the desired direction—is an indication that the proposed change is having the desired effect across time (see Figure 4.8). Rule 3 is commonly known as a trend and consists of minimally six data points that are moving consecutively either upward or downward. Similar to a shift, the trend is a favorable outcome and can indicate that true change is occurring within the process (see Figure 4.9) (Lloyd, 2019).

It is important to remember that all change visually depicted on a control chart is not special-cause variation; therefore, not every change in a process should be responded to or celebrated. Often in healthcare, leaders are quick to react to a downward or upward turn of one or two data points without having sufficient data to make an effective interpretation. The importance of the role of advance practice nurse leaders who can accurately interpret the data and contribute to these conversations can't be emphasized enough.

▨ SUMMARY

The APRN is in a pivotal role to direct QI in the practice setting. APRNs are equipped with the QI knowledge and skills to support quality care and patient safety in health systems. The common QI model/processes and tool used by APRNs to develop and lead QI project plans are reviewed in this chapter.

SUGGESTED LEARNING ACTIVITY

1. Complete the low-tech simulation exercise "Mr. Potato Head: A LEAN, Mean Quality Improvement Teaching Machine!" found on the QSEN website at https://qsen.org/ This exercise addresses each of the QSEN graduate RN competencies and ideally is completed in teams of seven to eight members.

2. The IHI website houses many valuable resources to assist with learning the QI process. Two specific resources to be aware of are the *IHI's QI Essentials Toolkit,* which provides templates for each of the common QI tools listed in Table 4.4, and *The Science of Improvement on a Whiteboard!* that features a collection of 20 short videos covering topics from Deming to control charts. Available on-line at www.ihi.org/

REFERENCES

American Association of Colleges of Nursing QSEN Education Consortium. (2012). *Graduate-Level QSEN Competencies: Knowledge, Skills, and Attitudes.* American Association of Colleges of Nursing. https://www.aacnnursing.org/Portals/42/AcademicNursing/CurriculumGuidelines/Graduate-QSEN -Competencies.pdf

American Association of Nurse Practitioners. (n.d.). *Standards of practice for nurse practitioners.* https:// www.aanp.org/advocacy/advocacy-resource/position-statements/standards-of-practice-for-nurse -practitioners

Barsalou, M. (2017). Square in the crosshairs. *Quality Progress, 50*(1), 24–28.

Batalden, P., & Stoltz, P. (1993). A framework for the continual improvement of health care: Build and apply- ing professional and improvement knowledge to test changes in daily work. *The Joint Commission Journal of Quality Improvement, 19,* 424–447. https://doi.org/10.1016/S1070-3241(16)30025-6

Berwick, D. M. (1989). Continuous improvement as an ideal in health care. *The New England Journal of Medicine, 320*(1), 53–56. https://doi.org/10.1056/NEJM198901053200110

Berwick, D. M., Godfrey, A. B., & Roessner, J. (1990). *Curing health care: New strategies for suality improve- ment.* Jossey-Bass.

Berwick, D. M., Nolan, T. W., & Whittington, J. (2008). The triple aim: Care, health, and cost. *Health Affairs (Project Hope), 27*(3), 759–769. https://doi.org/10.1377/hlthaff.27.3.759

Bodenheimer, T., & Sinsky, C. (2014). From triple to quadruple aim: Care of the patient requires care of the provider. *Annals of Family Medicine, 12*(6), 573–576. https://doi.org/10.1370/afm.1713

Brady, P. W., Tchou, M. J., Ambroggio, L., Schondelmeyer, A. C., & Shaughnessy, E. E. (2018). Quality improvement feature series article 2: Displaying and analyzing quality improvement data. *Journal of Pediatric Infectious Disease Society, 7*(2), 100–103. https://doi.org/10.1093/jpids/pix077

Burda, D. (1988). Providers look to industry for quality models. *Modern Healthcare, 18*(29), 24–26, 28, 30–32.

Cangany, M., Peters, L., Gregg, K., Welsh, T., & Jimison, B. (2018). Preventing falls: Is no toileting alone the answer? *MEDSURG Nursing, 27*(6), 379–382.

Centers for Medicare & Medicaid Services. (n.d.). *Quality Measure and Quality Improvement.* https:// www.cms.gov/Medicare/Quality-Initiatives-Patient-Assessment-Instruments/MMS/Quality-Measure -and-Quality-Improvement-

Chandrasekaran, A., & Toussaint, J. S. (2019, May 24). Creating a culture of continuous improvement. *Harvard Business Review.* https://hbr.org/2019/05/creating-a-culture-of-continuous-improvement? referral=03758&cm_vc=rr_item_page.top_right

Cleghorn, G. D., & Headrick, L. A. (1996). The PDSA cycle at the core of learning in health professions education. *Joint Commission Journal on Quality Improvement, 22*(3), 206–212. https://doi.org/10.1016/ s1070-3241(16)30223-1

Colton, D. (2000). Quality improvement in health care. *Evaluation & the Health Professions, 23*(1), 7–42. https://doi.org/10.1177/01632780022034462

Compton, J. J., & Carrico, C. (2018). *Development and implementation of an after-visit summary for COPD patients: A pilot QI project.* Unpublished manuscript, College of Nursing, Creighton University, Omaha, Nebraska, US.

Connelly, L. (2018). Statistical process control. *Medsurg Nursing, 27*(5), 331–332.

Cronenwett, L., Sherwood, G., Barnsteiner, J., Disch, J., Johnson, J., Mitchell, P., Sullivan, D. T., & Warren, J. (2007). Quality and safety education for nurses. *Nursing Outlook, 55*(3), 122–131. https://doi .org/10.1016/j.outlook.2007.02.006

Curtin, L. (2019). What you need to know about MIPS. *American Nurse Today, 14*(3), 48.

Dawson, A. (2019). A practical guide to performance improvement: Data collection and analysis. *AORN Journal. 109*(5), 621–631. https://doi.org/10.1002/aorn.12673

Donabedian, A. (1988). The quality of care. How can it be assessed? *Journal of the American Medical Association, 260*(12), 1743–1748. https://doi.org/10.1001/jama.1988.03410120089033

Donabedian, A. (2005). Evaluating the quality of medical care. *The Milbank Quarterly, 83*(4), 691–729. https://doi.org/10.1111/j.1468-0009.2005.00397.x

Florea, K. S., Novosel, L. M., & Schlenk, E. A. (2016). Improvement in colon cancer screening through use of a multilevel intervention: A QI initiative. *Journal of the American Association of Nurse Practitioners 28,* 362–369. https://doi.org/10.1002/2327-6924.12320

Fraire, M. L., & Whitehead, D. K. (2019). Reducing delirium in hospitalized older adults with a nursing prevention protocol. *MEDSURG Nursing, 28*(2), 114–118.

Fretheim, A., & Tomic, O. (2015). Statistical process control and interrupted time series: A golden opportunity for impact evaluation in quality improvement. *BMJ Quality & Safety, 24*, 748–752. https://doi.org/10.1136/bmjqs-2014-003756

Glasgow, J. M., Scott-Caziewell, J. R., & Kaboli, P. J. (2010). Guiding inpatient quality improvement: A systematic review of Lean and Six Sigma. *The Joint Commission Journal on Quality and Patient Safety, 36*(12), 533–540. https://doi.org/10.1016/s1553-7250(10)36081-8

Greiner, A. C., & Knebel, E. (2003). *Health professions education: A bridge to quality.* National Academies Press.

Grillo, D. M., Firth, K. H., & Hatchel, K. (2019). Implementation of purposeful hourly rounds in addition to a fall bundle to prevent inpatient falls on a medical-surgical acute hospital unit. *MEDSURG Nursing, 28*(4), 243–246, 261.

Heher, Y. K. & Chen. Y. (2017). Process mapping: A cornerstone of quality improvement. *Cancer Cytopathology, 125*(12), 887–890. https://doi.org/10.1002/cncy.21946

House, M., Stephens, K. P., Whiteman, K., Swanson-Biearman, B., & Printz, M. (2016). Cardiac medicine 30-day readmission reduction strategies: Do improved discharge transitions decrease readmissions? *MEDSURG Nursing, 25*(4), 251–254.

Institute for Healthcare Improvement. (n.d.). *The IHI timeline: More than 25 years of driving improvement.* http://www.ihi.org/about/Documents/IHI_Timeline_2019.pdf

Johnson, C., Miltner, R., & Wilson, M. (2018). Increasing nurse-driven heparin infusion administration safety: A quality improvement initiative. *MEDSURG Nursing, 27*(4), 243–246.

Kapu, A. N., & Kleinpell, R. (2013). Developing nurse practitioner associated metrics for outcomes assessment. *Journal of the American Association of Nurse Practitioners, 25*(6), 289–296. https://doi.org/10.1111/1745-7599.12001

Kazana, I., & Murphy, M. P. (2018). Implementing a patient-centered walking program for residents in long-term care: A quality improvement project. *Journal of the American Association of Nurse Practitioners, 30*(7), 383–391. https://doi.org/10.1097/JXX.0000000000000037

Kelly, D. L., Johnson, S. P., & Sollecito, W. A. (2013). Measurement, variation, and CQI tools. In W. A. Sollecito & J. K. Johnson (Eds.), *McLaughlin and Kaluzny's continuous quality improvement in health care* (4th ed., pp. 77–114). Jones & Bartlett.

Kennedy, C. M., & Jolles, D. R. (2019, November). Providing effective asthma care at a pediatric patient-centered medical home. *Journal of the American Association of Nurse Practitioners.* Advance online publication. https://doi.org/10.1097/JXX.0000000000000334

Kohari, A. N. (2018). Improving fall risk assessment and documentation: A QI project. *University of Kentucky DNP Projects.* 195. https://uknowledge.uky.edu/dnp_etds/195

Krueger, R. A., & Casey, M. A. (2015). *Focus Groups: A Practical Guide for Applied Research* (5th ed.). SAGE.

Langley, G. J., Moen, R. D., Nolan, K.M., Nolan, T. W., Norman, C. L., & Provost, L. P. (2009). *The improvement guide: A practical approach to enhancing organizational performance* (2nd ed.). Jossey-Bass.

Livesay, S., Zonsius, M., & McNett, M. (2020). Evaluating data to guide care delivery: Quality improvement methods and implementation science. In M. McNett (Ed.), *Data for nurses* (pp. 59–84). Elsevier.

Lloyd, R. C. (2019). *Quality health care: A guide to developing and using ndicators* (2nd ed.). Jones & Bartlett.

Loftus, K., Tilley, T., Hoffman, J., Bradburn, E., & Harvey, E. (2015). Use of six sigma strategies to pull the line on central line-associated bloodstream infections in a neurotrauma intensive care unit. *Journal of Trauma Nursing, 22*(2), 78–86. https://doi.org/10.1097/JTN.0000000000000111

Lopez, M., Blackburn, L., & Springer, C. (2018). Minimizing sleep disturbances to improve patient outcomes. *MEDSURG Nursing, 27*(6), 368–371.

Marjoua, Y., & Bozic, K. J. (2012). Brief history of quality movement in US healthcare. *Current Reviews in Musculoskeletal Medicine, 5*(4), 265–273. https://doi.org/10.1007/s12178-012-9137-8

Moen, R., & Norman, C. (2010). Circling back. Clearing up the myths regarding the Deming cycle and seeing how it keeps evolving. *Quality Progress, 43*(11), 22–28.

Nuzzo, R. L. (2016). Statistically speaking. The box plots alternative for visualizing quantitative data. *Physical Medicine and Rehabilitation Journal, 8*(3), 268–272. https://doi.org/10.1016/j.pmrj.2016.02.001

Nuzzo, R. (2019). Histograms: A useful data analysis visualization. *American Academy of Physical Medicine and Rehabilitation, 11*(3), 309–312. https://doi.org/10.1002/pmrj.12145

Perla, R. J., Provost, L. P., & Murray, S. K. (2011). The run chart: A simple analytical tool for learning from variation in healthcare processes. *BMJ Quality & Safety, 20*, 46–51. https://doi.org/10.1136/bmjqs.2009.037895

Provost, L. P., & Murray, S. (2011). *The Health Care Data Guide: Learning from Data for Improvement.* Jossey-Bass.

Re, R. N., & Krousel-Wood, M. A. (1990). How to use continuous quality improvement theory and statistical control tools in a multispecialty clinic. *Quality Review Bulletin, 16*(11), 391–397. https://doi.org/10.1016/s0097-5990(16)30398-0

Roy, R. E. (2018). *VCU Health Nursing inquiry process diagram (version 2).* https://scholarscompass.vcu.edu/libraries_pubs/52

Ruggiri, J. C., Milner, K. A., & Buonocore, D. (2019). Implementing post-discharge 48- hour scripted call for patients with heart failure: An evidence-based practice quality improvement project. *MEDSURG Nursing, 28*(3), 183–187.

Scoville, R., & Little, K. (2014). Comparing Lean and Quality Improvement. *IHI White Paper.*

Shaughnessy, E. E., Shah, A., Ambrogio, L., & Statile, A. (2018). Quality improvement feature series article1: Introduction to quality improvement. *Journal of Pediatric Infectious Disease Society, 7*(1), 6–10. https://doi.org/10.1093/jpids/pix061

Silver, S. A., Harel, Z., McQuillan, R., Weizman, A. V., Thomas, A. Chertow, G. M., Nesrallah, G., & Chan, C. T. (2016). How to begin a quality improvement project. *Clinical Journal of the American Society of Nephrology, 11*, 893–900. https://doi.org/10.2215/CJN.11491015

Spear, V. (2018). DNP student quality improvement proposal: Implementing suicide protocol in outpatient mental health clinic. *Scholar Archive, 4043.* https://digitalcommons.ohsu.edu/etd/4043

Tague, N. R. (2005). *The quality toolbox* (2nd ed.). ASQ Quality Press.

Takao, M. R. V., Woldt, J., & Bento da Silva, I. (2017). Six Sigma methodology advantages for small- and medium-sized enterprises: A case study in the plumbing industry in the United States. *Advances in Mechanical Engineering, 9*(10), 1–10. https://doi.org/10.1177/1687814017733248

Taylor, M. J., McNicholas C., Nicolay C., Darzi A., Bell, D., & Reed J. E. (2014). Systematic review of the application of the Plan-Do-Study-Act method to improve quality in healthcare. *BMJ Quality & Safety, 23*(4), 290–298. https://doi.org/10.1136/bmjqs-2013-001862

U.S. Department of Health and Human Services, & Health Resources and Services Adminstration. (2011). *Quality Improvement.* https://www.hrsa.gov/sites/default/files/quality/toolbox/508pdfs/qualityimprovement.pdf

Vejar, M. V., Makic, M. B. F., & Kotthoff-Burnell, E. (2015). Medication management for elderly patients in an academic primary care setting: A quality improvement project. *Journal of the American Association of Nurse Practitioners, 27*(2), 72–78. https://doi.org/10.1002/2327-6924.12121

Watts, S. A., & Nemes, D. (2018). Best practice nursing management of nosocomial hypoglycemia: Lessons learned. *MEDSURG Nursing, 27*(2), 98–102.

Wind, A., & van Harten, W. H. (2017). Benchmarking specialty hospitals, a scoping review on theory and practice. *BMC Health Services Research, 17*(1), 245. https://doi.org/10.1186/s12913-017-2154-y

ESTABLISHING AND SUSTAINING AN EVIDENCE-BASED PRACTICE ENVIRONMENT

ELIZABETH A. CARLSON, BETH A. STAFFILENO, AND
MARCIA PENCAK MURPHY

▪ INTRODUCTION

There are numerous reasons to establish an evidence-based practice (EBP) program for nursing staff at various practice sites. First, patients have complex needs, coupled with shortened in-patient lengths of stay and increases in new therapies used not only in acute settings but also in the community. Nurses must deliver care that is based on evidence of its effectiveness, safety, and currency. An EBP program is a proven way to move nursing care toward these desired outcomes (Black et al., 2015; Dols et al., 2019; Melnyk et al., 2016; Royer et al., 2018; Songur et al., 2018). In addition, use of EBP methods empowers nurses to address, in a systematic manner, questions and problems they encounter. Not only does it improve patient care, it also allows for dissemination both internally and to the broader nursing community (Brockopp et al., 2016).

Second, many organizations understand the positive influence that results from seeking accreditation. Ensuring that the processes and structure are in place to move toward positive outcomes allows an organization to establish, confirm, and codify goals and behaviors that result in exemplary practice. One such designation is the Magnet Recognition Program® awarded by the American Nurses Credentialing Center (ANCC). Magnet-recognized organizations have "strong leadership, empowered professionals and exemplary practice" as their "essential building blocks." EBP not only contributes to exemplary practice but also empowers nurses to provide strong leadership (ANCC, n.d.). The use of EBP and the supports and structures needed to improve practice and contribute to the profession results in an organization that values these contributions and those who make them.

Third, the American Nurses Association (ANA) Scope and Standards of Practice describes the who, what, where, why, and how of nursing practice activities (ANA, 2015). ANA Standard 13: Evidence-Based Practice and Research states, "The registered nurse integrates evidence and research findings into practice" (2015, p. 6). This standard serves both as a benchmark and as a clear delineation that EBP is a core competency for professional nurses. This is supported by the Quality and Safety Education for Nurses (QSEN). QSEN indicates that EBP is one of the six areas of knowledge, skills, and attitudes (KSA) necessary for pre-licensure students' education. These KSA are necessary for the nurse to use to continually improve the quality and safety of the healthcare systems in which they work. QSEN clearly defines EBP as the "integrat(ion) of best current evidence with clinical expertise and patient/family preferences and values for delivery of optimal healthcare" (Cronenwett et al., 2007).

Fourth, in 2001, the Institute of Medicine (IOM) report, *Crossing the Quality Chasm: A New Health System for the 21st Century,* presented the need to improve the healthcare delivery system by providing safe, effective, patient-centered, timely, efficient, and equitable care. One of the components of this needed redesign of healthcare was the use of "evidence-based decision-making" (p. 8). Coupled with the 2001 report is the IOM's report of 2011, *The Future of Nursing,* which stated that nursing is the key to improving healthcare. Three of the four key messages in the IOM report pertain to EBP. First, that nurses should practice to the full extent of their education and training, which includes the knowledge and skills needed to practice evidence-based care. Second, that nurses should attain higher levels of education and training, which addresses not only the world of academe but also the need for organizations to continually educate their staff. Third, that nurses should be full partners in redesigning healthcare, which again supports the need for nurses to be fluent in evidence-based approaches to problems.

As a result of these influencing factors, changes have occurred in both nursing education and nursing clinical practice. In academia, two key changes in educational preparation at the entry into practice level are evolving. At the baccalaureate level, the expectation of preparation for EBP is apparent as indicated by the American Association of Colleges of Nursing (AACN) Essential III: Scholarship for Evidence-Based Practice. "Baccalaureate education provides a basic understanding of how evidence is developed, including the research process, clinical judgment, inter-professional perspectives, and patient preference as applied to practice" (AACN, 2008). Thus, nursing programs have incorporated EBP into their curriculum as they focus on educating the student to use national standards based on evidence (Dols et al., 2019).

In addition, clinical nurse leader (CNL) has at its core the knowledge and ability to oversee the care coordination for a group of patients and provide direct patient care. As stated by the AACN, "this master's degree-prepared clinician puts evidence-based practice into action to ensure that patients benefit from the latest innovations in care delivery" (AACN, 2012). As more nursing programs offer this curriculum, organizations will have CNLs as staff members.

These key changes in the education of new graduates just entering practice affect where they look for their first job as a nurse. Literature supports the importance and benefits of new nurses working in an EBP environment that fosters skills for professional development (Dols et al., 2019). This results in new graduates having the expectation that the organizations at which they seek employment will incorporate an EBP approach to the delivery of care and would support their practice and leadership through an EBP approach. As a consequence of this organizational expectation, new graduates will expect the staff with whom they work to be conversant with and use EBP in their patient-care approaches. With the emphasis on EBP for recent graduates and their expectations of the EBP approach being used in organizations, it is critical that all members of the nursing staff who have not had the opportunity to learn the EBP approach during their educational programs obtain the necessary knowledge and skills. This is further supported by the increase in the number of DNP graduates who use EBP. As DNP students, they used evidence in the development of their doctoral project and scholarly work. They have similar expectations of the workplace as being a place where EBP is integrated into practice.

As the emphasis on teamwork and interprofessional approaches to care increases, it is important that a common approach to patient-care delivery is used. It is therefore incumbent upon the nurse leader to set the EBP vision for the organization.

■ INFRASTRUCTURE

Setting the Vision

EBP will not be successful unless it is clear that this is a priority of the organization and, most critically, the chief nursing officer (CNO) or equivalent nursing organizational leader (Brockopp et al., 2020a; Johantgen et al., 2017; Melnyk et al., 2016; Scala et al., 2016). The CNO must be the EBP champion for the organization. As with any program that is implemented, for EBP to be successful it must be part of the nursing vision for the organization. A strong and ongoing EBP program takes time to establish and integrate into the culture of how nursing functions. Without strong and visible support from the leadership, use of EBP and incorporation of the principles into the thought process of the nursing staff will not occur. The concept of continual inquiry and seeking to provide care that has been shown to result in improved patient outcomes must be interwoven into the structure and language of the organization for EBP to be successful. In addition, as indicated, the ANA (2015) describes that EBP is a core competency for professional nurses. Therefore, the use of EBP is not optional. The CNO must actively lead the organization to using an evidence-based approach to patient care.

An EBP program requires additional support from executive leadership throughout the organization. Merely including EBP as a goal is not sufficient for success. EBP needs to be a high priority in the nursing strategic plan and embedded into the organization's strategic plan. Farahnak et al. (2019) studied the role leadership plays in the implementation of innovation, specifically EBP. The role of transformational leadership and leader attitudes was influential on staff attitudes and on the success of implementation of new practices. Farahnak et al. (2019) suggest that leadership behaviors may be more critical to innovation implementation than the leader's attitude, thus supporting the key role the CNO plays in the implementation of EBP.

Before presenting the need for and benefits of EBP for inclusion in the organizational strategic plan, the CNO must get others on board with the vision. The creation of support requires a multipronged approach, and work at both the organizational executive level and the care deliverer's level is necessary. Not only does the organizational executive leadership's support need to be cultivated but nursing leadership and influential staff nurses need to be on board as well. Information and literature demonstrating the benefits of EBP must be discussed and provided to these key individuals. Multiple and disparate methods of communicating the benefits of EBP are required such as newsletters, town hall meetings, discussions with nursing staff, informational boards either electronic or paper, as well as cultivating the support and encouragement of any grassroots interest.

Having organizational executive support alone will not guarantee success, nor will strong nursing support alone result in success. Without the support of those who determine the strategic goals and what programs are funded, those who must enable the staff members to participate, and support from the caregivers who will be the ones implementing EBP, success is not ensured. All three legs to the stool need to be in place: (a) The CNO needs to establish the expectation, (b) the organizational executive leadership needs to support the use of resources for EBP, and (c) the staff need to see this as integral to how they practice nursing and not as a discrete action divorced from their professional practice. The CNO needs to present a logical and comprehensive assessment of the risk-to-benefit ratio resulting from care based on evidence. The benefits to the organization and thus to the key decision-makers must be presented and discussed. Concerns voiced during these discussions need to be considered and addressed. Organizational concerns may include the cost of the program, including needed personnel, support services, time away from patient care while learning, and any potential risks. Nursing leadership concerns may parallel these concerns and include issues of costs to the unit budgets, coverage for caregivers when in educational sessions, impact on staffing, seasoned staff responses, and the addition of "one more thing" to the nurses' workload. Influential nursing staff may voice concerns about obsolescence of their skills; impact on workload; expectations of accomplishment without support to be successful; and the impact on the evaluation, reward, and compensation systems. The CNO needs to be prepared to listen and address these concerns and offer mitigating solutions.

Subsequent to creating support for EBP and the costs and requirements involved, the CNO needs to have EBP included as an organizational goal within the strategic plan. Funds are allocated based on organizational priorities, and unless EBP is an organizational priority, funding may fall on nursing alone to provide or be nonexistent. Because EBP will improve not only nursing care but also patient outcomes, organizational support is the ideal. An EBP culture provides an opportunity for interdisciplinary dialogue and information exchange, thus leading to collaborative patient care. Organizational benefits include higher quality patient care, which contributes to greater patient and family satisfaction as well as decreased lengths of hospital stay (Wu et al., 2018). Many CNOs recognize the need for an EBP facilitator, but face resistance in acquiring the financial resources needed to support such services. Given the quality and financial benefits to the entire organization, the organization needs to support an EBP program and position. It is not appropriate for a program that benefits the organization to be the financial responsibility of nursing alone.

Loss of payments for hospital-acquired conditions (HACs) and proposed incentive pay for better outcomes should be the driving force to incorporate the EBP facilitator's role in healthcare settings as part of operational costs. The entire organization benefits by using EBP, for example by reducing the cost and rates of pneumonia, lengths of stay, and pain (Wu et al., 2018). Gilton et al. (2019) used evidence-based practice to change practice from routinely changing peripheral intravenous catheter sites to changing only when clinically indicated, all of which benefit the entire organization; thus, a case can be made that the cost of implementing and maintaining EBP is an organizational one.

Necessary Resources

Establishing and implementing an EBP environment requires essential resources, such as personnel, time, money, and space (Melnyk et al., 2018; McKinney et al., 2019). However, during times of cost containment, allocating these resources can be challenging and thereby may require creative and intentional planning (Christenbery, 2018a). The benefits of EBP include: nursing care driven by evidence improves patient care and clinical outcomes, nursing satisfaction increases as nurses become more empowered and engage in clinical inquiry to drive excellence and quality care, and the organization experiences improvement in reimbursement as patients experience fewer complications resulting in reduced resource utilization (Wu et al., 2018). Despite the well-documented benefits of EBP, nurses continue to experience difficulty incorporating EBP into daily practice because of insufficient time, lack of administrative support and mentoring, resistance to changing practice, and lack of education on the EBP process (McKinney et al., 2019; Melnyk et al., 2018).

Raising Awareness

Raising awareness and developing excitement about EBP often require a change in culture to move from tradition-based care to evidence-based care that is embraced by nurses at all levels of preparation. Several strategies can be implemented for building a foundation and stimulating enthusiasm for incorporating the EBP process. For instance, facilitating staff participation in EBP-related activities can be introduced through interactive sessions such as doing a version of the Great Cookie Experiment or conducting a mock trial. The original Great Cookie Experiment introduced concepts of the research process to nursing students by comparing two chocolate-chip cookies (Thiel, 1987). Student nurses gained insight into methodology, data collection, data analysis, and dissemination of research findings. Modifications of the Great Cookie Experiment have been done using other comparisons (such as hand sanitizers, lotions, breakfast bars, music, etc.) and with incorporating newer technology (Chanda, 2019; Lane et al., 2016). Nurses can become engaged in the experiment with "real-time" sequencing of events using online survey software (i.e., Survey Monkey) and data management tools (i.e., Excel), or by using audience response systems that allow for greater interaction, immediate feedback, and anonymous participation (Landrum, 2015; Thapar-Olmos & Seeman, 2018). Gaming systems, such as Kahoot (Kahoot, 2016) and Nearpod (Nearpod, n.d.) have recently emerged as alternative mobile approaches for engaging nurses in EBP educational opportunities (Calinici, 2017; Lane et al., 2016; Shatto & Erwin, 2016). Another interactive approach used to raise awareness about EBP is a mock trial. Mock trials have been used by other disciplines as an educational platform and more recently in nursing as a venue to highlight concepts of how to incorporate EBP into clinical practice (Harding et al., 2014; Mueller et al., 2017; White, 2015). For example, a mock trial can engage nurses to use available evidence when making clinical practice decisions. A topic that is relevant to all nurses, such as moral distress or safe patient handling, can be selected as a "case" to argue. To develop the pros and cons of the case, nurses gain experience reviewing literature, critiquing the evidence, and presenting an argument for or against the issue at hand. Thereby, nurses gain critical thinking skills using a problem-solving, systematic method for addressing clinical practice issues.

Education

Building an EBP infrastructure begins with staff education, which requires adequate personnel. Education promotes awareness and enables nurses to become professionally literate and develop necessary skills to critically appraise evidence before implementing findings into their practice. An advanced practice registered nurse, whether doctorally prepared or not, can serve as an EBP facilitator, whether employed by the organization or brought in as a consultant, and often has a dual appointment within a clinical and academic setting (Albert et al., 2019; Dols et al., 2019; Herron & Strunk, 2019; Lavenberg et al., 2019; Maneval et al., 2019; Monturo & Brockway, 2019; Saunders et al., 2019). The EBP facilitator enables others to initiate, conduct, and integrate EBP projects into clinical practice. The EBP facilitator serves as an educator, mentor, and change agent within the organization by (a) assessing the needs of nursing related to EBP; (b) raising awareness and developing excitement about EBP; (c) presenting EBP-related information and education in a way that is understandable and meaningful to direct-care nurses which may involve delivering content in "chunks" using micro-learning, just-in-time, or on-demand strategies; (d) building confidence and empowering nurses to engage in EBP-related activities; (e) assisting nurses with interpreting unit-specific data trends and facilitating EBP initiatives; (f) networking within the community and facilitating interdisciplinary collaboration; (g) facilitating the development of EBP proposals and project implementation; and (h) facilitating policy changes with intended plans for dissemination. Table 5.1 outlines an action plan that an EBP facilitator may use when establishing a foundation for an EBP environment.

TABLE 5.1 Evidence-Based Practice Action Plan

ACTIVITY	STRATEGY
1. EBP needs assessment	• Assess organizational readiness • Conduct a survey to assess staff knowledge and current state of EBP within the organization* • Conduct focus groups
2. Raising EBP awareness	• Gather an EBP team/committee and develop a campaign to market EBP culture • Create a logo to be displayed throughout the hospital and used as a screen saver on computer terminals • EBP team/committee review EBP models • Display posters/flyers/billboard
3. Information and education	• Executive meetings • Unit meetings • Brown-bag sessions • "How to" sessions (literature search, evaluating the evidence, critiquing research) • Emails/newsletters/announcements • Journal clubs (ejournal clubs) • Roving carts moving from unit to unit • Micro-learning environment to provide information in manageable bites (chunking) • Offer continuing education credit as educational programs
4. Building confidence	• Set goals that are realistic and attainable • Create EBP decisional algorithm showing the step-by-step process • Train the trainer and identify champions • Highlight accomplishments
5. Evaluating unit-specific data	• Review key metrics with unit managers and staff • Identify monthly and quarterly triggers
6. Networking	• Develop relations with local colleges and/or universities • Develop relations with the health department, senior citizen groups, etc.
7. Implementing EBP	• Develop a template and EBP protocol • Start with one EBP project to showcase the process and then build on it • Facilitate EBP practice change and evaluate
8. Disseminating	• Assist with presenting EBP projects internally (establish an annual EBP day) and externally (local, regional, and national meetings) • Assist with presenting educational programs

EBP, evidence-based practice.

*Examples of EBP assessment scales that can be used include: *BARRIERS: The Barriers to Research Utilization Scale* (Funk et al., 1991); *Evidence-Based Practice Beliefs Scale* (Melnyk & Fineout-Overholt, 2003a); and *Evidence-Based Practice Implementation Scale* (Melnyk & Fineout-Overholt, 2003b).

Depending on the needs of the organization, the EBP facilitator may assist with developing a formal EBP program that can be presented in one of two ways: (a) an EBP-condensed curriculum or (b) an EBP fellowship training (Brockopp et al., 2020b; Christenbery, 2018b; Hatfield et al., 2016; Lizarondo & McArthur, 2017). The EBP-condensed curriculum provides EBP education using a systematic approach and well-defined objectives (Table 5.2). The condensed curriculum can be offered using face-to-face classrooms, online modules, or podcast instruction. The curriculum can be designed with weekly content to include a review of EBP concepts, how to find

TABLE 5.2 Structured Evidence-Based Practice Programs

	CONDENSED EBP CURRICULUM	EBP TRAINING FELLOWSHIP
Format	Face to face or online	Face to face
Length	Approximately 8 weeks	Approximately 12–18 months
Content	• EBP concepts • Searching for evidence • Evaluating evidence • Managing/interpreting data • Applying evidence at the point of care	• EBP concepts and practical experiences • Identifying clinical questions • Forming a team • Proposal development • Project implementation • Dissemination and clinical practice changes
Continuing education	Awarded	Awarded
Outcome	• Ability to seek and critically evaluate evidence • Incorporate EBP into delivery of patient care	• Conduct an EBP project • Incorporate EBP project change to practice • Serve as EBP role model

EBP, evidence-based practice.

and evaluate available evidence, how to manage and interpret data, and how to apply evidence to practice changes. The EBP Training Fellowship offers a slightly different approach in that the program provides education and practical experiences. The EBP Training Fellowship provides an infrastructure for nurses, educators, and researchers to collaborate in promoting an evidence-based environment to improve the delivery of patient care. It offers nurses additional support and training that is needed for them to identify a clinical problem, develop a project proposal, and integrate an EBP change at the point of care. EBP fellowship programs can be implemented as a train-the-trainer approach whereby once nurses have completed the program, they can serve as EBP champions (Kauschinger, 2018; Storey et al., 2019). The scope of the EBP fellowship may vary depending on the organization, but can span 6 to 18 months. The key focus is to provide direct-care nurses with dedicated release time for education and facilitated time to implement an EBP change. Consistently, lack of time has been cited as a major barrier preventing nurses from implementing EBP in their daily practice (Christenbery, 2018c; McKinney et al., 2019). Therefore, providing dedicated time for EBP training and implementation sends a clear message supporting the importance of an EBP environment. Dedicated release time can range from 4 to 16 hours per month and may vary with respect to organizational setting. Interestingly, emerging evidence shows successful patient and financial outcomes with dedicated Training Fellowship programs (Hatfield et al., 2016). Continuing education certificates can be awarded as part of either of these EBP programs, which serve as incentive for nurses and demonstrate a professional development commitment on behalf of the organization.

Organizational Support

The success of an EBP environment requires organization-wide support involving personnel from various departments, such as executive leaders, nurse managers, information services (IS), operational development, and professional development (Brockopp et al., 2020a). Identifying key personnel is necessary for developing and implementing an EBP environment (Table 5.3). For

TABLE 5.3 Personnel Resources and Roles

Chief nursing officer	• Assess organizational need or gap analysis • Identify core EBP team • Set EBP vision to align with strategic plan • Establish EBP council/committee • Identify funding sources
Senior executives	• Support EBP infrastructure as part of the organization's mission • Endorse EBP culture
Nurse managers	• Provide active endorsement and accountability • Provide opportunities to learn about EBP and pose clinical questions • Identify EBP champions • Budget time and resources for creative EBP environment
Medical librarian	• Educate users on search methods • Serve as resource • Establish links to EBP websites, national guidelines, and specialty organizations • Assist with searches
Information services	• Assist with implementing interactive educational sessions • Coordinate with medical librarian to establish EBP links and resources on unit workstations for 24-hour access • Update electronic health record with practice changes
Operational development	• Implement new technologies to support EBP projects • Establish link to policy and procedures and mechanism for updating • Provide data management and statistical support • Establish a link to IRB education and processes
Professional development	• Offer EBP education and human subject training • Include EBP exemplars as part of performance appraisal and clinical ladder • Incorporate annual EBP competencies and skill appraisal • Incorporate evidence-based standards into policy and procedures • Review current practices and establish an audit and feedback system • Develop database to track and share house wide EBP projects, including ongoing and completed projects • Develop database posting conferences and call for abstracts

EBP, evidence-based practice; IRB, institutional review board.

example, the CNO is needed to support the EBP vision and align strategic goals with the organiza-tion's mission. The CNO and other senior executives are needed to garner support and financing for an EBP environment. Although initially creating an EBP infrastructure may require upfront expenditures for the organization, fostering an EBP environment increases patient safety and ultimately minimizes cost. The resultant EBP model of care helps improve the financial status of the organization by enhancing patient safety, improving patient outcomes and care efficiencies, and reducing the cost of care (Dols et al., 2019). Other key personnel resources needed include: (a) nurse managers to implement the EBP culture, support staff for EBP education, release time, and practice changes; (b) a medical librarian to assist with literature searches and using research databases, and identifying web-based resources; (c) information systems personnel to assist with interactive sessions and technological distribution of EBP-blasts, blogs, elogos, and update reminders; (d) operational development staff to assist with data management, statistical appli-cations, updates in practice in electronic health record, and coordination with the institutional review board process; and (e) professional development staff to integrate EBP skills and competencies, patient-care changes related to EBP project outcomes, documentation, and policy changes (Caramanica & Spiva, 2018; Wright & Brockopp, 2018).

Time, money, and space are additional resources necessary for successfully establishing an EBP environment. As noted previously, lack of time is a common and major barrier for nurses adopting EBP principles (Aljezawi et al., 2019; Christenbery, 2018d). Time is a commodity needed in all aspects of establishing an EBP environment. For example, time is needed by executive leaders to start the EBP transformation and identifying key stakeholders. Time is needed for mentoring, and nurses need time allocated for EBP training, integration, and evaluation. Nurse managers need to dedicate release time for nurses to attend educational sessions and for nurses to effectively implement EBP projects. There is a trickle-down time effect involving personnel whether it is the medical librarian providing instruction on doing a literature review, professional development staff providing EBP competency skills, or operational development staff assisting with data monitoring.

Money is another commodity necessary for establishing an EBP infrastructure and aligns hand in hand with personnel and time. However, many organizations are faced with limited resources, which pose challenges, especially for those nursing leaders interested in implementing EBP but who must do so while staying budget neutral. Frequently, the Division of Nursing underwrites the cost for initiating the EBP initiative; there is evidence showing a return on investment for the organization through adopting results/changes from nurse-driven evidence-based projects (Brockopp et al., 2016; Dols et al., 2019). As evidence for the financial benefits of an EBP environment increases, the CNO will have greater leverage to demonstrate why this is an organization-wide cost. Additionally, the CNO may consider alternative financial resources through both internal and external funding, such as identifying with foundation, philanthropic, community, or professionally related sponsorships. An ongoing process of EBP enables nurses' rapid adoption of scientific knowledge for the purpose of improving patient care. Moreover, using EBP standards in the delivery of care improves quality, increases healthcare value, and reduces costs (Dols et al., 2019).

Providing adequate space is a necessary resource for an EBP environment. Classrooms and conference centers are needed to conduct education, seminars, and presentations; provide one-on-one consultation; and support other EBP initiatives. Access to a medical library via hardcopy or electronic resources should be available within the organization and/or at the unit level. Nurses should have a designated area to store EBP-related supplies, toolkits, and equipment that may be associated with an EBP project. Some organizations may not be equipped with enough physical space to conduct education, therefore a virtual or web-based resource may be an alternative (Christenbery, 2018c) A web-based resource can serve as a central repository for EBP education and tools, and provides accessibility for nurses who may work off-site or varying shifts.

Interweaving Evidence-Based Practice Into the Organization's Structure and Culture for Sustainability

Implementing EBP into the organization is a beginning step of fully embedding the process into the environment. Sustaining EBP requires not only continuation of initial personnel and resources, as noted in Table 5.3, but also additional efforts and approaches are needed (Table 5.4). The key to sustainability and integration into the organization's culture is the demonstration of clinical and financial successes resulting from EBP. Therefore, evaluation of the outcomes must be

TABLE 5.4 Elements for Evidence-Based Practice Sustainability

EBP outcomes	• Maintain a database of EBP projects • Track EBP outcomes and trend results • Showcase projects and distribute clinical outcomes • Public recognition
Shared governance	• Structure to engage staff nurses • Promote staff accountability for practice
Reward and compensation	• Annual competencies and performance evaluation • Merit improvements • Individual and unit acknowledgments
Policy and procedures	• Update policy and procedures and track all EBP revisions
Interprofessional engagement	• Include healthcare members from various domains (physicians, pharmacists, physical and respiratory therapists, etc.)
Continuation of support and resources	• Regularly evaluate EBP implementation strategies and resources (as noted in Table 5.3) • Maintain momentum

EBP, evidence-based practice.

a primary component of any EBP project. Improvement in nurse-sensitive indicators, report card indicators, and cost savings is a way to demonstrate success. Nursing-initiated projects incorporating research and/or EBP processes can produce favorable outcomes for the organization (such as interventions to minimize the occurrence of pressure ulcers, which lead to decreased lengths of stay for patients or safe patient handling to reduce falls). A shared governance structure can be used to (a) engage nurses in conducting EBP and research projects, (b) communicate changes in practice, and (c) promote accountability for patient care and outcomes (Caramanica & Spiva, 2018). Therefore, this structure can serve as an effective strategy to integrate EBP into the culture of the organization.

Leadership includes incorporating EBP into the reward or compensation system. If use of EBP is not one of the aspects on which staff are evaluated, it will be seen by the staff as an add-on versus an integral aspect of how they practice nursing. In leading organizations, use of EBP in the care of the patient is an expectation for promotion via a clinical ladder system (Brockopp et al., 2020b). Behaviors are incorporated into the pertinent aspects of professional practice that are expected by the organization from its nursing staff. This links the rewards to the expectations and to the professional competencies. Documentation of how the nurse used an evidence-based structured approach to problem-solving and care given is required. Having EBP as one of the criteria on which a nurse is evaluated clearly sends the message that the organization values this approach and rewards employees who incorporate this behavior into their work.

Another leadership approach to incorporating, and thus sustaining, the use of EBP in the organization's way of doing business is to insist that both new and revised policies and procedures use EBP approaches as the underlying and determinant rationale. Because policy and procedures are the basis for how the care is delivered, or what the organizational standard is, having the policies and procedures based on evidence not only reinforces to the nursing staff that this is the expected approach to care and problem-solving, but also strengthens the policy and procedure. Because many policy and procedure committees are interprofessional, taking this approach also offers the benefit of demonstrating to all staff the benefits of EBP, thus increasing the likelihood that the organization will continue to use this approach and support it.

■ SUMMARY

Leadership, starting with the CNO, is essential for implementing and sustaining an EBP environment. Not only must the CNO provide leadership within nursing's domain, but engagement of the entire executive team is warranted as the accrued benefits of an EBP environment impacts the organization overall. Numerous resources and processes are required to implement and sustain a strong EBP infrastructure, and the deployment of these resources is an organizational responsibility. Continued efforts to: (a) minimize barriers that impede clinical inquiry, (b) implement strategies to enhance nurses' EBP knowledge and skills, (c) implement evidence-based project changes, and (d) acknowledge and reward EBP successes, will generate enthusiasm and maintain momentum for a sturdy EBP environment.

SUGGESTED LEARNING ACTIVITIES

1. Identify the key components needed to build an EBP infrastructure. Select three to four components and write a detailed plan that identifies who will be involved and what skills are needed to make the development of the infrastructure successful.

2. Based upon the elements for EBP sustainably, identify which elements are currently in place at your organization and which elements will need to be developed to sustain EBP.

REFERENCES

Albert, N. M., Chipps, E., Olson, A. C. F., Hand, L. L., Harmon, M., Heitschmidt, M. G., Klein, C. J., Lefaiver, C., & Wood, T. (2019). Fostering academic-clinical research partnerships. *JONA: The Journal of Nursing Administration, 49*(50), 234–241. https://doi.org/10.1097/NNA.0000000000000744

Aljezawi, M., Al Qadire, M., Alhajjy, M. H., Tawalbeh, L. I., Alamery, A. H., Aloush, S., & AlBashtawy, M. (2019). Barriers to integrating research into clinical nursing practice. *Journal of Nursing Care Quality, 34*(3), E7–E11. https://doi.org/10.1097/NCQ.0000000000000371

American Association of Colleges of Nursing. (2008). *The essentials of baccalaureate education for professional nursing practice.* http://www.aacn.nche.edu/education-resources/BaccEssentials08.pdf

American Association of Colleges of Nursing. (2012). *Clinical nurse leader (CNL).* http://www.aacn.nche.edu/cnl

American Nurses Association. (2015). *Nursing scope and standards of practice* (3rd ed.). Nursesbooks.org.

American Nurses Credentialing Center. (n.d.). Magnet Model—Creating a Magnet culture. https://www.nursingworld.org/organizational-programs/magnet/magnet-model/

Black, A. T., Balneaves, L. G., Garossino, C., Puyat, J. H., & Qian, H. (2015). Promoting evidence-based practice through a research training program for point-of-care clinicians. *Journal of Nursing Administration, 45*(1), 14–20. https://doi.org/10.1097/NNA.0000000000000151

Brockopp, D. Y., Hill, K. S., Bugajski, A. A., & Lengerich, A. J. (2020a). Developing a Research-Friendly Environment; strategies and resources. In D. Y. Brockopp, K. S. Hill, A.A. Bugajski, & A. J. Lengerich (Ed.), *Establishing a Research-Friendly Environment* (pp. 23–42). Jones & Bartlett Learning.

Brockopp, D. Y., Hill, K. S., Bugajski, A. A., & Lengerich, A. J. (2020b). Research-friendly environment; the future. In D. Y. Brockopp, K. S. Hill, A. A. Bugajski, & A. J. Lengerich (Ed.), *Establishing a research-friendly environment* (pp. 169–187). Jones & Bartlett Learning.

Brockopp, D., Hill, K., Moe, K., & Wright, L. (2016). Transforming practice through publication: A community hospital approach to the creation of a research-intensive environment. *The Journal of Nursing Administration, 46*(1), 38–42. https://doi.org/10.1097/NNA.0000000000000294

Calinici, T. (2017). Nursing apps for education and practice. *Journal of Health & Medical Informatics, 8*(3), 262. https://doi.org/10.4172/2157-7420.1000262

Caramanica, L., & Spiva, L. (2018). Exploring nurse manager support of evidence-based practice: Clinical nurse perceptions. *JONA: The Journal of Nursing Administration, 48*(5), 272–278. https://doi.org/10.1097/NNA.0000000000000612

Chanda, N. (2019). Using the great cookie experiment to teach qualitative and quantitative research concepts. *Journal of Nursing Education, 58*(10), 612–612. https://doi.org/10.3928/01484834-20190923-11

Christenbery, T. L. (2018a). Nursing leadership: The fulcrum of evidence-based practice culture. In T. L. Christenbery (Ed.), *Evidence-based practice in nursing: Foundations, skills, and roles* (pp. 293–306). Springer Publishing Company.

Christenbery, T. L. (2018b). Evidence-based practice: A culture of organization empowerment. In T. L. Christenbery (Ed.), *Evidence-based practice in nursing: Foundations, skills, and roles* (pp. 283–291). Springer Publishing Company.

Christenbery, T. L. (2018c). A prosperous evidence-based culture: Nourishing resources. In T. L. Christenbery (Ed.), *Evidence-based practice in nursing: Foundations, skills, and roles* (pp. 307–315). Springer Publishing Company.

Christenbery, T. L. (2018d). Using evidence to inform and reform clinical practice. In T. L. Christenbery (Ed.), *Evidence-based practice in nursing: Foundations, skills, and roles* (pp. 307–315). Springer Publishing Company.

Cronenwett, L., Sherwood, G., Barnsteiner J., Disch, J., Johnson, J., Mitchell, P., Sullivan, D., & Warren, J. (2007). Quality and safety education for nurses. *Nursing Outlook, 55*(3), 122–131. https://doi.org/10.1016/j.outlook.2007.02.006

Dols, J. D., Hoke, M. M., & Allen, D. (2019). Building a practice-focused academic-practice partnership. *JONA: The Journal of Nursing Administration, 49*(7/8), 377–383. https://doi.org/10.1097/NNA.0000000000000771

Farahnak, L. R., Ehrhart, M. G., Torres, E. M., & Aarons, G. A. (2019). The influence of transformational leadership and leader attitudes on subordinate attitudes and implementation success. *Journal of Leadership & Organizational Studies, 27*(11), 98–111. https://doi.org/10.1177/1548051818824529

Funk, S. G., Champagne, M. T., Wiese, R. A., & Tornquist, E. M. (1991). BARRIERS: The barriers to research utilization scale. *Applied Nursing Research, 4*(1), 39–45. https://doi.org/10.1016/S0897-1897(05)80052-7

Gilton, L., Seymour, A., & Baker, R. B. (2019). Changing peripheral intravenous catheter sites when clinically indicated: An evidence-based practice journey. *Worldviews Evidence-Based Nursing, 16*(5), 418–420. https://doi.org/10.1111/wvn.12385

Hatfield, L. A., Kutney-Lee, A., Hallowell, S. G., Del Guidice, M., Ellis, L. N., Verica, L., & Aiken, L. H. (2016). Fostering clinical nurse research in a hospital context. *Journal of Nursing Administration, 46*(5), 245–249. https://doi.org/10.1097/NNA.0000000000000338

Harding, M., Troyer, S., & Bailey, M. (2014). Using courtroom simulation to introduce documenting quality wound care to beginning nursing students. *Nurse Educator, 39*(6), 263–264. https://doi.org/10.1097/NNE.0000000000000078

Herron, E. K., & Strunk, J. A. (2019). Engagement with community partners to promote and enhance the transition of evidence-based nursing from the classroom to clinical practice. *Worldviews on Evidence-Based Nursing, 16*(3), 249–250. https://doi.org/10.1111/wvn.12365

Institute of Medicine. (2001). *Crossing the quality chasm: A new health system for the 21st century*. National Academies Press.

Institute of Medicine. (2011). *The future of nursing: Leading change, advancing health*. National Academies Press.

Johantgen, M., Weiss, M., Lundmark, V., Newhouse, R., Haller, K., Unruh, L., & Shirey, M. (2017). Building research infrastructure in Magnet® hospitals: current status and future directions. *The Journal of Nursing Administration, 47*(4), 198–204. https://doi.org/10.1097/NNA.0000000000000465

Kahoot. (2016). *Learn happy, learn loud*. https://kahoot.com/schools/how-it-works

Kauschinger, E. (2018). Advancing evidence-based practice through mentoring and interprofessional collaboration. In T. L. Christenbery (Ed.), *Evidence-based practice in nursing: Foundations, skills, and roles* (pp. 317–332). Springer Publishing Company.

Landrum, R. E. (2015). Teacher-ready research review: Clickers. *Scholarship of Teaching and Learning in Psychology, 1*(3), 250. https://doi.org/10.1037/stl0000031

Lane, S. H., Serafica, R., Huffman, C., & Cuddy, A. (2016). Making research delicious: An evaluation of nurses' knowledge, attitudes, and practice using the great American cookie experiment with mobile device gaming. *Journal for Nurses in Professional Development, 32*(5), 256–261. https://doi.org/10.1097/NND.0000000000000292

Lavenberg, J. G., Cacchione, P. Z., Jayakumar, K. L., Leas, B. F., Mitchell, M. D., Mull, N. K., & Umscheid, C. A. (2019). Impact of a hospital evidence-based practice center (EPC) on nursing policy and practice. *Worldviews on Evidence-Based Nursing, 16*(1), 4–11. https://doi.org/10.1111/wvn.12346

Lizarondo, L., & McArthur, A. (2017). Strategies for effective facilitation as a component of an evidence-based clinical fellowship program. *The Journal of Continuing Education in Nursing, 48*(10), 458–463. https://doi.org/10.3928/00220124-20170918-07

Maneval, R., Browne, K. P., Feldman, H. R., Brooks, C., Scuderi, D., Henderson, J., & Epstein, C. (2019). A collaborative academic-practice approach to meeting educational and workforce needs. *JONA: The Journal of Nursing Administration, 49*(10), 463–465. https://doi.org/10.1097/NNA.0000000000000788

McKinney, I., DelloStritto, R. A., & Branham, S. (2019). Nurses' use of evidence-based practice at point of care: A literature review. *Critical Care Nursing Quarterly, 42*(3), 256–264. https://doi.org/10.1097/CNQ.0000000000000266

Melnyk, B. M., & Fineout-Overholt, E. (2003a). *Evidence-based practice beliefs scale.* ARCC LLC Publications.

Melnyk, B. M., & Fineout-Overholt, E. (2003b). *Evidence-based practice implementation scale.* ARCC LLC Publications.

Melnyk, B. M., Gallagher-Ford, L., Thomas, B. K., Troseth, M., Wywngarden, K., & Szalacha, L. (2016). A study of chief nurse executives indicates low prioritization of evidence-based practice and shortcomings in hospital performance metrics across the United States. *Worldviews on Evidence-Based Nursing, 13*(1), 6–11. https://doi.org/10.1111/wvn.12133

Melnyk, B. M., Gallagher-Ford, L., Zellefrow, C., Tucker, S., Thomas, B., Sinnott, L. T., & Tan, A. (2018). The first U.S. study on nurses' evidence-based practice competencies indicates major deficits that threaten healthcare quality, safety, and patient outcomes. *Worldviews on Evidence-Based Nursing, 15*(1), 16–25. https://doi.org/10.1111/wvn.12269

Monturo, C. A., & Brockway, C. (2019). Micro-learning: An innovative strategy to cultivate a spirit of inquiry, step zero. *Worldviews on Evidence-Based Nursing, 16*(5), 416–417. https://doi.org/10.1111/wvn.12373

Mueller, R., Lind, C., McCaffrey, G., & Ewashen, C. (2017). A guide for using discussion-based pedagogy. https://taylorinstitute.ucalgary.ca/sites/default/files/discussion%20based%20learning%20TI%20guide_final.pdf

Nearpod. (n.d.). How it works. https://nearpod.com/how-it-works

Royer, H. R., Crary, P., Fayram, E., & Heidrich, S. M. (2018) Five-year program evaluation of an evidence-based practice scholars program. *The Journal of Continuing Education in Nursing, 49*(12), 547–554. https://doi.org/10.3928/00220124-20181116-05

Saunders, H., Gallagher-Ford, L., Kvist, T., & Vehviläinen-Julkunen, K. (2019). Practicing healthcare professionals' evidence-based practice competencies: An overview of systematic reviews. *Worldviews on Evidence-Based Nursing, 16*(3), 176–185. https://doi.org/10.1111/wvn.12363

Scala, E., Price, C., & Day, J. (2016). An integrative review of engaging clinical nurses in nursing research. *Journal of Nursing Scholarship, 48*(4), 423–430. https://doi.org/10.1111/jnu.12223

Shatto, B., & Erwin, K. (2016). Moving on from millennials: Preparing for generation Z. *The Journal of Continuing Education in Nursing, 47*(6), 253–254. https://doi.org/10.3928/00220124-20160518-05

Storey, S., Wagnes, L., LaMothe, J., Pittman, J., Cohee, A., & Newhouse, R. (2019). Building evidence-based nursing practice capacity in a large statewide health system: A multimodal approach. *JONA: The Journal of Nursing Administration, 49*(4), 208–214. https://doi.org/10.1097/NNA.0000000000000739

Songur, C., Özer, Ö., Gün, C., & Top, M. (2018) Patient safety culture, evidence-based practice and performance in nursing. *Systematic Practice and Action Research, 31*, 359–374. https://doi.org/10.1007/s11213-017-9430-y

Thapar-Olmos, N., & Seeman, S. R. (2018). Piloting classroom response systems in graduate psychology courses. *Journal of Educational Technology Systems, 47*(2), 193–204. https://doi.org/10.1177/0047239518794173

Thiel, C. A. (1987). The cookie experiment: A creative teaching strategy. *Nurse Educator, 12*(3), 8–10. https://doi.org/10.1097/00006223-198705000-00004

White, C. T. (2015). Using a mock trial method to enhance effectiveness of teaching evidence-based practice in nursing. *Journal for Nurses in Professional Development, 31*(6), E11–E14. https://doi.org/10.1097/NND.0000000000000214

Wright, L., & Brockopp, D. (2018). Exploring nurse manager support of evidence-based practice: Clinical nurse perceptions. *JONA: The Journal of Nursing Administration, 48*(5), 272–278. https://doi.org/10.1097/NNA.0000000000000612

Wu, Y., Brettle, A., Zhou, C., Ou, J., Wang, Y., & Wang, S. (2018). Do educational interventions aimed at nurses to support the implementation of evidence-based practice improve patient outcomes? A systematic review. *Nurse Education Today, 70*, 109–114. https://doi.org/10.1016/j.nedt.2018.08.026

BUILDING BLOCKS FOR EVIDENCE

CRITICAL APPRAISAL OF EVIDENCE

KAREN M. VUCKOVIC AND KATHERINE A. MAKI

■ INTRODUCTION

Whether one is reading a research article to translate findings into evidence-based practice (EBP) or as a building block for a proposed study, the process often begins with appraising a single research article. Advanced practice nurses frequently read evidence (research, guidelines, reviews) to answer questions related to diagnosis, therapeutic interventions, and prognosis of individual patients (Dale et al., 2019). One of the barriers to translating research findings (and therefore providing evidence-based care or guideline-directed therapy) into practice is a lack of confidence in one's ability to read and interpret research findings (Gray et al., 2017). The critical thinking skills nurses use in practice every day provide a foundation for developing the skill of reading and evaluating research.

Reading and evaluating literature is a *critical* skill in translating research into clinical practice. Previous chapters have addressed how to locate and retrieve evidence; chapters that follow detail the various elements and designs of collecting evidence and the reporting of results through publications. The purpose of this chapter is to review the sections of a single research article and to provide an organized approach to reading and interpreting the strength and relevance of the information presented in a data-based article.

The critical appraisal of the evidence determines the strengths, weaknesses, and usefulness of the findings for practice and future research. Using a published critical appraisal tool to evaluate the evidence guides the clinician through a comprehensive critique (Moralejo et al., 2017; Zuzelo, 2019). Clinicians must weigh the limitations and feasibility of the evidence with its strengths to evaluate if the evidence is usefulness to practice. One type of evidence clinicians appraise is a clinical research study. As a result, understanding the components of an article based on data and the important questions to consider while reading each section is needed.

All research articles are written with a standardized format. Components of an article based on data include the title, abstract, background or introduction and significance of the study, methods, data analysis, findings and results, discussion, limitations, and implications for practice. Minor variations in the formatting may be required by a journal for publication, for example, limitations may be included in the discussion. Even so, the logic of the researcher's thinking should be clear enough so that the reader has few questions about how and why the study was conducted. By the end of the article, the reader should be able to determine how the research results fit into current knowledge and how (or whether) the findings translate to the practice environment for implementation or necessitate further testing and validation. As the reader progresses through the article, each section builds on the previous information. Exhibit 6.1 summarizes key elements

EXHIBIT 6.1

EVALUATING A SINGLE RESEARCH ARTICLE—QUESTIONS TO CONSIDER

Abstract
Does the article fit your research question or purpose? Practice setting? Population?

Background and Significance
Literature Review
  Is the literature current and relevant?
  Is the research literature summarized and evaluated?
  Does the literature review introduce all concepts and variables proposed in the research?
  Are gaps in the literature noted? How likely is it that the current study will close the gaps in current knowledge?
Problem Statement/Purpose (appears at the end of the Background section)
  Are the aims of the study clearly stated? Is the research exploratory or hypothesis-testing?
  What is studied? What variables are measured (independent and dependent)?
  Does the purpose (or research question) clearly address the problem?

Method
Design
  What is the overall design of the study, quantitative or qualitative?
  Is the design a good match with the problem statement or purpose of the study?
Ethics
  How is the protection of human participants ensured?
Sample
  How is the sample identified? Do the participants have characteristics that can answer the research question? What are the inclusion and exclusion criteria?
Instruments
  Are the instruments used reliable and validated in the study population?
Study Procedure
  Is the procedure realistic?
  If an independent variable is manipulated, was it done so consistently?
  How are the instruments/tools administered, in what environment, and was the environment consistent?
  Over how much time are data collected?

Data Analysis
  How are the data analyzed?
  Are statistical tests used appropriately?
  If the research is a qualitative study, how are the themes and meaning elicited?

Findings/Results
  What are the outcomes of the study? Are the results valid?
  Are all aspects of the problem statement/purpose addressed?
  How do the findings fit with previous research? Are they supported or not supported?

(continued)

Discussion
   What conclusions did the researcher draw from the findings?
   Do the findings make sense? Relate to the problem?
   How do the findings compare with other research findings in the literature?
   Can the results be generalized to other populations and/or settings? Will the results help me care for
      my patients?

Limitations (may also be part of Discussion section)
   What limitations are noted? How will limitations affect generalizability of the findings?

Conclusion/Implications
   Are implications for practice and research noted?
   Do the conclusion/implications flow directly from the findings?

to consider when appraising a data-based article and may serve as a general guide or checklist in reading the literature. This exhibit is one example of an appraisal tool; several other guides and tools are available including online software to assist in critically appraising the data-based literature.

▦ TITLE

The title describes and explains what the article is about. The title may include information about the focus or outcome of the research, the population studied, and the study design (Polit & Beck, 2020).

▦ ABSTRACT

The first part of a research article is the abstract. The abstract is a brief, targeted summary of the full article that follows. Therefore a quality abstract presents a clear synopsis of the purpose, results, and research implications of the research manuscript. The abstract provides the reader with a succinct overview of the study and can be used to evaluate whether the study is of interest or applies to the reader's practice setting or population (Alspach, 2017). Most readers use the abstract as a screen to determine whether or not to read the entire research article.

▦ BACKGROUND (INTRODUCTION) AND SIGNIFICANCE

The background or introduction of a data-based article provides an overview of the current status of a specific field and a context for the research. The first few paragraphs provide the reader with an understanding of the background of the study, why the study was conducted, and why the study was important or significant. The reader should be able to identify gaps in current knowledge and how the proposed study specifically fills the gaps. Near the end of the section (or set apart), the purpose (also referred to as the aim) or problem statement of the study is presented. The purpose or problem statement is closely related. Both or only one may be included in an article. The purpose or problem statement should be clearly stated and provide the independent and dependent variables examined. The author may also include research questions, hypotheses tested in the study, or both. In any case, the reader will know the population (who) and the phenomenon (what) of interest. The reader uses this information to assess the remainder of the article.

■ LITERATURE REVIEW

In some cases, the background section includes a review of the literature. In other articles, the literature review is set apart as a separate section. The review of the literature should be appraised for both content and relevance. The literature presented should be relevant to the current study, relate to the variables that were studied, and be up to date. The literature review often includes reviews, theoretical and data-based sources. The previous research studies included in the background section should at the minimum address the purpose, sample, design, findings, and a brief critique of the study's strengths and weaknesses (Gray et al., 2017). Another approach in reporting the research literature is to review and synthesize numerous studies and evaluate the body of knowledge. Whichever approach is used, the reader should understand the existing knowledge and how the study may address gaps in knowledge or expand current knowledge. The research literature included in the review may be directly or indirectly related to the purpose of the study. Indirectly related studies should be linked for relevance.

The reader should check the publication dates of the literature cited and of the reference list to judge whether the references are (at least reasonably) current. Although some studies are considered classics, much of the cited literature should be recent and reflect up-to-date thinking and understanding of the study's focus. This is especially important in practice areas undergoing rapid change (e.g., genetics and genomics) and in areas that are time sensitive (e.g., attitudes and opinions). The reader's personal knowledge and level of expertise in the content area are valuable in determining the currency and strength of the literature review included in the research article.

■ METHODS

A large section of the research article is the methods section, which describes how the study was conducted. The methods section includes design, sampling, instruments, and specific procedures for data collection (Polit & Beck, 2020). The methods section is a critical part of a research article and deserves careful attention. While reading the methods section, the reader should be alert for any problems in the way the study protocol was implemented, such as sample bias, inconsistencies in data collection among participants, loss of participants or attrition, and weaknesses of the instruments or tools used to collect the data. The strength of the methods section helps the reader determine the overall usefulness and generalizability of the results that will follow.

Design

The study design is identified early in the methods section if it has not already been implied in the purpose or problem statement. The author should identify whether the study used a *quantitative, qualitative,* or *mixed methods* design. Quantitative studies use designs that result in numerical data that can be used in statistical (mathematical) analyses and assess the size of relationships among variables (Al-Jundi & Sakka, 2017). Variables in quantitative designs may be measured using physiologic instruments (e.g., blood pressure and weight), questionnaires with fixed responses (e.g., scale of 1 to 5), or variables that can be assigned a number (e.g., age). Quantitative research designs may be further identified as experimental, quasi-experimental, or nonexperimental (descriptive or correlational), depending on how participants were chosen, whether and how study variables were manipulated, and how the data to measure the variables were collected (Gray et al., 2017).

Qualitative studies use a nonnumerical study approach to collect data, often to describe a phenomenon (Melnyk & Fineout-Overholt, 2019). The most common qualitative designs are ethnographic, phenomenological, historical, and grounded theory approaches. Just as in quantitative designs, there are specific and distinguishing elements among the qualitative designs. The goal of studies that use qualitative designs is to explore or explain the phenomenon of interest from the perspective of individuals experiencing the phenomenon. As a result, qualitative designs yield descriptions that can then be analyzed and coded for themes, common elements, and shared meaning among participants (Lewis, 2019). The end result of a qualitative design may be new knowledge or the beginning of a theory, whereas the end result of a quantitative study is often acceptance or rejection of current knowledge or theory.

In some instances, the study design may include both qualitative and quantitative elements to examine a specific research question or hypothesis, resulting in a mixed methods design. How methods are mixed varies greatly but three major issues need to be addressed in this type of design, that of timing, weighting, and mixing (Moorley & Cathala, 2019). The analysis of a mixed-methods study design combines both numeric and narrative data (Moorley & Cathala, 2019). Quantitative and qualitative design approaches can differ greatly, with quantitative designs requiring large sample sizes and random selection or assignment to treatment groups, whereas some qualitative designs have small samples recruited from a narrow group of individuals. Thus, a mixed methods study may have a large or small sample depending upon which research design dominates. Ultimately, sampling decisions are based on the research questions (Eckhardt & DeVon, 2017).

The design of the study should be sufficiently detailed so that the reader can determine how the study was actually conducted. The timeline and sequence of the study procedures should be clear and concise so that the study can be replicated. Regardless of the overall research design, the key question for the reader to consider is how well the design used is likely to fulfill the purpose of the study and answer the research question.

Sample

The number of participants who participated in the study or sample size should be clearly stated and described in the article including the number of participants who do not complete the study. In addition, the authors should describe how the sample size was determined. In a quantitative study, sample size is determined by power analysis, a mathematical determination based on the researcher's desired level of statistical significance, estimates of variability, and effect size (Al-Jundi & Sakka, 2017). A power analysis is not included in a pilot study because a primary purpose of a pilot study is to collect information to justify and guide subsequent, larger studies (Lowe, 2019). In many qualitative studies, the researcher describes how the (often small) sample size was sufficient to answer the research question based on sufficient "saturation" of information obtained (Malterud et al., 2016; Polit & Beck, 2020).

The article should also provide details regarding specific inclusion and exclusion criteria for participants to be enrolled as participants. Careful attention to potential participants excluded from the study will assist in determining whether findings may be translated to clinical practice. The reader should be especially alert for any apparent bias in selecting the sample and exclusions that can limit generalizability of the findings beyond the study's individual sample and/or setting.

A description of potential participants who were approached for inclusion but refused to participate should also be included to determine how closely the study population represents the population of interest as a whole.

The demographic and clinical characteristics of study participants (e.g., age, gender, comorbidities) are usually presented and help the reader evaluate to what degree the study sample is congruent with the reader's population of interest. Sample characteristics are also important in determining whether or not the study findings might be applicable for translation into practice. Increased attention to include sex as a biological variable helps to prevent the generalization of findings obtained from studies lacking power to test for sex differences between males and females (Lee, 2018). The more closely the sample matches the reader's population, the more likely the reader is to implement the findings into practice if all other criteria are met (no contradictory study results and other supporting studies with similar results). In addition, the number of participants and a brief description of participants who did not complete the study or study procedures should be included so that the reader can make a judgment whether individuals who completed the study were different from those who did not complete the study, which is a potential source of bias called *attrition* (Kearney et al., 2017).

In quantitative studies, random selection of participants and random assignment of participants to treatment groups are ideal but often difficult to accomplish because of the constraints that accompany research on human participants in a clinical environment. As a result, a convenience sampling method is often used and is strengthened when the design incorporates random assignment to treatment groups. The reader needs to make a judgment regarding bias in the sample and the appropriateness of the sampling plan in answering the problem.

Research Instruments and Data Collection Tools

Each research tool or instrument used in the study should be described in detail. The instruments should measure the variables of interest. If an existing tool or instrument was used (e.g., depression scale), the number of items and a brief account of what the tool measures should be provided. Measures of reliability, the consistency of the tool or instrument, and validity (whether the tool actually measures the phenomenon under study) are important considerations and should be reported in the article (Vetter & Cubbin, 2019). It is imperative to include the reliability and validity information the first time a tool or instrument is implemented to study a specific population or demographic (Vetter & Cubbin, 2019). The choice of the specific tool used should be explained in the context of the study variables, previous research that used the tool(s), and any subject characteristics considered in choosing the tool (e.g., reading level and short administration time in a population likely to experience fatigue with a long tool). An advantage of using research instruments that have already been used is that reliability and validity data may already be established (Mayo, 2015; Polit, 2015). If the researcher had developed a tool for the study, a full description of the instrument and a discussion of how reliability and validity were established should be included. Whether an existing research instrument was used, or a tool was created for the study, a lack of information regarding reliability and validity leads to questions regarding whether or how well the variables in the study were actually measured (Vetter & Cuban, 2019).

Ethics

The methods section should also include a short description of how ethical considerations in conducting the study were addressed. Alternatively, the protection of human participants may be addressed as the first part of the description of the study procedure. In either case, a statement regarding review of the study by an institutional review board or research ethics board prior to the beginning of the study is generally included (Al-Jundi & Sakka, 2016). In addition, procedures for obtaining participants' consent to participate in the study and how consent was obtained should be detailed. If the participants were minors or were incompetent to provide informed consent personally, the author should fully describe assent (for minors) or consent procedures, mention whether any difficulties were encountered, and, if difficulties were encountered, how they were managed.

Study Procedures

The procedure section provides a detailed description of how the study was conducted, including exactly how and when data were collected and under what conditions. The information should be clearly presented so that the reader could replicate the study by following the description. The reader should see a logical flow in the data collection process and consider any extraneous variables in the setting that may affect the data.

▨ DATA ANALYSIS

By the time, the reader comes to the data analysis section of the research article, the reader will know a great deal about the study. The reader has formed beginning opinions about the strength and potential usefulness of the study and is looking forward to reading the findings and results. The data analysis section begins with a description of how the data obtained from the research instruments were summarized and analyzed. The intent of this section is to tell the reader how the data were analyzed and is a straightforward presentation of information. In a quantitative report, the data are analyzed using statistical methods and tests. There are numerous statistical procedures and tests available. The key issue in evaluating the statistical analysis is to determine that the method used was appropriate for the research question and how the data were measured (Melnyk & Fineout-Overholt, 2019). In a qualitative study, the data analysis approach is described and coded, including how themes or patterns were elicited from the data. For the novice reader, the data analysis section may be the most intimidating part of the research article (Jefferies et al., 2018). This discomfort is often due to limited exposure to and understanding of the statistical tests used and uncertainty about whether the appropriate test has been applied to the data. Resources that will aid the reader to develop their skills include a basic statistics book and colleagues with an understanding of data analysis techniques. As with any skill, the more the reader gains in understanding, the easier reading the analysis section becomes.

▨ FINDINGS AND RESULTS

For many, the most enjoyable section of a research article to read is the findings of the study. Each previous section has been laying the foundation for this part of the article. The findings tell the reader what the researcher discovered as a result of the data that were collected and analyzed. As the findings of a study are presented, whether a qualitative or quantitative design was used, the reader learns whether the research question was answered and how completely the question or problem statement was addressed. All results and data that address the research question or problem statement are included in a discussion of the findings. If the study was analyzed using statistical methods, the statistical significance (*p*-value or alpha) and confidence intervals of the results are reported. It is important to note that *p*-values do not measure the effect size or clinical significance of the results but convey the likelihood that the reported results were not achieved due to a false positive (or type I error) based on a predetermined alpha threshold, which is generally set to $p < 0.05$ (Wasserstein & Lazar, 2016). Therefore, confidence intervals can be more informative when interpreting results, especially when placed in a clinical context (Schober et al., 2018). In the results section, the data and outcomes of statistical analysis are presented but not explained or discussed. The intent of the results section is to present the factual outcome of data analysis, rather than explain the meaning of the data. Although this section may seem dry or unimaginative, the advantage of this approach is to allow the reader to make beginning judgments regarding the study outcomes in the absence of the opinion or interpretation of meaning from others. In addition to a narrative summary of the results, most articles present findings using tables, graphs, or figures for easier review. It can be helpful to carefully review and interpret the data presented in the manuscript's tables and figures before reading the results section in order to obtain a more comprehensive review of the data presented.

Qualitative study findings, depending on the specific qualitative design used in the study, are presented quite differently from quantitative results. In a qualitative study, direct quotes or summaries of participant responses are often included in the results section or may be presented in a combined results/discussion section (Cypress, 2019). The author may group the findings according to themes or patterns that became apparent during the data analysis (Moorley & Cathala, 2019). As a result, many qualitative studies provide data using a narrative approach and describe results in terms of richness and depth of the data.

Some readers prefer to read the results section immediately after reading the problem or purpose of the study. This may be due to curiosity about the outcome or to decide whether or not to read the entire article. The dedicated reader will then go back to the beginning of the article and read it entirely. There is nothing inherently wrong with reading the results out of sequence as long as the reader recalls that, in order to use the findings in practice or to build additional research studies, the previous sections of the article are critical in evaluating the strength of the findings. In addition, this approach may encourage a reader to fully read only those articles that report significance or that reinforce current ways of thinking. Studies that do not demonstrate statistical significance are often as revealing as those that do and encourage us to challenge existing perceptions. Finally, because the results section presents but does not discuss the findings, the reader may overlook studies with clinical (but not statistical) significance.

DISCUSSION

In the discussion section of an article, the author presents the conclusions drawn from the findings, acknowledges any limitations of the study, and suggests how findings may be generalized to individuals or groups beyond the study sample. In the discussion, the author describes how the results fit into the current body of general knowledge and specific previous research. The author should compare and contrast the study findings with those of the previous research that was cited in the review of the literature presented earlier in the article. A critical comparison by the author demonstrates to the reader that the researcher evaluated the findings with an open mind.

■ CONCLUSIONS

The author's conclusions provide the researcher's interpretation of the study findings. In contrast to the factual presentation of the study outcomes in the findings section, the conclusions present the meaning of the results from the author's perspective. The conclusions drawn by the researcher should flow from the scope of the study and directly relate to the purpose of the study; they should be confined to the variables that were studied. The reader should evaluate the author's perspective as well their own to determine whether the findings answer questions in the reader's clinical experience and/or provide information that explains phenomena previously unexplained.

■ LIMITATIONS

The author's identification of the study's limitations recognizes that, although no study is perfect, the results can contribute and provide valuable information for future researchers (Melnyk & Fineout-Overholt, 2019). At the same time, limitations cannot be used as an excuse for a poor design or flawed study procedures. Among the limitations often cited in research reports are problems with data collection (e.g., unexpected intervening variables that occurred during data collection), small sample size, problems with how the sample was obtained (e.g., convenience sample), and limitations inherent in the study's research design (e.g., non-random assignment of participants to groups; Melnyk & Fineout-Overholt, 2019). In most cases, the reader has already identified limitations and is not surprised by those noted by the author. The limitations will affect the reader's confidence in translating the findings into clinical practice.

■ GENERALIZABILITY

The generalizability of study findings is an essential evaluation of a study's outcome. Studies are conducted with participants who have specific characteristics and in settings with unique environments. In addition, manipulation of the independent variable and measurement of the dependent variable may be done in more than one way, and researchers may use comparable or divergent research instruments or tools. As a result, the meaning of the findings and how the findings may be implemented with other populations and in other settings must be addressed in the article. An understanding of the limitations of the study also affects generalizability. A study with numerous or key limitations results in findings that have minimal or narrow generalizability beyond the population or setting in the study. This is especially likely when bias is present in the sample. Bias may be a design flaw or may be unintentional and discovered during data analysis.

■ IMPLICATIONS

The final major aspect of a research article is its implications for practice and research. An important goal of research is to provide evidence to further explain phenomena, validate current thinking and practice, or change current practice and approaches. Depending on the purpose of the study, the strength of the study's design, and the statistical and clinical significance of findings, it is important for the author to suggest to the reader how the findings may actually be used. Useful clinical research should benefit patients and enhance wellness; the authors should provide transparency regarding how the results may be adapted for practice, education, or the delivery of healthcare services (Ioannidis, 2016). The implications should have direct links to the findings, be feasible and pragmatic, and be suggested within the limitations of the study as previously noted by the author (Hellier & Cline, 2016; Ioannidis, 2016). Again, the reader will critically evaluate the information presented, determine the extent to which the reader agrees or disagrees with the author's perspective, and decide whether or not to implement the findings into practice.

Implications for future research are similarly important. Authors commonly cite a need for replication of the study, recognizing that changes in clinical practice are rarely made on the basis of a single study. In addition, the author should make suggestions for further studies that might expand understanding of the phenomenon or problem studied. In the case of an article based on a pilot study, the author should make specific recommendations for a larger study that may incorporate additional variables, change the study design, or revise or change the research tools (McGrath & Brandon, 2018).

■ SUMMARY

Reading a single research article is the first step in progressing down the path of translating evidence into practice, planning a research study, or both. Like most skills in nursing, comfort and proficiency in reading research studies increase with diligent practice. The critical thinking skills that nurses use in clinical practice are the building blocks for critically evaluating each section of a research article.

SUGGESTED LEARNING ACTIVITIES

Read two research articles—one quantitative and one qualitative—in your area of expertise or interest. Compare and contrast the two studies in the following areas:

1. Evaluate the methods section of the articles and note the following:
   a. What specific type of design did the research use?
   b. Does the design "match" the purpose of the study? Will the design provide the information to achieve the purpose or answer the problem stated?
   c. How was the sample obtained? Based on the specific quantitative/qualitative design of the study, was the sampling plan appropriate?
   d. In the quantitative study, were the reliability and the validity of the research instrument(s) described? In the qualitative study, how did the researcher record and organize the data?
   e. Were data obtained in the same manner from all participants?
2. Evaluate how the data were analyzed.
   a. In the quantitative study, were the statistical tests appropriate to the type of data collected?
   b. In the qualitative study, were the data analyzed in a way consistent with the type of qualitative design?
3. In both studies, are conclusions consistent with the data? Are limitations identified?
4. How could the study's findings be used in practice and/or to plan further research?

REFERENCES

Al-Jundi, A., & Sakka, S. (2016). Protocol writing in clinical research. *Journal of Clinical and Diagnostic Research, 10*(11), ze10–ze13. https://doi.org/10.7860/JCDR/2016/21426.8865

Al-Jundi, A., & Sakka, S. (2017). Critical appraisal of clinical research. *Journal of Clinical and Diagnostic Research, 11*(5), je01–je05. https://doi.org/10.7860/JCDR/2017/26047.9942

Alspach, J. G. (2017). Writing for publication 101: Why the abstract is so important. *Critical Care Nurse, 37*(4), 12–15. https://doi.org/10.4037/ccn2017466

Buccheri, R. K., & Sharifi, C. (2017). Critical appraisal tools and reporting guidelines for evidence-based practice. *Worldviews on Evidence Based Nursing, 14*(6), 463–472. https://doi.org/10.1111/wvn.12258

Cypress, B. S. (2019). Qualitative research: challenges and dilemmas. *Dimensions of Critical Care Nursing, 38*(5), 264–270. https://doi.org/10.1097/DCC.0000000000000374

Dale, J. C., Hallas, D., & Spratling, R. (2019). Critiquing research evidence for use in practice: Revisited. *Journal of Pediatric Health Care, 33*(3), 342–346. https://doi.org/10.1016/j.pedhc.2019.01.005

Eckhardt, A. L., & DeVon, H. A. (2017). The MIXED framework: A novel approach to evaluating mixed-methods rigor. *Nursing Inquiry, 24*(4), e12189. https://doi.org/10.1111/nin.12189

Gray, J., Grove, S. K., & Sutherland, S. (2017). *Burns and Grove's the practice of nursing research: Appraisal, synthesis, and generation of evidence* (8th ed.). Elsevier.

Hellier, S., & Cline, T. (2016). Factors that affect nurse practitioners' implementation of evidence-based practice. *Journal of the American Association of Nurse Practitioners, 28*(11), 612–621. https://doi.org/10.1002/2327-6924.12394

Ioannidis, J. P. (2016). Why Most Clinical Research Is Not Useful. *PLoS Medicine, 13*(6), e1002049. https://doi.org/10.1371/journal.pmed.1002049

Jefferies, D., McNally, S., Roberts, K., Wallace, A., Stunden, A., D'Souza, S., & Glew, P. (2018). The importance of academic literacy for undergraduate nursing students and its relationship to future professional clinical practice: A systematic review. *Nurse Education Today, 60*, 84–91. https://doi.org/10.1016/j.nedt.2017.09.020

Kearney, A., Daykin, A., Shaw, A. R. G., Lane, A. J., Blazeby, J. M., Clarke, M., Williamson, P., & Gamble, C. (2017). Identifying research priorities for effective retention strategies in clinical trials. *Trials, 18*(1), 406. https://doi.org/10.1186/s13063-017-2132-z

Lee, S. K. (2018). Sex as an important biological variable in biomedical research. *BMB Reports, 51*(4), 167–173. https://doi.org/10.5483/BMBRep.2018.51.4.034

Lewis, L. (2019). Finding the stories: A novice qualitative researcher learns to analyse narrative inquiry data. *Nurse Researcher, 26*(2), 14–18. https://doi.org/10.7748/nr.2018.e1578

Lowe, N. K. (2019). What is a pilot study? *Journal of Obstetric, Gynecologic, & Neonatal Nursing, 48*(2), 117–118. https://doi.org/10.1016/j.jogn.2019.01.005

Malterud, K., Siersma, V. D., & Guassora, A. D. (2016). Sample size in qualitative interview studies: Guided by information power. *Qualitative Health Research, 26*(13), 1753–1760. https://doi.org/10.1177/1049732315617444

Mayo, A. M. (2015). Psychometric instrumentation: Reliability and validity of instruments used for clinical practice, evidence-based practice projects and research studies. *Clinical Nurse Specialist, 29*(3), 134–138. https://doi.org/10.1097/NUR.0000000000000131

McGrath, J. M., & Brandon, D. (2018). What constitutes a well-designed pilot study? *Advances in Neonatal Care, 18*(4), 243–245. https://doi.org/10.1097/ANC.0000000000000535

Melnyk, B. M., & Fineout-Overholt, E. (2019). *Evidence-based practice in nursing and healthcare: A guide to best practice* (4th ed.). Wolters Kluwer.

Moorley, C., & Cathala, X. (2019). How to appraise mixed methods research. *Evidence-Based Nursing, 22*(2), 38–41. https://doi.org/10.1136/ebnurs-2019-103076

Moralejo, D., Ogunremi, T., & Dunn, K. (2017). Critical Appraisal Toolkit (CAT) for assessing multiple types of evidence. *Canada Communicable Disease Report, 43*(9), 176–181. https://doi.org/10.14745/ccdr.v43i09a02

Polit, D. F. (2015). Assessing measurement in health: Beyond reliability and validity. *International Journal of Nursing Studies, 52*(11), 1746–1753. https://doi.org/10.1016/j.ijnurstu.2015.07.002

Polit, D. F., & Beck, C. T. (2020). *Nursing research: Generating and assessing evidence for nursing practice* (11th ed.). Phildadelphia, PA: Wolters Kluwer/Lippincott Williams & Wilkins.

Schober, P., Bossers, S. M., & Schwarte, L. A. (2018). Statistical significance versus clinical importance of observed effect sizes: What do *p*-values and confidence intervals really represent? *Anesthesia & Analgesia, 126*(3), 1068–1072. https://doi.org/10.1213/ANE.0000000000002798

Vetter, T. R., & Cubbin, C. (2019). Psychometrics: Trust, but verify. *Anesthesia & Analgesia, 128*(1), 176–181. https://doi.org/10.1213/ANE.0000000000003859

Wasserstein, R. L., & Lazar, N. A. (2016). The ASA's statement on *p*-values: context, process, and purpose. *The American Statistician, 70*(2), 129–133. https://doi.org/10.1080/00031305.2016.1154108

Zuzelo, P. R. (2019). Critically appraising research studies and reports: Tools to guide evidence evaluation. *Holistic Nursing Practice, 33*(6), 370–372. https://doi.org/10.1097/HNP.0000000000000356

ADDITIONAL RESOURCES

ANA's Research Toolkit. Retrieved from https://www.ahrq.gov/research/index.html

Critically Appraised Tool (CAT) maker and BestBETs. CATmaker is a software tool available through the Center for Evidence-Based Medicine. Retrieved from http://www.cebm.net

Review of CATs and Reporting Guidelines in Buccheri and Sharifi (2017).

IDENTIFYING A FOCUS OF PRACTICE INQUIRY

LEA ANN MATURA AND VIVIAN NOWAZEK

▣ INTRODUCTION

There are numerous sources of ideas for identifying the focus of an inquiry. The literature review presents what is currently known about the topic of interest and the gaps in the literature. Once a thorough search and evaluation of the available evidence have been conducted, the focus of the study can be defined in the form of a purpose, objectives, and specific aims, along with well-developed research questions. This chapter delineates the components needed to define a research topic. Examples are included to illustrate the concepts and to facilitate practice in critically evaluating material from an evidence-based perspective.

▣ SOURCES OF TOPICS AND PROBLEMS

When a researcher is identifying a topic of inquiry, several sources can provide guidance in determining the question or problem to investigate. Some areas previously identified as starting points include clinical practice, the research literature, professional organizations, and conferences (Polit & Beck, 2020). Likewise, there are multiple examples from varying clinical settings or domains of healthcare where ideas may be generated. Clinical problems or questions, the literature, regulatory agencies, new diagnoses, social media, sentinel events, and legislative issues are only a few possibilities, but these examples may stimulate thoughtful reflection on practice as we look forward to future studies. Once an idea is generated, a search of the literature is the next step in discovering what is already known and not known about the topic.

Clinical Problems or Questions

The clinical setting is an excellent place to generate research questions. For example, when a patient has an acute injury such as an ankle sprain, a commonly prescribed regimen is applying rest, ice, compression, and elevation (RICE) therapy within 72 hours of the injury (Ueblacker et al., 2016). However, is there sufficient evidence to support this therapy? We need data to support our interventions; perhaps RICE is an ineffective therapy, but more research is needed.

Another pervasive problem in healthcare is the prevention of pressure injuries. Standard practices recommend turning patients every 2 hours, but there continues to be little support for this practice or other measures to prevent pressure injuries. A recent literature review investigated turning frequency in adult bed-ridden patients to prevent hospital-acquired pressure injuries (Jocelyn Chew et al., 2018). The majority of studies could not reach a conclusion for frequency of turning. However, few studies have focused solely on frequency of turning and pressure ulcer prevention or development. One study using a descriptive correlational design analyzed the outcomes of a quality improvement project evaluating a turning intervention to prevent facility-acquired pressure injuries (Harmon et al., 2016). The study assessed a "turn team assignment" on pressure injury incidence in a surgical intensive care unit. Data were collected on cueing to turn, concurrent turning, independent turning in lieu of the cue, staff support, and possible barriers to turning and repositioning. Pressure injuries declined from 24.9% to 16.8% over 12 months. There was an association between verbal cueing and turning ($r = 0.82$; $p < .05$). A turn team using verbal cueing appears to be an effective intervention that decreases pressure injury occurrence. In another study the investigators implemented a multi-component intervention that included pressure-reducing beds; nutritional support; mandatory 2-hour change of posture; turning clocks; early surgical intervention; spot checks by the wound care nurse; and education to patients and caregivers (Lam et al., 2018). Over a 3-year period the incidence of hospital-acquired pressure injuries at the institution was initially 1.36%, which decreased to 0.98% in year 2 and to 0.39% in year 3 ($p = .002$).

Literature

Reading and critiquing the literature are other mechanisms for identifying gaps in what is known and not known in clinical practice. For example, in a randomized controlled trial, the investigators assessed the effectiveness of auricular acupressure on sleep in patients with breast cancer undergoing chemotherapy (Yoon & Park, 2019). Participants were randomized to auricular pressure on specific acupoints beneficial for sleep or a control group that received placebo auricular pressure on points not traditionally associated with improving sleep for 6 weeks. The quality of sleep was significant between the experimental and control groups ($F = 4.152$, $p = .048$). There were no significant differences in total sleep time, sleep efficiency, sleep latency, or number of times awakened during sleep. This study shows a non-pharmacological treatment for symptoms. However, more research is needed to determine if different doses produce different effects, how long the effects last, and can these results be translated to other disorders?

Regulatory Agencies

Regulatory agencies such as The Joint Commission (TJC) and the Centers for Medicare & Medicaid Services (CMS) are rich sources for research ideas (TJC, 2019). TJC collaborated with the American Heart Association and the American College of Cardiology to develop performance measures, or core measure sets, for acute myocardial infarction (AMI). These measures specify evidence-based interventions necessary to provide patients with quality care. These measures include such interventions as smoking-cessation education. Nursing is in an excellent position to test interventions that assist patients in their smoking-cessation efforts. Examples of other measures include pneumonia, stroke, and venous thromboembolism.

Technology

Mobile technology continues to expand in healthcare. In a randomized controlled trial of patients with irritable bowel syndrome, participants were randomized to telephone or web-based therapy or treatment as usual (Cook et al., 2019). Those in the treatment group received information on healthy eating patterns, managing stress, and reducing symptom severity. The telephone intervention received a self-help manual and 8 hours of telephone therapist support. The web-based participants received online access to an interactive website and 2.5 hours of telephone therapist support. All groups had a reduction of symptoms at 1 year. The telephone group had 84% greater adherence rates than the other groups. Conclusions and implications of this study show that traditional face-to-face cognitive behavioral therapy, web, and telephone delivered therapy still require trained therapist input. These results show the need to design and test technology that is easily deployed and used by providers and patients.

New Diagnoses

Discoveries in healthcare are frequent, including new diagnoses, especially because of research in genetics. As new syndromes are defined and new diseases and diagnoses are discovered, there will be an increasing need for research in these areas. Infectious diseases are continuing to emerge and evolve. For example, the Zika virus is spreading in the United States and can cause microcephaly and severe fetal brain defects (Baud et al., 2017). Zika is also associated with pregnancy loss and can cause issues with the infant's eyes and deformities of the joints. We do not know the long-term effects of the Zika virus, and currently there is no vaccine. Nursing can play a key role in assisting in the care of these infants and their families, which is a topic for investigation.

An example of a new genetic syndrome is a microdeletion of 15q13.3, which causes intellectual disabilities, epilepsy, and facial and digital dysmorphisms (Hassfurther et al., 2015). Although this disorder is thought to affect about three out of 1,000 individuals with intellectual disabilities, there is a need for further investigation to determine the impact of this syndrome on patients and their caregivers. This again gives nursing an excellent opportunity to investigate the impact of this syndrome and possible interventions to improve patient care.

Similarly, researchers discovered a new genetic syndrome, which revealed a microduplication of chromosome 22q11.2 in patients previously diagnosed with DiGeorge anomaly/velocardio-facial syndrome (DG/VCFS; Radio et al., 2016). The phenotypic features of this new syndrome are widely spaced eyes and superior placement of the eyebrows, with increased distance from the eyebrow to upper eyelid crease, downslanting palpebral fissures, and a long narrow face. These features are different from DG/VCFS, which led researchers to conclude that this is a new syndrome. Nursing would be especially poised to conduct research to improve the care and lives of these patients and their families.

Social Media

Social media represents another avenue for generating ideas for investigation. Examples of social media include Facebook, Twitter, and blogs. In a recent study, social media was used as a means to improve influenza vaccination rates at a private college (Monn, 2016). In addition to provider education and announcement of immunization clinics, a Facebook college web portal was used to increase immunization rates by announcing the time and place of the vaccination clinicals and distributing three wellness articles via the portal. Results of this strategy showed a 226% increase in the number of students vaccinated compared to previous years.

In a randomized controlled trial investigators aimed to determine the effectiveness of Facebook alone or with text messaging to encourage optimal calcium intake (Rouf et al., 2020). Results showed that at the end of the program there was no increase in milk consumption (odds ratio [OR] 1.51, 95% CI 0.61–3.75 Facebook; OR 1.77, 95% CI 0.74-4.24 Facebook plus text messages; $p = .41$) or calcium-rich foods ($p = .57$). Knowledge improvement did improve in the Facebook plus text message group ($p < .001$). Using social media shows promise in providing health education and promoting health and may be used in future research.

Sentinel Events

Unfortunately, untoward or sentinel events sometimes occur. TJC defines a sentinel event as "an unexpected occurrence involving death or serious physical or psychological injury, or the risk thereof. Serious injury specifically includes loss of limb or function" (TJC, 2019). These events may be related to system problems, knowledge deficits, equipment malfunction, or a variety of other related problems. Some examples of sentinel events captured by TJC's sentinel database in 2019 included delays in treatment; falls; postoperative complications; suicide; and wrong patient, wrong site, and wrong procedure. Nurses are well poised to study how these important occurrences happen and to develop effective interventions for prevention.

While the nursing bedside report has been suggested as a way to enhance patient safety, this is an example where little is known through research if this actually does keep patients safer. One study aimed to describe how bedside nurses can use bedside shift reports to keep patients safe (Groves et al., 2016). In this qualitative study it was found that the nursing bedside report is a storytelling mechanism at shift change that allows nurses to identify any patient risks that may potentially cause harm. The researchers speculated that shift report can actually prevent errors and improve patient safety, but more research is needed.

Legislative Issues

Other opportunities for nursing research are related to legislative and health policy issues. Nursing is an integral part of health policy discussions and should conduct research on legislative issues in order to promote and protect the public's health. There have been several states that have legalized recreational marijuana; however, we know little about changes in marijuana use and cannabis use disorder after recreational marijuana legalization. Investigators aimed to examine the associations between recreational marijuana legalization enactment and changes in marijuana use, frequent use, and cannabis use disorder in the United States between 2008 and 2016 (Cerdá et al., 2019). Results showed that among participants between 12 to 17 years, past-year cannabis use disorder increased from 2.2% to 2.7% after recreational marijuana legalization enactment, a 25% higher increase than that for the same age group in states that did not enact recreational marijuana legalization (OR, 1.25; 95% CI, 1.01–1.55). Therefore, more research is needed to assess how these increases occur and to identify subpopulations that may be especially vulnerable.

There have been several states that have implemented opioid prescribing mandates to help with the opioid epidemic. In 2016 Rhode Island passed a law that limited Rhode Island prescribers to a maximum of 30 mg equivalents per day, 20 total doses, or a total of 150 mg equivalents in the first opioid prescription for opioid-naïve patients. The legislation went into effect in April 2017. One study aimed to evaluate the prescribing opioids after orthopedic trauma before and after implementing opioid-limiting mandates (Reid et al., 2019). The post-law patients received less opioids (363.4 vs. 173.6 MMEs, $p < 0.001$) in the first postoperative prescription. They also received less cumulative levels of opioids during the 30-day postoperative period (677.4 vs. 481.7 MMEs, $p < 0.001$). Results of this show that opioid legislation reduces opioid prescriptions. More research is needed in this area especially as other states implement their own legislation. Additionally, research on the impact of patient care should be conducted to determine if there are any untoward consequences such as inadequate pain control for patients.

BACKGROUND

An exhaustive review of the literature is imperative to determine what is currently known about the subject or phenomenon. Well-written studies provide insight into the implications of the findings and suggestions for future research or directions for inquiry. A review of studies related to the topic helps to summarize the findings and thereby helps the reader to develop a sense of where the next inquiry should begin. The review also gives ideas on possible research designs, along with potential leads for experts or consultants for the study. The review should give a good suggestion of theories or conceptual models that have been applied or should allude to possible conceptual frameworks for future studies.

The background section of the proposal for the study should give a concise overview of the body of science under investigation and how the study contributes to knowledge development. The background should connect the literature and define the domains of the concepts under investigation. An explanation of how the literature search was conducted should also be provided. Common research databases include the Cumulative Index to Nursing and Allied Health Literature (CINAHL) and Medical Literature Analysis and Retrieval System Online (MEDLINE). CINAHL is primarily used by nurse scientists, but it is important not to limit oneself to only one research database as a tool for searches. MEDLINE is a search engine for biomedical research. It is important to use multiple databases when exploring a topic. Limiting oneself to one database may mean that one does not find all available research on the topic. Research fields for nursing overlap with those of other disciplines, such as medicine, pharmacy, physical therapy, nutrition, and psychology.

When searching for relevant studies, one should employ a variety of methods, including searches by subject, keywords, and author. A subject search is a broad search in which one is looking for general information on a topic. This may be a good starting point when determining the breadth of a particular topic or phenomenon. Depending on the topic, a subject search may reveal literally thousands of papers. At this point, it can be helpful to narrow the topic area by using limits. These limits may include gender, race, human subjects, or other areas. Selecting a particular article may be helpful to determine Medical Subject Heading (MeSH) terms as created by the National Library of Medicine (NLM). These terms are helpful in finding other studies on the topic once a good study has been found to provide an exhaustive search on a particular topic. Chapter 2, on general searching, includes ways of maximizing the effectiveness of the literature search.

When reviewing the literature, one should review primary, not secondary, sources; that is, publications written by those who conducted the study, not publications that report on and summarize studies conducted by others. Reviewing primary sources allows the reviewer to determine the validity of the study rather than relying on another person's interpretation of the study. An exception to this recommendation is the systematic review, the purpose of which is to summarize all the research on a topic to determine the outcome across a number of studies, populations, and clinical settings.

SIGNIFICANCE

Determining the significance of a study is vital to deciding whether the topic is worthy of investigation. Is the topic timely? Will the topic add significant information to a body of knowledge? Does it provide new information, or does it help confirm previous results by replicating a previously done study? Is the study innovative? Does it describe a new phenomenon or a new way of studying a problem? On the one hand, the section on significance should point out the limited amount of information currently available or determine whether no information is currently published. On the other hand, the section on significance may indicate that there is conflicting evidence on the topic and that further investigation is needed to clarify what is known or unknown. The significance of a study may be related to testing a theory or furthering scientists' understanding of how the research will help a particular patient population. Following are examples of how the significance of a study may be articulated.

Catheter-associated urinary tract infection (CAUTI) and catheter blockage are serious and significant challenges for patients living with long-term indwelling catheters. CAUTI and catheter blockages can be painful and interfere with normal daily activities. Researchers aimed to determine whether self-management strategies that focused on fluid intake could decrease CAUTI and/or catheter blockages (Wilde et al., 2016). This intervention, self-management of fluid intake, was found to have a positive effect on fluid intake, and fluid intake self-management predicted less frequent catheter blockages. This intervention has significant implications for decreasing costs related to CAUTI and/or catheter blockages and improving patients' lives.

Elderly patients who receive home healthcare may be at increased risk of mental health disorders that can impact morbidity, mortality, and recovery from illness. Therefore, this is a significant health issue that needs to be studied. Researchers sought to describe the prevalence and characteristics of mental health disorders in elderly adults in the United States (Wang et al., 2016). Forty percent of the elderly receiving home health had a health disorder, of which 28% had depression and 19% had anxiety. Those factors associated with mental health disorders were younger age, female, smoker, frailty, living alone, cognitively impaired, poor health status, and recent hospitalization. These data show the significance of screening for mental health disorders, especially anxiety and depression in older adults. This may have implications for healthcare costs and improving morbidity and mortality in this population.

■ PURPOSE, OBJECTIVES, AND AIMS

Once researchers have identified a topic of interest and conducted a thorough review of the literature, they can define the study further by developing its purpose, objectives, and specific aims. The purpose statement of a study is a statement of the essence of what the investigators are attempting to explore. The statement generally begins with, "The purpose of this study…." This statement will guide the development of the research project by denoting what the focus of the research is. Following is an example of a purpose statement. In a qualitative study investigators stated: "The purpose of this study was to explore the experiences and support needs of adult patients living with rheumatoid arthritis (RA) in Singapore" (Poh et al., 2017).

In another study, researchers stated: "The purpose of this study is to analyze mean differences in weekly time spent engaging in physical activity by level of perceived environmental resources, for adults with diagnosed coronary heart disease, at 3 and 6 months following graduation from cardiac rehabilitation" (Perez et al., 2016).

Another example of a purpose statement is: "The purpose of this study was to better understand whether and how readiness for hospital discharge varies by personal characteristics, including health literacy" (Wallace et al., 2016).

The objectives of a study are very closely related to the purpose. Although some researchers may use the terms *purpose* and *objectives* interchangeably, they are distinct components in the research protocol. Objectives are components of the study that can be measured. Although the objectives should flow from the purpose statement and are closely related to it, they are distinctly different. One study stated the objective of the study was "to compare equine-assisted therapy to exercise education on pain, range of motion, and quality of life in adults and older adults with arthritis" (White-Lewis et al., 2019). This objective helped identify the purpose of the study to compare the effects of an equine-assisted therapy intervention compared with an exercise educa-tion attention-control intervention on pain and mobility in the hips, knees, shoulders, and backs of adults with arthritis.

Similarly, the aim of a study and its purpose can be interchangeable. Although the purpose is the essence of what is being studied, the aim is more aligned with the goal of the study or what the researchers want to accomplish. Generally, the aim of the study is contained in a statement that begins like this: "The aim of this study...." In one study, the investigators aimed to increase non-supervised walking in patients with fibromyalgia (Peñacoba et al., 2017). They specifically outlined the following aims: (a) to analyze the prevalence of four walking beliefs in a sample of women with fibromyalgia; (b) to examine how much each one of those beliefs is associated with certain sociodemographic, clinical, comorbidity, and symptom variables; and (c) to evaluate whether the presence of these beliefs is associated with walking, according to clinical guidelines for this population.

The decision whether to use a purpose statement or to present an aim may be based on the personal preference of the researcher, the audience that the researcher is presenting to, or the funding agency. For example, thesis or dissertation committees may require specific wording related to aims in a research proposal or protocol. When writing for publication in journals, one may encounter similar requirements. When one is writing a grant proposal, one may be required to provide a list of objectives for the research project. Whatever the requirements, the researcher will need to state in some form the essence of the project and what the researcher wants to accomplish.

■ RESEARCH QUESTIONS

Once the topic of inquiry has been identified and the literature review conducted, the researcher can write the research questions. Research questions are interrogatives that bring out what is being stud-ied specifically. Not all studies have specific research questions; some studies may have a hypothesis or hypotheses, which are discussed in the next section. The research questions contain the indepen-dent variable (IV) and dependent variable (DV), which are also discussed in the "Variables" section of this chapter. Another important factor related to research questions is the way the question is stated. The wording of the question in a quantitative study drives the statistical analysis.

Research questions are often restatements of the purpose. For example, in a qualitative study the researchers' purpose was to explore the experiences and support needs of adult patients living with RA in Singapore (Poh et al., 2017). They identified two research questions. The first research question was "What are the experiences of patients living with RA?" and the second question was "What type of support needs do RA patients require or desire?" (Poh et al., 2017). In another study, the purpose was to investigate the effect of acupressure on quality of life of female nurses with chronic back pain (Najafabadi et al., 2019). The research question pertaining to the study was: What is the effect of acupressure on quality of life in female nurses with chronic back pain? Some researchers may decide to use hypotheses instead of research questions; these are discussed in the following section.

■ HYPOTHESES

A hypothesis is a prediction of outcomes between one or more variable(s) (Polit & Beck, 2020). Generally, in order to state a hypothesis, a researcher relies on previous literature or a theoretical framework to support the relationship between variables. Hypotheses can be directional, nondirectional, or null.

A directional hypothesis not only predicts the relationship between one or more variables but also states the direction of the relationship. Researchers were interested to determine if self-care using motivational interviewing in multimorbid heart failure patients would decrease hospital readmission rates and mortality (Riegel et al., 2016). The directional hypothesis was that patients with heart failure who were assigned to the motivational interviewing intervention would experience fewer readmissions than those assigned to the control group (Riegel et al., 2016). In this hypothesis, those who receive the motivational interviewing will have decreased hospital readmissions. Usually, theory or past findings enable the prediction. In this particular study their prior research determined the direction of their hypothesis.

In another study the researchers aimed to test the efficacy of a meridian cuffing exercise on functional fitness and cardiopulmonary functioning in older adults (Tung et al., 2020). Meridians in Chinese medicine are the pathways in the body where energy flows. Merdian cuffing unblocks these pathways via the Healthy Beat Acupunch (HBA). The HBA involves a serious of movements of the hands and feet in a rhythmic fashion. The investigators tested this directional hypotheses: after 6 months of the HBA regimen, the functional fitness and cardiopulmonary functioning would be significantly improved compared to baseline.

In contrast, a nondirectional hypothesis does not predict the direction of the relationship. An example of a nondirectional hypothesis is from investigators who wanted to better understand how readiness for hospital discharge varies by personal characteristics, including health literacy. The hypothesis was "patient characteristics, including patient health literacy, are associated with patient- and nurse-perceived readiness for hospital discharge" (Wallace et al., 2016). The investigators stated that there would be a relationship between the variables, but did not state the direction.

A null hypothesis or statistical hypothesis is a statement that predicts that there is no relationship between variables (Polit & Beck, 2020). The null hypothesis is not always explicitly written but can be derived from the hypotheses that are stated. The null hypothesis is what is accepted or rejected in relation to statistical procedures. A study hypothesized that those patients with higher levels of depressive symptoms would have poorer levels of cardiovascular health factors (McCarthy et al., 2019). The null hypothesis would be that those patients with higher levels of depressive symptoms will not have poor levels of cardiovascular health factors. In another study investigators hypothesized that self-efficacy for the human papillomavirus (HPV) vaccination would mediate the relationships between social-cognitive factors and intention to receive the HPV vaccine (Christy et al., 2019). The null hypothesis would be that self-efficacy for the HPV vaccination would not mediate the relationships between social-cognitive factors and intention to receive the HPV vaccine.

■ VARIABLES

A research question is written in terms of the dependent variables (DVs), also known as the observed outcome, and the independent variables (IVs), or the variable(s) hypothesized or thought to produce the DV. DV values depend on the IVs. Variables are operationally defined by what is measured, how the indicators are measured, and how the values are interpreted. In other words, an operational definition characterizes how the variable is measured.

Variables are classified according to the level or scale of measurement; the four scales are nominal, ordinal, interval, and ratio (NOIR). Knowing the level or scale of measurement provides the necessary information for readers to interpret the data from that variable. Certain statistical analyses are used only for data measured at certain measurement levels. The level of measurement of the IV, the question being asked, and the number of groups of the DV are key determinants for selecting the correct statistical test to analyze the research study data. In general, it is desirable to have a higher level of measurement (e.g., interval or ratio) than to use a lower one (e.g., nominal or ordinal). When in doubt as to the level of measurement, the rule of thumb is to treat the variable at the highest level of measurement that can be justified, that is, to use an interval rather than an ordinal scale and an ordinal scale rather than a nominal one. Statistics for higher levels of measurement are more powerful at detecting differences in the research data. Once the statistical test is determined, the sample size can be calculated.

■ SUMMARY

In summary, identifying a focus of study can be challenging. There are multiple sources for initially determining what to study, including, but not limited to, the literature and clinically derived questions. A thorough search of the literature will help determine what is already known on the subject and further define what the topic will be. Once the literature has been scrutinized, the purpose or aim of the study can be delineated. In conjunction with the purpose, research questions and/or hypotheses are then formulated. The hypothesis describes a relationship between the IV and the DV. The IVs and DVs determine the statistical test to be performed once the number of groups in the study and the level of measurement (NOIR) have been determined.

SUGGESTED LEARNING ACTIVITIES

1. Suppose you are interested in determining how to manage dyspnea in patients with heart failure. Write down your strategy for determining what information is currently known and formulate a research question(s).

2. For the following research questions, write a directional, a nondirectional, and a null hypothesis:

   a. Does massage decrease anxiety in patients undergoing cardiac catheterization?

   b. Does mouth care in intubated adult patients decrease ventilator-associated pneumonia?

   c. Are maternal–infant bonding behaviors affected by the performance of initial newborn infant physical examination?

REFERENCES

Baud, D., Gubler, D. J., Schaub, B., Lanteri, M. C., & Musso, D. (2017). An update on Zika virus infection. *The Lancet, 390*(10107), 2099–2109. https://doi.org/10.1016/S0140-6736(17)31450-2

Cerdá, M., Mauro, C., Hamilton, A., Levy, N. S., Santaella-Tenorio, J., Hasin, D., Wall, M. M., Keyes, K. M., & Martins, S. S. (2019). Association between recreational marijuana legalization in the United States and changes in marijuana use and cannabis use disorder from 2008 to 2016. *JAMA Psychiatry, 77*(2), 168. https://doi.org/10.1001/jamapsychiatry.2019.3254

Christy, S. M., Winger, J. G., & Mosher, C. E. (2019). Does self-efficacy mediate the relationships between social-cognitive factors and intentions to receive HPV vaccination among young women? *Clinical Nursing Research, 28*(6), 708–725. https://doi.org/10.1177/1054773817741590

Cook, R., Davidson, P., & Martin, R. (2019). Telephone or Internet delivered talking therapy can alleviate irritable bowel symptoms. *BMJ, 367*, l4962. https://doi.org/10.1136/bmj.l4962

Groves, P. S., Manges, K. A., & Scott-Cawiezell, J. (2016). Handing off safety at the bedside. *Clinical Nursing Research, 25*(5), 473–493. https://doi.org/10.1177/1054773816630535

Harmon, L. C., Grobbel, C., & Palleschi, M. (2016). Reducing pressure injury incidence using a turn team assignment. *Journal of Wound, Ostomy and Continence Nursing, 43*(5), 477–482. https://doi.org/10.1097/WON.0000000000000258

Hassfurther, A., Komini, E., Fischer, J., & Leipoldt, M. (2015). Clinical and genetic heterogeneity of the 15q13. 3 microdeletion syndrome. *Molecular Syndromology, 6*(5), 222–228. https://doi.org/10.1159/000443343

Jocelyn Chew, H. S., Thiara, E., Lopez, V., & Shorey, S. (2018). Turning frequency in adult bedridden patients to prevent hospital-acquired pressure ulcer: A scoping review. *International wound journal, 15*(2), 225–236. https://doi.org/10.1111/iwj.12855

Lam, C., Elkbuli, A., Benson, B., Young, E., Morejon, O., Boneva, D., Hai, S., & McKenney, M. (2018). Implementing a novel guideline to prevent hospital-acquired pressure ulcers in a trauma population: A patient-safety approach. *Journal of the American College of Surgeons, 226*(6), 1122–1127. https://doi.org/10.1016/j.jamcollsurg.2018.03.027

McCarthy, M. M., Whittemore, R., Gholson, G., & Grey, M. (2019). Diabetes distress, depressive symptoms, and cardiovascular health in adults with type 1 diabetes. *Nursing Research, 68*(6), 445–452. https://doi.org/10.1097/NNR.0000000000000387

Monn, J. L. (2016). An evidence-based project to improve influenza immunization uptake. *The Journal for Nurse Practitioners, 12*(4), e159–e162. https://doi.org/10.1016/j.nurpra.2015.11.030

Najafabadi, M. M., Ghafari, S., Nazari, F., & Valiani, M. (2019). The effect of acupressure on quality of life among female nurses with chronic back pain. *Applied Nursing Research, 51*, 151175. https://doi.org/10.1016/j.apnr.2019.05.020

Peñacoba, C., Pastor, M.-Á., López-Roig, S., Velasco, L., & Lledo, A. (2017). Walking Beliefs in women with fibromyalgia: clinical profile and impact on walking behavior. *Clinical Nursing Research, 26*(5), 632–650. https://doi.org/10.1177/1054773816646339

Perez, A., Fleury, J., & Belyea, M. (2016). Environmental resources in maintenance of physical activity 6 months following cardiac rehabilitation. *Clinical Nursing Research, 25*(4), 391–409. https://doi.org/10.1177/1054773815627277

Poh, L. W., He, H.-G., Chan, W. C. S., Lee, C. S. C., Lahiri, M., Mak, A., & Cheung, P. P. (2017). Experiences of patients with rheumatoid arthritis: A qualitative study. *Clinical Nursing Research, 26*(3), 373–393. https://doi.org/10.1177/1054773816629897

Polit, D. F., & Beck, C. T. (2020). *Nursing research: Generating and assessing evidence for nursing practice* (11th ed.). Lippincott Williams & Wilkins.

Radio, F. C., Digilio, M. C., Capolino, R., Dentici, M. L., Unolt, M., Alesi, V., Novelli, A., Marino, B., & Dallapiccola, B. (2016). Sprengel anomaly in deletion 22q11. 2 (DiGeorge/velo–cardio–facial) syndrome. *American Journal of Medical Genetics Part A, 170*(3), 661–664. https://doi.org/10.1002/ajmg.a.37503

Reid, D. B., Shah, K. N., Shapiro, B. H., Ruddell, J. H., Evans, A. R., Hayda, R. A., Akelman, E., & Daniels, A. H. (2019). Opioid-limiting legislation associated with reduced postoperative prescribing following surgery for traumatic orthopaedic injuries. *Journal of Orthopaedic Trauma, 34*(4), e114–e120. https://doi.org/10.1097/BOT.0000000000001673

Riegel, B., Masterson Creber, R., Hill, J., Chittams, J., & Hoke, L. (2016). Effectiveness of motivational interviewing in decreasing hospital readmission in adults with heart failure and multimorbidity. *Clinical Nursing Research, 25*(4), 362–377. https://doi.org/10.1177/1054773815623252

Rouf, A., Nour, M., & Allman-Farinelli, M. (2020). Improving calcium knowledge and intake in young adults via social media and text messages: Randomized controlled trial. *JMIR Mhealth Uhealth, 8*(2), e16499. https://doi.org/10.2196/16499

The Joint Commission (Producer). (2019). *Patient safety systems: Comprehensive accreditation manual for hospitals.* https://www.jointcommission.org/assets/1/18/CAMH_04a_PS.pdf

Tung, H.-T., Lai, C.-C., Chen, K.-M., & Tsai, H.-Y. (2020). Meridian cuffing exercises improved functional fitness and cardiopulmonary functioning of community older adults. *Clinical Nursing Research, 29*(1), 37–47. https://doi.org/10.1177/1054773818768021

Ueblacker, P., Haensel, L., & Mueller-Wohlfahrt, H.-W. (2016). Treatment of muscle injuries in football. *Journal of Sports Sciences, 34*(24), 2329–2337. https://doi.org/10.1080/02640414.2016.1252849

Wallace, A. S., Perkhounkova, Y., Bohr, N. L., & Chung, S. J. (2016). Readiness for hospital discharge, health literacy, and social living status. *Clinical Nursing Research, 25*(5), 494–511. https://doi.org/10.1177/1054773815624380

Wang, J., Kearney, J. A., Jia, H., & Shang, J. (2016). Mental health disorders in elderly people receiving home care: Prevalence and correlates in the national U.S. population. *Nursing Research, 65*(2), 107–116. https://doi.org/10.1097/NNR.0000000000000147

White-Lewis, S., Johnson, R., Ye, S., & Russell, C. (2019). An equine-assisted therapy intervention to improve pain, range of motion, and quality of life in adults and older adults with arthritis: A randomized controlled trial. *Applied Nursing Research, 49*, 5–12. https://doi.org/10.1016/j.apnr.2019.07.002

Wilde, M. H., Crean, H. F., McMahon, J. M., McDonald, M. V., Tang, W., Brasch, J., Fairbanks, E., Shah, S., & Zhang, F. (2016). Testing a model of self-management of fluid intake in community-residing long-term indwelling urinary catheter users. *Nursing research, 65*(2), 97. https://doi.org/10.1097/NNR.0000000000000140

Yoon, H. G., & Park, H. (2019). The effect of auricular acupressure on sleep in breast cancer patients undergoing chemotherapy: A single-blind, randomized controlled trial. *Applied Nursing Research, 48*, 45–51. https://doi.org/10.1016/j.apnr.2019.05.009

CONCEPTUAL AND THEORETICAL FRAMEWORKS

MARY E. JOHNSON

▤ INTRODUCTION

Advanced practice registered nurses (APRNs) may be involved in evidence-based practice (EBP), research, quality improvement (QI), and program evaluation projects (Cook & Lowe, 2012; Oberleitner, 2019; Raines, 2012). Although the purpose for each of these endeavors is different, the same methods can be used by the APRN to guide the project and expand nursing knowledge. Conceptual and theoretical frameworks provide important foundations for research, EBP, QI and program evaluation. They offer the APRN a structure for designing, implementing, and evaluating research and evidence-based and QI projects; designing and implementing program evaluation; interpreting the findings from these investigations; and designing interventions. Figure 8.1 depicts the relationship among conceptual and theoretical frameworks, research, QI, and program evaluation.

Conceptual and theoretical frameworks can be used to identify variables for study (e.g., Kamp et al., 2019; Kelley & Lowe, 2018; Lyttle et al., 2018), design measurement tools (e.g., Cleverley et al., 2018; Testa, 2017), and develop interventions (e.g., Lucas et al., 2019), which can then be tested through research (e.g., Lucas et al., 2019). Conceptual and theoretical frameworks can also be used to guide implementation of evidence-based interventions (e.g., Harvey & Kitson, 2016; Lazenby et al., 2019) and the evaluation of new or existing programs (e.g., Chao et al., 2015; Liska et al., 2018). Without a conceptual or theoretical framework, research, EBP, QI, and program evaluation projects lack coherence not only within the project, but also in relation to previous knowledge about a given topic.

The APRN who would like to use a theoretical or conceptual framework in practice-focused scholarship (American Association of Colleges of Nursing [AACN], 2015) is challenged with deciding which framework is most appropriate. Since there are many frameworks from which to choose (i.e., nursing grand theories, middle-range theories, and situation-specific theories; learning, leadership and management theories; and theories from the sociological, behavioral, and biomedical sciences; McEwen & Wills, 2019), the APRN must be able to evaluate the appropriateness and applicability of the theoretical or conceptual framework. This chapter includes a discussion of the relationships among theories, theoretical/conceptual frameworks, practice, and research; the characteristics of theory; and the criteria for evaluating a theory and its use in research, EBP, QI, and program evaluation.

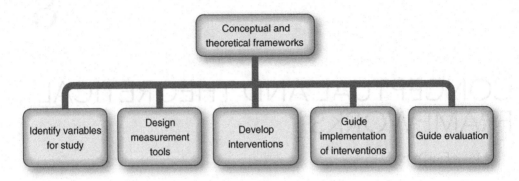

FIGURE 8.1 The roles of conceptual and theoretical frameworks.

▪ THEORETICAL AND CONCEPTUAL FRAMEWORKS

There has been considerable debate about the definition of the different terms—theory, theoretical framework, and conceptual framework, with Risjord (2019) proposing that "model" be used instead of "theory" for middle-range theories. The consensus among authors is that theoretical and conceptual frameworks are more abstract than theories. Conceptual frameworks link concepts in meaningful ways but are usually not considered to be as fully developed as theoretical frameworks. This leads some to assert that the development of conceptual frameworks is a necessary step in the development of theories (Meleis, 2018). Other nurse theorists view conceptual frameworks as analogous to grand theories (McEwen, 2019b). Still others use the terms interchangeably (Meleis, 2018). In the end, Meleis proposes that the debate over the meaning of these terms is an academic issue of "semantics" (p. 123), which not only has led to confusion within the discipline, but also has delayed progress in the development of theories useful to research and practice. Meleis suggests that the use of the term "theory" is sufficient.

A theory (or theoretical framework) is a "set of logically interrelated concepts, statements, propositions, and definitions" (McEwen, 2019a, p. 28), which presents a systematic view of a phenomenon from which one may ask questions and specify relations among variables in order to describe, explain, and/or predict phenomena and prescribe actions (McEwen, 2019a; Peterson & Bredow, 2017). Theories help define and differentiate a discipline, explain events, structure, and organize knowledge, guide APRNs by identifying the goals and outcomes of practice, and contribute to a rational practice that questions and validates intuition and assumptions.

Over time, there has been considerable debate about whether nursing should only use theories developed by and for nursing or could also use theories that were developed in other disciplines. The rationale for the former is that theories help define the boundaries of a discipline. In other words, theories developed by and for nurses articulate the purpose of nursing and identify nursing interventions and research that use theories developed within nursing that contribute to the development of nursing knowledge. The widespread use of non-nursing theories in research and practice lends support to the assertion that the origin of the theory is less important than the theory's pragmatic utility. Those who find the use of theories developed in disciplines other than nursing (borrowed theories) acceptable assert that knowledge is not confined to a particular discipline, but rather is available to all. Moreover, in this day of interdisciplinary research and practice, knowledge and theories are shared within a team; theories provide a common language to frame research and practice. As an applied discipline, nurses use knowledge from the physical and social sciences. Likewise, theories developed within nursing may also contain concepts shared by other disciplines. In other words, the boundaries that separate disciplines may not be rigid and impenetrable. When theories from other disciplines are used in research or practice, they should be consistent with a nursing perspective, and regardless of the term used or whether nursing or borrowed theories are employed, a theory must be meaningful and relevant (McEwen & Wills, 2019).

■ CLASSIFICATION OF THEORIES

There are two major ways of classifying theories. The first is by scope and the second is by purpose (McEwen, 2019b). This section focuses on these two major classifications.

Scope

Scope refers to the breadth of phenomena encompassed by the theory and is correlated with the degree of theoretical abstractness. In terms of scope, a theory may be classified as grand, middle-range, or practice/situation specific. Grand theories focus on broad areas of a discipline. In nursing, the grand theories explain phenomena of central concern to nursing, such as the meta-paradigm concepts of person, health, nursing, and environment. Grand theories incorporate highly abstract concepts that often lack operational definitions. Therefore, the propositions are not considered to be accessible to testing (McEwen, 2019b). However, there is evidence that grand theories are used as frameworks for nursing research (Im & Chang, 2012). Some examples include the Neuman Systems Model (Yarcheski et al., 2010), Watson's Theory of Human Caring (Gillespie et al., 2012), and Orem's Self-Care Theory (Peters & Templin, 2010).

Middle-range theories are more focused and limited in scope than grand theories. Middle-range theories encompass a limited number of concepts that tend to be more concrete than those found in grand theories. Thus, the concepts can usually be operationally defined. The theoretical properties are more specific and accessible to testing than those found in grand theories (McEwen, 2019b). There has been a significant growth in the development of middle-range theories (Peterson & Bredow, 2017). One reason may be their applicability to both research and practice. One theory that has been used in research and practice is the Transitions Theory (e.g., Stixrood, 2019). Briefly, Meleis and colleagues describe the types and properties of transitions people experience, the conditions that facilitate or inhibit movement through transitions, process and outcome indicators, and nursing interventions (Meleis et al., 2000).

Middle-range theories may be developed in several ways (Im, 2018; Liehr & Smith, 2017; Peterson & Bredow, 2017). They may be developed from grand theories (e.g., Pickett et al., 2014), non-nursing theories (e.g., Pender et al., 2011), reviews of the literature (e.g., Spratling & Weaver, 2012), research (e.g., Baydoun et al., 2018; Walter, 2017), a combination of research and literature reviews (e.g., Siaki et al., 2013), or clinical practice (Liehr & Smith, 2017; Peterson & Bredow, 2017). For example, a theory of weight management was developed from Orem's Theory of Self-Care (Pickett et al., 2014). Major components of this middle-range theory of weight management are weight management contextual factors, weight management agency, and weight management behaviors Spratling and Weaver (2012) developed a theoretical framework of resilience in medically fragile adolescents from reviews of the risk and resilience literature in this population. Sanford et al. (2011) developed a theoretical model of decision-making in heart failure from their grounded theory study of the ways caregivers of people with heart failure make decisions. Siaki et al. (2013) constructed a middle-range theory of risk perception from their synthesis of the literature and qualitative and quantitative data from a study of Samoan Pacific Islanders who were at high risk for developing diabetes and cardiovascular disease. Finally, Riegel et al. (2019) expanded their Middle-Range Theory of Self-Care of Chronic Illness by incorporating knowledge from models and theories related to illness symptoms.

Situation-specific or practice theories are the most focused and least complex theories. Situation-specific theories contain a limited number of concepts that are easily defined and explain a small aspect of reality. Situation-specific theories tend to be prescriptive (McEwen, 2019b). Unlike grand or middle-range theories that are generalizable across populations and situations, situation-specific theories are most applicable in specific contexts. Situation-specific theories are limited to specific populations or particular areas of interest and take sociopolitical, cultural, and historical contexts into consideration (Im & Meleis, 2018). Situation-specific theories may be developed from middle-range theories, research, and practice (Peterson & Bredow, 2017). An example of a situation-specific theory is the Asian Immigrant Menopausal Symptom (AIMS) theory (Im, 2010). This theory was developed using an integrative approach of literature synthesis and research and describes the process by which Asian women progress through menopause and the factors that influence how Asian women experience menopause and the symptoms they experience.

Purpose

Theories may be classified as descriptive, explanatory, predictive, or prescriptive. Descriptive theories describe or name concepts, properties, and dimensions, but do not explain how the concepts in the theory are related. Descriptive theories tend to be generated from descriptive research such as concept analyses, case studies, literature reviews, surveys, phenomenology, or grounded theory research (McEwen, 2019b). Explanatory theories describe associations or relationships among concepts or propositions, explaining how and why these concepts are related. These studies are developed using correlational research or in-depth reviews of the literature (McEwen, 2019b). Predictive theories describe the relationships between concepts and the conditions under which particular outcomes will occur. These theories are generated and tested using research designs such as pretest, posttest, quasi-experimental, and experimental designs (McEwen, 2019b). Prescriptive theories prescribe interventions that will achieve a particular outcome and are thought to be the highest level in theory development (McEwen, 2019b).

■ COMPONENTS OF THEORIES

Theoretical and conceptual frameworks are characterized by concepts that are organized in a coherent manner. Concepts are considered to be the building blocks of theories, and relational statements provide coherence within a theoretical framework. In other words, relational statements describe how concepts are related to each other. This section focuses on the components of theories.

Concepts

Concepts are mental representations of experiences, people or things, images, interactions, feelings, or attitudes (Chinn & Kramer, 2015). Concepts may be a single word, two words, or a phrase and are generally regarded as the building blocks of theories. Concepts may be classified as abstract or concrete, variable or nonvariable, and theoretically or operationally defined (Wills & McEwen, 2019). Concrete concepts are directly observable, whereas abstract concepts are inferred indirectly. Examples of concrete concepts include height or weight, which are directly measured. Highly abstract concepts such as pain, hope, or caring are more difficult to measure. The continuum from concrete to abstract is important to researchers because concepts that are more concrete are not only easier to measure, but are also less prone to measurement error than abstract concepts.

Variable concepts are those that exist on a continuum and are measured using an instrument that reflects the range of possibilities for the concept. For example, participants in a research study might be asked to rate pain on a scale from 1 to 10 or they might be given a validated self-report tool that indicates the degree to which the person feels hopeful or height or weight might be recorded. On the other hand, nonvariable concepts are discrete concepts for which there is no range of possibilities; for example, one is either pregnant or not pregnant and one is either male or female. In research, important discrete variables are often recorded as demographic data.

When researchers use a theory to underpin a research study, they decide which concepts are useful for the study and how they are going to measure the concept. For example, in their study of patient satisfaction with postpartum teaching methods (Wagner et al., 2011), the researchers used a middle-range theory, the Interaction Model of Client Health Behavior (IMCHB), as their theoretical framework. Although there are many concepts in the theory, the authors selected patient satisfaction as the main outcome concept. This concept was measured using a client satisfaction tool, which was determined to be both reliable and valid. This tool also contained measures of subconcepts that are central to the theory: affective support, health information, decisional control, professional competencies, and overall satisfaction with care.

Theoretical definitions of concepts indicate the meaning of a concept in the context of a theory. Theoretical definitions may be highly abstract, which entails the need for operational definitions and indicate how the concept is defined and measured in the context of a particular research study. Operational definitions form the bridge between the theoretical and the empirical worlds. Because of the close relationship between theoretical and operational definitions, they need to be consistent. In other words, the link among theoretical definitions, operational definitions, and the measurement tools should be clear and congruent. For example, the study by Alhusen et al. (2012) of the relationships between maternal–fetal attachment and health practices on neonatal outcomes in low-income urban women was grounded in two theoretical frameworks, Maternal Role Attainment (MRA) and an expansion of MRA, Becoming a Mother (BAM). Maternal–fetal attachment is a primary theoretical concept, which was defined as behaviors that indicate an affiliation between the woman and her unborn child. Maternal–fetal attachment was measured using the Maternal–Fetal Attachment Scale and although it was not directly stated, one can infer that maternal–fetal attachment was operationalized as the score on the Maternal–Fetal Attachment Scale.

Relational Statements

Relational statements describe the direction, shape, strength, symmetry, sequencing, probability of occurrence, necessity, and sufficiency of concepts within a theory (Polit & Beck, 2017). Understanding and articulating relational statements are important because these statements can form the basis for the hypotheses in research studies. Further testing will confirm the accuracy of these relational statements and will also determine the strength of the relationship and whether the nature of the relationships among concepts is positive or negative, linear or curvilinear, or symmetrical or asymmetrical. Positive relationships mean that as the strength or volume of one concept changes, the strength or volume of another concept will change in a similar direction. For example, if the number of calories one consumes increases, one's weight will also increase. Negative relationships indicate that as the strength or volume of one concept changes, the strength or volume of another concept will change in the opposite direction. That is, a significant drop in blood pressure is often accompanied by an increase in heart rate.

In Mishel's Uncertainty Theory, which Jiang and He (2012) used as the framework for their study of the effects of an uncertainty management intervention on uncertainty, anxiety, depression, and quality of life in persons with chronic obstructive pulmonary disease (COPD), uncertainty increases when patients have a lack of information that is important to them. Also, when uncertainty increases because of exacerbations of symptoms, patients use behavioral strategies to manage the uncertainty. The authors proposed that their uncertainty intervention would decrease uncertainty experienced by those with COPD, which would consequently increase the participants' quality of life and decrease their depression and anxiety.

■ THEORY EVALUATION

Over time, multiple methods for describing and evaluating a theory have been proposed (Meleis, 2018; Peterson & Bredow, 2017). This section will focus on evaluating a theory for use in research (Peterson & Bredow, 2017) and evaluating theories for their use in published studies (Polit & Beck, 2017). Theory evaluation is an important step in evaluating the strength of a research study. Overall, when selecting a theory to frame research or other scholarly projects, the choice of theory should be clear and there should be a clear link among the theory, the research or project design, hypotheses, the measures used, and the interpretation of the findings.

When selecting a theory for use in research or other scholarly projects or reviewing a theory in a published research study, the theory should be evaluated for clarity and consistency. If an APRN wants to use a theory for research or practice, it is recommended that the investigator return to the theorist's original works.

Internal Criticism

Internal criticism refers to internal coherence of the theory's components. Questions the reviewer should ask regarding internal criticism pertain to the clarity, consistency, adequacy, logical development, and level of theory development (Peterson & Bredow, 2017).

- **Clarity:** Are the theory's main components clearly stated and easily understood?
- **Consistency:** Are definitions of the key concepts consistent? Is the use of terms, interpretations, principles, and methods consistent?
- **Adequacy:** Does the theory cover all that it purports to cover? Are there gaps? Does the theory require further development?
- **Logical Development:** Has the theory been logically developed over time? Are statements and conclusions well supported or are assumptions and premises unsubstantiated?
- **Level of Theory Development:** What is the stage of development of the theory? Is the theory consistent with the level of development (grand, middle, or situation specific)?

External Criticism

External criticism refers to the coherence between the theory and external factors such as the social context or nursing's meta-paradigm (Peterson & Bredow, 2017). Questions the reviewer should ask regarding external criticism pertain to the theory's relation to the real world, significance, scope, and complexity (Peterson & Bredow, 2017).

- **Reality Convergence:** Is the theory consistent with the reader's experience of the world of nursing? Do the assumptions seem logically coherent?
- **Utility:** Is the theory useful to the APRN in terms of explaining a phenomenon, guiding a project, or guiding interventions?
- **Significance:** To what extent does the theory address issues important to nurses? Will the findings from the study impact healthcare?
- **Discrimination:** Does the theory generate hypotheses that are not adequately addressed by other theories?
- **Scope:** Is the focus of the theory narrow enough to produce relational statements that are testable? Is the theory applicable to practice?
- **Complexity:** How complex is the theory? Is the theory parsimonious, using as few concepts as possible to explain it? Can the theory be easily understood?

When evaluating the use of a theory in a QI or evaluation project, a research study, or a published study, the following questions can be used to evaluate the use of the theory (Polit & Beck, 2017):

- *Determine the use of the theory.* Was a theory used to frame the study or project? If so, is the theory described in sufficient detail to make it understandable? If not, does the study or project lack coherence because of the lack of a theoretical or conceptual framework?
- *Appraise the logical structure of the theory.* Are the variables reflective of the major theoretical concepts? Are the conceptual definitions supported by the literature? Are the relational statements logical?
- *Evaluate the relationship between the theory and the methodology.* Are the conceptual and theoretical definitions consistent? Are the hypotheses, questions, or objectives consistent with the relational statements in the theory? Is the fit between the relational statements and research design appropriate?
- *Appraise the findings.* Are the findings interpreted in relation to the theory? Are the implications linked to the conceptual or theoretical framework?

THEORY/PRACTICE/RESEARCH

There is a cyclical relationship among theory, practice, and research in that theory can provide a framework for or be generated from research and provide a framework for or be generated from practice (McEwen & Wills, 2019; Meleis, 2018). Theory that is generated from practice may be validated through research and, based on the findings from research, modified for continued use in practice. Theory lends structure to practice by enabling the APRN to "see" what is happening in a particular way and directing the APRN toward improving practice through targeted interventions (Bartholomew & Mullen, 2011). Theories also enable clinicians to make sense of seemingly disparate pieces of clinical data and help identify areas for practice improvement.

For example, in the COPD study previously cited, Jiang and He (2012) found that their uncertainty intervention significantly decreased the uncertainty, anxiety, and depression and increased the quality of life experienced by persons with COPD. Thus, an APRN who works primarily with this population might be interested in implementing this intervention. However, the APRN should also be aware of limitations of the study. For example, the sample included people who had moderate to severe COPD for less than 2 years. The population also consisted of outpatients in China. Thus one can see that further research is needed to determine whether the intervention is effective with a wider range of the population. In other words, this intervention seems very promising, but the APRN who will use the findings in practice needs to ask whether it would also be effective with people who have had COPD longer than 2 years or who live in the United States or Europe. The need for further research does not preclude the use of the intervention in practice, but further research would potentially increase one's confidence that the intervention would produce positive outcomes.

■ SUMMARY

A theoretical or conceptual framework is constituted by concepts (words or terms) that represent abstract ideas, which are linked in a manner that represents the relationship between the concepts. The scope and purpose of the theory may vary. Theories might be grand, middle-range, or practice/situation specific. Theories are useful in describing, explaining, and predicting phenomena. Depending on the scope and purpose, the theory may provide only general guidelines for practice or may provide new knowledge suitable for specific guidelines (Fawcett & DeSanto-Madeya, 2012).

Theories comprise concepts and relational statements that indicate how the concepts are related to each other. When evaluating a theory for use in research or evaluating a theoretically grounded research study for use in practice, it is important to scrutinize whether the selected theory is congruent with the research design and whether the theory and the findings are useful and applicable to the APRN's particular practice setting.

SUGGESTED LEARNING ACTIVITIES

1. Debate whether nurses should only use theories developed within nursing or whether it is acceptable to use theories developed in other disciplines and used in research conducted by nurses.

2. Select an article that focuses on a clinical intervention that has been implemented as part of a research study or QI project. Identify the theory that was used to guide the study. Use the guidelines presented in this chapter to determine the fit between the focus of the study and the selected theory.

3. Select an article that focuses on program evaluation. Identify the theory that was used to guide the study. Use the guidelines presented in this chapter to determine the fit between the focus of the project and the selected theory.

4. Select a theory and illustrate how it can be used to describe, explain, or predict a phenomenon.

REFERENCES

Alhusen, J. L., Gross, D., Hayat, M. J., Woods, A. B., & Sharps, P. W. (2012). The influence of maternal-fetal attachment and health practices on neonatal outcomes in low-income, urban women. *Research in Nursing & Health, 35*(2), 112–120. https://doi.org/10.1002/nur.21464

American Association of Colleges of Nursing. (2015). *The doctor of nursing practice: Current issues and clarifying recommendations. Report from the task force on implementation of the DNP.* Author.

Bartholomew, L. K., & Mullen, P. D. (2011). Five roles for using theory and evidence in the design and testing of behavior change interventions. *Journal of Public Health Dentistry, 71*, S20–S33. https://doi.org/10.1111/j.1752-7325.2011.00223.x

Baydoun, M. Barton, D. L., & Arslanian-Engoren, C. (2018). A cancer-specific middle-range theory of symptom self-care management: A theory synthesis. *Journal of Advanced Nursing, 74*, 2935–2946. https://doi.org/10.1111/jan.13829

Chao, M. T., Abercrombie, P. D., Santana, T., & Duncan, L. G. (2015). Applying the RE-AIM framework to evaluate integrative medicine group visits among diverse women with chronic pelvic pain. *Pain Management Nursing, 16*(6), 920–929. https://doi.org/10.1016/j.pmn.2015.07.007

Chinn, P. L., & Kramer, M. K. (2018). *Knowledge development in nursing. Theory and process* (10th ed.). Elsevier.

Cleverley, K., Bartha, C., Strudwick, G., Chakraborty, R., & Srivastava, R. (2018). The development of a client care needs assessment tool for mental health and addictions settings using a modified *Nursing Leadership, 31*, 52–65. https://doi.org/10.12927/cjnl.2018.25603

Cook, P. F., & Lowe, N. K. (2012). Differentiating the scientific endeavors of research, program evaluation, and quality improvement studies. *Journal of Obstetric, Gynecologic, and Neonatal Nursing, 41*(1), 1–3. https://doi.org/10.1111/j.1552-6909.2011.01319.x

Fawcett, J., & DeSanto-Madeya, S. (2012). *Contemporary nursing knowledge* (3rd ed.). F. A. Davis.

Gillespie, G. L., Hounchell, M., Pettinichi, J., Mattei, J., & Rose, L. (2012). Caring in pediatric emergency nursing. *Research and Theory for Nursing Practice, 26*(3), 216–232. https://doi.org/10.1891/1541-6577.26.3.216

Harvey, G., & Kitson, A. (2016). PARIHS revisited: From heuristic to integrated framework for the successful implementation of knowledge into practice. *Implementation Science, 11*, 33. https://doi.org/10.1186/s13012-016-0398-2

Im, E. O. (2010). A situation-specific theory of Asian immigrant women's menopausal symptom experience in the United States. *Advances in Nursing Science, 33*(2), 143–157. https://doi.org/10.1097/ANS.0b013e3181dbc5fa

Im, E. O. (2018). Theory development strategies for middle-range theories. *Advances in Nursing Science, 41*, 275–292. https://doi.org/10.1097/ANS.0000000000000215

Im, E. O., & Chang, S. J. (2012). Current trends in nursing theories. *Journal of Nursing Scholarship, 44*(2), 156–164. https://doi.org/10.1111/j.1547-5069.2012.01440.x

Im, E. O., & Meleis, A. (2018). Developing situation-specific theories. In A. I. Meleis (Ed.). *Theoretical nursing. Development and progress* (6th ed., pp. 390–401). Wolters Kluwer Health/Lippincott Williams & Wilkins.

Jiang, X., & He, G. (2012). Effects of an uncertainty management intervention on uncertainty, anxiety, depression, and quality of life of chronic obstructive pulmonary disease outpatients. *Research in Nursing & Health, 35*(4), 409–418. https://doi.org/10.1002/nur.21483

Kamp. K. J., Luo, Z., Holmstrom, A., Given, B., & Wyatt, G. (2019). Self-management through social support among emerging adults with inflammatory bowel disease. *Nursing Research, 68*, 285–295. https://doi.org/10.1097/NNR.0000000000000354

Kelley, M. N., & Lowe, J. R. (2018) Strong cultural identity effects stress levels among Native American youth at risk for obesity. *Journal of Cultural Diversity, 25*, 127–131.

Lazenby, M., Ercolano, E., Tan, H., Ferrucci, L., Badger, T., Grant, M., Jacobsen, P., & McCorkle, R. (2019). Using the RE-AIM framework for dissemination and implementation of psychosocial distress screening. *European Journal of Cancer Care, 28*, e13036. https://doi.org/10.1111/ecc.13036

Liehr, P., & Smith, M. J. (2017). Middle-range theory. A perspective on development and use. *Advances in Nursing Science, 40*, 51–63.

Liska, C. M., Morash, R., Paquet, L., & Stacey, D. (2018). Empowering cancer survivors to meet their physical and psychosocial needs: An implementation evaluation. *Canadian Oncology Nursing Journal, 28*, 76–81. https://doi.org/10.5737/236880762827681

Lucas, R., Berrnier, K., Perry, M., Evans, H., Ramesh, D., Young, E., Walsh, S., & Starkweather, A. (2019). Promoting self-management of breast and nipple pain in breastfeeding women: Protocol of a pilot randomized controlled trial. *Research in Nursing and Health, 42*, 176–188. https://doi.org/10.1002/nur.21938

Lyttle, D., Montgomery, A. J., Davis, B. L., Burns, D., McGee, Z. T., & Fogel, J. (2018). An exploration using the Neumann Systems Model of risky sexual behaviors among African American college students: A brief report, *Journal of Cultural Diversity, 25*, 142–147.

McEwen, M. (2019a). Overview of theory in nursing. In M. McEwen & E. M. Wills (Eds.), *Theoretical basis for nursing* (5th ed., pp. 23–48). Wolters Kluwer Health.

McEwen, M. (2019b). Concept development. In M. McEwen & E. M. Wills (Eds.), *Theoretical basis for nursing* (5th ed., pp. 72–93). Wolters Kluwer Health.

McEwen, M., & Wills, E. M. (2019). *Theoretical basis for nursing* (5th ed.). Wolters Kluwer Health.

Meleis, A. I. (2018). *Theoretical nursing: Development and progress* (6th ed.). Wolters Kluwer Health/Lippincott Williams & Wilkins.

Meleis, A. I., Sawyer, L. M., Im, E.-O., Messias, D. K. H., & Schumacher, K. (2000). Experiencing transitions: An emerging middle-range theory. *Advances in Nursing Science, 23*(1), 12–28. https://doi.org/10.1097/00012272-200009000-00006

Oberleitner, M. G. (2019). Theories, models, and frameworks from leadership and management. In M. McEwen & E. M. Wills (Eds.), *Theoretical basis for nursing* (5th ed., pp. 376–408). Wolters Kluwer Health.

Pender, N. J., Murdaugh, C. L., & Parsons, M. A. (2011). *Health promotion in nursing practice* (6th ed.). Pearson.

Peters, R. M., & Templin, T. N. (2010). Theory of planned behavior, self-care motivation, and blood pressure self-care. *Research and Theory for Nursing Practice, 24*(3), 172–186. https://doi.org/10.1891/1541-6577.24.3.172

Peterson, S. J., & Bredow, T. S. (2017). *Middle range theories: Application to nursing research* (4th ed.). Wolters Kluwer.

Pickett, S., Peters, R. M., & Jarosz, P. A. (2014). Toward a middle-range theory of weight management. *Nursing Science Quarterly, 27*, 242–247. https://doi.org/10.1177/0894318414534486

Polit, D. F., & Beck, C. T. (2017). *Nursing research: Generating and assessing evidence for nursing practice* (10th ed.). Wolters Kluwer.

Raines, D. A. (2012). Quality improvement, evidence-based practice, and nursing research. Oh my! *Neonatal Network, 31*(4), 262–264. https://doi.org/10.1891/0730-0832.31.4.262

Riegel, B., Joarsma, T., Lee, C. S., & Strömberg, A. (2019). Integrating symptoms into the middle-range theory of self-care of chronic illness. *Advances in Nursing Science, 42*, 206–215. https://doi.org/10.1097/ANS.0000000000000237

Risjord, M. (2019). Middle-range theories as models: New criteria for analysis and evaluation. *Nursing Philosophy, 20*, e12225. https://doi.org/10.1111/nup.12225

Sanford, J., Townsend-Rocchicciolli, J., Horigan, A., & Hall, P. (2011). A process of decision making by caregivers of family members with heart failure. *Research and Theory for Nursing Practice, 25*(1), 55–70. https://doi.org/10.1891/1541-6577.25.1.55

Siaki, L. A., Loescher, L. J., & Trego, L. L. (2013). Synthesis strategy: Building a culturally sensitive mid-range theory of risk perception using literary, quantitative, and qualitative methods. *Journal of Advanced Nursing, 69*(3), 726–737. https://doi.org/10.1111/j.1365-2648.2012.06096.x

Spratling, R., & Weaver, S. R. (2012). Theoretical perspective: Resilience in medically fragile adolescents. *Research and Theory for Nursing Practice, 26*(1), 54–68. https://doi.org/10.1891/1541-6577.26.1.54

Stixrood, B. (2019). Reducing 30-day readmissions through nursing science. An application of transitions theory with best practice guidelines. *Advances in Nursing Science, 43*, 2–14. https://doi.org/10.1097/ANS.0000000000000259

Testa, D. (2017). Development and psychometric evaluation of the nurse's perception of the relationship-based care environment scale. *International Journal for Human Caring, 21*, 193–199. https://doi.org/10.20467/HumanCaring-D-17-00025

Wagner, D. L., Bear, M., & Davidson, N. S. (2011). Measuring patient satisfaction with postpartum teaching methods used by nurses within the interaction model of client health behavior. *Research and Theory for Nursing Practice, 25*(3), 176–190. https://doi.org/10.1891/1541-6577.25.3.176

Walter, R. R. (2017). Emancipatory nursing praxis: A theory of social justice in nursing. *Advances in Nursing Science, 40*, 223–241. https://doi.org/10.1097/ANS.0000000000000157

Wills, E. M. & McEwen, M. (2019). Concept development. In M. McEwen & E. M. Wills (Eds.), *Theoretical basis for nursing* (5th ed., pp. 49–71). Wolters Kluwer Health.

Yarcheski, T. J., Mahon, N. E., Yarcheski, A., & Hanks, M. M. (2010). Perceived stress and wellness in early adolescents using the Neuman Systems Model. *The Journal of School Nursing, 26*(3), 230–237. https://doi.org/10.1177/1059840509358073

QUANTITATIVE DESIGNS FOR PRACTICE SCHOLARSHIP

SUSAN WEBER BUCHHOLZ

■ INTRODUCTION

In a quantitative approach, research questions are explored using numerical data for analysis and interpretation to provide an objective means to answer study questions and test hypotheses. Quantitative methods involve determining the purpose of the research that can be addressed with a measurable question, determining an appropriate study design, study implementation, and statistical analysis. Study implementation involves carrying out study procedures in a particular setting, collecting study data, and data management. Statistical analysis of data enables the investigator to determine whether findings were likely to occur by chance alone rather than due to a proposed relationship between variables or effect of an intervention.

This chapter provides an overview of quantitative methods, including defining key variables, measurement, data types, sampling concepts, overall study design, and analysis considerations. Practical aspects in planning and implementing quantitative research in clinical settings are briefly reviewed. Approaches to evaluate clinical as well as statistical significance of quantitative findings are briefly discussed.

■ STUDY VARIABLES

Every quantitative research study begins with identification of a topic area that can be addressed with a measurable *study question*. A clear question forms the foundation for study design, is measurable, identifies the population that is being studied, and identifies key variables of interest about that population. Variables are the building blocks of the study. Studying different variables can help determine relationships and/or differences in a population. Suppose, for example, that a nurse researcher is interested in the effect of a smoking cessation program on oncology patients' smoking habits. The question posed is: Will a smoking cessation program for oncology patients reduce daily tobacco use? Key *variables* in this question are *smoking cessation program* and *tobacco use*. The researcher will also decide who comprises the sample, which is a subset of the population. The research question can be easily transformed to a *hypothesis*, which predicts the relationship between these two variables. In this example the hypothesis would be: A smoking cessation program will reduce tobacco use in oncology patients. However, it is also important to determine the **null** *hypothesis*, which in this case would be: A smoking cessation program does **not** reduce tobacco use in oncology patients. It is useful to understand how a question can be linked to a hypothesis and null hypothesis in order to later understand how statistical analysis is interpreted.

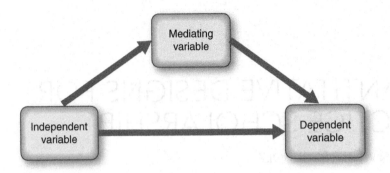

FIGURE 9.1 Mediator Model.

There are different types of variables that influence the subject of research, including *independent, dependent, mediating,* or *moderating variables* (Polit & Beck, 2020). Interrelationships among possible types of variables are shown in Figures 9.1 and 9.2. An *independent variable* is what the researcher manipulates, and is the presumed cause in the study. A *dependent variable* is the presumed effect in the study, and may also be termed the *outcome variable*. A *mediating variable* is an intervening variable. Mediating variables are factors that affect the interaction between the independent and dependent variables and facilitate, augment, or reduce the effects of the independent variable. The *moderating variable* influences or affects the relation between variables. Moderating variables are factors that create an interactive effect between the independent and dependent variables. In the previous example, the smoking cessation program would be the *independent* variable. Tobacco use would be the *dependent* variable, because the question posed suggests that amount of tobacco used would depend on provision of the smoking cessation program.

In the proposed research study with the smoking cessation program, the astute clinician can determine from a clinical, theoretical and existing literature perspective, about the role that mediating and moderating variables play in tobacco use by an oncology patient. For example, the patient's confidence in their ability to quit, or the benefits that they perceive from stopping smoking, as well as the barriers that they perceive, could act as mediating variables. The effect of the smoking cessation program on tobacco use may also be mediated by the way in which the program is delivered. Say, for example, the program is provided as a web link that the patient can view at home on their phone or computer, prior to a visit with their healthcare provider. The effectiveness of the program might be mediated by the number of times the patient views it or whether the patient views it with family members and discusses the information provided with

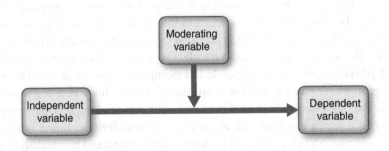

FIGURE 9.2 Moderator Model.

the program. The participant's age, type of cancer, and prognosis could influence or moderate the response of the patient to the program. The effects of the program might also be moderated by the patient's mental state. Statistical analyses are used to analyze the effects of mediators and moderators on an intervention.

There are other variables that can have an effect on the outcomes of the study. These are *extraneous variables* (Gray et al., 2017; Vogt & Johnson, 2016). Extraneous variables represent a condition that is not part of the study design and that the researchers are not interested in measuring, but can still affect the outcome of the study. If an extraneous variable is recognized prior to the study beginning, but the researchers are unable to control for it, or the variable is not recognized until after the study has been initiated, then these represent *confounding variables*. Randomization is useful in limiting the impact of confounding variables, and statistical techniques such as analysis of covariance can be used to account for the effect of variables. If the design of the study and the statistical analysis cannot account for a confounding variable, then the researcher must note that as a limitation.

■ MEASUREMENT PROPERTIES

Measurement is the process of assigning numbers to variables. Methods used for measurement are referred to as *instrumentation*. Data can be obtained through physical measurements, biomedical data, use of questionnaires, and use of patient rating scales, diaries, or responses in structured interviews. Whatever instrumentation is used, major characteristics of measurement that determine its quality and utility include the properties of *validity, reliability, sensitivity,* and *specificity* (Gray et al., 2017; Polit & Beck, 2020; Waltz et al., 2017). In planning research, the objective is to select measurement methods that provide valid and reliable results that are also sensitive and specific.

- **Validity** is a broad term that is used to describe the degree to which the instrument used is truly measuring what the researcher intends to measure. The researcher needs to take adequate time to review potential measures to determine if the measure provides sufficient validity for their specific study question. One way to understand the scope of validity is to review it within four different categories: *construct validity, statistical conclusion validity, internal validity* and *external validity* (Cook & Campbell, 1979).
  - **Construct validity** assesses how adequate an instrument is in measuring the main construct. Construct validity is comprised of *translation validity* and *criterion validity*.
    - **Translational validity** assesses how well the construct is translated and includes *face validity* and *content validity*. Face validity is based on looking at an instrument and determining if it measures what it is supposed to be measuring according to an expert in the field. Content validity assesses if the content adequately represents the "universe" of what is being measured.
    - **Criterion validity** assesses the correlation between what the instrument measures and another criterion. There are multiple methods that can be used to assess criterion validity, including concurrent validity, predictive validity, convergent validity, and discriminant validity. With *concurrent validity*, a researcher will assess the correlation between the instrument and a criterion that is related. With *predictive validity*, a researcher will assess how well the scores predict a score on another future criterion. With *convergent validity*, a

researcher uses different methods to measure the same attribute to assess if they obtain the same results. With *discriminant validity,* a researcher assesses how easy or difficult it is to be able to differentiate between the construct that they are measuring and a similar construct.

- **Statistical conclusion validity** assesses how accurate to reality the conclusions are about decisions made regarding findings on relationships and differences, based on the statistical evidence.

- **Internal validity** assesses if the independent variable actually was the cause of the observed effect in the dependent variable. Because of the complex nature of human research, there are multiple threats to internal validity that should be addressed as needed. These threats to internal validity are discussed later in the chapter.

- **External validity** is often spoken of as "generalization." External validity answers the question to what degree the results of the study can be generalized to a specific population. There are several threats to external validity that should be addressed as needed and are also discussed later in the chapter.

- **Reliability** *assesses measurement consistency.* Reliability evaluates how dependable an instrument is in the measurement of a variable. If a measure is reliable, then it will report the same value for the same item being measured successively. There are three categories of reliability: *stability, internal consistency* and *equivalence.* The type of reliability that matters most is related to the study design. For example, in a repeated-measures design, test–retest reliability is important. In a study plan in which multiple observers collect data, it is important to be sure that different people using the same instrument in the same observation would obtain the same result, meaning the tool has good inter-rater reliability.

  - **Stability** assesses if the instrument measures the same results repeatedly. Stability is comprised of two measures: *test–retest reliability* and *parallel forms.* Test–retest reliability refers to whether or not the same person using the instrument would get the same result with multiple uses. Parallel forms assess the consistency of the results of two tests that are constructed both in the same way and with the same content domain.

  - **Internal consistency** is applicable to measurement instruments such as questionnaires and multiple item rating scales. Internal consistency shows the degree to which items on an instrument actually measure a single thing. If internal consistency is high, it suggests that the set of questionnaire items is measuring the same concept or variable. If internal consistency is low, it suggests that individual items within a questionnaire may be measuring different concepts. While interpretation of internal consistency values can be somewhat arbitrary, it can be said that higher values reflect greater reliability. Three different measures for internal consistency include: *Cronbach's alpha, split-half,* and *Kuder-Richardson.* Cronbach's alpha is a correlation coefficient that estimates internal consistency. Cronbach's alpha is the statistic used frequently to measure internal consistency. The higher the value for alpha, the greater the internal consistency. Split-half assesses for consistency when a set is divided into two sets, administered separately, and then compared. Kuder-Richardson assesses inter-item consistency by examining the adequacy of content sampling and heterogeneity of the domain that is being sampled.

  - **Equivalence** assesses how different observers rate an instrument. Equivalence can be assessed with these three measures: *inter-rater reliability, kappa statistic,* and *intraclass correlation*. Inter-rater reliability is the degree to which different observers would achieve the same result using the instrument. If different people, using the same tool or making the same observation, come up with very different results, confidence in the measurement and the resulting accuracy of results would be questionable. Kappa statistic assesses an index which compares the agreement against that which a researcher might expect by chance. The value of kappa can be interpreted as the proportion of agreement in results among raters that did not occur by chance alone. Intraclass correlation assesses consistency for a data set when there is more than one group present.

- **Sensitivity** is defined as the number of true positive decisions divided by the number of actual positive cases (the true positives plus the false negatives). It indicates the ability to identify positive results and the degree to which a measurement method is responsive to changes in the variable of interest. Sensitivity also refers to the magnitude of a change that a measure will detect. The more sensitive a measure, the better it will reflect small changes and detect positive findings.

- **Specificity** is the degree to which a result is indicative of a single characteristic and can accurately detect negative results. Mathematically, specificity is the number of true negative decisions divided by the number of actual negative cases (the true negatives plus the false positives). In clinical settings, a receiver operator curve (ROC) is often used to display sensitivity and specificity (Janssens & Martens, 2020).

In addition to validity, reliability, sensitivity, and specificity, assessing a measurement's *feasibility* properties is also important. There are a number of factors to consider when examining feasibility. Assessing the actual number of questions including the length of the questions, will allow the researcher to determine if there is undue participant burden in answering questions. Assessing the types of questions that are asked (e.g., multiple choice or open-ended) is important in determining if the type of data received will be useful and meaningful in the analysis. It is useful to assess if the participant is able to complete the questionnaire or if someone else is required to complete it, such as the researcher or a family member. The participant needs to know prior to starting, how long it will take to complete the instrument. If the information is not given at the appropriate literacy level for the population intended, the researcher risks obtaining inaccurate answers. It is also important to assess if an instrument needs to be translated. If an instrument has been translated, the researcher needs to document how the instrument was assessed for language accuracy. Two other important feasibility considerations include ease of administration and scoring, as well as availability of the instrument, and potential cost associated with using the instrument.

There is increased emphasis on inclusion of *patient-reported outcomes* (PROs) in clinical research and practice. PROs are the patient's direct report of their own condition, behavior, or experience, without interpretation by a clinician or someone else. The word "patient" is inclusive of not only patients, but also their families and caregivers, as well as consumers. The term is also used to encompass anyone that receives support services. There are four key PRO domains, and these include health-related quality of life, symptoms and symptom burden that are experienced, how people experience care, and specific health behaviors (National Quality Forum, 2020). These domains are measured by a range of various tools that assess how a patient reports their physical, mental, and social well-being. There are different measurement concepts to consider when using PROs (National Quality Forum, 2013). PRO as already noted is the patient-reported outcome. PROMs is the instrument, tool, and/or single-item measure that is used to assess the outcome. PRO-PM is the PRO-based performance measure.

In appraising research for application in the clinical setting, the quality of measurement methods is a factor that contributes to the confidence in overall results. The type of data that is generated with measurements used will also influence the type of analysis that can be done.

■ UNDERSTANDING DATA

Data are the discrete values that result from measurement of study variables. Quantitative data are one of four types in terms of numerical scale: *nominal, ordinal, interval,* or *ratio.* These scales indicate a hierarchical structure for the data type, where the ratio scale is the highest scale level (Polit & Beck, 2020).

- **Nominal** scale data assign a "name" to each observation. Gender is an example of a nominal scale variable. Examples of nominal scale variables encountered in the clinical setting are gender, diagnosis-related group (DRG) designation, diagnosis codes, and procedure codes. Nominal data are the lowest scale level.

- **Ordinal** scales provide numerical data that have an "order." The most common examples of ordinal scale data are Likert-type scales, in which one rates an item on a scale such as (a) "poor," (b) "fair," (c) "good," (d) "very good," or (e) "excellent." Responses have an order in relationship to each other, such that "fair" is better than "poor," "very good" is better than "good," and so on. However, there is no mathematical relationship in this order. One cannot say that "good" is twice the value of "poor" or that "excellent" is twice the value of "very good." Results from typical patient satisfaction questionnaires used in the clinical setting are examples of ordinal scale data. Ordinal data are above nominal data on the scale hierarchy.

- **Interval** scales provide data in which distances on the numerical scale are equal. The distance between the numbers 1 and 2 is the same as the distance between 2 and 3. The Fahrenheit temperature scale is an example of an interval scale. The difference between a temperature of 100°F and 90°F is the same as the difference between a temperature of 90°F and 80°F. One cannot, however, say that 100° is exactly twice the temperature of 50°. Interval scales refer to equal distances, not a mathematical relationship. Patient ratings on a standard numerical pain symptom distress scale and patient severity scoring systems are examples of interval scales. Interval data are above ordinal data on the hierarchy of data scales.

- **Ratio** scales provide the same information as interval scales, but in addition, have an absolute zero point. This means that mathematically, on a ratio scale, "20" is exactly twice "10," and "30" is exactly three times "10." Volume, length, weight, and time are examples of ratio scales.

The scale of the measurement has implications for the type of analysis that is most appropriate. The higher the scale level, according to the hierarchy as described earlier, the broader the range of statistical procedures one can employ. The scale of measurement also determines if you will need nonparametric or parametric statistics. Nonparametric statistics are appropriate when dealing with nominal and ordinal data. Because the sampling distribution of means should produce a normal curve, interval and ratio scale data can be analyzed with parametric statistical procedures.

There is some disagreement about the appropriate statistics that one can use with Likert-type rating scales and questionnaire scores. In some instruments, multiple Likert-type responses can be summed to provide total attribute scores or subscale scores. Some argue that resulting data simply order responses, whereas others contend that such scores truly represent the magnitude of the variable being measured, and that items summed for analysis approach the interval scale level. It has been suggested that the statistical analysis used should be driven by the nature of the clinical question, rather than focused on the level of the data (Waltz et al., 2017). One way to determine appropriateness of dealing with such data as interval level is to examine the frequency distribution of responses. If results approximate a normal curve, then parametric statistics may be appropriate.

▪ SAMPLING

Given the many factors that can affect the dependent variable, quantitative research is designed to control, reduce, or account for as many of these factors as practical. This can be done by establishing study sample inclusion and exclusion criteria, including measurement and analysis of potential confounding variables, and overall study design to reduce threats to validity. When a researcher wants to use randomization to select participants for their research, they can employ *simple randomization*, where, for example, participants can be selected using a random number table. In addition to simple random sampling, there are other sampling strategies that the researcher can use, including *systematic, stratified,* and *cluster* sampling techniques (Pedhazur & Schmelkin, 1991; Waltz et al., 2017). Systematic sampling chooses every Kth case, from a list of individuals within a population. Stratified sampling involves subdividing a population into homogeneous groups, in respect to a specific characteristic, and from that group participants are randomly selected. With primary cluster sampling, an inclusive unit of a population is determined, and a sample of those units is then randomly selected.

In planning to study the effects of an intervention on patient anxiety, one might exclude patients who have a major anxiety disorder or cognitive impairment to reduce variation in study findings that could be attributed to these variables. Other variables that experience suggests might affect results, such as age, physical symptoms, diagnosis, and so on, can be measured and included in analysis and interpretation of findings. Selecting a homogeneous sample of patients for a research study is helpful to reduce effects of confounding variables. However, studying a very narrowly defined group of patients limits generalizability of findings to other types of patients.

Sampling decisions can also introduce bias into the study, because the characteristics of patients included can influence results. Selection of a random sample of patients would be expected to provide a sufficient random distribution of characteristics to reduce such bias; however, random sampling is usually not always possible or practical in prospective clinical research.

▪ STUDY DESIGN

The study design is the structure of the research that defines the timing of observations and interventions and strategies used to ensure objectivity. Study designs generally fall into one of three broad categories: *nonexperimental, quasi-experimental,* and *experimental*. With a nonexperimental design, the researcher is observing and measuring what is occurring for participants without changing or controlling their situation. With a quasi-experimental design, a researcher manipulates an independent variable, but cannot or does not use random assignment. With an experimental design, the researcher delivers an intervention, and also uses randomization in the assignment of participants to different groups.

◼ NONEXPERIMENTAL DESIGNS

Nonexperimental designs are used when a researcher wants to observe and describe what is occurring with a group or group of participants. The researcher does not intervene in manipulating the independent variable for these participants. Nonexperimental designs include descriptive, correlational, and observational designs.

- ◼ **Descriptive designs** are used in studies where the researcher seeks to observe and describe what is occurring within a sample from a population. Descriptive studies provide information about commonalities and differences within a defined group of patients. These types of studies are used to identify the incidence or prevalence of conditions, describe a phenomenon, or evaluate relationships among variables explored. The design may be *cross-sectional*, where data are collected at one specific point in time; *retrospective*, with information collected from prior participant records or other preexisting sources of data; *prospective*, with information collected after the study starts; or *longitudinal*, with data collection at time points in the future as well. For example if a researcher wants to assess how many hospitalizations occur in children due to a diagnosis of respiratory syncytial virus at varying times throughout the year in the same set of hospitals, then they would prospectively and longitudinally track those data.

- ◼ **Correlational designs** are used to evaluate relationships or associations among variables. Statistical analysis such as regression and other multivariate techniques can be done to evaluate those variables that may predict or influence results in patient outcomes. Correlational designs can be viewed as a type of descriptive design, because use of this design does not involve the attempt to evaluate causality or effects of an intervention. For example, a researcher might explore the correlation between literacy levels and following a specific procedure on a handout. While the researcher can note if there is or is not a correlation, they cannot infer a causal relationship between those two variables.

- ◼ **Observational designs** are used in studies where the outcomes of interest are analyzed between groups of patients that received different interventions. In this design, interventions are not controlled and patients may not be specifically sampled or assigned to treatments. Patients, interventions, and results are described and statistical analysis of data is used to determine differences in outcomes. There are two major types of observational designs: *cohort* and *case control*.

  - ◼ **Cohort designs** involve a group or groups of patients that have one or more common defined characteristics. Cohort designs may be prospective or retrospective. In a prospective cohort study outcomes from a group of patients receiving an intervention, or exposed to some factor, are compared to outcomes from a group of patients who do not receive the intervention, receive a different intervention, or are not exposed. In a retrospective approach, patients receiving an intervention would be compared to a previous group of patients who did not receive the intervention being tested. This is referred to as a group of historical controls. This type of design can be used when usual clinical care varies, or standard approaches for care have changed over time. For example, routine testing procedures for methicillin-resistant *Staphylococcus aureus* (MRSA) have changed over time in hospitals and a researcher could observe the number of diagnoses made related to MRSA in regard to how the procedure was carried out over time, or in comparison to a group of participants who were not routinely tested.

■ **Case-control designs** examine outcomes from a study group of patients who are exposed to an intervention, or are identified by an outcome of interest, and are compared to a group of patients from the same source population who are not exposed, or do not have the same outcome. In a *matched* case-control study, study patients are individually matched with patients who have the same characteristics that may influence outcomes, for example disease, age, and gender. This approach reduces the bias introduced as a result of potential confounding variables in an attempt to ensure comparability between cases and controls. For example, if a researcher is studying osteoporosis treatments, they could match participants who received different treatments by age, gender, and history of a specific type of fractures.

In situations in which the independent variable cannot be manipulated, observational studies may be the only option to begin to answer clinical questions about the results of a specific intervention. In this case, it is important to measure and analyze potential intervening and extraneous variables insofar as possible, attempting to rule out other variables that may have produced the results. Clear sample inclusion and exclusion criteria are also essential. Although a single observational type of study cannot provide evidence of cause and effect, it does provide evidence that is stronger than case study level evidence, and if multiple observational studies provide the same conclusions, the synthesis of that information provides stronger evidence about the findings.

■ QUASI-EXPERIMENTAL STUDIES

Quasi-experimental designs can be constructed with single or multiple groups, and may involve pretest and posttest or posttest-only measurement (Cook & Campbell, 1979; Polit & Beck, 2020). There are several different quasi-experimental designs. Presented here are three of the more common quasi-experimental designs, including *one-group pretest–posttest design, nonequivalent control group posttest-only design,* and *nonequivalent control group pretest–posttest design.*

■ With a **one-group pretest–posttest design** measurement of the dependent variable is done prior to and then again after an intervention in the same subject or group. Changes in the dependent variable from pre- to postintervention in each subject are compared. In this design, the individual patient essentially functions as their own control. The difference between pre- and postintervention measurement is analyzed to evaluate the impact of the intervention. However, in this type of quasi-experimental design, without comparison to a group that did not have the intervention, there is no way to tell whether changes in the outcome would have occurred in any case. An example of this phenomenon is seen with the trajectory of patient anxiety levels in the course of treatment for cancer. A substantial body of research has shown that over time during active antitumor treatment, in the general population of patients with cancer, levels of anxiety tend to decline. If an intervention aimed to reduce anxiety is given to a single group of patients and then anxiety is later measured, it is possible that any decline in anxiety observed would have occurred anyway, without the intervention.

■ With a **nonequivalent control group, posttest-only design,** the intervention is provided and the dependent variable is measured only after the intervention. With this design, the lack of a pretest points to the possibility that any differences between groups may be due to selection bias rather than an intervention effect. If a weight loss intervention is offered at a community center, and a group of participants receive the intervention while another group does not, and no pretest measures are done with the groups, it is possible that findings where the group that received the intervention lost more weight may be related other factors. For example if those that did not sign up for the study didn't know about it because they did not regularly attend the community center health-related activities, they may not have been as invested in their health, or perhaps had other barriers that prevented them from losing weight.

■ With a **nonequivalent control group, pretest–posttest design**, participants are assigned to study groups by the researcher or by participant self-selection of the group in which they want to participate. The key limitation to this approach is the fact that patients in the intervention or control groups may have different characteristics that influence the outcome. This can be addressed to some extent in analysis by examination of the differences between the groups at the onset of the study; however, it is likely that the researcher may not have data to compare all of the potential characteristics that function as intervening variables. Another approach is to match patients in an intervention group to those in the control group, either through sample selection or in the analysis of results, based on key characteristics that might influence outcomes. This approach can help reduce unexplained variability; however, it is still unlikely that the researcher can account for every characteristic that might be important. Also, sufficient analysis within subgroups of patients based on these characteristics would require a large overall sample size in order to detect statistically and clinically significant differences.

■ EXPERIMENTAL DESIGNS

Experimental designs allow researchers to examine a cause-and-effect relationship between the independent and dependent variables (Gray et al., 2017; Polit & Beck, 2020). Participants are randomly assigned to a treatment or control group. This design allows for comparison of outcomes that can overcome the limitations seen in a quasi-experimental design. Random assignment of participants in a *randomized controlled design* is the generally accepted way to attempt to spread the effect of intervening and extraneous variables across study groups by chance alone. An experimental design typically requires a highly structured and controlled environment. There are multiple procedures that have to be carefully followed when conducting a randomized controlled trial, including allocation concealment. The research team members who are doing the assessments should not be aware to which group the participant has been assigned. Without random assignment there is a potential for *selection bias*, resulting in selection of particular types of patients to receive particular treatments. There are different types of experimental randomized designs. Presented here are four common experimental designs including the *basic pretest–posttest design, multiple intervention design, crossover design,* and *factorial design.*

■ The **basic pretest–posttest design** is used when change is being assessed. Participants are measured before and after delivery of an intervention, and are assigned to either a group that receives the intervention or a control group. This design is relatively simplistic for a randomized control trial, and allows the researcher to assess differences in both groups. However, the pretest can potentially influence the outcome variable. This is a good design to use when usual care is adequate, but the researcher wants to test an intervention that they have hypothesized will be more effective than usual care. For example, this design could be used to test the effectiveness of giving diabetic participants in the intervention group counseling sessions with a registered nurse in addition to educational handouts on lifestyle modification, as compared to the control group who receives the usual care delivery of educational handouts.

- With a **multiple intervention design**, participants are again assessed pre- and postintervention, but different interventions or combinations of interventions are tested, requiring a larger sample. When a researcher is examining multiple components of an intervention, or a complex intervention, this design allows the researcher to test different intervention components. As stated, this design may require a larger sample size than the basic pretest–posttest design. If a researcher has tested two different interventions that were bundled together, and found that they had significant changes, but is uncertain which of the interventions had an impact, then the researcher could disentangle those intervention components and test them separately. For example, this design could be used if a researcher had positive significant results when they tested a multi-component intervention that involved providing group sessions as well as phone calls to help decrease the stress of family members who were taking care of a family member with a chronic illness. If they are uncertain which component was most effective, they could use a multiple intervention design to test the components of group sessions and phone calls separately.

- A **crossover design is** a type of experimental design used to provide an even stronger basis for comparison between study interventions or conditions. Even with well-controlled randomized designs, it is understood that human experience and outcomes can be affected by a huge number of personal, environment, social, and other factors. In a crossover design, individual patients are exposed to both the control and experimental conditions, and results from each condition in all patients are compared. Subjects are usually randomly assigned to the sequence in which the intervention or control condition will be provided. One of the major threats in this design is contamination due to continued effects of either treatment condition. The degree of threat depends on the nature of the intervention. In clinical trials involving medications, patients have a "wash-out" period between study conditions, so that the effects of one medication are no longer present before the patient is exposed to the other medication. With other types of interventions, an appropriate amount of time needed to eliminate intervention effects may not be clear, or may not be possible.

- In a **factorial design** two interventions are tested for simultaneously. This is a useful design for testing interaction effects. A factorial design allows the researcher to test for two different interventions at the same time. However, a large sample size may be required, as compared to testing each intervention separately. A factorial design is particularly useful for a researcher who is expecting that combining different intervention components together will have a synergistic effect. If, for example, a researcher has developed four different interventions for improving handwashing in the hospital by healthcare professionals, and theorizes that when combining them together in sets of two, one of the four combinations is more likely to be effective, then they could use a factorial design to test these different combinations.

The **randomized controlled trial (RCT)** is generally viewed as the most valid approach and the only true experimental design. Certain types of studies, such as pharmaceutical studies, consistently use an experimental design. It is important, however, to recognize that not all study questions can be subjected to this approach. Nonexperimental or quasi-experimental designs are often more practical in the clinical setting.

Representation of Study Designs

The study design can be visually represented to show the sequence of observations and interventions in a variety of ways. The X–O model uses an "X" to indicate the intervention, or independent

TABLE 9.1 Example Representations of Research Designs

DESIGN		REPRESENTATION		
Nonexperimental descriptive repeated measures design		O_1	O_2	O_3
Quasi-experimental one-group pretest–posttest design		O_1	X	O_2
Quasi-experimental nonequivalent control group posttest-only design			X	O_1
				O_1
Quasi-experimental nonequivalent control group pretest-posttest design		O_1	X	O_2
		O_1		O_2
Experimental basic pretest–posttest design	R	O_1	X	O_2
	R	O_1		O_2
Experimental multiple intervention design	R	O_1	X_A	O_2
	R	O_1	X_B	O_2
	R	O_1		O_2
Experimental crossover design	R	O_1X_A	O_2X_B	O_3
	R	O_1X_B	O_2X_A	O_3
Experimental factorial design	R	O_1	X_{A1B1}	O_2
	R	O_1	X_{A1B2}	O_2
	R	O_1	X_{A2B1}	O_2
	R	O_1	X_{A2B2}	O_2

O, observation (measurement); R, random assignment to groups; X, intervention (where multiple interventions are used, subscripts show the different interventions)

variable, and an "O" to indicate the observation to measure the dependent outcome variable. Although this is not an exhaustive list, shown in Table 9.1 are more the commonly used examples of the X–O model that illustrate study designs.

Control Conditions

The nature of the control condition used in a controlled trial is also important. Studies trials may use a *placebo control, active control,* or *attentional control.*

- In a **placebo-control trial** individuals in the control group receive an inactive treatment that appears exactly like the intervention being tested. This approach is most often associated with trials of new medications, but is not limited to that type of intervention. In some cases, use of a placebo would be inappropriate, unethical, or impractical. For patients who require medications for a health condition, use of a placebo rather than an active medication would be inappropriate. With interventions that involve invasive procedures, one would not unnecessarily expose patients to risks without any expected benefit, and there may be limited ability to provide an inactive version of the intervention.

- An alternative to a placebo-controlled trial is using an **active-control trial.** In this approach, the control group receives a different intervention for the same problem, and outcomes between the two groups are compared. Active controls may be a current standard treatment or "usual care" for the problem or a different experimental intervention. Designs with active control conditions may be aimed at testing a new intervention or aimed at comparing the effects of alternate treatments. While most randomized controlled trials are *superiority trials*, where the researcher has hypothesized that the intervention they are delivering to a control group is more effective, some studies that use an active control are *noninferiority trials*. A noninferiority study design aims to show that an experimental intervention is not *less* effective than a known treatment. This information is beneficial in the case where another treatment may, for example, be less costly, more available, or easier to administer. This design requires the investigator to establish a planned margin of effect between the new and experimental treatments that is clinically acceptable. The margin is generally determined from the clinically acceptable difference between interventions tested, known effect size of the comparison treatment, or the minimal clinically important change of the instrument used. Statistical analysis is done to test the hypothesis that results are not significantly different from the margin used (U.S. Department of Health and Human Services, 2016). Positive results are interpreted to demonstrate that the experimental intervention is not less effective than the alternative. One consideration in interpretation of an inferiority design study is whether or not the margin established is clinically meaningful. For example, if studies in the effectiveness of various antiemetic regimens to prevent nausea and vomiting in patients receiving emetogenic chemotherapy have established a margin of 15% difference in the proportion of patients who obtain complete control of the symptom, then it is up to the clinician evaluating these results to judge whether or not that 15% difference is acceptable to say that interventions are essentially equally effective.

■ *Attentional control* is a concept that needs to be considered in studies that involve examination of psychosocial, educational, and supportive types of interventions. For many types of patient outcomes it can be expected that providing additional attention alone to the patient can result in the patient feeling better. For example, if the researcher is examining the effect of a nursing supportive intervention on patient anxiety, it is likely that giving more attention and spending more time with the patient can reduce anxiety. For valid comparison, the control group should be given similar time and attention as the experimental group. In this area, researchers can provide some kind of "neutral" time and attention to patients as a control condition. Attention control delivery can take on many different formats, including given a general handout, or broad text messages, or a non-descript audio message in comparison to an intervention group that receives tailored information on a handout, very specific text messages, or a focused audio message about management of a specific health condition or health goal.

■ MIXED METHODS

Quantitative methods can be used alone, or in combination with qualitative techniques for a mixed methods approach. In a mixed methods study design, qualitative results are used to provide additional depth and context to results. Qualitative and quantitative results can also be triangulated to demonstrate whether or not findings from both methods converge to support each other. There are different study designs for collecting and studying qualitative and quantitative results, and these designs are beyond the scope of this chapter. However, there are many excellent references available to inform researchers on how to conduct a mixed methods approach (National Institutes of Health Office of Behavioral and Social Sciences, 2018).

■ OTHER DESIGN CONCEPTS

Longitudinal Designs

Longitudinal designs involve some duration of follow-up after an intervention to determine longer term effects over time. It is not clear how long the follow-up needs to be for us to term it a "longitudinal" design, and study follow-up periods can be decades, as seen in some epidemiological research. Depending on the study question, the duration of effect may be of interest, and necessitate some follow-up period for evaluation. In clinical situations or patient problems that last for months or years, the effect of an intervention at a single point in time immediately after an intervention or 2 days later is not sufficient to address the clinical problem. Measurement of outcomes at subsequent times is used to evaluate duration of effect. Longitudinal studies often involve repeated measures. Major problems encountered in longitudinal studies are patient loss to follow-up or subject attrition and the fact that other events can occur between the intervention and the follow-up measurement that are unknown and can affect results.

In any design to evaluate the effects of an intervention, the meaningful duration of an effect should be a consideration in the timing of postintervention measures. In addition to longitudinal designs that evaluate longer term results, one may be interested in knowing shorter term duration of effects. This depends on the nature of the dependent variable of interest. For example, if one wants to know whether provision of therapeutic touch can relieve acute pain, an immediate postintervention measurement can answer that question. However, if one wants to know whether therapeutic touch can relieve a more chronic and lasting symptom, a single immediate post-measurement provides insufficient information to address the question. In this type of situation, one may consider using a repeated-measures design to see how long an effect lasts.

Repeated-Measures Design

Repeated-measures design refers to measurement of variables multiple times. This approach can be used within any type of descriptive or interventional research. Measurement of dependent variables at multiple points in time enables evaluation of trends and timing of effects. There is no rule to guide the exact timing of repeated measures. Clinical judgment and review of findings from other research in the area can guide this decision.

Adaptive Designs

An adaptive study design uses accumulating study findings to modify aspects of the study as it continues. Study modifications can be such things as changes in randomization procedures, sample size re-estimation, and adaptation of the intervention. Two specific adaptive designs gaining popularity among scientists are the multiphase optimization strategy (MOST) and the sequential multiple assignment randomized trial (SMART) designs (Wilbur et al., 2016). The MOST methodology involves a preparation phase of literature review and establishing a hypothesis about how an intervention may work, an optimization phase involving empirical research to estimate effects of various components of an intervention, and an evaluation phase consisting of a standard randomized controlled trial. In this method, the optimization phase involves adaptive experimentation to identify the most effective intervention components to later evaluate in an RCT. In a SMART design, a set of optional interventions that have been shown to be effective, a set of known variables that may influence desired outcomes, and a sequence of decision rules that are used over time to adjust interventions are combined to identify how to best tailor and sequence interventions to achieve outcomes (Buchholz et al., 2019). It has been suggested that these approaches are particularly helpful to study multicomponent interventions, and are well aligned with clinical practice since they involve treatment modifications according to patient responses. In contrast to clinical practice where modifications may be intuitive or ill-defined, SMART research provides evidence about the efficacy of such modifications and associated decision rules.

A unique type of adaptive design is the N-of-1 trial approach. This type of study is a multiple crossover trial conducted in a single patient. Usually interventions are randomized and blinded. N-of-1 trials are suggested when there is uncertainty about the comparative effectiveness of treatments considered for an individual patient or existing evidence is conflicting. This approach is most applicable in chronic or stable conditions that are amenable to deliberate experimentation, situations in which all other intervention options have not worked, or highly experimental trials. N-of-1 trials can be a pragmatic approach in clinical practice and provide potential for patient-centered care along with an objective approach to determine patient responses to interventions (Kravitz, Duan, [Eds.], and the DEcIDE Methods Center N-of-1 Guidance Panel, 2014). N-of-1 trials may be useful for research of nursing interventions for which there is little evidence and for interventions such as psychoeducational approaches for which the most effective "dose" is unclear. This approach is one that enables individualized and patient-centered clinical care while evidence is collected to advance knowledge.

The design concepts reviewed here can be combined in various ways. Randomized controlled trials often involve pre- and postintervention measurement of dependent variables. Study groups may be included that provide several types of control conditions. Any type of study may be designed to include long-term patient follow-up with a longitudinal approach. Clinicians may find the adaptability in a SMART design congruent with their practice. Across all types of studies, the design needs to be planned to reduce potential bias and threats to the internal validity of the study.

■ SOURCES OF BIAS IN QUANTITATIVE METHODS

Bias is a relatively broad term, and includes any aspect of a study that produces systematic error in regard to the study findings (Gray et al., 2017; Waltz et al., 2017). Bias in a study can cause results that are inaccurate and distorted, and can occur knowingly or unknowingly. However to the extent possible for a researcher, potential biases need to be thought through carefully prior to the execution of a research study. Study biases can have an effect on a small number of participants, or on a large number of participants in a study.

It is at the point of designing the study that the researcher needs to consider potential biases, including *common biases that can occur with the researcher, measures, participant, and the intervention*. The researcher needs to maintain objectivity as much as possible, and needs to consider if they have a biased view that may influence the design of the study. Measurements need to be assessed to make sure that they do not automatically examine a variable from a perspective that will, for example, only favor positive results, or not completely address central facets of the study variables. Also, how measurements are delivered needs to be standardized, so that, for example, in the case of a measure that requires a research team to rate a variable, it is done the same with each participant, or in the case of using an objective measure, that the instrument is calibrated. How participants are recruited for a study so that all potential participants have an equal opportunity to be enrolled, needs to be carefully considered. Measures need to be put in place to analyze differences between the intervention group and control group, and between those individuals who participate fully, and those that drop out. If an intervention is flawed, or it is not delivered correctly or delivered inconsistently by the research team, then that can impact the study, and act as a bias.

▪ THREATS TO INTERNAL AND EXTERNAL VALIDITY

Both research design and implementation affect the validity of the study. Validity can be expressed as the degree of confidence that changes seen in a dependent variable are the result of the independent variable studied, rather than some unknown extraneous variables. In purely descriptive studies, internal validity refers to the accuracy and quality of the study. In studies that are done to evaluate effects of interventions, there are a number of specific threats to internal and external validity that have been described (Cook & Campbell, 1979; Gray et al., 2017; Pedhazur & Schmelkin, 1991; Polit & Beck, 2020).

Internal Threats to Validity

Extraneous variables that can reduce internal study validity are outlined in the following. Although these are discussed as unique issues, multiple threats can be present, can interact, and can have a cumulative effect on the validity of the study. Random assignment to study groups addresses many of these threats, because it allows one to reasonably expect that the distribution of extraneous variables would be similar across groups and has similar effects on outcomes in all study groups. A list of threats to validity, aspects of study design and implementation that are likely to produce the threat, and some approaches to avoid or reduce the threat are shown in Table 9.2.

- **History** refers to an event that occurs during the point of measurement of pretest to posttest, due to something other than the intervention and intervening or mediating variables. This type of threat involves an event that has an effect on what is being observed, the dependent variable. This threat is more common with longitudinal designs than those in which data are collected over shorter time periods. Analysis of potential intervening and mediating variables as covariates in analysis can facilitate interpretation of the role of history in findings.

- **Maturation** results in natural changes over time as subjects change; for instance as they become older, gain experience, become stronger or weaker, become more or less motivated, and so on. This type of threat is associated with longitudinal designs, particularly those that involve children or individuals with diseases that naturally progress over time. Analysis of potential covariates to illuminate maturation effects can be helpful.

TABLE 9.2 Threats to Internal Validity: Designs and Risk and Management Approaches

THREAT	STUDY DESIGNS AT RISK FOR THREAT	MANAGEMENT APPROACHES TO DECREASE RISK
History	Longitudinal studies Studies using repeated measures Long time period between pre- and post-measures One group pretest–posttest	Measure intervention and control groups simultaneously Measure potential intervening variables and include in analysis Limit time between pre- and post-measures Random group assignment

(continued)

TABLE 9.2 Threats to Internal Validity: Designs and Risk and Management Approaches (*continued*)

THREAT	STUDY DESIGNS AT RISK FOR THREAT	MANAGEMENT APPROACHES TO DECREASE RISK
Maturation	Longitudinal studies, especially involving children, individuals with conditions that naturally progress One group pretest–posttest	Measure for disease progression and other factors Measure intervention and control groups simultaneously Random group assignment
Testing	Repeated-measures and pretest–posttest design, especially if the same tool is used repeatedly Test battery administration	Multiple measures and different tool versions Consider mixed methods design Limit measurement burden Random group assignment
Instrumentation	Studies with biomedical instruments and calibration needs Studies with biological samples that have to be obtained, stored, and tested Studies using measures with untested or minimally tested validity and reliability	Select instruments with known reliability and performance Ensure relevant instrument calibration Educate data collectors in instrument use Blind of data collectors/investigators Logically score groupings in analysis to account for floor and ceiling effects
Statistical regression	Pretest–posttest design Repeated-measures design Design that uses sample with extreme high or low scores	Observe changes in extreme scores Random group assignment
Attrition, high dropout rate, mortality	Longitudinal designs Lack of placebo, active, or attentional control	Intent-to-treat design Analyze characteristics of dropouts and compare to remaining sample Plan for attrition in sample size Use appropriate control conditions Minimize participation burden
Contamination/diffusion of treatment	Studies involving two or more groups in the same location Crossover designs involving patient psychoeducation and behavior change interventions	Plan approaches to minimize study group interactions Use of attentional control condition Plan appropriate "washout" period
Compensatory equalization of treatment	Two or more group trials with no active or attentional control and comparison is to usual care only	Blinding of group assignment Use of active and attentional control conditions
Compensatory rivalry	Two or more group trials with no active or attentional control—comparison to usual care only	Blinding of group assignment Use of active or attentional control conditions
Resentful de-moralization	Two or more group trials with no active or attentional control—comparison to usual care only	Blinding of group assignment Use of active and attentional control conditions
Selection	Nonrandom group assignment Time series – with population changes over time	Random group assignment Analyze differences within and between groups in key intervening variables
Lack of treatment fidelity	Multiple intervention providers Complexity and interactive nature of the intervention	Observe and analyze delivery and receipt of intervention sessions to assess fidelity Train providers in the intervention Use clear processes and directions for both the research team and the participants

■ **Testing** can be an issue when measurement methods involve repeated use of the same patient questionnaires, testing, and self-report measures. Familiarity with a test can enhance performance because "desired" answers can be learned. Effects of testing can also be an issue in studies in which a large battery of questionnaires is administered to patients, where patient fatigue can affect responses. Triangulation of results from several instruments and using alternative forms of a test can address this threat. Use of a mixed methods design can also be employed to confirm quantitative results with qualitative findings.

■ **Instrumentation** is a threat when there is a change in the measurement instrument or scoring between pre- and postintervention points. Observer judgment or experience can change over time. With biomedical and technical instrumentation, calibration and instrument reliability should be confirmed. Instrumentation is also an issue with measurement tools that perform differently at the ends of a scale than they do at the midpoint. This situation results in what are termed "floor" or "ceiling" effects in measurement. With ceiling or floor effects, changes in the variable being measured may not be observable if the value is already at the high or the low end of the possible scale. This type of threat is of concern when measurement is done by a single observer, when data are collected in person, and in studies in which pretest values are already at extreme high or low values. Selection of valid and reliable instruments with known normative ranges can assist the researcher in determining whether this is a threat in the study.

■ **Statistical regression** is a natural statistical phenomenon in which individuals who have extreme results (either high or low) will have scores that move toward the mean on a repeated test, and the resulting group mean will change. The magnitude of regression depends in part on the test–retest reliability of measurement. The potential for statistical regression is greatest when a study sample demonstrates extreme scores on the instrument used.

■ **Attrition** is a threat when individuals who drop out of a study, or are lost to follow-up, are different from those who remained in the study in ways that influence results. This can create an artifact in results if study groups are different kinds of people at the posttest time point compared to those who completed a pretest. Attrition is a problem in longitudinal studies and studies that may require substantial effort or impose burden on participants. Obtaining a sample size that accounts for possible attrition should be considered in planning the study. Analysis of key characteristics of those who withdraw versus those who complete the study enables one to determine whether significant differences between those individuals may have influenced results. Attrition also says something about the utility of the intervention. If large numbers of patients drop out of an experimental group, the intervention being tested may not be acceptable to patients, may create too much of a burden to participate, or may be associated with more negative side effects than benefits. Another approach to address study attrition is *intention-to-treat* analysis. Intention-to-treat analysis includes all study subjects regardless of conforming to inclusion criteria, treatments actually received, or withdrawal from the study. This prevents overoptimistic estimates of effectiveness of an intervention. This approach necessitates conducting clinical research to avoid missing data and to continue to follow up as much as possible with individuals who may withdraw (Gupta, 2011).

■ **Contamination** occurs if treatment is diffused to subjects in different study groups because participants interact and learn from each other. This can happen in crossover designs in which subjects who initially receive an education or behavioral intervention continue strategies learned in subsequent observations. This can also be a problem with studies involving two or more study groups in the same location. Implementing the study in such a way that groups will not be in contact with each other is one way to avoid this problem.

- **Compensatory equalization of treatments** can occur when staff or administrators feel that persons who do not receive the intervention are lacking a benefit and compensate for this perceived lack. This threat is most likely in studies in which group assignment is known to others and no placebo, active, or attentional controls are used.

- **Compensatory rivalry for participants with the less desirable treatment** is a situation in which subjects in the control group feel neglected or see themselves as underdogs, and are motivated to compete or perform in an attempt to reverse expected effects of an intervention. This is most problematic with study designs in which subjects know they are in the control group and where intact units of staff are assigned to interventions. Blinding study subjects to group assignment and provision of placebo, active, or attentional control conditions can reduce this type of threat.

- **Resentful demoralization of no-treatment groups** can be an issue if individuals who are not receiving what is seen as a more desirable treatment become discouraged and perform at a lower level in retaliation or because they feel dejected. This is a potential threat in study designs in which group assignment is known and those in which no appropriate control conditions are provided. This may also be more expected in studies involving work or other settings, where individuals may retaliate for lack of a perceived advantage by lowering productivity. Blinding subjects to group assignment and use of appropriate active or attentional control conditions help to address this problem.

- **Selection** can be a threat when there is a difference between participants in the study groups. This can occur because subjects choose to be in a certain group, or they are chosen for a certain group. This occurs when there is a lack of random assignment, for example in a quasi-experimental two-group study, where there is a lack of equal probability for being chosen for the different study groups.

- **Lack of treatment fidelity** occurs when the intervention is not provided in a consistent manner to all study subjects. This may be an issue when complex study interventions are provided by several different people, or where the intervention is provided by patients for self-care, where patient adherence is important. Provider training, provision of clear guidelines, references, and treatment algorithms can enhance performance of the intervention consistently. When the intervention is dependent on patient use, patient reminders can be used, and patient diaries or posttest interviews can be used to assess patients' adherence to interventions. In clinical drug trials, documentation of protocol violations is used to evaluate treatment fidelity. The Behavior Change Consortium's Model of Treatment Fidelity provides recommendations for incorporation of treatment fidelity (Bellg et al., 2004). In this model, there are five different categories that need to be addressed regarding intervention delivery including study design, training of the research team, treatment delivery by the research team, receipt of the intervention delivered by the research team to the participant, and enactment of different aspects of the intervention by the participant.

External Threats to Validity

External threats to validity refer to the extent to which findings can be generalized to and across different people, time, settings, and conditions. This involves potential statistical interactions that may not be readily discernible from specific study data and are best understood through deductive reasoning. Experience in relevant clinical care and knowledge of the field of study enable judgment of the applicability of findings in larger contexts. There are several common threats to external validity (Cook & Campbell, 1979).

- **Interaction of selection and treatment** occurs when the researcher is recruiting participants for the study. It may be challenging for the researcher to get a representative sample dependent on the nature of the study and the mode of recruitment. One method of handling this threat is to ensure that taking part in the study is as convenient as possible, so as to attract not only people who can handle the inconveniences that being in a study can cause, but to also be more inclusive of those who for example have limited time to participate in a study.

- **Interaction of setting and treatment** can be a threat to external validity if a limited number of settings are used that limit generalizability to other settings. This can be challenging if sites are limited or resources to recruit at a number of different sites are not available. Consideration in using these study findings to apply to other settings has to be carefully thought through in regard to applicability of these findings. For example, if participants are recruited at a work site for a health promotion intervention where it is conveniently held for them before and after work and on their lunch hour, would participants also participate at the same rate if they had to drive or take public transportation to a separate site for the same health promotion intervention?

- **Interaction of history and treatment** can be a threat as well, to external validity. Events that took place prior to and during an intervention can have an effect on study outcomes in an untended direction, and that the intervention itself did not fully contribute to. If for example a researcher is studying how to prevent a common infectious disease with a respiratory mode of transmission, and is using an intervention to decrease droplet transmission with sneezing and coughing, and ends up conducting the studying during a global pandemic that is transmitted via a respiratory mode, then the results of that study may in part be due to what participants are reading in the news regarding prevention of the pandemic. The researcher in this case would need to conduct this experiment at a different time.

IMPLEMENTING RESEARCH IN THE CLINICAL SETTING

Implementing research involves performing interventions as planned according to the study design and collecting study data. Operationalizing the study in a clinical setting requires a design that is practical and also well-constructed to minimize threats to validity. The workability of providing the intervention as planned in the specific setting is an important initial consideration. It is valuable to obtain expert opinion, and perform a feasibility study to test the study plan, methods, and acceptability to patients, before conducting a large clinical trial in the clinical setting.

Providing the Intervention

Studies held in clinical settings provide their own set of challenges. Although it can be more of a controlled environment than a community-setting environment, there are also many factors that have to be taken into account in the design of the intervention, including the patient, other patients, family members, healthcare providers, other hospital employees, environmental resources, and determination on how and when care delivery occurs when there are multiple patients to take care of at the same time. For example if sleep is being studied in an intensive care unit, and proximity of the patient's bed to the nurse's station is not accounted for, then the intervention could be complicated by a higher level of noise and activity, and possibly lack of privacy, when a patient is closest to the nurse's station.

If study interventions involve use of specific psychoeducational, supportive, or behavioral interventions, it is important to ensure that the key underlying principles in the approach are used as desired. In addition to general approaches to ensure treatment fidelity, reliability of the intervention can be analyzed by observation of a random sample of interventions directly, or through review of randomly selected video- or audio-taped sessions of delivery of the intervention.

Interventions need to be practical, accessible, and acceptable to study participants. If study subjects need to travel great distances, find it difficult to participate in scheduled activities, or do not adhere to self-care interventions, the actual delivery of the intervention may be questionable. For example, if the intervention is a program of group exercise and education classes, and subjects only attend 10% of the planned classes, it would be difficult to argue that the planned intervention was actually delivered to the patients. If the intervention being studied is not received, its efficacy cannot really be examined.

Data Collection

Providing healthcare to individuals generates a wealth of data. Clinical settings maintain computerized data sets for purposes of electronic health records, results reporting, quality reporting, and billing. Clinical practice generates information about individual patient demographic and biomedical information. Specific admission data on patient functional status and other factors are routinely obtained on patient admission to rehabilitation units and home care agencies as required by Medicare and other insurance companies for reimbursement. Hospital administrative and financial data sets contain information such as admission and discharge dates, lengths of stay, diagnosis codes, and procedure codes. Intensive care setting data often include patient severity scores, and emergency departments may generate triage and trauma scores. There has been a rapid conversion of many quality measures to *e-measures*, which can be collected as part of the electronic health record. These data can be used for descriptive analysis, measurement of outcomes, and incorporated into interventional studies to provide data about the characteristics of the subjects studied.

Many of the phenomena of interest to nursing are not readily available from existing data sets or incorporated in an easily usable form into electronic health records. Relevant data must be obtained through review and coding of verbal documentation or directly obtained by patient observation or patient responses on a questionnaire or rating scale. There are many different instruments available to use for patient rating of symptoms, and measurement of attributes such as anxiety, depression, resilience, quality of life, and so forth. Internet and literature searches can be used to identify instruments designed to measure a wide variety of patient attributes and symptoms.

Data can also be generated from abstraction and coding of health record documentation. Suppose one wants to determine whether nurses routinely assess patients for e-cigarette use, or vaping, and consideration of cessation of those habits, and current practice does not include use and documentation of any formal screening tool. Intake notes can be used to collect data from what is documented regarding e-cigarette or vaping habits. However, to do so, the researcher needs to predefine how to document these data, for example by daily or weekly use. One of the challenges in this method is to ensure that all individuals who abstract data to interpret verbal documentation do so in the same way. The investigator would need to decide how documentation would be coded or counted to generate numerical data for use in analysis. Another challenge with data collection from health record review comes from the fact that open-ended documentation may not routinely capture information about the variables of interest. Just because a clinician did not ask a patient about their e-cigarette or vaping habits or document those habits does not mean that the patient doesn't have them, or hasn't considered stopping. Validity and reliability of abstracted data can be evaluated by auditing a random sample of cases to ensure acceptable interpretation of documentation and data collected. There also has to be an organized way to collect and manage that information. For this type of data collection, creation of an electronic data collection tool is essential.

Consideration of practicality and time involved in data collection and data management are important components of planning clinical research. When possible, repurposing existing data for study purposes can address the barrier of time. It is helpful to collaborate with key individuals in an organization to identify what information already exists that can be captured and used to answer study questions. Managers and directors of various clinical departments can identify the type of information that is contained in their systems. Health record coding professionals can provide insight into how items such as diagnosis and procedure codes can be used to define patient characteristics and outcomes. Infection control and quality professionals can identify the type of information that is available from their work that may already reside in computer systems. Librarians can provide assistance in searching for existing measurement tools and approaches in the area of interest for study. Information systems professionals can assist in efforts to extract data from existing computer systems for analysis.

■ DATA ANALYSIS

There are two types of statistical analysis—*descriptive* and *inferential* (Gray et al., 2017; Polit & Beck, 2020). Descriptive statistics illustrate characteristics within a defined set of data. In contrast, inferential statistics are used to extrapolate findings beyond a single data set to determine the probability that results are applicable beyond the individual sample.

Descriptive Statistics

Descriptive statistics are used whenever the researcher wants to describe the findings within a sample of observations. Data can be described and communicated more easily if they are organized and summarized. The first step in organizing data is a *frequency distribution.* A frequency distribution provides a method to arrange observed values from lowest to highest, noting how often each value was counted. Numbers can be listed in order from lowest to highest, with the amount of times they were observed, and a percentage obtained. Also, histograms or a frequency polygon can be used to display the data. There are three important characteristics with frequency distributions, and these include the *shape of the distribution of values,* the *central tendency,* and *variability.*

- **Shape of the distribution of values** can occur in different configurations. If a distribution is symmetric then the two halves are equal to each other. If a distribution is asymmetric, then the two halves are not equal to each other and the data are skewed, resulting in a longer tail on the right or the left of a pictorial representation of the data. If a distribution has more than one peak then it has a multimodal distribution. However, many human attributes are symmetric and unimodal.

- **Central tendency** of the sample in a given attribute is one way to demonstrate what is common in a set of scores—how things look on average. Measures of central tendency are the mean, median, and mode. The *mean* is the sum of scores divided by the number of scores The mean can be used more easily in further statistical analysis, but extreme scores in the distribution will affect it, and it may not be the most accurate representation of the average The *median* is the 50% percentile of distribution—the point at which one half of the scores are lower, and one half of the scores are higher. The *mode* is the score that occurs most frequently. There is no clear answer as to which of these measures is the best. The measure that can be used also depends upon the scale of the data gathered. If the data are nominal scale, only the mode is meaningful.

- **Variability** in a set of scores includes the range, standard deviation, and variance. The *range* is the difference between the lowest and highest scores. The *standard deviation* and *variance* are calculated from the deviation, or distance, of all scores from the group mean. As such, these provide a view of the overall dispersion of results. The standard deviation is a linear measure. The variance is calculated as the standard deviation squared, providing a more three-dimensional picture of the overall difference in the variable being represented by the data. The standard deviation and variance can be compared between groups to evaluate the magnitude of differences. For example, if one has two samples or two groups with the same mean, but the standard deviation in group 1 is 3 and the standard deviation in group 2 is 6, one can conclude that the variability in group 2 is greater. Just as study design aims to reduce the potential for unexplained variability, analysis attempts to objectively account for the amount of variance found.

There are a number of different measures for *assessing relationships and associations among variables*. The strategy used depends on the scale and nature of the data. There are a variety of correlation statistics that can be used with nominal, ordinal, and interval data. For example, if the researcher is interested in determining if a characteristic is associated with an age, one could calculate a correlation coefficient such as the *Pearson product moment* between the raw values of age and the measure of the characteristic. The relationship between age and some characteristic could also be evaluated with a procedure such as *chi-square* by using age groups and determining if the average characteristic score, or if the percentage of patients who have the characteristic, differs significantly across age groups. Both approaches would yield the same conclusion. The use of a statistical decision tree can guide the researcher in choosing the recommended statistic dependent on the nature of the research question (Gray et al., 2017).

Inferential Statistics

The term *inferential* comes from the fact that these statistical procedures enable the researcher to draw inferences about populations from sample findings. We are used to talking about whether something is "statistically significant" based on the *p*-value of findings, but what does that actually mean? Clear interpretation of meaning necessitates a clear study question or hypothesis and an understanding of basic concepts of error and probability that apply to inferential statistics. Inferential statistics are either parametric or nonparametric. With a parametric statistical analysis, the parameters are normally distributed. The level of measurement with a parametric statistical analysis is interval, or if it is ordinal than there has to be an approximate normal distribution. As the name suggests, with nonparametric statistical analyses, studies do not meet the assumption of having a normal distribution. However nonparametric statistical analyses can also be used with nominal and ordinal data, as well as interval data that present as skewed.

HYPOTHESIS TESTING AND ERROR

Inferential statistics use the scientific method, posing a hypothesis that is then tested using probability theory. By convention, one poses a *null hypothesis*, and then calculates the probability of error in concluding that the null hypothesis is false. The underlying principle is that the researcher's theory or proposition is considered false until proven to be true beyond reasonable doubt (Nesselroade, 2019). It is useful to have a clear statement of the null hypothesis to clearly interpret the statistical findings. The null hypothesis is derived from the study question. For example, if the study question is: "Is there a relationship between anxiety and pain?" the corresponding null hypothesis would be: "There is *no* relationship between anxiety and pain." To support the researcher's actual theory that there is some relationship between these variables, the researcher has to show that the opposite conclusion, the null hypothesis, is not true.

In probability theory, there are two types of errors in hypothesis testing that can occur, *type I* and *type II*. These are displayed in Exhibit 9.1. As shown, a type I error occurs if one concludes that the null hypothesis is false, when it is actually true. In contrast, a type II error occurs if one concludes that the null hypothesis is true, when it is actually false. The probability of a type I error is termed alpha (α), and the probability of a type II error is beta (β). Using the preceding example, a *p*-value (α) of .05 means that the probability of incorrectly concluding that there *is* a relationship between anxiety and pain (making a type I error and incorrectly rejecting the null hypothesis) is 5%. Another way of stating this is that a *p*-value of .05 shows that there is a 5% chance that the results occurred by chance alone.

Another approach for hypothesis testing is the use of a *confidence interval* (CI) rather than calculating an actual *p*-value (Nesselroade, 2019). For example, if one obtains a Pearson product-moment correlation coefficient between anxiety and pain of 0.46, and obtains a 95% CI of 0.23 to 0.7, the results obtained are significant at the 0.05 level. If the statistic obtained falls within the CI, and the actual CI does not include 0, the finding is statistically significant, and the null hypothesis can be rejected. In this example the value of 0.46 is within the interval and the CI does not contain 0, so it is significant at the $\alpha = 0.05$ level. The CI does not indicate that 95% of the time the correlation coefficient in individuals will be between those values. This CI indicates that there is 95% confidence that the coefficient in the *theoretical* population, rather than an individual or a single sample, would be contained within this range. To some extent, one can also say something about the precision of the finding. If the CI is very large, the finding is not very precise.

The actual probability and testing for β (type II error) is not generally done due to the degree of specificity that would be required for the researcher to test the alternative to the null hypothesis. For such testing, it would be necessary to know the possible values of the dependent variable in the theoretical population that underlies the statistical testing. In the real world, this information is not known. To minimize the risk of a type II error, the researcher needs to choose the largest sample size available.

POWER

Another important statistic to consider is *power*. Power indicates the degree of assurance one can have in the statistical conclusions, considering that, even with a low *p*-value and probability of a type I error, there is also still the possibility of a type II error. Statistical power findings give further information about the reliability of conclusions. Power analysis is generally used to determine the sample size that is needed, at a specified level of alpha, to have confidence in the

---

EXHIBIT 9.1

ERROR TYPES AND POWER

Actual situation	Conclusion drawn	
	When the Null Hypothesis Is True	When the Null Hypothesis Is False
Fail to Reject the Null Hypothesis	Correct → $1 - \alpha$ (95%)	Type II error β (20%)
Reject the Null Hypothesis	Type I error α (5%)	Correct → Power $1-\beta$ (Power) (80%)

---

findings. Power analysis can also be used in adaptive study design to make changes in sample size. Usually researchers calculate sample sizes needed to achieve results at least at 80% power. Power at the level of 0.8 indicates that the researcher can expect that 80% of the time the study would yield the correct conclusion in terms of rejecting the null hypothesis. The interpretation of power is shown in Exhibit 9.1 (Nesselroade, 2019).

Four components make up a power analysis that is used to calculate a sample size (Polit & Beck, 2020). The researcher needs to first determine the significance, the effect size, and the power. The significance criterion α needs to be preset, noting that the smaller the α value, the lower the power. The effect size demonstrates the relationship between the independent and dependent variables. The equation for determining the effect size between two means is to find the difference between the two population means and divide that number by the standard deviation. Power is conventionally set at .80. The higher the sample size, the higher the power. Using existing tables, the researcher can approximate a sample size if the significance, effect size, and power are predetermined (Polit & Beck, 2020).

■ EFFECT SIZE

It is important to remember that statistical significance does not necessarily indicate clinical significance, or results that are meaningful for actual clinical practice. There are a number of additional statistics that can be helpful to clinicians in drawing conclusions about potential effects or benefits of interventions. In addition to providing information for power analysis, the concept of effect size can tell us something about how meaningful findings might be in real clinical situations. Effect size is a concept that indicates the magnitude of the relationship observed between variables (Vogt & Johnson, 2016). Strength of effect can be evaluated in research results from statistics such as the *Pearson product–moment* and other correlation coefficients, *standard mean difference (SMD), odds ratio (OR), relative risk (RR) ratio,* and statistics such as Cohen's *d* and Hedges's *g*.

The Pearson product–moment correlation, designated by *r*, has a possible effect size between +1 and -1. The correlation coefficient squared (r^2) shows the proportion of the total variance in the dependent variable that is explained by the independent variable. For example, if the correlation between anxiety and severity of pain is 0.4, this says that 16% (0.4^2) of the total variance

---

EXHIBIT 9.2

MATRIX FOR CALCULATION OF ODDS RATIO AND RELATIVE RISK RATIO

OBSERVATION*	TREATMENT GROUP (NUMBER OF CASES)	
	STANDARD CARE	NEW INTERVENTION
Event happens/desired outcome occurs	a	b
Event does not happen/desired outcome does not occur	c	d

*The observation can be a positive event, such as improvement in a symptom, or a negative event, such as development of a complication.

---

in pain severity is explained by anxiety. Clinician judgment can be applied to evaluate whether explaining 16% of total variance in pain severity is meaningful or not in the clinical context.

The SMD can be calculated for effect size when results are based on population means and standard deviations. The SMD is calculated as the difference between population means divided by the variance. Cohen's d is also based on means and standard deviations as the difference between two population means. It is important to note that effect size measures that use means are not just the average difference between pre- and post-results. In thinking about effect size, both the mean and the variability in results need to be considered together.

An OR is used when one of two possible outcomes is evaluated in response to an intervention or exposure to some event. The OR can be constructed with a 2×2 or larger table as [OR = $(a \times d)/(b \times c)$] as shown in Exhibit 9.2. The OR is a practical measure that can be calculated by hand in a clinical setting to determine the odds of a particular event or response for a patient or groups of patients. However, interpreting the OR is not completely straightforward. It is the ratio of the odds of success to the odds of failure. An OR of 1 would mean that the odds are the same for both groups. An OR of 4 would mean that one group had four times the *odds* of the results seen compared to the other group, not four times the *likelihood* of having the results seen in another group. Making decisions based on OR alone is more akin to betting on horse racing than it is to making risk-based decisions.

Equations for OR and RR, based on this matrix are:

$$OR = (a \times d) \div (b \times c).$$
$$RR = [a \div (a + b)] \div [c \div (c + d)].$$

RR ratio is similar to the OR but can be interpreted more easily. An RR less than 1 would mean that the result, or event, is less likely to occur, and an RR greater than 1 would mean that the event or outcome is more likely to occur in one group compared to the other. RR is calculated as the incidence of an outcome in one group divided by the incidence of that outcome in another group, as shown in Exhibit 9.2. In research reports, it is important that the direction of RR and OR results be clearly stated so that the direction of odds and risk difference is clearly tied to the study groups analyzed.

These types of effect size calculations have been used most often in meta-analyses, but they are also now being reported in individual research study reports. For the clinician to evaluate applicability and clinical meaningfulness of study findings, it is important to understand how to interpret these results.

DATA MANAGEMENT

Once research data are collected, they need to be stored and prepared for analysis. These processes are generally referred to as *data management*. Data management needs to address how and where raw data will be stored or accessed in study implementation and analysis to protect subject confidentiality, how data will be coded and computerized, how data will be cleaned, and the software that will be used for analysis. Cleaning data is often not given sufficient attention, particularly when data sets extracted from computerized databases are used. It should be remembered that just because data come from a computerized database does not mean they are accurate. For example, large data sets that are generated from administrative and insurance claims data can contain many errors.

Data cleaning involves identifying errors or extreme values in the data set. Extreme values and potential errors can be identified by looking at frequency distributions to identify aberrant results, and by various data-mining techniques to evaluate the degree to which the data reflect known relationships. For example, an analysis involving the use of hospital administrative data, including length of stay and cost per case, showed that one individual had a length of stay of 2 days and a total cost of $200,000. This cost for such a brief length of stay would be highly unlikely, suggesting that one or both of these values are incorrect. Such findings should be verified, or if not verifiable, can be treated as missing in data analysis.

There are a variety of statistical software packages that can be used for research analysis, meta-analysis procedures, and power calculations. There are also a number of applications for OR and RR calculation that are freely available on the internet. When conducting research, the researchers may choose to use a separate database for tracking participant data, for example Access, and another database to obtain and house results from the study, such as REDCap. By doing this, there is a clear separation between identified data that occurs with tracking (e.g., name and phone number) and de-identified data obtained from assessments (using subject ID numbers).

USING CLINICAL RESEARCH

If one understands how to plan and conduct good quality research, one also understands how to appraise research to determine quality and applicability in the clinical setting. The same principles of consideration of key variables to reduce unexplained variance, design to avoid bias and threats to validity, instrumentation, and interpretation of statistical results in terms of statistical significance as well as magnitude of effect, guide the evaluation of applicability of study findings.

Use of a research planning checklist, such as that shown in Exhibit 9.3, can be used to both plan research and evaluate some aspects of published research for clinical application. As seen here, planning quantitative research in the clinical setting involves many different factors to produce valid and meaningful results. It can be helpful to have a concrete tool to check off various aspects

EXHIBIT 9.3

QUANTITATIVE STUDY DESIGN AND PLANNING CHECKLIST

Study Planning Aspect	
1. Published research in the area of interest has been reviewed, and methods and measurement approaches are reviewed.	☐
2. The study question and the related null hypothesis are clear.	☐
3. Independent and dependent variables are clearly identified.	☐
4. Critical intervening, extraneous, and mediating variables have been identified.	☐
5. The study sample inclusion and exclusion criteria are defined. Criteria used will reduce potential extraneous variables that can impact the dependent variable.	☐
6. An appropriate sample size is identified with power analysis.	☐
7. Measurement methods have been identified that are valid and reliable.	☐
8. Measurement instruments have been developed or obtained, and directions for use and scoring have been reviewed.	☐
9. Existing data sources that are relevant for study have been identified and steps to obtain these data are in place if relevant.	☐
10. The type of data generated from measurement is known, and implications for planned statistical analysis are identified.	☐
11. The overall study design, sequence, and timing of observations and/or interventions are planned. The design has been reviewed for potential threats to internal validity, and steps have been taken to prevent or reduce these threats.	☐

12. Implementation of the design is planned, including:
    a. How the planned sample will be obtained
    b. An appropriate setting for the conduct of the study
    c. How data will be collected
    d. Who will be involved in data collection
    e. Who will provide interventions, if applicable
    f. Education, training, guidelines, and procedures for data collection and coding, and delivery of interventions have been provided
    g. What steps will be taken to avoid missing data
	☐
	☐
	☐
	☐
	☐
	☐
	☐
	
	☐

13. Methods to ensure intervention fidelity have been identified and are in place, if applicable.	☐
14. Methods for data storage and computer data entry are planned. Individuals involved in data entry and data management are trained in procedures needed.	☐
15. Statistical analysis is planned, and appropriate statistical software is available. Statistical consultation and support are available as needed.	☐

of study design and implementation, to ensure consideration of appropriate variables, measurement, and consideration of sources of bias and validity threats.

The movement from the idea of research utilization to concepts of evidence-based practice points to the need to use the best quality evidence available, and to the value of combining results from multiple studies to provide such evidence. Given the complexity of providing healthcare to individuals, as well as the many facets of research design and implementation, it is easy to see how different studies involving the same types of observations can yield conflicting or uncertain results. It is only by considering the full range of findings from a body of work, as well as the quality of research design and conduct, that one can determine the utility of research findings.

■ SUMMARY

Conducting and using quantitative research involves all aspects of a study, from initially forming a clear research question, through implementation, to analysis and interpretation of results. Understanding variables, the nature of data, measurement properties, study design, data management, and the ability to correctly use and interpret statistics are essential to generating good quality evidence for use in clinical practice.

Collaboration with others is vital in planning and conducting quantitative research. The input of experienced researchers and statisticians facilitates the work of identifying appropriate measurement methods, designing the study, sample selection, data collection and management approaches, statistical analysis, and accurate interpretation of findings. Collaboration with library science professionals facilitates review of the literature to inform the process and identify measurement instruments. Seeking the input of clinical professionals and others who work in the clinical setting enables determination of both theoretical and practical aspects that need to be considered in implementation and study design. Working with others in the clinical setting can also identify existing data sources that can be used for research purposes.

SUGGESTED LEARNING ACTIVITIES

1. Determine a study question that reflects an intervention you want to examine in your clinical setting.
   a. Determine the independent and dependent variables.
   b. Write out the hypothesis and null hypothesis.
2. Describe the level of data that are needed to test this intervention (nominal, ordinal, interval, and/or ratio).
3. Choose a study design that is feasible for you to use to examine this intervention.
4. Address one potential threat to internal validity and the approach you would use to reduce or eliminate that threat.
5. Consider how you might collect data in the clinical setting.
6. Discuss how you would use descriptive and inferential statistics with this study.

REFERENCES

Bellg, A. J., Borrelli, B., Resnick, B., Hecht, J., Minicucci, D. S., Ory, M., Ogedegbe, G., Orwig, D., Ernst, D., Czajkowski, S., & Treatment Fidelity Workgroup of the NIH Behavior Change Consortium. (2004). Enhancing treatment fidelity in health behavior change studies: Best practices and recommendations from the National Institutes of Health Behavior Change Consortium. *Health Psychology: Official Journal of the Division of Health Psychology, American Psychological Association, 23*(5), 443–451. https://doi.org/10.1037/0278-6133.23.5.443

Buchholz, S. W., Wilbur, J., Halloway, S., Schoeny, M., Johnson, T., Vispute, S., & Kitsiou, S. (2019). Study protocol for a sequential multiple assignment randomized trial (SMART) to improve physical activity in employed women. *Contemporary Clinical Trials, 89*, 105921. https://doi.org/10.1016/j.cct.2019.105921

Cook, T. D., & Campbell, D. T. (1979). *Quasi-experimentation design and analysis issues for field settings.* Houghton Mifflin Company.

Gray, J. R., Grove, S. K., & Sutherland, S. (2017). *The practice of nursing research: Appraisal, synthesis, and generation of evidence* (8th ed.). Elsevier.

Gupta, S. K. (2011). Intention-to-treat concept: A review. *Perspectives in Clinical Research, 2*(3), 109–112. https://doi.org/10.4103/2229-3485.83221

Janssens, A. C. J. W., & Martens, F. K. (2020). Reflection on modern methods: Revisiting the area under the ROC curve. *International Journal of Epidemiology, 49*(4), 1397–1403. https://doi.org/10.1093/ije/dyz274

Kravitz, R. L., Duan, N., & eds, and the DEcIDE Methods Center N-of-1 Guidance Panel (Duan N, Eslick I, Gabler NB, Kaplan HC, Kravitz RL, Larson EB, Pace WD, Schmid CH, Sim I, Vohra S). (2014). *Design and implementation of N-of-1 trials: A user's guide. AHRQ publication no. 13(14)-EHC122-EF.* Agency for Healthcare Research and Quality.

National Institutes of Health Office of Behavioral and Social Sciences. (2018). *Best practices for mixed methods research in the health sciences* (2nd ed.). National Institutes of Health. https://www.obssr.od.nih.gov/wp-content/uploads/2018/01/Best-Practices-for-Mixed-Methods-Research-in-the-Health-Sciences-2018-01-25.pdf

National Quality Forum. (2013). *Patient reported outcomes in performance measurement.* https://www.qualityforum.org/Publications/2012/12/Patient-Reported_Outcomes_in_Performance_Measurement.aspx

National Quality Forum. (2020). *Patient-reported outcomes.* https://www.qualityforum.org/Patient-Reported_Outcomes.aspx

Nesselroade, K. P. (2019). *Statistical applications for the behavioral and social sciences* (2nd ed.). John Wiley & Sons, Inc.

Pedhazur, E. J., & Schmelkin, L. P. (1991). *Measurement, design, and analysis: An integrated approach.* Lawrence Erlbaum Associates, Inc.

Polit, D. F., & Beck, C. T. (2020). *Nursing research: Generating and assessing evidence for nursing practice* (11th ed.). Wolters Kluwer.

U.S. Department of Health and Human Services. (2016). *Non-inferiority clinical trials to establish effectiveness: Guidance for industry.* https://www.fda.gov/media/78504/download

Vogt, W. P., & Johnson, R. B. (2016). *The SAGE dictionary of statistics and methodology.* SAGE.

Waltz, C. F., Strickland, O. L., & Lenz, E. (2017). *Measurement in nursing and health research* (5th ed.). Springer Publishing Company.

Wilbur, J., Kolanowski, A. M., & Collins, L. M. (2016). Utilizing MOST frameworks and SMART designs for intervention research. *Nursing Outlook, 64*(4), 287–289. https://doi.org/10.1016/j.outlook.2016.04.005

QUALITATIVE APPROACHES FOR PRACTICE SCHOLARSHIP

BETH RODGERS

▦ INTRODUCTION

Qualitative research methods constitute a vital part of nursing knowledge development and provide information that is essential for evidence-based practice (EBP). Researchers frequently use methods of this type to address problems relevant to aspects of nursing practice and human existence that cannot be reduced to isolated variables or captured in numerical form. Some of the aspects are critical to the holistic aspect of nursing practice—the feelings and subjective experiences of the people with whom nurses interact and the ways in which people go through their lives and redefine their daily world through various challenges and successes. There also are many areas of nursing for which we have little information and may function on the basis of personal experience or habit. Qualitative methods can be useful to create a solid foundation for future study.

Historically, formal hierarchies that rank different levels of evidence tend to place qualitative research at a lower level than any of the quantitative approaches. These rankings reflect a continuing reverence for controlled trials more than they provide an accurate assessment of the actual value of qualitative research. In fact, the artificiality of many controlled trials could easily call into question the value of those studies and it is not uncommon that real-world results often achieve different outcomes than those obtained through controlled settings. Effective nursing care must include evidence that addresses aspects of the human experience, and many of these cannot be studied using controlled means. More recent systems for evaluating levels of evidence show qualitative research typically at about a midpoint, above opinion and anecdote, but still below quantitative approaches. Such ranking systems overlook the fact that different types of research are done for very different purposes, thus one-to-one comparison of types of research is unrealistic. The goal of the research, and the need for the research to enable informed decisions, makes a difference in determining the value of the evidence provided.

There are many different types of research, each with its own rules and criteria for quality, and also a variety of research that involves a combination of methods. In this context, nurses must have the skills to evaluate all types of evidence to make the most informed decisions that affect their practice. The ability to assess evidence means that nurses must understand the processes involved in qualitative research and be able to evaluate the quality of evidence derived from such studies if the goal is to use the best evidence available as a basis for nursing practice. The advanced practice nurse also is likely to want to explore opportunities for change and innovation in the practice setting, and such studies may require the ability to understand an array of options available for generating quality evidence, not just for using work that has been done by others.

When reading reports of qualitative studies, it is immediately apparent that the designs and procedures for qualitative research differ considerably from those of quantitative studies. A question that is raised often when discussing different types of research is whether different approaches are sufficiently scientific and, therefore, have a legitimate place in the research base of nursing. For many people, the mention of science conjures an image of a laboratory setting or, at least, an environment where the researcher carefully controls the conditions for the investigation by isolating the phenomenon being studied from other elements that might interfere with the results. The researcher, in this view of science, also is presumed to be "objective," observing the results of the experiment without preconceived ideas or biases. As such, the results are considered to be some form of truth regarding the situation being studied. There is a belief that science, conducted in such a way, provides answers about cause and effect, definitive explanations that serve as proof about what happens in certain situations and, in regard to clinical practice, a clear understanding of what is the best thing to do in a particular circumstance. Compared to this idea of science, qualitative research certainly does seem quite unorthodox.

Educational systems, particularly at the early levels where students generally are first introduced to science, perpetuate this idea; society, in general, extends it as well through communication and media that refer to proof as if it were the appropriate goal and could be achieved definitively. It becomes clear with just a little review of research, however, that very little about actual research is consistent with this idea of science. Finding one absolute, indisputable answer to questions is unreasonable in any context, much less where humans are involved. As humans interact with their environment, they change, the environment changes, and so does the phenomenon being studied.

Objectivity, in a complete and unbiased sense, is not something that can be achieved by any scientist, or by any human being, nor is it necessarily desirable in every situation. The mere identification of something as a problem involves judgment on the part of the researcher. The researcher's existing biases are integrated throughout the conduct of inquiry and, in fact, often are useful in the research situation as they provide the researcher with important tools for research such as language, concepts, theories, and mechanisms for interacting with human subjects of study. These are all biases in a sense, yet research would not be possible without them. Complete objectivity, therefore, is not possible without dispensing with all that has been learned through both education and development in a social context and without dispensing with some basic facts of how human beings function. Rather than seeing the possibility of one absolute answer or truth, objectivity, and control as necessary ingredients for science, recent philosophers of science (those who explore what makes science work and what constitutes good science) provide a contemporary view of science as an attempt to solve problems, to generate solutions that work, to exercise creativity and innovation in the interest of discovery and development of knowledge, and to tie research to a broad interest in the good of society (Rodgers, 2005). Outcomes of science sometimes point to what it is appropriate to do in a situation. In other cases, they point to enlightening and empowering people to be active participants in their own lives and health-related situations. This shift in perspective is associated with a philosophy known as postmodernism, and the growth of such research spurred energetic debate about the evidence in general and various ranking systems earlier in the movement toward EBP (Porter & O'Halloran, 2009).

The evolving idea of what constitutes science fueled a substantial increase in the acceptance and, consequently, the volume of qualitative research being conducted in a variety of disciplines. Qualitative research, although a mainstay of inquiry in the social sciences for more than a century, ultimately blossomed in acceptance and use in a broad array of disciplines. In nursing, evidence of considerable growth in this area can be seen starting particularly in the 1980s, although there was some discussion of its utility even earlier than that. Quint (1967), for example, produced a seminal work demonstrating the importance of qualitative research in theory development at the dawning of the theory movement in nursing, decades before qualitative research developed any noticeable foothold in nursing. Acceptance of such methods in the research enterprise was slow at first, but it has become an essential aspect of nursing's knowledge base, providing valuable information on aspects of human health and illness that are best explored using the capabilities of qualitative methods. The role of qualitative research results in regard to evidence-based practice is still the subject of some debate, although qualitative research appears on Level of Evidence tables with increasing regularity (Melnyk & Fineout-Overholt, 2019) and there is no question that nurses understand the importance of patient experiences in determining the appropriateness of various interventions and practices in healthcare. It is the relationship that nurses develop with people in the context of health and wellness that differentiates nursing care from other aspects of health and illness work. These connections with individuals and groups create a strong need for evidence and a scientific base such as is obtained through qualitative research.

◼ WHY QUALITATIVE RESEARCH?

As noted previously, qualitative research is appropriate for inquiry that addresses a number of aspects relevant to nursing and provides an important part of the evidence base essential to nursing practice. Qualitative research approaches the study of phenomena in a natural setting. Rather than attempt to control elements of the research situation, such as by manipulating variables (e.g., an intervention presented in a controlled setting), a qualitative study typically is designed to capture experiences or events as they naturally occur. Qualitative research also excels at capturing people's thoughts and feelings, which are not easily reduced to numbered responses to questions on paper and pencil instruments. Qualitative research offers insights important to viewing situations and people holistically and, therefore, is ideal to answer broad questions that warrant in-depth description. Some examples of research questions that might be used for qualitative studies are provided in Box 10.1.

The broad questions presented in the samples reveal some of the specific purposes and functions of qualitative research. Qualitative research can be used to describe, providing both a deep and rich description of a situation or experience. Qualitative research also helps to provide information about aspects that might be missed with a quantitative study. For example, quantitative research is appropriate for determining if one intervention is more effective than another in a way that is statistically significant. Such a study, however, will not provide information about what it is like for an individual to live with the intervention. In such a situation, qualitative research makes it possible to capture information that is essential to gaining a complete picture of a situation or experience. Qualitative research can also be very sensitizing, raising awareness of aspects of an

---

BOX 10.1 Common Questions for Qualitative Research

- ◼ What is happening here?
- ◼ What is it (a particular situation or condition) like for people who experience this?
- ◼ What are the experiences of people with X (the phenomenon of interest)?
- ◼ What is the meaning of X (the phenomenon of interest)?

experience that might not have been recognized previously. By doing so, nurses are better able to anticipate patients' needs and concerns and understand their perspectives when confronted with a health-related situation. Obviously knowledge of these types is important for nursing practice where nurses need to be able to individualize care and work with psychological, social, and emotional aspects as well as the physiologic components of health and illness situations. Qualitative research is ideal for understanding what people think, feel, believe, and live through as they encounter situations related to their health and well-being.

Before continuing, it is important to note that some studies that are primarily quantitative in nature may also include qualitative data, or data in the form of words. Qualitative data can be an important adjunct to an otherwise quantitatively focused study capturing elements that otherwise would be overlooked or providing important detail to provide a more complete picture of what is being studied. For example, a study focused on an educational intervention to promote adherence to a prescribed regimen for treating hypertension could include some important numerical data regarding knowledge, medication use, and diet and exercise changes adopted by the participants. Such numerical data are ideal for making comparisons across groups such as to determine whether the intervention was effective in promoting changes in knowledge and behaviors. A study of this type can be more complete, however, if the researcher also collects data regarding what people thought about the intervention, what they saw as challenges in acting on the information received, and whether they feel capable of continuing with the recommended changes. Such data regarding perceptions and experiences are best collected in a qualitative form based on the words and narratives provided by the participants. In such a situation, the researcher clearly is using qualitative data but the primary focus of the study is on the quantitative testing of effectiveness in regard to the outcomes. This is an important distinction because studies that are completely qualitative in nature are conducted and evaluated according to very different guidelines and criteria.

The inclusion of qualitative data does not make the study a qualitative one by design. It is necessary to determine the primary focus of the study and use appropriate criteria to guide the design, evaluation, and critique of the inquiry. In general, a study is referred to as a qualitative study when the primary focus is on gathering narrative descriptions of experience; those narratives are, of course, expressed in the form of words and the results are presented through words as well. While there may be some quantitative data in a qualitative study, those data generally are limited to describing the participants. As a general guide, the criteria for conducting or evaluating a qualitative study apply when there is a focus on words both as data and as words in the reporting of results. This focus will apply to the remainder of this chapter when the reference is made to a qualitative study.

Numerous examples of specific types of qualitative studies, including different questions and applications, can be found throughout the nursing literature. A worthwhile activity for anyone interested in research of any type is to explore the literature and read reports of completed research that have been conducted using different designs. In qualitative research, this is particularly important as there are multiple types of qualitative studies, each with its own specific question, procedures, and manner of presenting results, as evident in the following section.

■ TYPES OF QUALITATIVE RESEARCH

As noted earlier, qualitative research typically is focused on words as data rather than numbers and the qualitative researcher reports results in the form of words. Some qualitative studies also can involve other forms of communication such as dramatizations or the use of photos. There has been considerable growth in the use of visual forms of data and of expression, although such research is much less common than research focused on verbal accounts (Banks, 2018). Even in cases of visually oriented research, word descriptions typically accompany and elucidate the other components of data. In spite of this common characteristic among all the qualitative approaches, there are distinct methodologies for qualitative research, each of which has its own unique philosophical underpinnings, history, and procedures for the conduct of a study.

On a very basic level, there is a general type of qualitative research that often appears in the literature. A study might be described as merely "qualitative," "descriptive," "qualitative descriptive," "exploratory," "naturalistic," "field research," or "ethnographic." All of these refer to the collection of data directly from subjects (referred to as participants in acknowledgment of their active role in the process) and are typically in the form of words. Such studies are similar in that they tend to rely on either individual or group interviews and, occasionally, observation, and general forms of analysis that identify patterns and similarities in the data. Qualitative studies can be conducted quite well without being associated with a more specific methodology that has unique requirements regarding the question and the collection and analysis of data. Note that descriptive research can be quantitative as well, so seeing a study characterized as "descriptive" in a report of research requires a closer look at the nature of the data and the report of results to determine if it is qualitative or quantitative. The term "ethnographic," similarly, can have multiple meanings, referring most generally to research in a natural setting. There also is a distinct methodology known as ethnography, which is discussed later.

More specific methodologies for qualitative research are found in the literature. In nursing, some of the more common types of qualitative studies are grounded theory, phenomenology, hermeneutic (most often hermeneutic phenomenology), narrative inquiry, and, as noted earlier, ethnography. A brief definition of each of these primary methodologies is provided in Table 10.1.

Grounded theory research was introduced formally in the 1960s based on the work of noted sociologist Anselm Strauss and colleague Barney Glaser (Glaser & Strauss, 1967). This method is guided by the theoretical viewpoint of symbolic interactionism (Blumer, 1969), although the essential nature of the link to symbolic interactionism has been questioned in recent years. In general, symbolic interactionism holds that people create their sense of self, their reality, societies,

TABLE 10.1 Common Qualitative Methodologies

METHODOLOGY	GENERAL DESCRIPTION
Grounded theory	Focused on the social and psychological processes associated with an experience. Results provide a substantive theory that describes that experience.
Phenomenology	Experience is conceptualized as "lived experience" based on the idea that people construct their experiences and those experiences, in turn, shape the individual and the response. Results provide insight into "meaning," which is defined uniquely in this methodology.
Narrative inquiry	Emphasizes the stories that people construct about their lives to bring order to experience. Results provide insight into the ways in which such stories are constructed as people make sense of their lives.
Ethnography	Focused on the study of culture, which can be any group or setting where there is learned behavior and shared ideas. Results presented as detailed and extensive descriptions of that culture.

and so on, through interaction with other people. How an individual experiences some event or process in life is heavily influenced by those interactions. In a grounded theory study, the researcher seeks information about the overall experience of people in specific situations of interest to the researcher. The researcher conducting an investigation using the methodology of grounded theory will have a research question such as "what is it like to . . . " or "what is the experience of people with. . . . " The experience that is the focus of research will involve the thoughts, feelings, actions, interactions with others, and interpretations of events associated with the situation being studied as described by the people who are going through that experience.

Grounded theory research has a unique end product in that it is used to construct a substantive theory that provides a detailed depiction of the experience being studied that is derived from (grounded in) the data obtained from participants. This theory is organized around a central idea referred to as the core variable (Charmaz, 2014; Glaser, 1978; Glaser & Strauss, 1967), which represents the primary focus of the experience. This core variable represents the Basic Sociopsychological Process involved in the experience and reflects the symbolic interactionism foundation regarding interaction being important in the shaping of experience. Since Glaser and Strauss pioneered this method in the late 1960s, other variations have been introduced, including a version by Strauss and Corbin (1998). The underlying principles are the same, although the Strauss and Corbin version imposes more structure on the data analysis process and on the reporting of results. Other adaptations have been created as well, most notably the constructivist orientation provided by Charmaz (Bryant & Charmaz, 2019; Charmaz, 2000, 2005, 2008, 2014). From the standpoint of the advanced practice nurse who needs to critique and evaluate research for implications for practice, reports of grounded theory studies can be evaluated similarly, keeping in mind the foundations of this approach and the expected outcome of a substantive theory, regardless of the specific variation a researcher used in a study.

The qualitative method known as *phenomenology* is also used to study experiences, but is focused on the meaning of the lived experience of the people in the study. Phenomenology was derived originally from the philosophies of Edmund Husserl (1960) and Merleau-Ponty (1962/1999), and its origins contributed to the extensive foundation in philosophy that is evident in this method. Based on this foundation, modifications to the method were presented by existentialist philosopher Martin Heidegger, and the method was adapted further as a means of study in psychology. There are numerous unique approaches that are all justifiably referred to as phenomenology, including a variation called *hermeneutic phenomenology* (Crowther et al., 2017; Matua & Van Der Wal, 2015; Spence, 2017), which is fairly common in nursing. All of these approaches have some elements in common, however. Whereas grounded theory is focused on social interaction and processes, phenomenology is a method to study the individual and how the individual ascribes meaning to an experience. A significant underpinning of this research method is the idea that humans create their own realities and these realities, in turn, have a strong influence on creating the individual. This idea is referred to as co-constitution, capturing the notion that people, and their realities have an influence on the construction of each other. Experiences and events have their own essence or what might in common language be referred to as the facts of the situation, or what actually happened. A person is diagnosed with a chronic illness, for example, and there is solid evidence to support that diagnosis and the fact that it was communicated to the individual. In phenomenology, however, the focus is on the layers of meaning or interpretation that the individual gives to the situation. It is not even necessary that there be facts to support the interpretation.

As an example for phenomenology, consider an individual who has a family history of a condition associated with cognitive decline. That person might have occasional feelings of being distracted or forgetting to do a particular task and interprets those as a symptom of the impending hereditary decline, even though there is no substantive or documented reason to make that association. The interpretation or meaning the individual assigns to what he or she is experiencing will have a profound influence on the sense of self and the willingness to share the experiences with others. While all qualitative methods are focused on people's experiences and their own individual realities, the phenomenological researcher typically goes beyond the actual words spoken by an individual to describe the experience in an attempt to interpret these words and identify underlying meaning. For that reason, phenomenology sometimes is referred to as an interpretive method (Horrigan-Kelly et al., 2016; Van Manen, 1997) rather than a descriptive one. The product of phenomenological research is a discussion of significant ideas or meaning statements derived through analysis of the participant's words and interpretation of the meanings the experience being studied has for the individual. Phenomenology is a complex and highly variable qualitative method and the sample sizes, analytic approaches, and results will differ depending on the particular orientation employed by the researcher.

Narrative inquiry is another form of qualitative research that is common in nursing. Narrative inquiry (Clandinin, 2020; Holstein & Gubrium, 2012; Riessman, 1993) is grounded in the premise that people typically construct stories about their various life experiences including stories that form their own identities. These stories represent the individual's way of weaving together elements of the event into their story of their experience. According to Riessman (1993), the purpose of narrative inquiry is "to see how respondents in interviews impose order on the flow of experience to make sense of events and actions in their lives" (p. 2). These stories involve all the typical aspects of a story including players, supporting players, settings, sequencing of events, and outcomes. Using the techniques of narrative analysis, the researcher examines these stories to uncover an underlying narrative that characterizes the stories associated with an experience (Riley & Hawe, 2005). Narrative inquiry emphasizes the dimensions of temporality, sociality, and place in gaining understanding of an experience. According to this methodology, events involve a temporal timeline, or a past, present, and future. Sociality refers to the interplay of personal and social aspects of experience. This includes personal elements of feelings and hopes as well as cultural and social conditions. The relationship that develops between the researcher and the participants also is a part of the experience. Finally, the element of place refers to physical boundaries (Connelly & Clandinin, 2006). These elements are not considered on their own; for example, a simple reporting of when or where something happened. Instead, these are considered to be related components of the complex experiences in people's lives. These elements are interwoven in the stories people create about their lives and the way they use language to construct these narratives.

The final form of qualitative research that will be discussed here is *ethnography*. Ethnography as a specific method (in contrast to the more generic use of the term "ethnographic" to refer to research that takes place in a natural setting or in the field) originated in the discipline of anthropology. Ethnography is focused on the study of culture. For purposes of this type of research, a culture is "the total way of life of a group and the learned behavior that is socially constructed and transmitted" (Wolf, 2012, p. 295). In conducting research using the methodology of ethnography, the researcher typically spends extensive time in the setting being studied. In addition to "getting in," the process of becoming accepted by the group being studied, a goal in the early phase of such a study is the identification of key informants or people who are particularly familiar with the setting or experience and whose perspectives are important to understanding the workings of the setting. The researcher will observe the group and interactions among the group, keep extensive notes, and talk with individuals in addition to the key informants whose input is particularly important to the study. Ethnographies are found much less frequently in the nursing literature than are examples of the other methods, perhaps because of the extremely time-intensive nature of the research. In addition, ethnographies typically are so extensive and detailed that they can be reported only partially through the usual format of a journal article.

■ CONDUCTING A QUALITATIVE STUDY

Before attempting the critical evaluation of qualitative studies, it is necessary to understand how qualitative research is conducted. In spite of the differences in the foundation and the development of the various traditions, the overall procedures for conducting a qualitative study are quite similar. Those procedures differ considerably from those used in conducting quantitative studies (Wu et al., 2016), and a review of the steps in the process, comparing qualitative and quantitative types of research, can be helpful to identify important differences.

It is important to remember that the intent in any type of qualitative research is to capture the individual realities of the participants and to provide a detailed description of those realities and the experiences of the people studied. Therefore, elements of research that involve ideas such as control, theoretical frameworks, hypothesis testing, reliability, and generalizability, for example, are either inappropriate or take on an entirely different meaning in the context of a qualitative study. The following sections describe the sequence of steps typically pursued in conducting a qualitative study. Ideas about what to look for in the critique of qualitative studies are included as well to develop skill in assessing the quality of published reports of qualitative research.

Research Problem and Question

As with any type of research, the process of qualitative inquiry begins with identification of a problem and a research question. Problems appropriate for qualitative research exist when there are new ideas or situations to explore and little is known about the phenomenon. In such a situation, studies aimed at broad discovery are appropriate. A change in a treatment modality might warrant a study that explores the experiences of people who receive that treatment; staffing patterns for nurses might be explored in regard to the experiences of the nurses who live with that pattern on a regular basis or might lead to exploration of other aspects of the care delivered by the nursing staff. Problems appropriate for qualitative research also exist when there are significant gaps in knowledge. A long-standing procedure might have been studied extensively regarding its effectiveness, yet there may be very little information about what patients think or feel about the treatment and how it affects their daily lives. A problem amenable to qualitative research can be just about anything that can be answered through in-depth discovery and descriptions of the experiences, thoughts, and feelings of people who have encountered the situation being studied.

Questions for qualitative studies appear to be similar in spite of the specific tradition of inquiry that underlies the research. There are subtle differences in wording, however, that clue the reader as to the specific tradition being explored. Phenomenology, for example, involves the phrase "lived experience" or the word "meaning" as a specific focus of the research question for that type of study. Beyond some seemingly minor variations in wording, questions for a qualitative study in general address the broad experience or the reactions (including thoughts, feelings, interpretations, and meanings) regarding a life encounter.

Researchers often do not state a specific research question in their report of qualitative studies; the absence of an actual question is not a weakness in a research report. The purpose of the study and the problem situation that led to the development of the research, however, should be clear to the reader and, ideally, these are presented early in the published report. The question or problem should be one that is appropriate to qualitative inquiry as well. Questions about what should be done in a situation or what is better are not amenable to any type of research as they call for judgments that go beyond the actual data gained through the study. A researcher can, however, address a question about what people report, what characteristics are identified, how people describe their feelings, and how they live with some situation or experience as a step toward developing conclusions about what is better and why that is the case.

Review of Literature

Another step in the typical research process involves a review of the literature. It is a bit misleading to consider this a separate step, as with any type of study the review of the literature can be very helpful in refining the original problem. The iterative process of reviewing the literature and rethinking the original problem helps the researcher to gain clarity and important perspectives that give direction to the subsequent research. In a quantitative study, the literature review typically provides an important foundation for the research by revealing what is already known about the situation of interest. On this basis, the researcher can determine the appropriate next steps for inquiry and, depending on the type of research, can develop a theoretical foundation for the study and possible hypotheses. At this point, qualitative and quantitative studies differ considerably. The qualitative researcher does not intend to build on existing research but typically embarks on an attempt to explore, discover, and describe areas and experiences about which little already is known. In this spirit, the researcher wants to remain as open as is plausible to the many possibilities that can exist in any situation. Using the literature review to frame the study would put some boundaries around what is explored and what might be seen in the data that are collected.

Some discussions of qualitative research present the argument that there is no need for any type of literature review before embarking on a qualitative study (Glaser & Strauss, 1967). Avoiding contact with existing information is believed to enable the researcher to be more open and unbiased about what might be encountered through the study. While the idea of being as unbiased as possible is appealing, this approach is faulty on a couple of levels. First, it is never possible to be completely open and unbiased about anything. The researcher is making judgments from the very beginning of a study by identifying something as a problem and by naming phenomena; in other words, by using certain words to label what is being studied. The researcher also inherently possesses some bias due to the researcher's own experience as a human interacting with others and with the knowledge they already have accumulated. Individual values influence all research, so the idea of objectivity being enhanced by avoiding a literature review is not defensible; yet, this is not the same as the researcher actively seeking a foundation in the literature on which to build the new study.

Diminishing bias in a study is a desirable goal to the extent possible and typically the researcher does not want to skew the study in any particular direction to avoid placing limits on what might be discovered. Seeking possible explanations or hypotheses in the literature would add specific direction to the research that is counter to the openness that is such a strength in qualitative research. In qualitative studies, therefore, there often is a literature review but it takes on a unique form. The qualitative researcher typically does a thorough literature review prior to the start of the study, but that review is oriented toward substantiating that a problem does exist, that qualitative methods are appropriate to address that problem, and, in some cases, to gain direction and support for the methods chosen for the study. Rather than provide a foundation for the research, the literature review in a qualitative study enables the researcher to justify the need for the research and the chosen form of qualitative inquiry.

The literature review section that appears relatively early in a report of a qualitative study should be thorough and give good background information about the problem. Since the researcher usually is not building on this existing information for further inquiry in an area, the literature review sometimes is more broad, discussing a wide variety of studies that have been done and often identifying gaps in knowledge rather than focusing on a select few items or articles to provide underpinnings for the research. Ultimately, the researcher uses the literature review to make a clear case for the fact that a researchable problem exists and that it is important to generate information that will fill this gap. As noted earlier, the appropriateness of qualitative methods to address the problem should be apparent as well.

The use of an initial literature review to substantiate the problem and methods is one difference between qualitative and quantitative studies. Similarly, in quantitative research, the initial literature review is used to tie the study to previous work, showing how the study presented in a published report relates to other research. In qualitative studies, this connection to existing work is made near the end of the study rather than at the beginning. As themes and patterns are identified in the data obtained during the study, the researcher will conduct an extensive literature review late in the conduct of the study to determine how the ideas that have been discovered relate to extant knowledge. For example, in a study of the experiences of people living with obstructive sleep apnea (OSA) (Rodgers, 2013), the researcher returned to the literature to gather information about several aspects of the experience that arose during the study. While dependence on technology associated with sleep apnea could be expected to be an issue in this study, the researcher did not find the machine aspect to be a pronounced aspect of the experience, although that has been a focus of experience with other technology-dependent conditions. People expressed some distress about having to use a mask, but expressed little concern about the role of a machine in their lives or managing the technology. The impact was felt far more in the area of adjustment to diagnosis with a chronic illness and feeling supported throughout the process. Technology-dependent conditions often come with considerable training and support which was not the case for the people in this study. This raised questions about the interconnections of variables in this study that might help to understand the different experiences. Ultimately, this led to an extensive literature review to examine associations among these concepts as a means of connecting the findings from the study with existing knowledge, particularly in regard to other conditions in which technology is a significant factor in health status. If the study had been based on a framework focused on technology, other key findings might have received much less emphasis as they might have fallen outside the framework used to explain the findings. This example demonstrates the value of a more broad and open approach in qualitative studies and what can be accomplished without a predetermined framework that narrows the inquiry.

Theories provide an important foundation and guide for research but also can place limits on how something is studied and how the results are interpreted. When reading published reports of qualitative research, the literature review component needs to be evaluated in regard to the initial review that is used to substantiate the problem as well as in the discussion section at the end of the report. In this latter section, the researcher discusses the findings of the current study in the context of previous research and theoretical literature. This use of the literature enables additional clarification of the findings of the study as well as a means to tie the findings to what is already known. As a result, there are benefits both to the current research and to expanding the knowledge base. The researcher can compare findings from the study to those already in the literature as a step toward expanding the findings as well as to demonstrate how the research contributes to what has been presented previously in the literature. The elements of any good literature review are appropriate for use in evaluating this component of a qualitative study: use of primary sources, evidence of a thorough search, and use of current sources that are appropriate in any literature review. The results of the literature review that is done later in the study to expand findings and make connections with existing knowledge are presented in the discussion section of the research report. In this section, the researcher is expected to use relevant literature in discussion of major findings as a means to enhance understanding of the findings and demonstrate a clear connection to prior theory and research.

■ DESIGN OF QUALITATIVE STUDIES

In qualitative studies, the researcher has a broad problem of interest and specific variables are not identified in advance. As a result, the researcher develops the design for the study based on the problem, the initial literature review, and the purpose—what the researcher intends to accomplish with the study. The typical form of design for a qualitative study is referred to as an *emergent design*—the design actually emerges as the study proceeds. In qualitative studies, the researcher not only has flexibility to make changes in the design but, in the course of doing the study, actually is expected to make changes in the design to pursue new ideas and areas of inquiry as they are determined to be important. It is not possible to plan all of the elements of the research design in advance and, in fact, the quality of the study often requires that some changes be made if the researcher is to do a thorough investigation of the phenomenon being studied. This is in stark contrast to how quantitative research typically is conducted. In a quantitative study the researcher plans every element of the design in advance and then follows that plan closely. In some studies, there may be minor modifications, but not of the magnitude that may be encountered in a qualitative study. In quantitative research, a pilot study often is conducted to determine if any changes in the original design are needed and the researcher generally follows the plan for the study that is created before the study actually begins.

A qualitative study, as with any research, needs a clear purpose, but the study will benefit from some flexibility in the path to achieve that purpose. This is not a limitation of qualitative research but should be seen as a benefit as it offers the opportunity to explore ideas that were not evident at the start of the study. New information, including things that the researcher could not anticipate, often arises in the course of collecting data from participants. As new information is obtained through data collection, the astute researcher will realize that there are new avenues to be explored, people with different characteristics that need to be investigated, and new questions to ask in interviews.

A study of women's experiences with myocardial infarction conducted by the author provides an example of how unanticipated occurrences can be followed to enrich the outcome of the research. Early in this study the investigator was surprised to learn that none of the women interviewed had gone to the hospital by ambulance in spite of recognizing that they probably were having a heart attack at the time. This was an unanticipated finding and certainly something that needed to be explored to provide a meaningful and comprehensive description of the experiences of these women. Merely reporting this to be the case would have been interesting but would have been a lost opportunity for full description. The benefits of the research, also, would have been diminished considerably as what could be a key element in their experience was not explored sufficiently. Realizing this aspect of the experience, the investigator made a couple of changes in the study. The investigator began explicitly gathering information from each woman about the actual transportation to receive healthcare after recognizing she was having an MI. This constituted a change in the interview process. The researcher also added a new site for subject recruitment as those interviewed up to that point in the study had been in a comfortable position economically and the researcher was interested in determining whether this observation persisted in different socioeconomic groups. In one sense, this following of leads sometimes is thought of as a form of hypothesis testing; for example, does the mode of transportation to the hospital differ with socio-economic status, age, or living situation? The ability to follow a relevant path wherever it may lead in the inquiry is important to achieving the depth and scope of understanding of the situation that is sought in qualitative research and accounts for the need for elements of design to *emerge* in the course of a study. It also is a good example of how it is not always clear at the start of a study what data are relevant to answer the research question. Adhering to a predetermined set of variables from the beginning of a study can result in unnecessary restrictions on what is being studied and, consequently, gaps in fully understanding the phenomenon or situation of interest.

Sample Selection

Qualitative researchers often view their research as an interactive process involving the people who are involved in a study. Rather than view them as subjects of the study, they can be thought of as having an active role in the research; this active role often involves sharing sensitive aspects of their lives and is recognized in researchers commonly referring to them as participants or informants rather than subjects. Participants help to construct the study in a way by offering information about their experiences and this information, in turn, is used by the researcher to determine the appropriate direction of the research. Although some aspects of design can change throughout the conduct of a qualitative study, many elements can be determined in advance. The specific sample typically is not determined in advance and probability samples usually are not appropriate for qualitative research. That does not mean, however, that the researcher simply takes into the study anyone who comes along and is willing to participate. The researcher must establish clear eligibility criteria for selection of participants, and these criteria typically involve competence to provide informed consent to participate, the ability to speak and understand the language of the researcher, and an adequate amount of engagement with the experience being studied. Other factors can be included as appropriate to determine eligibility for a study and there may be some differences in sampling technique and sample size across the different traditions of qualitative research, though the general approach is remarkably similar (Gentles et al., 2015).

Studying the experiences of women with MI, for example, obviously requires the participants to have experienced an MI. Similarly, for the study of people's experiences with OSA, the people included in the study were those who had some encounter or awareness with a diagnosis of OSA. Beyond the criterion of having experience with the situation or phenomenon being studied, the researcher can impose more specific requirements appropriate to the nature of the study. The MI study was focused on women's concurrent experiences rather than on a retrospective account of their situations. Therefore, eligibility criteria included a time frame for the occurrence of the MI relative to data collection. For this study, the participant also could not have had a diagnosis of MI previously as the researcher was interested in each woman's experience of first becoming aware that she had experienced an MI. For the OSA study, the researcher was interested in the experience of OSA from the time of early recognition that the person might have OSA through various experiences with actual treatment. Therefore, the sampling criteria were intentionally broad to capture people at all stages of the condition including awareness, but per-diagnosis.

Because of the existence of specific criteria for eligibility, the usual sample for a qualitative study is described as purposive. Occasionally the samples are described as samples of convenience, meaning whoever is available, willing, and accessible to the researcher. For some studies, such a broad sampling plan may be acceptable. Many qualitative studies, however, require a sample that involves a bit more selectivity in which there are relevant and distinct criteria that enable the researcher to purposefully recruit participants who are in the best position to provide data needed for the study. Regardless of the specific type of sampling procedure employed, it is important that the qualitative researcher have participants in the study who are willing and capable of describing their experiences with the situation being studied, that those people actually have experience with the situation being studied, and that they have sufficient experience to provide meaningful descriptions and insights.

Sample size is a concern in any type of research, and qualitative research is no exception. Researchers using quantitative designs have the ability to determine appropriate sample sizes using statistical procedures such as power analysis in many cases. In qualitative research there is no ability to predict in advance precisely how many participants are needed to produce meaningful results. It is also the case that in qualitative research the amount of data that are generated has bearing on determination of the appropriate sample size. One hour of an audio-recorded interview generally produces as many as 30 pages of single-spaced transcribed text, an incredible amount of data. All of the data in an effectively conducted interview need to be analyzed. As a result, the amount of data available for analysis can be quite large with even a small group of participants. Qualitative research also can place a high demand on time and other resources. These factors in combination contribute to qualitative studies typically having relatively small sample sizes, but those smaller samples also are due to the fact that large samples are not necessary to generate meaningful and credible results due to the volume of data generated. There is no rule for what constitutes an adequate sample size in a qualitative study. Rather than counting participants, it is important that the researcher make a strong case that the study involved a considerable volume of data of high quality and that the data were sufficient to provide a cohesive and defensible answer to the research question.

Determination of an adequate sample, therefore, is based on several factors including the quantity and quality of data generated, the characteristics of the participants, the procedures employed in the study to maximize diversity in the participants and their experiences, and the ability to answer the research question with the data that are generated through the research. In planning to do a qualitative study the researcher can anticipate approximately how many people will be needed in the sample to reach this desired outcome. Because this is not an absolute number, proposals for qualitative research often include a range for the number of participants who will be recruited for the study. Published reports may show sample sizes ranging from 10 to 30 or more. In evaluating these studies, as noted earlier, there are several factors that need to be considered beyond the actual number of people involved.

A common practice in qualitative research is to use the criterion of saturation (Morse, 1991) or redundancy (Lincoln & Guba, 1985; Patton, 2001) to determine when the sample size is adequate. The word "saturation" is found in many published reports of qualitative studies with the researcher justifying the sample size by saying that saturation was achieved. Saturation typically is defined as the point at which the researcher is not hearing anything new in the data; in other words, the descriptions provided by participants are sufficiently similar that there is no need to continue with subject recruitment. For reasons that should be obvious, this can be a very troublesome criterion. First, the researcher is making a fairly bold assumption that talking with additional people will not provide anything new. Second, the failure to obtain new insights through the data collection processes that are being used could be a function of the data collection process itself and not necessarily a reflection of the experiences of the participants. If the researcher is asking leading questions during the interviewing or becomes fixated on certain aspects of the experience, this could lead to a premature sense that there is nothing new being learned through data collection. Finally, the researcher has to avoid the development of bias in interpreting things in a particular way. Such bias could give the false impression that there is nothing new in the data. It is important in qualitative research, as in any study, that the researcher be open to new ideas and insights that arise through data collection and analysis, and recognize that there is always the possibility of learning something new. A better justification of sample size is if the data are of high quality, the study rigorous, and the results are based on sufficient data to support that the answer to the research question is credible and comprehensive without any obvious gaps or leaps in the conclusions.

Data Collection for Qualitative Research

Any non-numerical data can be used for purposes of qualitative research. This can include notes written when making observations, a review of existing documentation and records such as patient medical records, print media such as books or popular literature, participant-generated journals or diaries, or video recordings. The majority of data collection for qualitative studies occurs through the use of interviews with individuals or in focus groups. Typically, interviews are conducted on a face-to-face basis, although telephone and email or web-based interviews with individuals have been used in qualitative research. Focus groups ideally consist of small groups and are organized in a way that the group setting promotes thoughtful discussion of the experience being explored in the study.

Interviews can have any degree of structure, ranging from specific questions that are asked consistently of each participant to an interview that is very open-ended and non-structured. The amount of depth and richness of the data tend to vary inversely with the degree of structure imposed on data collection: More structure generally leads to less richness and depth, while less structure facilitates greater depth. This may seem counterintuitive at first. Consider asking a friend about some recent travel. If the conversation progresses according to a series of structured questions – where did you go, how long were you there, how did you travel, what did you do, did you have a good time – the answers likely are limited to the scope of those questions and there will be less opportunity for the person you are talking with to bring up what they thought was most important about the travel. In a non-structured interview, there is more opportunity to learn what is most important to the person describing the experience, which is ideal in a qualitative study. The researcher helps to guide the interview by thinking about the research question of interest, for example, what is it like for people to live with OSA? After starting with a broad opening question, the researcher allows the participant to talk, presenting their experience in whatever way is comfortable so the conversation flows naturally for the participant. This might be as broad as "I understand you have been diagnosed with OSA. What has that been like for you?" This allows the participant to reveal things that are of greatest concern or interest regarding the experience without the researcher providing too much direction or imposing restraint on the conversation. The researcher focuses on listening, delicately guiding the conversation to ensure that relevant aspects are covered and participants provide a thorough account of their experiences, but without abruptly redirecting the interview or otherwise imposing constraints on the conversation. The researcher will have some specific questions that they want to address with each participant, such as symptoms, timeline of events, treatments received, and family history as just a few possibilities. Questions about these aspects of the experience can be incorporated into the interview at appropriate times if this information does not arise naturally during the interview.

The emphasis on listening and facilitating the participants' elaboration about their experiences can be challenging for nurses who are accustomed to collecting information from patients or clients relevant to a health situation. Nurses are very skilled at eliciting specific information and then formulating conclusions and determining the actions that are appropriate. It is easy for the novice qualitative researcher to interject suggestions, make decisions, or prematurely assume understanding of the participant's situations. In an interview for qualitative research, however, the investigator must learn to listen very attentively and to tolerate some gaps and silence in the interview while the participant is reflecting and forming next statements. The researcher needs to be able to track the conversation and return to significant items in the conversation when appropriate, and gently redirect when appropriate. While participants need to be allowed to present their experiences as they perceived them, introducing aspects and ideas they found to be important, the researcher needs to be careful that participants do not stray completely off topic. If the interview turns into a rambling conversation the participant can become fatigued and the quality of the interview will be compromised. This also is a long time to listen with great focus, thus the researcher may miss important points as attention fades. People also have busy lives and typically cannot dedicate unlimited time to an interview. The typical in-depth interview lasts about 90 minutes to 2 hours, and the researcher does need to make sure that the interview is sufficiently on track so that the desired information is obtained within a reasonable time frame.

An interesting feature of qualitative research is that some of the data in the study actually come from (or are generated by) the researcher. Data usually are thought of as information that is collected from the people who are being studied, in other words, the subjects of the study. In qualitative studies, however, it is important that the researcher generate some of the data. Such data include notes about the researcher's actions, thought processes, and decisions made throughout the course of the investigation. The researcher also will prepare documentation that is helpful to understanding and, later, analyzing the interview data. Notes about the setting or context for an interview as well as observations made during the process of data collection, such as notes about a participant's behaviors or nonverbal communication, are referred to as field notes. These notes provide insights that are valuable in the analysis of data as they facilitate understanding the situation being studied (Rodgers & Cowles, 1993).

Evaluating the quality of data collection procedures in a qualitative study involves looking at a number of factors related to the subjects as well as the researcher. The researcher must have gathered data from participants who have had the experience of being studied, who are able to articulate their experiences, who feel comfortable and unconstrained in sharing their experience, and who have adequate opportunity to share the experiences of interest. Accomplishing this places a considerable burden on the researcher who must develop effective rapport with participants, to ensure confidentiality necessary to protect their identity when discussing matters that can be sensitive to the individual, and to use effective interviewing techniques to obtain comprehensive and clear data that can be analyzed appropriately to answer the research question. In reading a qualitative study, it is important to consider the situation in which the data collection took place; for example, provisions for privacy during the interview; the amount of time allowed for an interview; efforts made by the researcher to establish rapport; other factors such as gender, culture, ethnicity, language, or age that might affect the researcher–participant relationship; means to ensure accuracy of the data collected such as by audio-recording of interviews; and any other information the researcher provides about strategies used to enhance the quality of the data collected. The researcher also should provide an account of notes that were taken during the data collection session and how these were used to supplement the data collection process and enhance the quality of the data.

Data Analysis in Qualitative Research

Data analysis can be an intimidating process in any study. In qualitative research the volume of information, along with the lack of any prescribed structure for organizing and analyzing it, can be overwhelming, particularly for investigators new to the process. It is also the case that this process can be the most enjoyable part of the research. This is the part of the research process where the inquisitive mind, the puzzle-solver, the curious and the creative aspects of the nurse are allowed to grow and thrive.

There are many approaches to the analysis of qualitative data with some specific guidelines that are unique to each tradition of research. Grounded theory, for example, involves a process of analysis that leads toward the identification of a core variable, a central concept that describes the experience being studied, and then categories of information or themes that contribute to that core of the experience. Phenomenology involves a search for significant statements and meaning in the data, and narrative research focuses on stories. In spite of these variations, however, all qualitative procedures have in common a similar process of reducing the data to manageable units and then constructing a description of the experience being studied by putting back together the pieces of the data into a coherent whole.

Some common steps in the process of data analysis are presented in Exhibit 10.1. It is important to recognize that not only is the process different for each methodology, but the process also is not linear. There are, however, some aspects of data analysis that are fairly common across methods. When interviews are done in a study, one of the first steps is preparing the data for analysis. This involves getting verbatim transcripts of the interviews and checking those for accuracy. The process of analysis then begins with a stage of general data reduction. Typically, the researcher

---

EXHIBIT 10.1

EXAMPLE OF ASPECTS OF DATA ANALYSIS THAT ARE COMMON IN QUALITATIVE RESEARCH

1. Prepare data for analysis, typically a verbatim transcript of interviews, and review transcript for accuracy.

2. Organize researcher notes and observations to review along with transcript.

3. Code to capture the central notion of each phrase or sentence. This also reduces longer passages to short words or phrases for analysis.

4. Review ideas in the broader context of the interview to ensure credible interpretation.

5. Organize codes to identify categories of experience that apply across participants.

6. Revise, reorganize, and rename the system of codes to capture all aspects of the experience being studied.

7. Use an iterative process, back and forth between categories and codes and the original data and context, to generate a system of themes appropriate to answer the research question.

Note: Each methodology has its own specific analysis process. However, many use a process of data reduction and coding, and then organizing codes into patterns in order to answer the research question. Analysis is not a linear process.

will read through the data (assume an interview transcript here for this purpose) identifying statements or parts of statements that carry a unique idea, and will label or code those statements using some term that captures the essence of that statement. This process of coding, carried out with all of the data collected in the study (including data generated by the researcher), reduces the large volume of data in the transcripts to smaller segments that then become the focus of further analysis. Working with these codes, the researcher begins to organize the codes into a meaningful structure with common ideas grouped together. The researcher is looking for patterns or recurrent ideas in the data (sometimes called themes) and the data are organized and reorganized into categories until clear patterns or themes can be identified. This process of organizing and categorizing is continued until the researcher can identify the particular themes or categories that account for and reflect the data that have been gathered without leaving any gaps in the resulting cluster of categories (Knafl & Webster, 1988). It is not necessary to account for every element of data in identifying themes or patterns. There will always be more questions, new avenues to explore, ideas of where research is needed, and so on. There should not, however, be major pieces of data that are ignored or left out of this categorizing process or major gaps in the themes that are identified.

The physical management and organization of data are accomplished using a technique that is best described using the metaphor "cut and paste." Historically, researchers would make multiple photocopies of the data (typically the interview transcripts) and cut the transcript into small segments, each segment containing a distinct idea relevant to the focus of the study. The researcher then would paste the segment onto a card (specific cards were developed just for this purpose) and sort those cards according to patterns that were identified in the data. Researchers made various adaptations in this approach to reflect their own style of data organization and analysis. Miles et al. (2019) offered a variety of ways to display and organize data to facilitate analysis, some of which are quite complex. Some researchers have used word processing software in which they could write or paste the data into large spreadsheet-type formats, or different categories could be identified directly on the transcript pages and coded using unique colors. This led to the development of software specifically designed for qualitative research. One of the early programs developed for this purpose was The Ethnograph (Qualis Research, 1984), which was first released in 1984. This was very early in the development of computers for personal use. It is no surprise, then, that programs and capabilities have expanded as technology has evolved and computers have become ubiquitous. Some of the currently popular programs are NVivo (QSR International Pty Ltd., 2018) and an earlier version of this software named NUD*IST, ATLAS/Ti (Scientific Software Development, 2019), HyperResearch (Researchware, 2019), MaxQDA (VERBI Software, 2019), Dedoose (2016), and others. In reviewing a report of qualitative research, these will be mentioned by the researcher, and the nurse reading the report should recognize that these are simply software programs that help with aspects of data management and organization. Software programs do not analyze the data for the researcher, but are very useful in organizing data and facilitating the researcher's cognitive processes of data analysis. The use of software does not enhance the quality of the study, nor does the absence of it detract. While there are considerable benefits to software when used by a researcher skilled in the program, the process of analysis ultimately depends on the diligence and cognitive effort of the researcher.

Reporting the Results of a Qualitative Study

The results of a qualitative study are presented in a manner appropriate to the specific method employed. Grounded theory research, for example, produces a type of theoretical construction that presents a substantive description of the experience that was studied. Regardless of the specific approach, results generally consist of a detailed discussion of patterns that were evident in the data collected in the study. Patterns can be organized around a specific concept, such as the core variable in grounded theory research, in a hierarchical manner with themes and subthemes, or as categories of descriptive ideas.

A well-written report of a qualitative study reads like a good story regardless of the specific approach employed in the study. Acknowledging this characteristic of qualitative studies initially may seem to minimize the importance of this type of research. Quite the contrary—the fact that a well-written study reads a bit like a good story points out the richness of this type of research. A well-written report captures the reader's attention and draws the reader into the experiences presented in the report of the study. The subjects come alive and the reader may begin to feel as if they actually know the participants or at least can relate to their experiences. As the researcher is presenting results based on the analysis of the data, quotations using the actual words of the participants provide examples that support the researcher's conclusions. The reader, therefore, does not merely have to rely on the interpretations of the researcher but is presented with evidence that supports these conclusions. Reading these examples not only adds considerable credibility to the findings but also increases the richness and provides detail that is not evident in other types of research. The researcher may use some quantitative data to present demographic information; it is the words of the participants and the researcher's weaving of these words with detailed analysis that make qualitative research so sensitizing and illustrative of individual experiences.

Trustworthiness and Rigor

The qualitative study report that is written well gives the reader a strong sense that the results are believable. The voices of the participants seem alive and it is easy to grasp their experiences. While this can be a valuable observation in assessing the quality of a qualitative study, there are additional criteria that must be considered. In quantitative research the criteria that are used to evaluate the quality of a study overall are referred to as validity and reliability, and these have been discussed elsewhere in this text. Qualitative studies are carried out to accomplish different purposes and are completed using very different procedures. Consequently, a different set of criteria, referred to as using a unique vocabulary, is used to evaluate the varied aspects of a qualitative study.

Noted researchers and methodologists Lincoln and Guba (1985) presented a framework in the mid-1980s that has been accepted widely as offering appropriate criteria to ensure a quality investigation. As new methodologies have gained in popularity that involve different approaches, particularly those with an interpretive focus, there has been some variation and refinement of the criteria appropriate to different processes and foci of the research (Hays et al., 2016; Rettke et al., 2018). The criteria created by Lincoln and Guba (1985), however, has provided a foundation that has endured for decades for the assessment of quality in qualitative research.

In an effort to avoid confusion with the criteria of reliability and validity that are used for quantitative research, Lincoln and Guba proposed a broad framework organized around the key concept of "trustworthiness" to evaluate the rigor and overall quality of a study. It is interesting to note that the aspects of research addressed by these criteria could be applied to any type of research: The primary concern in any study is whether the results are believable and worthy of attention. Specific terminology has been adopted for qualitative research to acknowledge differences in how this type of research is done and the unique concerns associated with these methods.

The terminology and ideas adopted from Lincoln and Guba (1985) include the essential concerns of "truth value" or credibility, "applicability" or transferability, "consistency" or

TABLE 10.2 General Criteria for Trustworthiness in Qualitative Research

CRITERION	DEFINITION
Truth value	Can the results be believed?
Applicability	To what extent can the results apply in other settings or contexts?
Consistency	Could the results be repeated if the research were done again with the same or similar people?
Neutrality	To what extent do the results reflect the experiences of the participants rather than the interests or bias of the researcher?

Source: From Lincoln, Y. S., & Guba, E. G. (1985). *Naturalistic inquiry.* SAGE.

dependability, and "neutrality" (p. 290). Key points for each of these criteria are provided in Table 10.2. As noted previously, there are some variations in criteria for rigor or trustworthiness that have been developed specific to different contexts for qualitative research (Davies & Dodd, 2002; Hall & Stevens, 1991; Im et al., 2004). For general critique purposes, however, the principles explicated by Lincoln and Guba are worth remembering because of the extent to which they reflect the unique strengths of qualitative research. These criteria provide useful general guidelines for evaluating the quality of qualitative studies and continue to be used extensively in nursing as well as in other disciplines.

According to Lincoln and Guba (1985), the first criterion, truth value, addresses an extremely important concern in any research, the concern about whether or not it is reasonable to believe or have faith in the results. For qualitative research, this means that there needs to be confidence that the results are an accurate reflection of the participants and the experiences that were studied. There are numerous techniques that qualitative researchers can use to increase the likelihood that results will be credible. Researchers need, first, to spend sufficient time with participants to be able to fully understand their realities and how they describe their experiences (a technique referred to as prolonged engagement). Sufficient contact also is necessary to establish rapport with participants to increase their comfort with the researcher and, consequently, their willingness to share important details. A technique known as triangulation sometimes is used to enhance credibility or trustworthiness. The term "triangulation" is adopted from a process for navigation in which several location points are determined and the intersection of lines drawn from these points is determined. Using simple principles of geometry, it is possible for an individual at sea to pinpoint their specific location. When applied to a qualitative study, triangulation means the corroboration of information using multiple sources, multiple methods, different investigators, or even the perspective provided by different theories (Denzin, 1978). In a health-related study, participants' descriptions of their experiences might be triangulated with the accounts of nurses or family members or even with the health record.

It is worth noting that whether a participant's description of an experience is factual or not is not always a concern. People construct their viewpoints and the experiences are shaped by what they believe happened, whether or not such beliefs are based in fact. Someone who experienced major trauma and believes they died and were brought back to life will, undoubtedly, relate to that experience in a way that is shaped by that belief. Whether or not, clinically, the described events actually took place may be of little consequence. For occasions where different perspectives or the need to determine actual events are important in the study, triangulation is a very effective technique.

Other techniques can also be used to enhance the trustworthiness of results. A process referred to as peer debriefing provides an opportunity for the researcher to talk through aspects of the study with a colleague (peer) who is not invested in the study. This simple act of talking through parts of the study can be helpful in bringing to light some of the thoughts and ideas of the researcher that might not have been recognized otherwise or, in other words, might have stayed hidden in the recesses of the researcher's mind. The peer debriefer asks probing questions, challenges assumptions, encourages exploration, and, overall, helps the researcher become aware of any potential misinterpretation, missed clues in the data, and personal value orientation or bias. Complete objectivity in any study is not possible; yet, while it is not possible to be completely devoid of bias in any study, peer debriefing helps the researcher to recognize what bias exists and how it might affect the study. Through this awareness, the researcher can make a conscious effort to limit the influence of bias in the research.

Occasionally researchers will use a technique known as a "member check" to ensure the credibility of findings. In doing a member check, the researcher returns to the participants, or to a subset of participants, and shares findings with them so that they can verify that the researcher correctly understands the views and experiences presented in the interview. A member check can also be done at the conclusion of an interview, with the interviewer giving the participant a brief summary of the interview for their feedback; and can be done near the conclusion of a study by taking study results back to some of the participants for their consideration and review. Using this technique, the researcher is able to verify with study participants that the results accurately reflect the experiences that were described to the researcher. In other words, the researcher knows the results are credible because they asked the participants themselves to ensure that they are. Member checks are not possible in all studies and research situations and there is debate as to their utility (Birt et al., 2016). When appropriate and consistent with the methodology employed, they may be a useful means to support that the results of a study are credible or trustworthy in that they reflect the experiences of the participants, but the absence of a member check is not a threat to the trustworthiness of the study overall.

The second criterion is referred to as "applicability" and addresses an issue similar to generalizability. As noted previously, there is no expectation or desire on the part of qualitative researchers that their results are, in fact, generalizable. Generalizability always has to be considered with great caution and, in qualitative studies, where the emphasis is on depth and richness, it would minimize the role of each unique individual to assume or stipulate that results actually will be generalizable simply by virtue of some feature of how the study was conducted. In contrast, the researcher in a qualitative study acknowledges that the consumer of the research is in the best position to evaluate whether or not results are applicable in other settings. For nurses in practice settings, this means that the nurse is in the best position to determine to what extent results are likely to be useful for clients in the setting in which the nurse works with these individuals. How similar are the contexts and the individuals in the study to those with whom the nurse works? Rather than stipulate that results are generalizable, the obligation of the qualitative researcher is to provide sufficiently detailed description of the research situation to enable the reader of the research to make the determination whether the results are likely to transfer to other settings.

The two remaining criteria for conducting rigorous qualitative inquiry and for evaluating the rigor of studies that have been reported in the literature are consistency (dependability) and neutrality (confirmability). Consistency is similar to the concept of reliability for quantitative studies. In a quantitative study, there is an expectation that repeated use of an instrument will provide comparable results with each administration. In a qualitative study, however, things cannot be expected to be the same with repeated episodes of data collection or with repeated collection of information from different groups. People often change their perspective as they talk about experiences, the act of talking providing an opportunity for reflection with new insights and memories emerging. Similarly, a different investigator might elicit different descriptions from people based on the focus of the interview, whatever cognitive or emotional processing has gone on within the individual, changes in context for data collection, and other factors that can influence what is obtained in a qualitative study. Consequently, it is unreasonable to expect an occurrence comparable to stepping on a bedside scale and receiving the same results each time. What is important, however, is that all aspects of a qualitative study, including the collection of data and the analytic techniques that are employed and the insights generated, are conducted in a way that is dependable or confirmable. The process must be rigorous and comprehensive and the product must be supported by appropriate data. The question, therefore, is not whether another researcher would find the same thing if someone else did the research. The appropriate question is whether the results obtained by the researcher who did the study are appropriate and reasonable, and the processes can be traced and documented so the results are defensible.

Both of these aspects of quality can be assessed using an audit trail (Halpern, 1983; Rodgers & Cowles, 1993). Qualitative researchers keep records about all the steps in the process of conducting the study including procedures, methodological changes that are instituted, insights generated during data analysis, and observational or field notes. These records can be reviewed by other investigators who serve as auditors to ensure the processes and procedures are carried out in a rigorous manner. All of the steps in the conduct of the study can be retraced and evaluated for quality. While audits can be conducted on a large-scale basis just as a financial audit of a large company might be conducted, more often a researcher will engage a colleague to serve as a peer reviewer to evaluate aspects of the study on an ongoing basis while the research is being conducted and results are being prepared for dissemination.

■ SUMMARY

Qualitative research contributes vital information necessary to effective work with human beings. It is valuable in exploring areas about which little is known, in developing theory, and in generating rich and detailed descriptions about the lives of people with whom nurses work. Understanding the human element of health situations, the thoughts, feelings, and perceptions of individuals, is essential to providing sensitive care that is provided in a manner appropriate to the people with whom nurses work. This aspect of human experience also contributes essential information for EBP, illuminating the personal experience associated with various health situations and events. Recognizing the roles and contributions of qualitative research and understanding and critiquing published studies is an important ability for nurses who strive to base their practice on quality evidence relevant to the populations and situations that nurses encounter.

SUGGESTED LEARNING ACTIVITIES

1. Complete a thorough critique of a published report of a qualitative study.
2. Retrieve journal articles presenting the results of qualitative studies using different qualitative methods. Analyze the similarities and differences in the studies in regard to the major components including research question, sample, data collection strategies, data analysis techniques, report of findings, and discussion.

3. Identify a problem significant for research. Describe how research questions and procedures would vary if the problem is addressed using quantitative methods in comparison to qualitative methods. What are the strengths of each approach in addressing the problem?

REFERENCES

Banks, M. (2018). *Using visual data in qualitative research* (2nd ed.). SAGE.

Birt, L., Scott, S., Cavers, D., Campbell, C., & Walter, F. (2016). Member checking: A tool to enhance trustworthiness or merely a nod to validation? *Qualitative Health Research, 26*(13), 1802–1811. https://doi.org/10.1177/1049732316654870

Blumer, H. (1969). *Symbolic interactionism: Perspective and method.* Prentice-Hall.

Bryant, A., & Charmaz, K. (2019). *The SAGE handbook of current developments in Grounded Theory.* SAGE.

Charmaz, K. (2000). Grounded theory: Objectivist and constructivist methods. In N. Denzin & Y. Lincoln (Eds.), *Handbook of qualitative research* (2nd ed., pp. 509–535). SAGE.

Charmaz, K. (2005). Grounded theory in the 21st century: Applications for advancing social justice studies. In N. Denzin & Y. Lincoln (Eds.), *Handbook of qualitative research* (3rd ed., pp. 507–535). SAGE.

Charmaz, K. (2008). The legacy of Anselm Strauss in constructivist grounded theory. *Studies in Symbolic Interaction, 32,* 127–141. https://doi.org/10.1016/S0163-2396(08)32010-9

Charmaz, K. (2014). *Constructing grounded theory (2nd ed).* SAGE.

Connelly, F. M., & Clandinin, D. J., (2006). Narrative inquiry. In J. Green, G. Camilli, P. Elmore (Eds.), *Handbook of complementary methods in education research* (pp. 375–385). Lawrence Erlbaum.

Clandinin, D. J. (2020). *Journeys in narrative inquiry: The selected works of D. Jean Clandinin.* Routledge.

Crowther, S., Ironside, P., Spence, D., & Smythe, L. (2017). Crafting stories in hermeneutic phenomenology research: A methodological device. *Qualitative Health Research, 27,* 826–835. https://doi.org/10.1177/1049732316656161

Davies, D., & Dodd, J. (2002). Qualitative research and the question of rigor. *Qualitative Health Research, 12,* 279–289. https://doi.org/10.1177/104973230201200211

Dedoose. (2016). *Web application for managing, analyzing, and presenting qualitative and mixed method research data, Version 7.0.23.* SocioCultural Research Consultants, LLC.

Denzin, N. K. (1978). *Sociological methods.* McGraw-Hill.

Gentles, S. J., Charles, C., Ploeg, J., & McKobbon, K. A. (2015). Sampling in qualitative research: Insights from an overview of the methods literature. *The Qualitative Report, 20,* 1772–1789.

Glaser, B. (1978). *Theoretical sensitivity.* Sociology Press.

Glaser, B., & Strauss, A. (1967). *The discovery of grounded theory.* Aldine.

Hall, J. M., & Stevens, P. E. (1991). Rigor in feminist research. *Advances in Nursing Science, 13*(3), 16–29. https://doi.org/10.1097/00012272-199103000-00005

Halpern, E. S. (1983). *Auditing naturalistic inquiries: The development and application of a model.* Indiana University. University Microfilms International AAT 8317108.

Hays, D. G., Wood, C., Dahl, H., & Kirk-Jenkins, A. (2016). Methodological rigor in *Journal of Counseling & Development* qualitative research articles: A 15-year review. *Journal of Counseling & Development, 94,* 172–183. https://doi.org/10.1002/jcad.12074

Holstein, J. A., & Gubrium, J. F. (2012). *Varieties of narrative analysis.* SAGE.

Horrigan-Kelly, M., Millar, M., & Dowling, M. (2016). Understanding the key tenets of Heidegger's philosophy for interpretive phenomenological research. *International Journal of Qualitative Methods, 15,* 1–8. https://doi.org/10.1177/1609406916680634

Husserl, E. (1960). *Cartesian meditations: An introduction to phenomenology* (D. Cairns, trans.). Martinus Nijhoff.

Im, E. O., Page, R., Lin, L. C., Tsai, H. M., & Cheng, C. Y. (2004). Rigor in cross-cultural nursing research. *International Journal of Nursing Studies, 41*(8), 891–899. https://doi.org/10.1016/j.ijnurstu.2004.04.003

Knafl, K. A., & Webster, D. C. (1988). Managing and analyzing qualitative data: A description of tasks, techniques, and materials. *Western Journal of Nursing Research, 10*(2), 195–218. https://doi.org/10.1177/019394598801000207

Lincoln, Y. S., & Guba, E. G. (1985). *Naturalistic inquiry*. SAGE.

Matua, G. A., & Van Der Wal, D. M. (2015). Differentiating between descriptive and interpretive phenomenological research approaches. *Nurse Researcher, 22*(6), 22–27. https://doi.org/10.7748/nr.22.6.22.e1344

Melnyk, B. M., & Fineout-Overholt, E. (2019). *Evidence-based practice in nursing and healthcare* (4th ed.). Lippincott Williams and Wilkins.

Merleau-Ponty, M. (1999). *The phenomenology of perception*. Routledge. (Original work published 1962.)

Miles, M. B., Huberman, M., & Saldana, J. (2019). *Qualitative data analysis: A methods Sourcebook* (4th ed.). SAGE.

Morse, J. M. (1991). Strategies for sampling. In J. M. Morse (Ed.), *Qualitative nursing research: A contemporary dialogue*. SAGE.

Patton, M. Q. (2001). *Qualitative research and evaluation methods* (3rd ed.). SAGE.

Porter, S., & O'Halloran, P. (2009). The postmodernist war on evidence-based practice. *International Journal of Nursing Studies, 46*, 740–748. https://doi.org/10.1016/j.ijnurstu.2008.11.002

QSR International Pty Ltd. (2018). *NVivo* [Computer software]. Doncaster, Victoria, Australia.

Qualis Research. (1984). *The ethnograph*. Colorado Springs, CO.

Quint, J. C. (1967). Research—How will nursing define it? The case for theories generated from empirical data. *Nursing Research, 16*(2), 109–114. https://doi.org/10.1097/00006199-196701620-00003

Researchware. (2019). *HyperResearch* [Computer software]. Randolph, MA.

Rettke, H., Pretto, M., Spichiger, E., Frei, I. A., & Spirig, R. (2018). Using reflexive thinking to establish rigor in qualitative research. *Nursing Research, 67*, 490–497. https://doi.org/10.1097/NNR.0000000000000307

Riessman, C. K. (1993). *Narrative analysis*. Sage.

Riley, T., & Hawe, P. (2005). Researching practice: The methodological case for narrative inquiry. *Health Education Research, 20*(2), 226–236. https://doi.org/10.1093/her/cyg122

Rodgers, B. L. (2005). *Developing nursing knowledge: Philosophical traditions and influences*. Lippincott Williams & Wilkins.

Rodgers, B. (2013). Breaking through Limbo: Experiences of adults living with obstructive sleep apnea. *Behavioral Sleep Medicine, 11*, 1–15. https://doi.org/10.1080/15402002.2013.778203

Rodgers, B. L., & Cowles, K. V. (1993). The qualitative research audit trail: A complex collection of documentation. *Research in Nursing & Health, 16*(3), 219–226. https://doi.org/10.1002/nur.4770160309

Scientific Software Development. (2019). *Atlas.Ti* [Computer software]. Berlin, Germany.

Spence, D. G. (2017). Supervising for robust hermeneutic phenomenology: Reflexive engagement within horizons of understanding. *Qualitative Health Research, 27*(6), 836–842. https://doi.org/10.1177/1049732316637824

Strauss, A., & Corbin, J. (1998). *Basics of qualitative research: Techniques and procedures for developing grounded theory*. SAGE.

Van Manen, M. (1997). *Research lived experience: Human science for an action sensitive pedagogy* (2nd ed.). Althouse.

VERBI Software. (2013). *MAXQDA* [Computer software]. Berlin, Germany.

Wolf, Z. R. (2012). Ethnography: The method. In P. L. Munhall (Ed.), *Nursing research: A qualitative perspective* (5th ed., pp. 285–338). Jones & Bartlett.

Wu, Y. P., Thompson, D., Aroian, K. J., McQuaid, E. L., & Deatrick, J. A. (2016). Commentary: Writing and evaluating qualitative research reports. *Journal of Pediatric Psychology, 41*, 493–505. https://doi.org/10.1093/jpepsy/jsw032

SAMPLING METHODS

MARY D. BONDMASS

▨ INTRODUCTION

One of the first and most frequent questions asked in any discussion of sampling is, "How many participants do I need in my sample?" The first and most frequent answer to this question usually is, "It depends." Many contemporary authors agree that sampling decisions contribute critically to a study's internal validity (truthfulness or accuracy) and external validity (generalizability or applicability; Fain, 2017; Gray et al., 2017; Marshall, 2020; Polit & Beck, 2020; Torre & Picho, 2016). Asking or answering the question of sample size as the first discussion point about sampling is analogous to the adage of "putting the cart before the horse," that is, reversing the order of addressing an issue or problem. Although it is essential, sampling is about more than just about how many participants you need; decisions and processes such as a study's design and a study's data source(s) are related and need to be considered sequentially in planning research (Amatya & Bhaumik, 2018; Beavers & Stamey, 2018; Show-Li & Shieh, 2018; Tam et al., 2020; Vanderlaan et al., 2019). A study's design is its general structure, and its data source is the actual sample. More specifically, the individual elements or basic units that make up that sample are not necessarily people, although in healthcare research, this is often the case. Ethical issues in sampling also need to be considered and must be part of any discussion and/or decisions on a type or number included in a sample (Hunter et al., 2018; Sasso et al., 2018). These factors are all considered in an a priori approach to answering *"How many participants do I need in my study?"*

This chapter is primarily intended for those advanced practice registered nurses (APRNs) and novice researchers who need basic information to critically appraise the sample section of a research article and for those who may be contemplating conducting research or a quality improvement project, either of whom may need clarification on the earlier *"it depends"* answer. However, before addressing the sample size question, for either of the two intended audiences of this chapter, it is essential to understand the logic and fundamental principles and concepts related to sampling. Therefore, a description of basic terminology and definitions of terms used in the subsequent discussions of the underlying theory and logic of sampling are presented. This basic terminology will hopefully provide you with some context to answer the question of sample size question. A summary of the central limits theorem, as well as of the concept of power and power analysis, will also aid in addressing sample size determination. A section on the critical appraisal of sampling in published research has been added to address the crucial need for APRNs or anyone involved in advanced nursing practice to thrive in an evidence-based practice (EBP) environment. Suggested activities are also included at the end of the chapter for you to self-assess your understanding of the content.

■ TERMINOLOGY

Exhibit 11.1 defines terms that are used throughout this chapter. Many of you have probably heard these terms used in research discussions but might not have fully understood them. Whether you are conducting research or critically appraising the research of others, an understanding of research terminology is foundational for EBP. You are referred back to this section and the exhibit for clarification when a term is used, but the context is not fully understood.

EXHIBIT 11.1

GLOSSARY OF TERMS

Cluster sampling refers to a type of sampling method wherein the researcher divides the population into separate groups, called clusters. Then a simple random sample of clusters is selected from the population. The researcher analyzes data from the sampled clusters. Compared to simple random sampling and stratified sampling, cluster sampling has advantages and disadvantages. For example, given equal sample sizes, cluster sampling usually provides less precision than either simple random sampling or stratified sampling. On the other hand, if travel costs between clusters are high, cluster sampling may be more cost-effective than the other methods.

Convenience sampling is nonprobability sampling, sometimes called an accidental sample, wherein members of the population are chosen based on their relative ease of access. Friends, coworkers, or shoppers at a single mall are all examples of convenience sampling. Such samples are biased because researchers may unconsciously approach some kinds of respondents and avoid others, and respondents who volunteer for a study may differ in unknown but essential ways from others; representativeness of the target population is often questionable.

A ***mean*** is an average; often, the mean is a score or other interval level characteristic that can have an average.

Nonprobability sampling is the process wherein population elements are selected based on their availability or a personal judgment or determination that they are representative.

A ***parameter*** is a measurable characteristic of a population, such as a mean or a standard deviation.

Probability sampling is the process wherein all elements in the population have some opportunity of being included in the sample.

Purposive sampling is a nonprobability sampling strategy, sometimes called *judgmental* sampling in which the researcher chooses the sample based on who the researcher thinks would be appropriate for the study.

Quota sampling is nonprobability sampling, sometimes called strat-based sampling or ad hoc quotas wherein a quota is established (say 65% women), and researchers are free to choose any respondent they wish as long as the quota is met.

Random error or *sampling error* is the difference between sample estimates and the population parameters.

Randomization refers to the practice of using chance methods (random number tables, flipping a coin, etc.) to assign participants to treatments or groups.

(continued)

Representativeness is the quality of a sample having the same distribution of characteristics as the population from which it was drawn.

Sampling bias or non-representative sampling bias is also known as selection bias as this inaccuracy is caused due to not implementing random methods during the selection process, which results in either inadequate or excess representation of some elements in the population.

Sampling design or sampling plan is a combination of the sampling process and the estimation or inferences made to the entire group from the sample data. The design/plan also outlines the strategies used to obtain the sample.

A *sampling distribution* is essential in statistics because it provides a major simplification on the route to statistical inference. Important information can be determined from the shape of the distribution, which can be obtained using a histogram.

Simple random sampling refers to any sampling method that has the following properties: (a) The population consists of N objects, (b) the sample consists of n objects, and (c) if all possible samples of n objects are equally likely to occur. An important benefit of simple random sampling is that it allows researchers to use statistical methods to analyze sample results. For example, given a simple random sample, researchers can use statistical methods to define a confidence interval around a sample mean. Statistical analysis is not appropriate when nonrandom sampling methods are used.

Snowball sampling, also called *network* sampling, is a nonprobability sampling method, primarily used in qualitative research, but sometimes is used in quantitative research. This type of sampling relies on participants referring other participants to increase the sample size via a snowball effect. Insight and understanding of a population that is often difficult to access is the main reason for using snowball sampling.

The *standard deviation* is a numerical value used to indicate how widely individuals in a group vary. If individual observations vary greatly from the group mean, the standard deviation is large, and vice versa. It is essential to distinguish between the standard deviation of a population and the standard deviation of a sample. They have different notations, and they are computed differently. The standard deviation of a population is denoted by σ and the standard deviation of a sample by s.

The *standard error* is a measure of the variability of a statistic. It is an estimate of the standard deviation of a sampling distribution. The standard error depends on three factors including (a) the number of observations in the population, (b) the number of observations in the sample, and (c) the way that the random sample is chosen.

The *standard error of the mean,* also called the standard deviation of the mean, is a method used to estimate the standard deviation of a sampling distribution.

A *statistic* is a characteristic of a sample. Generally, a statistic is used to estimate the value of a population parameter.

Statistics is a discipline that allows researchers to evaluate conclusions derived from sample data.

Stratified sampling refers to a type of sampling method wherein the researcher divides the population into separate groups called strata. Then a probability sample (often a simple random sample) is drawn from each group. Stratified sampling has several advantages over simple random sampling. For example, using stratified sampling, it may be possible to reduce the sample size required to achieve a given precision, or it may be possible to increase the precision with the same sample size.

(continued)

With **systematic random sampling,** a list of every member of the population is created. From the list, one randomly selects the first sample element from the first *k* elements on the population list. After that, one selects every *k*th element on the list. This method is different from simple random sampling since every possible sample of *n* elements is not equally likely.

A **variable** has two defining characteristics: (a) *t* is an attribute that describes a person, place, thing, or idea, and (b) the value of the variable can "*vary*" from one entity to another.

Sources: Many of the above definitions are taken directly from Stat Trek. (2020). *Statistics and probability dictionary.* https://www.stattrek.com; others provide similar definitions (Fain, 2017; Gray et al., 2017; Marshall, 2020; Polit & Beck, 2020).

Population Versus Sample

Other terms critical to the understanding of sampling and sampling methods include *target population, accessible population, sampling frame,* and *sample.* The *theoretical* or *target population* (often simply just referred to as the *population or population of interest*) is an aggregate of people, groups, objects, or things that meet a designated set of criteria. The population of a particular study is the group of interest that a researcher wishes to make generalizations about. The individual units of a population are referred to as *elements.* Since it is generally impossible to reach an entire population, an accessible population is delineated. An *accessible population* is a subset of the population that is reasonably accessible to a researcher. A *sampling frame* is the listing of people, groups, objects/things, or a procedure developed for drawing a sample from the accessible population. The sampling frame becomes the methodological "how to" related to the actual drawing of your sample. Lastly, the *sample* consists of those people, groups, or objects that a researcher selects from the accessible population using the sampling frame. Theoretically, a study's actual or true sample usually ends up being a subsample due to non-respondents and attrition; however, for a more practical discussion, the subsample will simply be referred to here as the study sample. In theory, if error and bias are eliminated or minimized, the study sample should be representative of the population, and thereby generalizations can be made about the population from the sample (Fain, 2017; Gray et al., 2017; Marshall, 2020; Polit & Beck, 2020).

As an example, let's say you plan to conduct a study involving an intervention that would decrease salt in the diets of hypertensive African American women; the desired result of your study is blood pressure control. In your study design, you already have in mind that your *target population* will be African American women with hypertension, but this could include millions of women; there is no way to intervene and collect data on this entire population. You will need to limit your participant search to those hypertensive African American women that you can reasonably access yet still have them belong to, and be representative of, your original *target population.* Your *accessible population* may depend heavily on the logistics of where you plan to carry out your study. For this example, let's say you work at an urban medical center in Chicago, wherein many hypertensive African American women are treated. You may, therefore, define your *accessible population* as hypertensive African American women attending a particular clinic(s) in Chicago. Lastly, your *sample* is the number of consenting participants selected (randomly or otherwise) from your *accessible population* to be included in your study. The study sample, in theory, then serves as a surrogate or proxy for your originally targeted population of hypertensive African

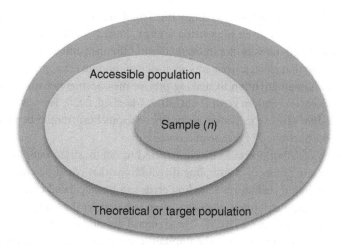

FIGURE 11.1 Relationship between theoretical/target population, accessible populations, and sample.

American women. Figure 11.1 graphically depicts the relationship between the theoretical/target population, accessible population, and the study sample.

A sample is drawn from the accessible population that is derived from somewhere within the theoretical or target population. The sample always has a number associated with it, often represented as a lower or uppercase N. The lowercase n usually refers to groups within a sample and the uppercase N to the total sample; however, generally within a well-written article, the reader can easily surmise which value the author(s) is referring to without further explanation, be it a lowercase or uppercase value. The uppercase N has also been used to represent the number of cases in the sampling frame.

Sampling Theory and Logic

The definition of sampling has not changed over the decades; many recent references can be found that similarly define sampling as the process of selecting a subset of observations from an entire population, such that the characteristics of the subset (e.g., the sample) will be representative enough to draw conclusions or make inferences about the population (Fain, 2017; Gray et al., 2017; Marshall, 2020; Polit & Beck, 2020).

Central Limit Theorem

The central limit theorem (CLT), credited initially to Simon–Pierre Laplace in the early 1800s, provides the theoretical foundation for sampling and probability theory. The CLT states that given certain conditions, the mean of a sufficiently large number of independent random variables will be approximately normally distributed (Burgess, 2019; Marshall, 2020). Put simply, the CLT tells us that if we take the mean of multiple samples and plot the frequencies of the means, we will get a normal distribution (e.g., a bell curve).

The logic of sampling, then, is rather simple; it is efficient and accurate. The efficiency of sampling relates to gaining information about a large group from a small group; that is, your population of interest (large group) can be studied via a sample (small group), thereby obtaining the information that is sought at an acceptable cost. Accuracy is assumed because of the CLT, but only when sampling errors are minimized (Burgess, 2019; Marshall, 2020).

Random error, also called sampling error, is incidental and has to do with expected fluctuations among samples from a given population and/or unpredictable fluctuations in the readings of a measurement apparatus or the interpretation of the instrumental reading made by the researcher. Considering that all measurements are prone to random error, precision in any instrumentation used and human attention to making precise measurements with those instruments would be a way to decrease random error (Fain, 2017; Marshall, 2020; Terry & ProQuest, 2018). Conversely, nonrandom error (e.g., conscious or unconscious bias) should be avoided or minimized to decrease the likelihood of erroneous conclusions.

A small sampling distribution could be constructed to demonstrate sampling error. Still, in theory, there are infinite numbers of sampling distributions that could be created, so we never really see a true sampling distribution. Sampling error can be calculated even though we never actually see the sampling distribution; the calculation is based on the standard deviation of the sample (standard error of the mean [SEM]). The standard deviation of the sampling distribution of the mean is called the standard error; the standard error is called sampling error (Fain, 2017; Marshall, 2020; Terry & ProQuest, 2018). Rather than try to reteach the whole of sampling theory here, when reading a research article, keep the following two statistical 'pearls' in mind related to error:

- The greater the sample's standard deviation, the greater the standard error (and the sampling error).
- The standard error is also related to the sample size; therefore, the greater the sample size, the smaller the standard error (because, the greater the sample size, the closer the sample is to the actual population itself).

Another way of looking at this last bullet point is that when you know that values are likely to be different, increase your sample size. This last point should be useful, regardless if you are conducting the research or critically appraising a study.

Again using the example of the study of hypertensive African American women, if you were to include only 15 women in the study sample, the standard error would theoretically be much larger than if your sample included 150 hypertensive African American women. The likelihood of 150 versus 15 participants being representative of the target population increases with the sample size and therefore decreases the standard error.

■ METHODS: SAMPLING PROCEDURES

Before beginning a specific discussion on the types of samples, it is important to know the procedures involved; this varies depending on whether your research or project is quantitative or qualitative. Quantitative researchers are interested in statistical conclusions about validity and generalizability, and they start with a sampling plan. Conversely, qualitative researchers often do not begin with a sampling plan, but rather make sampling decisions at the same time as they collect data (Fain, 2017; Marshall, 2020; Polit & Beck, 2020; Terry & ProQuest, 2018). This chapter focuses primarily on sampling procedures for a quantitative study or project, but will also reference qualitative issues at times.

Fain (2017) and Marshall (2020) both opine that initial decisions about the sample plan are often related to how much error can be tolerated and the cost involved. An interventional drug study or a study related to biomarkers, for example, would have little room for error. The cost of data collection (personnel and/or testing procedures) also needs careful consideration during the sample planning stage. A combination of the sampling process and the estimation or inferences made to the entire group from the sample data may need careful consideration when obtaining the sample. Polit and Beck (2020) also note that a key issue for EBP is information about the population of interest, which should be determined early on as part of the sample plan. Sampling units (elements or groups forming the basis of sample selection) and sampling lists (inventories of the units in a population) are also important as you plan your sample.

Eligibility or inclusion criteria also need to be considered in your sample plan. These criteria specify defining population characteristics and, whenever possible, should be driven by theoretical considerations with implications for the interpretation of the results and external validity of the findings. Conversely, exclusion criteria will also need to be decided a priori and often mirror the inclusion criteria (Fain, 2017; Marshall, 2020; Polit & Beck, 2020; Terry & ProQuest, 2018).

The goal of sampling in the quantitative world is to select cases that will represent an entire population, thereby allowing one to make population inferences from a study's results. It is important to remember at all times that the sample of a study is simply a subset of the population of interest (see Figure 11.1).

Among other issues involved in the sampling plan that may affect the researcher, the participants, and the critical appraiser, are recruitment, incentives, benefits (to participants and society), convenience, endorsements, and assurances to the participants (Fain, 2017; Polit & Beck, 2020). Sampling designs are discussed in the following sections, and critical appraisal or evaluation of sampling methods in published research is addressed at the end of this chapter.

▦ PROBABILITY AND NONPROBABILITY SAMPLING

There are two classifications of sampling designs: probability and nonprobability sampling. Each method can have several different sample types within the respective classification. While probability sampling could theoretically be used in both quantitative and qualitative research, nonprobability sampling is more frequent with qualitative research (Fain, 2017; Polit & Beck, 2020).

Probability Sampling

Probability samples are those samples selected utilizing some component of probability theory, typically involving some sort of randomization features such as random selection or random assignment. While addressing the general concept of randomization, I am always reminded of a quote that I heard in my very first statistics course that is, "*If you don't believe in random sampling, the next time you have a blood test, tell the phlebotomist to take it all*" (unknown author). I have seen this quote attributed to several people, including former presidential candidate Thomas E. Dewey, a U.S. Census deputy, and Confucius. While I doubt it is the latter or any of the former for that matter, I will leave the credit to an unknown author, and ask that you just take a moment to reflect on the underlying meaning of the quote.

In probability samples, all the elements of the population theoretically have an equal chance of being included in a particular sample. While some may argue the blood test example could be interpreted as convenience sampling, I contend it is a random sample and representative of the whole population of blood components in the donor's blood vessels. When research demands precise, statistical descriptions of large populations, probability sampling is used. Generally, all large-scale survey research and clinical trials use probability sampling methods. The fundamental premise of probability sampling is to provide useful descriptions of the total population. Therefore a sample from that population must demonstrate the same variation as in that population, yet this concept is not as straightforward as it may appear. If you recall the previous discussion on error, you can probably imagine the multiple ways that either random or nonrandom error can affect the ability of a probability sample to perform as expected, that is, to be a representative sample of the population. The major advantage of probability sampling is fairness; the major disadvantage is the possibility of flaws in the randomness model. Some common probability samples include *simple random, stratified, cluster, and systemic samples.* As a self-assessment of your understanding of probability samples, design a sampling method for each of the common probability sample types listed here using the hypothetical study of hypertensive African American women. See Exhibit 11.1 for the description of each of the probability sample types to assist you in this learning activity.

Nonprobability Sampling

When nonprobability sampling methods are used, every element in the population does not have an equal chance of being in a study sample; therefore, nonprobability samples are less likely than probability samples to be representative of the population. Moreover, nonprobability samples may be more predisposed to error. There are advantages, however, to nonprobability sampling, primarily the ease of implementation. Additionally, with control strategies, nonprobability methods can produce credible samples. Also, keep in mind that the purpose and design of a particular study using nonprobability methods might not be to demonstrate population representativeness. Many qualitative studies are not interested in representativeness to a population, but rather an in-depth description of the lived experience of the individual elements of a sample. The four common types of nonprobability sampling include purposive (judgmental), snowball (network), quota (strata based), and convenience (accidental) samples; the latter of the four is the most commonly used. See Exhibit 11.1, Glossary of Terms, for a description of each of the nonprobability sample types.

▪ RELATED CONCEPTS

Sample Size

At the beginning of this chapter, the question "*How many participants do I need in my sample?*" was posed. The answer was given as "*it depends*," and this last portion of this chapter discusses why. The number of participants in a study is part of the overall design process as well as the sampling plan; it should be determined before beginning any research, recognizing that there are advantages to both large and small sample sizes. Aside from methodological design issues and conclusion validity, a priori determination of sample size may have both economic and ethical considerations. Research is a costly enterprise; the more participants recruited for and ultimately retained in a sample, the more money your research will generally cost in dollars and institutional and human resources. Moreover, the researcher has an ethical responsibility to the participants of human and even animal research not to expose them to any more procedural processes, which may include, pain or possible inconvenience, than needed. A larger sample is not necessarily better and may be unethical when statistical significance can be demonstrated by a predetermined and possibly smaller sample size than an arbitrarily larger number that just seems large enough (Hunter et al., 2018; Sasso et al., 2018).

Despite the importance of sample size determinations, there is no universally agreed-upon method for this within the healthcare professions; however, APRNs who lead or participate in research teams, as well as nurses who critically appraise research for practice, require a basic understanding of the factors involved in sample size determination. Study and population characteristics, measurement issues, effect size, and practical issues are all factors affecting sample size determination (Amatya & Bhaumik, 2018; Beavers & Stamey, 2018; Copsey et al., 2018; Show-Li & Shieh, 2018; Tam et al., 2020; Vanderlaan et al., 2019). Generally, more complex studies, with multiple variables and relationships being explored, require larger samples. While there are others, one relatively simple method of determining sample size determination is presented below with a discussion of statistical power and power analysis.

Statistical Power and Power Analysis

Statistical power is the probability of a statistical test finding a significant difference if such a difference indeed exists; it is the probability of rejecting the null hypothesis when it is false (Aberson & ProQuest, 2019; Nuzzo, 2016). Simply put, it is the probability of not committing a Type II error, or a false-negative result (β). As power increases, the likelihood of making a false-negative decision related to your study's results decreases.

Power is statistically represented as $1 - \beta$ and 0.80 is generally accepted as adequate statistical power for a study (Aberson & ProQuest, 2019; Nuzzo, 2016). Others have opined that statistical power is analogous to the sensitivity of a diagnostic test, and one may mentally substitute the word sensitivity for the word power to assist in understanding the concept (Miciak et al., 2016; Tavernier et al., 2016).

Power is affected by four major factors (Aberson & ProQuest, 2019; Anderson et al., 2017; Nuzzo, 2016), including the significance criterion (α), the magnitude of the effect (effect size), the sample size, and the study design. Two clinical *'pearls'* related to power and power analysis include:

- As the effect size increases, you may be able to decrease your sample size, because if the effect of the intervention is large, it should be able to be detected easily in a smaller sample.

- Conversely, if you have a small effect size, you would need to increase your sample size to be able to detect that effect.

Power analysis can be used to calculate the minimum sample size required to reasonably detect the effect of a given size. Power analysis can also be used to calculate the minimum effect size that is likely to be detected in a study using a given sample size. More and more publishers now encourage researchers to calculate and publish the effect size for each variable in their study, so others can be more exact in their power analysis calculation when utilizing a similar intervention or treatment. However, if hand calculating your power and/or effect size is not something you choose to do (not sure why you would want to), there are open (free) online power calculators that can decrease work and stress levels for the average healthcare practitioner tasked with determining sample size for a study or quality improvement project. The best online power analysis tool I have found, available for both Mac and Windows, is called G*Power 3.1.9.6 (Faul et al., 2009). This application is available from the Department of Experimental Psychology, Heinrich-Heine-University in Düsseldorf, Germany (www.psychologie.hhu.de/arbeitsgruppen/allgemeine-psychologie-und-arbeitspsychologie /gpower.html). Much of the website is in German, but instructions are also in English.

Once again, using the hypothetical study of African American women, let's assume you plan to have two groups of randomly assigned participants to receive or not receive (i.e., a control group) your intervention. For this example, your outcome or dependent variable is systolic blood pressure only; a literature search indicates that interventions similar to yours have demonstrated small (0.20) to medium (0.50) effect sizes. In designing your study, you want to determine how many participants will reasonably be needed (power of 0.80) to demonstrate a statistical difference between the intervention and control groups, given a specific effect size (Aberson & ProQuest, 2019; Nuzzo, 2016). The following are examples of the results of a priori power analysis to make this determination. Since the effect size is not definitive, you choose to do a power analysis using multiple effect sizes to cover the range of small to medium. You are asked to pay particular attention to the sample size requirement (to achieve 0.80 power) when the effect size changes. What does this tell you about the desired effect size?

- Using a two-tailed independent t-test, with an α error probability of 0.05, and a medium effect size of 0.50, 64 participants per group ($N = 128$) would be needed to achieve 0.80 power to detect statistical differences between the groups if such differences exist.

- Using a two-tailed independent t-test, with an alpha error probability of 0.05, and an effect size of 0.35, 130 participants per group ($N = 260$) would be needed to achieve 0.80 power to detect statistical differences between the groups if such differences exist.

- Using a two-tailed independent t-test, with an alpha error probability of 0.05, and a small effect size of 0.20, 394 participants per group ($N = 788$) would be needed to achieve 0.80 power to detect statistical differences between the groups if such differences exist.

See Exhibit 11.2 for G*Power 3.1.9.6's five different types of statistical power analysis offered.

EXHIBIT 11.2

FIVE DIFFERENT TYPES OF STATISTICAL POWER ANALYSIS

G*Power 3.1.9.6 (2020):

1. A priori (sample size N is computed as a function of power level $1 - \beta$, significance level α, and the to-be-detected population effect size).

- Compromise (both α and $1 - \beta$ are computed as functions of effect size, N, and an error probability ratio $q = \beta/\alpha$).

- Criterion (α and the associated decision criterion are computed as a function of $1 - \beta$, the effect size, and N).

- Post hoc ($1 - \beta$ is computed as a function of α, the population effect size, and N).

- Sensitivity (population effect size is computed as a function of α, $1 - \beta$, and N).

Sources: From Faul, F., Erdfelder, E., Buchner, A., & Lang, A.G. (2009). Statistical power analyses using G*Power 3.1: Tests for correlation and regression analyses. *Behavior Research Methods, 4*(4), 1149–1160. https://doi.org/10.3758/BRM.41.4.1149; Faul, F., Erdfelder, E., Lang, A. G., & Buchner, A. (2007). G*Power 3: A flexible statistical power analysis program for the social, behavioral, and biomedical sciences. *Behavior Research Methods, 39*(2), 175–191. https://doi.org/10.3758/BF03193146; Heinrich-Heine-Universität Düsseldorf. (2020). G*Power: Statistical power analyses for Windows and Mac. http://www.psychologie.hhu.de/arbeitsgruppen/allgemeine-psychologie-und-arbeitspsychologie/gpower.html

CRITICAL APPRAISAL OF SAMPLING IN PUBLISHED RESEARCH

Many nursing authors would agree that critical appraisal of published research to determine the quality of evidence is part of the responsibilities of advanced nursing practice (Gray et al., 2017; LoBiondo-Wood & Haber, 2018; Melnyk & Fineout-Overholt, 2019). Specific to this chapter, the evaluation of sampling methods of a study needs to be part of any study's critical appraisal, and the sampling plan, in particular, requires scrutiny. Polit and Beck (2020) contend two issues, in particular, are needed. First, one should determine if the sampling strategy of the study is adequately described. This determination includes the sampling approach or the type of sampling used, the population of interest, eligibility criteria for the sample, the sample size and rationale with power analysis, a description of the resultant sample's main characteristics (e.g., age, gender), and the number and characteristics of any potential participants who declined participation. Next, the appraiser has to determine if adequate sampling decisions were made to be able to conclude the use of the evidence for practice. Unfortunately, without an adequate description of the sample, one cannot conclude the quality of the evidence for practice. In the end, as in the beginning, a key criterion when assessing a sampling plan takes one back to the purpose of sampling in the first place, that being to obtain a true representation of the population being studied. Others echo the contentions of Polit and Beck (2020) and add that a description of institutional review board (IRB) approval and the informed consent process is readily apparent (Gray et al., 2017; LoBiondo-Wood & Haber, 2018).

Melnyk and Fineout-Overholt (2019) take a slightly different perspective than both Polit and Beck (2020) and others in calling for rapid critical appraisal using a checklist and evaluation and synthesis tables as a key step in the EBP process; believing these provide efficient critical appraisal methods for both quantitative and qualitative evidence for clinical decisions. A rapid critical appraisal checklist, according to Melnyk and Fineout-Overholt (2019), would include a general description of the study and, related to this discussion, would cover *the sampling technique, size, and characteristics* only.

Evidence supporting the best method to critically appraise research (or for our discussion, critical appraisal of sampling methods) by either the more extended narrative version or, the more contemporary rapid checklist version, is lacking. Still, one might assume the level of expertise of the appraiser and the clinical question being asked in the research would play a large part in determining the most appropriate method to critically appraise research in general, and sampling plans specifically.

SAMPLING FOR RESEARCH VERSUS QUALITY IMPROVEMENT PROJECTS

Much has been written about the similarities and differences between a research study and quality improvement projects. The main difference is the inference that can be drawn from a systematic research study compared to a quality improvement project. Specific to sampling and samples the concepts are generally similar to the information presented above, including the importance of the planning involved before the start of any quality improvement project; however the issue of statistical power and sample size may not become an unsurmountable barrier (Baker, 2017; Hain, 2017; Jang et al., 2018; Pimentel et al., 2019; Polit & Beck, 2020; Sarff & O'Brien, 2020). Additionally, when an APRN is conducting a quality improvement project, without the availability of statistical software or statistical skill, outcomes from a clinical intervention may be easily demonstrated using a percent change formula ([y2-y1]/y1x100). Many free websites are available to insert your project-specific numbers to arrive at percent change easily; my preferred site is www.percentage-change-calculator. com. Moreover, descriptive statistics such as frequencies and percentages can be calculated without special programs with only an Excel application. The reader is referred to the chapter of this text focused on quality improvement for a more in-depth discussion of quality improvement projects.

■ SUMMARY

In summary, sampling is the process of selecting a subset of observations from an entire population, such that the characteristics of the subset (i.e., the sample) will be representative enough to draw conclusions or make inferences about the population. Sampling decisions contribute critically to a study's internal and external validity and need to be made thoughtfully and judiciously. Decisions and processes depending on such things as a study's design and a study's data source(s) are related and need to be considered sequentially in planning research. Economic and ethical issues in sampling also need to be considered and are part of any discussion and/or decisions on a type or number included in a sample. Choosing between probability and nonprobability sampling and the kind of sample within each category are key to the validity of a study's conclusions. Determining sample size can be made easier, and likely to be more accurate when one has an understanding of the underlying logic and principles related to sampling. Established strategies such as CLT theory, and applications like G*Power 3.1.9.6., are useful for sampling plans. Lastly, the evaluation or critical appraisal of sampling methods are varied, and no one specific method is suggested; relying on the expertise of the appraiser seems most appropriate.

You are reminded that this chapter discussed the theory and a bit of the mathematics of sampling, but it is not inclusive of all the concepts which clinicians or researchers need to be aware of. Simply finding statistical differences does not always correlate with clinical significance or relevance. It is very satisfying when an intervention is found to be both clinically and statistically significant, but this is not always the case; an advanced practice nurse is expected to be able to discern the difference. Additionally, statistical significance does not prove that the results demonstrated are generalizable to the target population, but may only be suggestive of this at best. Multiple studies and rigorous systematic reviews presenting synthesized results are also needed for researched interventions to become part of an EBP.

SUGGESTED LEARNING ACTIVITIES

You are interested in differences related to three variables, including systolic blood pressure, HgbA$_{1C}$ levels, and weight for African American patients with type 2 diabetes seen at your clinic. You want to determine if there are differences in patient outcomes after three months of treatment by a family nurse practitioner compared to the family medicine physician. You also are interested in three variables, but in two groups of patients to see if the provider had an effect.

Complete the following exercises:

1. What type of sampling method and sample type would you use?
2. Using the central limit theorem, determine the sample size needed for your study.

3. For the same patients described earlier, but this time using G*Power 3.1.9.6., determine the sample size needed per group to have 0.80 power, with a 0.25 effect size, α of 0.05, and using a *t*-test for mean independent samples.

4. Repeat No. 3, keeping everything the same but change the effect to size to 0.50. What happens to the sample size? Why? Try an effect size of 0.10; now, what happens to the sample size?

Although Nos. 3 and 4 may seem beyond the scope of this chapter, following the instruction on the G*Power 3.1.9.6. website and the information given in this exercise, you may surprise yourself and any colleagues you may be working on a quality improvement study.

REFERENCES

Aberson, C. L., & ProQuest (2019). *Applied power analysis for the behavioural sciences.* (2nd ed.). Routledge.

Amatya, A., & Bhaumik, D. K. (2018). Sample size determination for multilevel hierarchical designs using generalized linear mixed models. *Biometrics 74*(2), 673–684. https://doi.org/10.1111/biom.12764

Anderson, S. F., Kelley, K., & Maxwell, S. E. (2017). Sample-size planning for more accurate statistical power: A method adjusting sample effect sizes for publication bias and uncertainty. *Psychological Science, 28*(11), 1547–1562. https://doi.org/10.1177/0956797617723724

Baker, D. J. (2017). Nursing research, quality improvement, and evidence-based practice: The key to perioperative nursing practice. *AORN Journal, 105*(1), 3–5. https://doi.org/10.1016/j.aorn.2016.11.020

Beavers, D. P., & Stamey, J. D. (2018). Bayesian sample size determination for cost-effectiveness studies with censored data. *PLoS ONE, 13*(1), E0190422. https://doi.org/10.1371/journal.pone.0190422

Burgess, C. (2019). Distribution of data: The central limit theorem. *Pharmaceutical Technology, 43*(10), 62–64. https://search.proquest.com/docview/2315904536?accountid=3611

Copsey, G., Thompson, J. Y., Vadher, K., Usama, A., Dutton, S. J. Fitzpatrick, R., Lamb, S. E., & Cook., J. A. (2018). Sample size calculations are poorly conducted and reported in many randomized trials of hip and knee osteoarthritis: Results of a systematic review. *Journal of Clinical Epidemiology, 104*, 52–61. https://doi.org/10.1016/j.jclinepi.2018.08.013

Fain, J. A. (2017). Selecting the sample and setting. In J. A. Fain (Ed.), *Reading, understanding, and applying nursing research.* (5th ed.). (pp. 133–152). F. A. Davis Company.

Faul, F., Erdfelder, E., Buchner, A., & Lang, A. G. (2009). Statistical power analyses using G*Power 3.1: Tests for correlation and regression analyses. *Behavior Research Methods, 4*(4), 1149–1160. https://doi.org/10.3758/BRM.41.4.1149. See also http://www.psychologie.hhu.de/arbeitsgruppen/allgemeine-psychologie-und-arbeitspsychologie/gpower.html

Faul, F., Erdfelder, E., Lang, A. G., & Buchner, A. (2007). G*Power 3: A flexible statistical power analysis program for the social, behavioral, and biomedical sciences. *Behavior Research Methods, 39*(2), 175–191. https://doi.org/10.3758/BF03193146

Gray, J., Grove, S. K., & Sutherland, S (2017). *Burns and Grove's the practice of nursing research: Appraisal, synthesis, and generation of evidence* (8th ed.). Elsevier.

Hain, D. J. (2017). Focusing on the Fundamentals: Comparing and contrasting nursing research and quality improvement. *Nephrology Nursing Journal, 44*(6), 541–543. https://drive.google.com/file/d/1RxdN6qEhlugCg0c4-bsWSbYvAOKWHFDn/view?usp=sharing

Hunter, R., Gough, A., O'Kane, N., McKeown, Fitzpatrick, A., Walker, T., McKinley, M., Lee, M., & Kee, F. (2018). Ethical issues in social media research for public health. *The American Journal of Public Health, March, 108*(3), 343–347. https://ajph.aphapublications.org/doi/10.2105/AJPH.2017.304249

Jang, H. J., Weberg, D., & Dowere, C. (2018). Nursing partnerships in research and quality improvement within a large integrated health care system. *Nursing Administration Quarterly, 42*(4), 357–362. https://drive.google.com/file/d/1-g-sGbBW1XnFs25XLM3J-fp8-3dMBvIZ/view?usp=sharing

LoBiondo-Wood, G. & Haber, J. (2018). *Nursing research: Methods and critical appraisal for evidence-based practice* (9th ed.). Elsevier.

Marshall, B. (2020). *Fast facts to loving your research project: A stress-free guide for novice researchers in nursing and healthcare.* Springer Publishing Company.

Melnyk, B. M., & Fineout-Overholt, E. (2019). *Evidence-based practice in nursing and healthcare: A guide to best practice* (4th ed.). Wolters Kluwer.

Miciak, J., Taylor, P. W., Stuebing, K. K., Fletcher, J. M., & Vaughn, S. (2016). Designing intervention studies: Selected populations, range restrictions, and statistical power. *Journal of Research on Educational Effectiveness 9*(4), 556–569. https://doi.org/10.1080/19345747.2015.1086916

Nuzzo, R. L. (2016). Statistical power. *American Academy of Physical Medicine and Rehabilitation, 8*(9), 907–912. https://www.clinicalkey.com/#!/content/journal/1-s2.0-S1934148216308413

Pimentel, C. B., Mills, W. L., Palmer, J. A., Dillon, K., Sullivan, J. L., Wewiorski, N. J., Snow, A. L., Allen, R. S., Hopkins, S. D., & Hartmann, C. W. (2019). Blended facilitation as an effective implementation strategy for quality improvement and research in nursing homes. *Journal of Nursing Care Quality, 34*(3), 210–206. https://drive.google.com/file/d/1RxdN6qEhlugCg0c4-bsWSbYvAOKWHFDn/view?usp=sharing

Polit, D. F., & Beck, C. (2020). Sampling in quantitative research. In D. F. Polit & C. Beck (Eds.), *Nursing research: Generating and assessing evidence for nursing practice* (11th ed.). Wolters Kluwer/Lippincott Williams & Wilkins.

Sarff, L., & O'Brien, R. (2020). Evidence-based quality improvement training programs: Building staff capability and organizational capacity. *Journal of Nursing Care Quality, 35*(2), 95–101. https://doi.org/10.1097/NCQ.0000000000000416

Sasso, L., Delogu, B., Carrozzino, R., Aleo, G., & Bagnasco, A. (2018). Ethical issues of prison nursing: A qualitative study in Northern Italy. *Nursing Ethics, 25*(3), 393–409. https://doi.org/10.1177/0969733016639760

Show-Li, J., & Shieh, G. (2018). The Bland-Altman range of agreement: Exact interval procedure and sample size determination. *Computers in Biology and Medicine, 100*(1), 247–252. https://doi.org/10.1016/j.compbiomed.2018.06.020

Stat Trek. (2020). *Statistics and probability dictionary.* https://www.stattrek.com

Tam, W., Lo, K., & Woo, B. (2020). Reporting sample size calculations for randomized controlled trials published in nursing journals: A cross-sectional study. *International Journal of Nursing Studies, 102*, 103450. https://doi.org/10.1016/j.ijnurstu.2019.103450

Tavernier, E., Trinquart, L., & Giraudeau, B. (2016). Finding alternatives to the dogma of power based sample size calculation: Is a fixed sample size prospective meta-experiment a potential alternative? *PLoS One, 11*, e0158604. https://www.doi.org/10.1371/journal.pone.0158604

Terry, A. J., & ProQuest. (2018). *Clinical research for the doctor of nursing practice* (3rd ed.). Jones & Bartlett Learning.

Torre, M. D., & Picho, M., K. (2016) Threats to internal and external validity in health professions education research. *Academic Medicine, 91*(12), e21–e21. https://journals.lww.com/academicmedicine/Fulltext/2016/12000/Threats_to_Internal_and_External_Validity_in.54.aspx

Vanderlaan, J., Dunlop, A., Rochat, R, Williams, B., & Shapiro. S. E. (2019). Methodology for sampling women at high maternal risk in administrative data. *BMC Pregnancy and Childbirth, 19*(364), 1–7. https://doi.org/10.1186/s12884-019-2500-7

12

DESIGNING QUESTIONNAIRES AND DATA COLLECTION FORMS

ROSEMARIE SUHAYDA AND UCHITA A. DAVE

▦ INTRODUCTION

Survey methods have advanced over the decades, enhanced by technology and the experience of researchers and analysts. Questionnaires are the most commonly used survey method because they are cost-effective, easily administered to large numbers of people, and subject to robust statistical analyses. They can be used for research, quality assurance, administrative decision-making, and determining the characteristics, attitudes, and preferences of respondents. Although seemingly easy, constructing a questionnaire that conforms to rules for good questionnaire design can be challenging.

This chapter provides general guidelines that can be applied to questionnaires developed for structured interviews and mailed or electronic surveys. The content can be applied to the simplest data collection form or to the most elegant study. Most situations require the development of a data collection instrument specific to the topic under investigation; in other cases, there may be a standardized or commercial instrument available. Published series such as *Instruments for Clinical Health-Care Research* (Frank-Stromborg & Olsen, 2004), *Measures for Clinical Practice and Research: A Sourcebook* (Corcoran & Fisher, 2014), and *Assessing and Measuring Caring in Nursing and Health Sciences: Watson's Caring Science Guide* (Sitzman & Watson, 2019) give examples of instruments that can be used in clinical healthcare research. Internet and library searches focused on specific topics might also include bibliographies and sources of measurement tools.

▦ GENERAL CONSIDERATIONS

Let us address some general considerations about questionnaires and surveys. The most important questions to ask yourself before developing a survey is, "Why is the survey being conducted?" You must have a clear understanding of the survey's purpose, what you hope to learn from the data, how the information will be used, and what types of decisions will be made based on the results.

The process for designing questionnaires should be orderly and systematic, beginning with clearly defined survey objectives. Early consideration should be given to the feasibility of administering a questionnaire based on time, budgetary constraints, and access to subjects. The amount and type of data needed, timing of data collection, and the intended analysis should be carefully planned before the questionnaire is finalized. If an item cannot be analyzed or will not influence a decision, then it should not be included in the questionnaire. Time should also be allotted for pretesting the instrument to obtain feedback on the clarity and wording of items, subjects' willingness to respond to each item, and time required to complete the questionnaire. A survey design matrix (see Table 12.1) can help illustrate some of the factors that should be considered in questionnaire development.

TABLE 12.1 Survey Design Matrix

SURVEY OBJECTIVES	SURVEY ITEMS	SAMPLING STRATEGY	DATA COLLECTION METHOD	DATA ANALYSIS
Determine the number of part-time and full-time employees who desire to have company-provided child care	Do you work a. Part time? b. Full time? Do you desire the company to provide child care? a. Yes b. No	A convenience sample of 500 employee names obtained from agency records	Electronic survey sent to selected employees' email addresses in the spring prior to beginning of the new school year	Frequency data described by number and percent of total respondents in each category Chi-Square analysis to determine association between employment status and desire for child care
Determine the potential numbers and ages of children needing company-provided child care	For each age range, indicate the number of your children who would be enrolled in the company-sponsored child care program. Select all that apply. Column options: a. <1 year old b. 1–2 years old c. 3–4 years old d. 4–5 years old e. >5 years old Row options: none, 1, 2, 3, >3			Contingency table displaying number of children by age range

The goals of a well-designed questionnaire are to engage the respondent in the process, make the respondent feel that the task is important, reduce respondent burden, and increase response rates. Low response rates will reduce the amount of confidence that can be placed in the survey results. Begin with a well-written cover letter. In many cases, the cover letter will determine whether or not the respondent completes the questionnaire. The cover letter should be written in a conversational tone. It should include the survey purpose, who is conducting the survey, how the data will be used and reported, how the respondent will benefit from the results, and who to contact should the respondent wish to ask questions about the survey. It should convey respect for the respondents and their privacy and explain your confidentiality/anonymity policy, particularly if the survey asks for sensitive information. The cover letter and the questionnaire need to look "official." People are not motivated to respond if the questionnaire looks like it was produced on a printer low on toner. Some software packages can give a very official appearance with little effort. Use of institutional letterhead for the cover letter lends an official nature to the survey. Give the questionnaire a short, meaningful, and descriptive title. Include clear and concise instructions on how to complete and return the questionnaire. If the questionnaire is to be returned by mail, then include a preaddressed and stamped envelope.

Item types should be interesting and nonthreatening to the intended audience; otherwise respondents are less likely to participate in the survey. Keep the order of the items in mind. Include the most important items in the first half of the questionnaire and items such as demographics at the end. Be aware that earlier items might influence responses to later items. Keep the questionnaire short to reduce respondent burden. Many investigators fail to differentiate between necessary and "interesting" data. The "interesting" information unnecessarily lengthens the questionnaire and may actually discourage someone from completing the questionnaire. The novice investigator may wallow in the large amounts of data only to find that the "interesting" data may not even enter into the final analysis. Such items are a waste of time for both the respondent and the investigator and should not be included in the survey.

■ APPEARANCE AND FORMAT

The initial appearance of the questionnaire is important, regardless of whether the questionnaire is in an electronic or print format. Attending to the appearance of a page is more important than attending to the number of pages. Many investigators think that reducing a five-page questionnaire to a three-page questionnaire makes the task seem less overwhelming. Crowding the page with black print, however, reducing the font size, and using reduction techniques in photocopying do not fool respondents and may actually discourage them from completing the questionnaire. Consider, also, the black-to-white ratio on a page. White should be more prominent than black. For printed questionnaires, the size of the page is also important. Consider possibilities other than the default size of 8.5″ × 11″. If the questionnaire is to be printed professionally, many sizes are available. One option is to use a centerfold approach, creating the appearance of a booklet. How the questionnaire will be mailed is one consideration that will affect the investigator's decision on what size of paper to use. The size of the envelope may be another limiting factor. When mailing a questionnaire, use an envelope that's unique. Colored envelopes that are individually hand addressed are more impressive than bulk mail.

Spacing

Spacing throughout the questionnaire is important. Spacing between questions should be greater than the spacing between the lines of each question, allowing the respondent to quickly read each question. Also, the spacing between response options should be sufficient to make it easy to determine which option was selected, especially if the task of the respondent is to circle a number. When material is single spaced, it can be difficult to determine which number was circled. Following these suggestions enhances the overall black-to-white ratio as well.

Typeface

The typeface should be chosen carefully for readability and appearance. Script typeface should be avoided. The size of the typeface should be selected with the reader in mind. For example, if the questionnaire is to be read by the elderly, the typeface should be larger than would be required for a younger adult. A good test is to have a few individuals close to the intended respondents' average age answer the planned questionnaire and describe the ease of completion.

Color and Quality of Paper

Although white or near-white paper may give the best appearance, the investigator may choose another color for several reasons. For instance, when potential respondents need to be separated by groups, the use of different colors for each group will make the task easier. Using a color other than white also makes it less likely that the questionnaire will get lost on the respondent's desk. The use of dark colors should be avoided since black print on dark colors is hard to read. The weight of the paper can give the impression of cheapness if it is too light; on the other hand, a heavy paper may increase the cost of postage. Physically feel the paper stock before printing questionnaires, and weigh the number of pages required along with the envelope and the return envelope to determine if a slight reduction in weight will avoid the need for additional postage.

Respondent Code

Another consideration is the place for a respondent code number. A code number is typically assigned to each respondent to facilitate tracking completion of the questionnaire and sending reminders. Usually an underscore line is placed at the upper-right corner on the first page. Although code numbers are essential if follow-up is anticipated, respondents are sometimes troubled by these numbers and either erase or obliterate them. This concern is particularly true when respondents fear an administrator's reaction to their answers or worry about lack of privacy. An explanation for the use of a code number in the cover letter may alleviate this concern but may not be sufficient if any of the information is at all revealing. When no respondent code is used, it is not possible to follow up on the non-respondents because they cannot be separated from those who have responded. Not using a code number means that everyone will need to get a second and third contact, increasing costs of the study.

When respondent codes are not used on questionnaires, different colors of paper can be used to represent separate subgroups. In this instance, response rates can still be determined for the entire sample, as well as for each subgroup. Selective follow-up without code numbers can be done on everyone in the subgroup with a low response rate if funds and time permit.

Subjects who receive electronic surveys linked to their email address can be tracked and reminded through that address. Subjects cannot be tracked when the online survey link is embedded in an email message or placed into social media.

■ SECTIONS OF THE QUESTIONNAIRE

Questionnaires are structured with several components. These include the title, directions for the respondents, questions to be answered, transition statement(s) when sections change, and a closing statement. Avoid labeling the survey as "Questionnaire." The title should be descriptive and relate to the content of the questionnaire. Directions for completing the questions follow the title. For example, the direction may be that the respondent is to select the best possible option and circle a response code. The implication here is that there is only one option per question and that all options selected require a circle around a number or letter by that option. Directions would be different if they were to select as many as apply. Specific directions may be required for each section of the questionnaire, and these should be explained in a conversational manner. The closing statement should thank the respondent for the time and effort taken to complete the task.

Types of Survey Items

Survey items can be written as a question or statement, referred to as the stem, followed by possible response options. Items can be either open-ended or close-ended. Open-ended items ask respondents to write a response in their own words. Close-ended items ask them to select among predetermined response choices. Choosing between open-ended and close-ended items depends on several factors. The *nature of the question to be answered* by the data is one factor. For example, if the item is requesting subjects to elaborate about their feelings, attitudes, or opinions, then an open-ended format would be appropriate. When detail and elaboration are not required, then close-ended items should be used. If the desired outcome is a set of statements from respondents, open-ended questions should be chosen. If a quick count of responses in different categories is desired, close-ended items will make the task easier.

Another factor that influences the choice between open- and close-ended questions is *how much is known about the possible responses.* If all possible responses are known, then they can be listed as response options, allowing the respondents to choose among them. If only some response options are known, then open-ended questions might be more appropriate. In instances when only some of the response options are known and the format calls for a close-ended item, then the use of "Other (please specify)_____" gives respondents a chance to answer if their response does not match the response options given.

One of the most important factors in selecting between the two types of survey items is the *sample size.* When dealing with a small number of questionnaires (fewer than 30), the investigator can use either option. With larger surveys (e.g., an entire hospital or institution or a national survey), close-ended items are preferable because of the work effort involved in reading, analyzing, and summarizing the written responses.

There are trade-offs with either choice. Richness of responses and freedom of expression are lost with close-ended questions. Ease of analysis and time are lost when open-ended questions are used unnecessarily. The investigator's burden is different with each. The time spent on designing the close-ended items can be significant, but their analysis is relatively quick. Open-ended items are quicker to design but may take significantly longer to analyze. Where the time is spent—up front in design or later in analysis—may be an additional factor in the investigator's decision-making.

Wording of the Survey Items

Carefully select the words used when writing survey items. Avoid jargon, slang, technical terms, abbreviations, vague imprecise language, or words that have several meanings. Define terms that might be unfamiliar to the respondents. Pretesting the items with several people who are similar to the intended audience will help establish clarity of the items. During the pretesting phase, probe the respondents to draw out any additional meanings or potentially confusing items. Interview the participants to solicit their interpretation and understanding of the items and establish any difficulties they had in completing the questionnaire. It is helpful to time these pretests, because that information can then be included in the cover letter to help the final respondents estimate how long it will take them to complete the questionnaire.

Guidelines for Well-Written Questions

1. Use a conversational tone. The tone of the questions and of the entire questionnaire should be as if the respondent were present. For example, the item:

    Ethnicity

    Hispanic   1

    Non-Hispanic   2

    Revision: What is your ethnicity? Are you

    Hispanic   1 or

    Non-Hispanic   2

2. Avoid leading questions that suggest the expected response, for example:

    Most mothers ensure that their infants receive immunizations as infants. Has your child been immunized?

    Yes   1

    No   2

    Revision: Has your child been immunized?

    Yes   1

    No   2

3. Avoid double-barreled questions that ask two questions at the same time, for example:

    Do you prefer learning about your illness in a group format, or would you rather use written material?

    Yes   1

    No   2

    Revision: Do you prefer a group format for learning about your illness?

    Yes   1

    No   2

    Do you prefer written materials for learning about your illness?

    Yes   1

    No   2

Or, consider this option:

Which format do you prefer for learning about your illness? Select all that apply.

Group format   1

Written materials   2

4. Try to state questions simply and directly without being too wordy. For some questions, the respondent wonders, "What was the question?" after reading wordy sections. A direct approach is more likely to yield the desired information.

5. Avoid double negatives.

Should the nurse not be responsible for case management?

Yes   1

No   2

Revision: Who should be responsible for case management?

The physician   1

The nurse   2

An administrator   3

Other (please specify) _____

6. Do not assume that the respondent has too much knowledge, for example:

Are you in favor of care for walk-ins in the clinic?

Yes   1

No   2

Revision: In the clinic, walk-ins are individuals who arrive without prescheduled appointments. These walk-ins will be seen for short appointments on the same day they call in with questions, rather than being scheduled for appointments later in the week. There will be a block of 1-hour appointments in both the morning and the afternoon left open for these walk-ins.

Are you in favor of receiving walk-ins in the clinic?

Yes   1

No   2

Guidelines for Writing Response Options

Response options are developed for close-ended questions. The designer of the questionnaire needs to have an idea about what the common options could be. When not all options are known, there should be an open-ended opportunity for the respondent to give an answer. Some options are categorical, such as "yes" and "no." Others may involve numerical scales that are continuous. As a reminder, it is important to consider the level of measurement needed to conduct the final analysis before constructing response options. For example, if continuous data such as age are categorized by range, then data can only be reported by frequencies and percentages within each category. If, on the other hand, the respondents are asked to record their exact age, then an arithmetic mean can be calculated. Statistical techniques specify whether categorical or continuous data are more appropriate for the analytic technique. Continuous data, such as age in years, can be reduced to categories; however, if age is collected in categorical form only, then those data cannot revert to a continuous form. Further discussion on levels of measurement of data is provided in Chapter 13 on analyzing quantitative data.

The most common guidelines for writing response options are listed here.

1. Do not make response options *too* vague or *too* specific.
   Problem (too vague): How often do you call in sick?

Never	1
Rarely	2
Occasionally	3
Regularly	4

   Revision: How often did you call in sick in the past 6 months?

Never	1
1–2 times	2
3–4 times	3
More than 4 times	4

   Problem (too vague): Which state are you from? _____

   Revision: In which state do you currently live? _____

   In which state do you work? _____

   Problem (too specific): How many total books did you read last year? _____

   Revision: How many books did you read last year?

None	1
1–3	2
4–6	3
More than 7	4

2. The categories should be mutually exclusive, that is, there should be no overlap. This can become a problem when ranges are given. For example:
   Problem: How old are you?

20–30 years	1
30–40 years	2
40–50 years	3
50 or older	4

   The person who is 30 years of age does not know whether to circle "1" or "2."

   Revision: How old are you?

20–29 years	1
30–39 years	2
40–49 years	3
50 or older	4

3. The categories must be inclusive and exhaustive.

   In the previous example, the categories would be inclusive of all respondents only if all of the respondents contacted were at least 20 years old. The last response, "50 or older," exhausts the upper age limit. To be more inclusive, the lower limit should be "20 or younger." The only caution in the use of broad ranges at the lower and upper ends is that such a grouping loses detail if the number of respondents at either end is extensive. If only a few respondents are expected to fall into these categories, then collapsing the upper or lower limits as described in the example may be adequate.

4. The order of options given is from *smaller* to *larger* or from *negative* to *positive*.

   As an example: For a 5-point scaled item ranging from "not at all" to "a great extent," the value for "not at all" is scored as "0" or "1" and "a great extent" is scored as "5." In the analysis and explanation of the findings, it is easy to explain that higher numbers mean more of something. A mean satisfaction score that is higher than another mean satisfaction score would then be a more desirable finding. It would be counterintuitive to associate a high mean value with a response of "not at all" or a low mean value with a response of "to a great extent." If response options are categorical, for example, race, then consider alphabetizing them. Another option is to order responses chronologically. Alphabetizing or numerically ordering lists of response items helps the respondent read through them more quickly to find their preferred choice.

5. The balance of the options should be parallel.

   Problem: To what extent do you agree that nurses are fairly compensated for the work they do?

Very strongly disagree	1
Strongly disagree	2
Agree	3
Strongly agree	4

   Revision: To what extent do you agree that nurses are fairly compensated for the work they do?

Strongly disagree	1
Disagree	2
Agree	3
Strongly agree	4

6. Limit the number of different types of response options chosen for use in the same questionnaire.

   Whenever possible, the same response options across questions are preferred. For example, common response options include levels of approval (approve–disapprove), agreement (agree–disagree), satisfaction (satisfied–dissatisfied), or evaluation (very good–very poor). The respondent's task becomes more difficult when it is necessary to adjust to multiple types of options within the same questionnaire. The respondent feels required to constantly "change gears," and the burden is increased.

7. Limit the number of response options and weigh carefully the inclusion of a neutral option.

    Response options or scales can range from as few as two to as many as ten. Generally shorter scales place less burden on the respondent, while longer scales are more reliable and allow for greater discrimination or variability in the scoring of items. The usual recommendation is to have between four and seven options per survey item. Giving more than seven options, however, makes the task of discriminating among options more difficult for the respondent and perhaps meaningless for both the respondent and the data analyst. In all cases, the investigator must weigh the trade-off between brevity and reliability.

    An internet search using the keywords "survey response scales" results in examples of the various types of response options. Some examples include:

    Two options: Yes–No; False–True

    Three options: Unimportant–Somewhat important–Very important

    Four options: Never–Seldom–Often–Always

    Five options: Very dissatisfied–Dissatisfied–No opinion–Satisfied–Very satisfied

    Seven or more options:

    Excellent   Poor

    (1)   (2)   (3)   (4)   (5)   (6)   (7)

    There is controversy over whether or not to include a neutral or middle option. Some fear that the neutral option will become the preferred choice. Others (Newcomer & Triplett, 2016) have not found that to be the case. Still others suggest placing the neutral (undecided, uncertain, neither agree/disagree) item outside of the scaled values, for example, to the right. If a neutral middle response is desired, then five responses should be used, with the third or middle response being the neutral one. If there is an even number of responses, the respondent is forced to choose one side or the other, which might cause some to avoid the item. In some cases, the respondents may feel that neither agreement nor disagreement is the best choice for them. If decisions need to be made on the basis of the degree of agreement obtained, then the surveyor may wish to force the respondent to choose a side. Using the items in a focus group and pretesting items may help determine the best arrangement.

8. The responses should match the question.

    If the question is about how satisfied the respondent is with the services, then the options should not be "agree/disagree." Options should also not be mixed within the same item, that is, using both "agree/disagree" and "satisfied/dissatisfied." Although these suggestions seem obvious, such violations are sometimes seen in poorly designed surveys.

Ordering of the Survey Items

There should be a logical flow to the sequencing of survey items. Early items are critical and should be related to the main topic and the title of the questionnaire. These items serve to engage the respondents and encourage them to initiate the task of completing the survey. For that reason, items should be interesting, nonthreatening, easy to answer, and devoid of sensitive material. Sensitive items should be placed near the middle of the questionnaire, at a point where some rapport with the respondent has been developed. If they appear too early, this intrusion can lead some respondents to decide not to complete the entire questionnaire. On the other hand, if sensitive questions are placed too close to the end, the respondent may feel an abrupt ending to a difficult conversation. If the entire topic of the questionnaire is sensitive, the reader will be informed by reading Waltz et al. (2016) who wrote about researching sensitive topics. Demographic questions should always appear at the end. They are the least interesting to the respondent and will be completed only if the respondent feels that a commitment has been made to finish the task.

Another factor to consider in the ordering of questions is the chronology of events. For example, if information about the health of a child is to be obtained, the first question should pertain to the child's birth, and later questions should focus on infancy and childhood.

Whenever possible, items of similar format should be grouped together. For example, if there are several clusters of "agree–disagree" items, these should be grouped. Items of similar content or focus should be grouped as well. Possible reasons for not grouping items include a major shift in content or a particular task that is required. In all cases, a transitional sentence or paragraph should precede a change or shift in focus.

Using Skip Logic

If all respondents answer all questions sequentially, then the logistics of navigating the questionnaire are simple to set up. Some survey items, however, might not apply to all respondents. In these cases, it is advisable to include skip logic in sequencing the items. Skip logic allows respondents to navigate through a survey by reading and responding only to items that pertain to them, thereby reducing the reading burden and the length of time it takes to complete the survey. To be effective, however, skip logic must be carefully applied. In written surveys, the directions to skip an item should be placed close to the response option. For example,

1. Do you work in an intensive care unit?

    Yes

    No (skip to item 7)

For electronic surveys, carefully test skip logic before sending the surveys out. If the skip logic is incorrectly developed, then entire sections of the survey will not be available to respondents. This results in unintentional loss of data.

Web-Based Surveys

Web-based surveys offer many advantages relative to cost, speed, candor, and format when compared to traditional survey formats. Web-based surveys are less expensive; allow for quick distribution; support flexibility in format and design; give a sense of confidentiality; and provide automated data input, handling, analysis, and reporting. There is an increased risk, however, of selection bias attributed to socioeconomic status, internet access, and internet literacy. Sampling of email addresses may also be difficult, and response rates are generally lower than those for traditional survey formats.

The principles of good survey design discussed throughout this chapter apply to electronic web-based surveys. The advantage of using a web-based service, however, is that most have preprogrammed formats and prompts that help in designing the survey. These include editing capabilities, moving and copying survey items, and selecting item formats. Surveys can also be preprogrammed to send reminder messages to non-respondents.

Various services are available that can be used to create web-based surveys and viewing reports online. Popular services include SurveyMonkey, Qualtricks, Crowdsignal, REDCap, and Google Forms. Table 12.2 compares the price and features of these four services.

Table 12.2 Comparison of Fiver Popular Services for Creating Web-Based Surveys and Reports

	SURVEYMONKEY	QUALTRICS	CROWDSIGNAL	REDCAP	GOOGLE FORMS
Basic Free Package Includes	10 questions per survey; 100 responses per survey.	10 questions per survey; 100 responses per survey.	Unlimited questions; unlimited responses	Unlimited questions; unlimited responses	Unlimited questions; unlimited responses
Plans/Pricing	Advantage Annual $32/Month; Premier Annual $99/Month	Plans start at $1,500 a year and go up to $5,000 a year.	Pro ($17/Month/User); Corporate ($75/Month/User)	No charge and no limit on users	No charge and no limit on users
Quick/Easy Sign Up	√	√	√	✗	√
Get Responses Via	Web, social media, email	Web, social media, email	Web, social media, email	Web, email	Web, social media, email
Export Response Data to	CSV, XLS,SPSS, PDF	CSV, XLS,SPSS, PDF	CSV, XLS, PDF, XML	XLS, SPSS, STATA, SAS, R	Google spreadsheet, CSV
Apply Filter to Survey Reports	√	√	√	√	✗
Question and Page Skip Logic	√	√	√	√	√
Custom Logos, Colors, and More	√	√	√	√	√
Themes	√	√	√	√	√
Track Email Response	√	√	√	√	√
Available in Mobile App/Tablet	√	√	√	√	√

There are some differences among these services. For example, SurveyMonkey's free package includes very limited features and does not allow exporting results or reports. Qualtrics free trial plan offers access to certain tools including summary reports and filtering, online reporting, and survey logic. Crowdsignal does not allow exporting of data into SPSS and has a limited number of email invites per month. While REDCap is completely free, there are some infrastructure requirements to set up the software. It is not as user-friendly and requires training before you are able to start building surveys. Google Forms offers many good features that are free; however, summaries cannot be modified and data cannot be exported; also, individual response data are only available to export in CSV format and Google spreadsheet.

Clinical Data Collection Forms

There are a few additional comments to be made about tools used for recording clinical data or chart information in contrast to tools used for asking questions. Data collection forms are used in clinical studies to record observations or in quality improvement activities to record compliance with standards. Most of the previous comments still apply.

In order to reduce the amount of writing, units of measurements should be written out where information is to be entered (e.g., _____mmHg). The use of checks or circles to complete a selection when the options are known will also reduce the amount of writing required.

When data are to be collected from various sections of a chart or in a series of steps, the data entry spaces should be placed in the order in which they occur, whether the data are on paper or screens. For example, if the order sheet is first in the paper chart, followed by progress notes, nursing notes, and graphs, the data collection should be ordered in that manner. When screens need to be navigated, the order of appearance should be taken into account.

The instructions about pretesting apply to data collection forms as well. By pretesting on a real chart or an electronic record, one can determine whether the order has been reversed and whether placement of items is optimal. When the order of data collection is not preserved, there is a greater tendency to skip an entry, resulting in missing data.

▣ FOLLOWING THE DEVELOPMENT OF THE QUESTIONNAIRE

Many questionnaires are analyzed by simply counting the number of respondents for each category of response. If more complex analysis is desired, the data analyst should be involved in designing the questionnaire and the data collection procedures. If consultation on the proposed analysis is needed, the consultant should review the questionnaire before the questionnaire is printed or administered. Revisions may be necessary solely for analytic reasons.

Optimizing Response Rates

Plans should be made for optimizing the response rates to your surveys. Some investigators recommend that a response rate of 50% is adequate, whereas others recommend at least a 70% response rate for successful surveys. A 30% to 40% response rate for electronic questionnaires is considered highly successful. A major challenge in improving return rates is persuading the respondent to complete the survey. The Tailored Design method is one of the more popular data collection procedures aimed at optimizing response rates (Dillman et al., 2014). This method follows a three-step format: (a) included in the first mailing is the questionnaire, cover letter, and prepaid return envelope; (b) follow-up reminder postcard sent within 10 days emphasizing importance of the study; and (c) a repeat mailing of another questionnaire with a shorter cover letter sent 2 weeks later.

Contact procedures for web-based surveys are similar to those for traditional surveys. The timing of the contact, however, is shortened. The initial survey is typically sent out with a short email invitation. Follow-up reminders should be sent when a significant drop-off in response rates is noticed, typically within a few days. Final reminders should be sent when another drop-off is noticed, within approximately 8 to 10 working days. Additional suggestions for improving response rates to web-based surveys include optimizing the survey for all devices, i.e., desktop PCs to mobile devices and adding a progress bar to show respondents how much longer the survey will take.

Phone follow-up has the additional advantage of permitting the respondent to clarify their reasons for not responding. The first mailing might not have been received, for example, especially in a complex organization. Questions that are answered in the phone call may permit the respondent to reply.

■ CODING THE RESULTS

This section considers issues in coding quantitative data resulting from surveys. Directions for coding qualitative data are found in Chapter 10.

The plans for analysis need to be made according to the amount of data, the intended level of analysis, and the method planned. If there will be a large data set or if a complicated analysis is anticipated, computer entry of the data is a necessity. With smaller data sets and when simple counts are planned, a manual system might be faster, although more errors are possible this way.

Entry of the data into the computer can be done in several ways. All of the responses can be entered onto a scantron sheet with response bubbles. Although this method is easy for the investigator, it is cumbersome for the respondent, who has to be sure that the response is placed on the right numbered line. If the questionnaire is complicated and/or multiple sources of data are used, it may be easier to enter responses into an Excel spreadsheet or an Access database. These products facilitate the calculation of descriptive and some inferential statistics that may be sufficient for analytic purposes without the investigators having to export the data to a statistical program.

If the questionnaire is precoded and simple, the numbers circled by the respondent may be directly entered into the appropriate Excel column. In this case, each subject will be a row and each answer will be found in one column. One should plan to check for errors, especially if a high degree of accuracy is needed.

TeleForm is a software package that converts paper forms into usable data. It consists of several functions:

- **Form Designer:** Design forms/surveys optimized for automated computer recognition.
- **Reader:** A service that waits for incoming forms whether from scanned papers, email, fax, or other means.
- **Verifier:** A program an operator can open to view processed forms and, if needed, make decisions on character recognition that could not be read with the specified confidence level.
- **AutoMerge Publisher:** Print forms with unique IDs, barcodes, or any number of data premerged onto the form at the time of printing.

This expensive software is available from Cardiff and is probably available only in larger survey centers or major industries. If scanned questionnaires are planned, then the need for a scanner that has an automated data feeder will add to the costs of the initial setup. For subsequent surveys, costs of data entry, time required, and error rates are all reduced with this system. Another option to consider is Qualtrics Research Suite, an enterprise online survey software solution that collects, analyses, and acts on relevant data.

The first run of the data should include a count of all the values for each variable. That allows numbers out of the expected range, illegal values, to be detected. For example, a yes-or-no question that was coded "1" and "2" would not have response numbers from "3" to "8." A "9" might be a legitimate value if the convention of inserting a "9" where there are missing data was followed. If illegal values are found, the ID number for the questionnaire containing the incorrect value needs to be determined. Then the original questionnaire for that subject should be reviewed to look for the correct value, and the spreadsheet should be corrected. This process, called data cleaning, should be done before any meaningful statistics are calculated.

▇ SUMMARY

Multiple decisions about questionnaire design, the items to be developed, and the responses that are anticipated influence the quantity and the accuracy of the data that will be collected. The response rate will partially determine the value of the results to the intended audience. Development of well-designed data collection forms is vital in collecting accurate evidence for practice.

SUGGESTED LEARNING ACTIVITIES

1. Select a topic that allows both open-ended and close-ended responses. Develop three to four questions in each format. Discuss with a partner the advantages and disadvantages of each format.

2. Select a quality improvement topic from your clinical setting. Describe how you would design a tool to collect data, the process you would use to collect the data, and how you would feed back the results to those involved.

REFERENCES

Corcoran, K., & Fisher, J. (2014). *Measures for clinical practice and research: A sourcebook* (5th ed.). Oxford University Press.

Dillman, D. A., Smyth, J. D., & Christian, L. M. (2014). *Internet, phone, mail, and mixed-mode surveys: The Tailored Design method* (4th ed.). Wiley & Sons.

Frank-Stromborg, M., & Olsen, S. J. (2004). *Instruments for clinical health-care research* (3rd ed.). Jones & Bartlett.

Newcomer, K. E., & Triplett, K. (2016). In H. P. Hatry & J. S. Wholey (Eds.), *Handbook of practical program evaluation* (4th ed.). Wiley & Sons.

Sitzman, K.L., & Watson, J. (2019). *Assessing and measuring caring in nursing and health sciences: Watson's Caring Science guide* (3rd ed.). Springer Publishing Company.

Waltz, C. F., Strickland, O. L., & Lenz, E. R. (2016). *Measurement in nursing and health research* (5th ed.). Springer Publishing Company.

ADDITIONAL READINGS

DeVellis, R. F. (2017). *Scale development: Theory and applications* (4th ed.). SAGE.

Hohwü, L., Lyshol, H., Gissler, M., Jonsson, S. H., Petzold, M., & Obel, C. (2013). Web-based versus traditional paper questionnaires: A mixed-mode survey with a Nordic perspective. *Journal of Medical Internet Research, 15*(8), e173. https://doi.org/10.2196/jmir.2595

Robinson, S., & Leonard, K. (2019). *Designing quality survey questions*. SAGE.

Walford, G., Tucker, E., & Viswanathan, M. (Eds.). (2010). *The SAGE handbook of measurement*. SAGE.

PHYSIOLOGICAL AND PSYCHOLOGICAL DATA COLLECTION METHODS

SUSAN K. FRAZIER AND CAROL GLOD

▦ INTRODUCTION

Evidence-based practice (EBP) is the clinical application of research findings that have been synthesized, replicated in appropriate populations of patients, evaluated for scientific rigor, and found to be the most effective approach to a clinical problem; clinical expertise and patient preferences also contribute to EBP. The intent of EBP is to optimize outcomes, whether individual clinical outcomes, or system-wide outcomes, or community outcomes. It is essential that clinicians are skillful in the interpretation, evaluation, and critique of quality research studies to determine their scientific soundness and appropriateness for application to clinical practice. This requires a rigorous evaluation of the physiological and psychological instruments used for data collection.

▦ PHYSIOLOGICAL DATA COLLECTION METHODS

Biomedical instruments collect data about individual physiological status, biological functions and processes, and the consequences of disorders, injuries, and malfunctions. Clinicians use biomedical instrumentation daily in practice to acquire data about patient condition, to monitor patient progress, and to evaluate the efficacy of management. However, biomedical instruments used in the clinical setting and in research studies must be an accurate reflection of reality. Research data and investigator interpretation may be doubted when instruments used to collect physiological data were inappropriate. Thus, published reports must include information about physiological instruments to demonstrate the appropriateness, accuracy, and reliability to ensure sufficient research rigor. Evaluation of these data requires a clear understanding of the principles of biomedical instrumentation, the physiological variables measured, the characteristics of biomedical instrumentation, the procedures for measurement of biological variables, and the criteria for evaluation of accuracy and precision of biomedical instruments.

Biomedical instruments extend human senses by measurement of physiological variables, detection of changes over time in these variables, and amplification and display of these data so our senses can detect them. Many physiological changes are miniscule and not detectable with our senses. For example, the electrocardiogram (EKG) captures millivolt changes in electrical activity that occur in cardiac myocytes, amplifies the signal to volts, and displays the signal audibly as a sound, or visually as a waveform on a screen or a printout from a computer.

■ CLASSIFICATION OF BIOMEDICAL INSTRUMENTS

Biomedical instruments are broadly classified as in vivo and in vitro. In vivo (within the living) instruments are applied directly on or within a living organism. In vitro (in the glass) instruments study living cells or tissues after removal from the body, most often in a laboratory. A cardiac monitor is an in vivo instrument, as sensing electrodes are applied directly to the individual. In vitro instruments may measure intracellular activity in cells once they are removed from the body. For example, blood samples removed from an individual are analyzed for electrolyte concentrations.

In vivo instruments are further categorized as invasive or noninvasive. Invasive instruments enter a body cavity or break the skin barrier for measurement. An arterial catheter connected to a pressure transducer for measurement of arterial blood pressure is an invasive measure, while a 12-lead EKG and a bedside cardiac monitor with electrodes applied to the skin surface are noninvasive biomedical instruments.

The selection of an invasive or noninvasive instrument is a central consideration in clinical practice and research. The use of noninvasive instruments is often preferred because they are associated with fewer patient risks like tissue ischemia, hemorrhage, infection, and subsequent sepsis that may be associated with the intra-use of arterial or IV catheters. Another important consideration for instrument selection is the type and number of potential mechanical issues associated with the instrument and measurement technique, such as proper placement, potential infection, or possible obstruction.

Prior to selection of a biomedical instrument, the investigator or clinician should consider the necessary frequency of data collection, either intermittent or continuous. Intermittent or cross-sectional measures provide data at only one point in time, and rapid and clinically important alterations in a variable may be missed. For example, indirect measures of arterial blood pressure using an automated oscillating blood pressure cuff provide intermittent data; the frequency can be altered by reprogramming the instrument. However, continuous measurement of arterial blood pressure with an intra-arterial catheter connected to a transducer provides a continuous direct measure of intra-arterial pressure with beat-to-beat responsiveness to rapid alterations in blood pressure that could be clinically important. Thus, the frequency of data capture is a major consideration in selection of an instrument.

The choice of an indirect measurement technique requires the investigator or clinician to select the most accurate and reliable technique available for data collection. For example, indirect blood pressure measurement may be obtained by auscultation, oscillometric technique, finger probe technique using photoplethysmography to evaluate pressure fluctuations in the finger, an ultrasound technique, and tonometry (Muntner et al., 2019). The accuracy of indirect blood pressure measures is dependent on the technique used and the fidelity to recommended measurement procedure. Indirect blood pressure measurement by auscultation using a mercury sphygmomanometer is the gold standard indirect measurement for research and clinical care (Muntner et al., 2019); however, the use of mercury has decreased and in some countries has been banned because of its toxic nature and potential environmental contamination (O'Brien, 2000).

Oscillometric measures of blood pressure with automated cuffs are common in clinical practice but often vary considerably from auscultory measures (Wohlfahrt et al., 2019). Investigators identified systolic pressure was 1 to 26 mmHg higher and diastolic was 1 to 25 mmHg higher when oscillometric technique was compared with auscultation; differences were greater in individuals older than 65 years. Because of questionable validity of oscillometric measures of blood pressure, an independent database (www.dableducational.org/sphygmomanometers) provides validation data for review and evaluation by consumers. Devices are evaluated using established standards and categorized as recommended, not recommended, or questionable. Unfortunately, this type of database is not available for other instruments. Clinicians and researchers must evaluate the manufacturer's specifications and research findings focused on the validity, accuracy, precision of the biomedical measure needed.

Errors in measurement may occur and invalidate physiological data. For example, the American Heart Association guidelines for measurement of auscultory blood pressure recommend measurements made with the cuff placed over the bare arm (Muntner et al., 2019). Prior investigators suggested that measures taken over clothing are also valid (Pinar et al., 2010), but Ozone et al. (2016) found that accurate measurements were made only over the bare arm. Recently investigators found that when compared to auscultory measures, automated systolic measures were on average 10 mmHg lower, and prevalence of hypertension varied from 31.5% with the automated technique versus 40.1% with the auscultory technique (Wohlfahrt et al., 2019). Thus, the investigator or clinician should select the most accurate technique and validated equipment and follow the established procedure for valid measurements.

Although in vitro biomedical instrumentation does not pose direct risks to an individual in clinical practice or research, there must be consideration of the sample required for measurement. Sampling techniques may be associated with complications like bleeding, hematoma formation, pain, infection, and disability. The burden to the individual clearly will vary depending on the type of sample needed, and the instrument that provides the most accurate measurement with the least burden to the individual should be the first choice.

In vitro measures are also be categorized as direct or indirect measures. For example, a direct measurement of catecholamine concentration uses blood or plasma, whereas an indirect measure evaluates the breakdown products of catecholamines in urine; and elevated carbon monoxide (CO) levels due to cigarette smoking are directly measured in blood with a CO-oximeter, and indirectly measured in exhaled air using an ecolyzer.

CATEGORIES OF PHYSIOLOGICAL VARIABLES DETECTED BY BIOMEDICAL INSTRUMENTS

Physiological variables are commonly measured in hospitals, clinics, and community and home settings to evaluate health status, diagnose diseases, determine efficacy of therapeutic regimens, and provide metrics for goal setting. To ensure accuracy of physiological data, the components of the organism–instrument system, the subject, stimulus, and biomedical instrument, must be understood. A variety of physiological variables can be measured using biomedical instrumentation.

COMPONENTS OF THE ORGANISM–INSTRUMENT SYSTEM

The components of the organism–instrument system include the participant, the stimulus, the sensing equipment, the signal conditioning equipment, the display equipment, and the recording and data-processing equipment (Figure 13.1). Each component requires evaluation to ensure that the data obtained are an authentic reflection of reality. However, these components must function together as a system to produce high-quality, accurate, and reliable data.

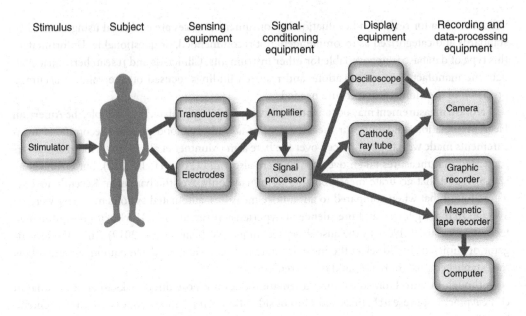

FIGURE 13.1 The organism–instrument system.

Source: From Polit, D. F., & Hungler, B. P. (1987). *Nursing research: Principles and methods* (3rd ed.). Lippincott.

Subject

The subject is the individual, either healthy or ill, from whom data will be obtained. The demographic and clinical characteristics of the individuals included in a study are dependent on the research purpose and specific aims, and careful attention to the selection of demographic and clinical variables is essential in any research study. A number of nursing science studies also test interventions intended to improve health outcomes in a group of individuals with selected characteristics. However, there are research purposes and specific aims that cannot be studied in humans because of the need for invasive in vivo measures that would be inappropriate and/or unethical in humans, as well as associated with high potential for serious adverse reactions and risks. These studies may be performed in animal models, in vitro cell cultures, or with computer models.

Stimulus

The specific aims of a research study will determine the variables to measure. Once the variables to measure are identified, an experimental stimulus may be selected. This could be a nursing care procedure like endotracheal suctioning or position change, which alters the physiological variables to be measured. Other stimuli might include minute electric shocks to elicit an electromyogram (EMG), auditory stimuli like environmental noise in critical care, or tactile stimulation by touching the skin of a premature infant. In these examples, a stimulus elicits a response in selected physiological variables, which is then measured by biomedical instrumentation. In an experimental study, the stimulus can be altered by changing its duration, intensity, or frequency. For example, the effect of environmental noise in an intensive care unit lasting for 5, 10, or 15 minutes (duration) can be measured at 20 and 50 decibels (intensity) every 30 minutes (frequency) in a number of physiological variables that might include heart rate, blood pressure, intracranial pressure, respiratory rate, and catecholamine concentration in the blood.

Sensing Equipment

Sensing equipment is required to detect alterations in a physiological variable. Transducers and recording electrodes are types of sensing equipment commonly used in research and clinical practice for the measurement of physiological variables. Transducers sense a nonelectrical signal and convert it to an electrical signal; electrodes sense an electrical signal.

Transducers

A transducer is a device that converts one form of energy, like pressure, temperature, or partial pressure of gases, and simultaneously produces an electrical signal in volts proportional to the change in the variable. Conversion to volts is required because a biomedical instrument is an electronic device that will only respond to changes in electrical output. There are a number of different types of transducers.

There are several considerations when using a transducer to collect physiological data to ensure accuracy and reliability of the measures. Pressures must be measured using specific reference planes. The right atrium, the reference plane for blood pressure measures, is located in the supine position at the fourth intercostal space in the midaxillary line (Figure 13.2). The pressure transducer balancing port is positioned so that it is perfectly horizontal to the right atrium of the individual using a level (Avellan et al., 2017; Jacq et al., 2015). Leveling a transducer using the appropriate reference point is vital; for each inch (2.5 cm) of difference between the balancing port and the right atrium, the blood pressure varies 2 mmHg (Jacq et al., 2015). If the position of the individual is changed, then the transducer must be releveled to the reference position to obtain valid measures. The right atrium is also the reference for indirect blood pressure measurement; the middle of the blood pressure cuff on the upper arm should be at the level of the right atrium (the midpoint of the sternum) for valid measures (Muntner et al., 2019). The reference point for intracranial pressure measurement is the level of the ventricles of the brain, which is in line with the foramen of Monro (Thompson, 2011). In the supine position, the foramen is level with the tragus of the ear or the outer canthus of the eye; in the lateral position, the foramen is level with the midsagittal line between the eyebrows. Position change again requires releveling for accurate measurement (Song et al., 2016).

After the appropriate level of the pressure transducer is achieved, it must then be balanced and zeroed by opening the balancing port and exposing the sensing diaphragm to atmospheric pressure. This procedure establishes the strain gauge at zero voltage with respect to atmospheric pressure. In the transducer, four strain gauges, or resistances, are mounted to a sensing diaphragm; these resistances are connected to form a Wheatstone bridge circuit. In the strain gauges, as

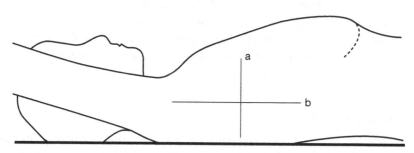

FIGURE 13.2 Right atrial reference plane for cardiac pressure measures.

pressure increases, two stretch and two contract; the sensitivity of the transducer is then increased fourfold. When the balancing port is exposed to atmospheric pressure, the strain gauges are balanced or equal, and the voltage output is set at zero. When the balancing port is closed and the arterial catheter connected to the pressure transducer, the actual pressure changes occurring in the blood vessel cause the sensing diaphragm to move inward and outward, which changes the resistance in the wires and the voltage output. Transducers that are not correctly zeroed may systematically add or subtract from the actual values, and introduce an error into each measure made.

Pressure transducers must also be calibrated against a column of mercury (Hg) or water (H_2O), depending on the range of pressures to be measured. Known values of pressure in increments of 50 to 250 mmHg for arterial pressure, 5 to 50 mmHg for pulmonary arterial pressure, or 5 to 25 cm H_2O for central venous or intracranial pressure are applied to the transducer to determine whether the electrical output is linear. Linearity is the extent to which an input change is directly proportional to an output change. Thus, for every 1 mmHg change in pressure there is a 1 mmHg change in the measurement; this linear response must be consistent through the range of possible pressures. This procedure verifies that changes in blood pressure are proportional to the voltage output. To ensure the accuracy and reliability of research data, the transducer should be calibrated before, during, and after data collection. The same principles of balancing, zeroing, and calibrating apply to temperature and biochemical transducers.

Recording Electrodes

Recording electrodes sense naturally occurring electrical signals, most often from the heart (EKG), the brain (electroencephalogram or EEG), and muscle (electromyogram or EMG). Natural electrical signals occur because of ion currents produced when positive and negative ion cellular concentrations change, as during a cardiac action potential (Kennedy et al., 2016). There are three types of electrodes: surface electrodes, indwelling macroelectrodes, and microelectrodes. Surface electrodes are most commonly used in clinical practice and in research with humans. An example of indwelling macroelectrodes is a needle electrode, where a needle is placed in subdermal tissue to detect electrical signals. Microelectrodes are often placed in a single cell outside of the body to measure ionic currents directly at the cellular level. Surface electrodes placed on the skin surface record the sum of electrical potentials.

Signal Conditioning Equipment

Signals produced by a transducer or detected by electrodes are usually measured in millivolts, and must be amplified to volts to drive a display unit. Amplification of the signal is referred to as "increasing the gain." Once a signal has been amplified, the frequency of the signal in cycles per second is modified to eliminate noise or artifact. An example of artifact is the muscle movement seen on an EKG or 60-cycle (Hz) noise from environmental electrical interference. Electronic filters are a component of the signal conditioning equipment that controls this noise or artifact by rejecting the unwanted signals. Artifact can also be separated, diluted, or omitted by adjusting the sensitivity control on a biomedical instrument.

Display Equipment

Display units may be an oscilloscope, a computer, or a graphic recorder. Most display units require an input voltage of 5 to 10 V (Enderle & Bronzino, 2012). Once a physiological signal has been modified and amplified by signal conditioning equipment, the display equipment converts the electrical signals into visual or auditory output that our senses can detect and evaluate. In the clinical setting, computers and computer screens display the voltage change or waveforms by time, and most often display multiple measured variables. Heart rate, cardiac rhythm, blood pressures, respiratory rate, and oxygen saturation are common physiological variables that may be displayed continuously and simultaneously on a computer screen. These data are automatically stored, and can be retrieved to evaluate trends over time, and to compare changes in physiological variables at different points in time. Computers with specialized software acquire, store, and analyze a wide variety of research and clinical data. However, the rate of data acquisition must be sufficient to ensure that sufficient values of physiological data are captured. Software systems also convert analog signals into digital values that can be transported into a data spreadsheet.

▨ CHARACTERISTICS OF BIOMEDICAL INSTRUMENTS

Measurement of physiological data using biomedical instruments is fundamental to many nursing science studies. However, not every instrument functions equally well for all circumstances, and inattention to any one component of the organism–equipment system may result in the collection of data that are not an accurate reflection of reality. Thus, there are basic characteristics of the data collected that must be considered for every physiological variable. These include the validity, accuracy, and precision or reliability of the measure.

Validity is the extent to which the biomedical instrument measures the actual variable of interest, and accuracy is the degree to which the measured value reflects the actual value. For example, the validity of cardiac output measure taken with bioimpedance can be evaluated by inspection of the waveform obtained by the instrument, and the degree of accuracy by comparison with a "gold standard" measure like the Fick equation or a thermodilution measure. Reliability refers to the accuracy of the measure over time. When using new measures and new biomedical instruments, validity, accuracy, and reliability should be evaluated using a gold standard measure and reported.

Biomedical instruments also have specifications that demonstrate their ability to measure the variable of interest. These specifications are important in the decision-making process for selection of the instrument and are typically reported in the instrument specifications provided by the manufacturer. Important characteristics of an instrument include the range, the frequency response, specificity, stability, linear response, and the signal-to-noise ratio (Table 13.1).

▨ USING BIOMEDICAL INSTRUMENTATION FOR RESEARCH PURPOSES

Any biomedical instrument used to obtain physiological data for research purposes must be thoroughly evaluated prior to selection and use for research purposes, as it directly influences the rigor of the study and the value of the findings. Bedside pulse oximetry is described as an illustrative example that considers the required characteristics of biomedical instrumentation.

Oxygen Saturation

The gold standard measure of oxygen saturation is obtained with an invasive arterial blood gas sample and determined in vitro using a CO-oximeter. An alternative noninvasive measure of

TABLE 13.1 Specifications to Determine the Accuracy and Validity of Biomedical Measures

SPECIFICATION	DEFINITION	EXAMPLES
Range	Complete set of values that an instrument can measure	Scale range 0 to 100 grams Cardiac monitor 1–250 beats per minute Thermometer 0 to 60° C
Frequency response	Capacity of the instrument to respond equally well to rapid and slow components of a signal	EKG 0.5–100 Hz Pulse oximeter 0.66–15 Hz
Sensitivity	Degree of change in the physiological variable that the instrument can detect	Instrument chosen for a study should have the degree of sensitivity that responds to the research purpose Scale may weigh within 1 gram or within 0.01 gram
Stability	Ability to maintain calibration over a given time interval Biomedical instruments develop gradual loss of calibration or calibration drift	Equipment specifications describe stability over time, and indicate manufacturer's recommendation for recalibration frequency
Linearity	Extent to which an input change is directly proportional to an output change Linearity should be evaluated for the entire range of the instrument	For every 1 degree of actual change in temperature, there is a 1-degree change recorded by the thermometer
Signal-to-noise ratio	Relationship between the signal strength and the amount of noise or artifact detected	The higher the signal-to-noise ratio, the fewer the artifacts and the clearer the signal obtained

oxygen saturation is obtained by pulse oximetry (SpO_2). A clear understanding of the instrumentation and technique of these two measurement techniques is vital to ensure that the data obtained with a pulse oximeter are appropriate for a study and are an accurate reflection of reality.

Measurement of Oxygen Saturation

Measurement of hemoglobin saturation may be either a fractional or a functional measurement. A fractional measurement of hemoglobin saturation requires a blood sample and is performed with a CO-oximeter, typically associated with a blood gas analyzer. The fractional oxygen saturation is the ratio of oxygen-saturated hemoglobin or oxyhemoglobin (HbO_2) to the *total* number of hemoglobin molecules. Thus, the status of total hemoglobin is evaluated with a fractional measurement.

A pulse oximeter provides a functional measurement of hemoglobin saturation, which is the ratio of oxygen-saturated hemoglobin to the total amount of hemoglobin *available for binding* to oxygen. This type of measurement *does not include* evaluation of hemoglobin that is not available for binding with oxygen, either carboxyhemoglobin (HbCO) or methemoglobin (Hbmet).

Newer pulse-oximetry technology uses eight wavelengths of light and is capable of making noninvasive fractional measures of HbCO and Hbmet. The primary use of these instruments is rapid detection of carbon monoxide poisoning. Compared with CO-oximetry values, this technology has a reported bias and precision for HbCO of 0.1% and 2.5%, respectively; thus, compared with gold standard measures, measures will be between –6% and 4% of actual value. Thus, an actual measure of HbCO of 10% could range between 4% and 14% using this noninvasive technique (Zaouter & Zavorsky, 2012).

Validity of Oxygen Saturation Measurement by Pulse Oximetry

The fractional measurement of oxygen saturation by a CO-oximeter using four or more wavelengths of light is the gold standard measure of oxygen saturation. Numerous studies have compared functional values obtained by pulse oximetry with simultaneous fractional measurement of oxygen saturation by CO-oximeter. In the range of 70% to 100% oxygen saturation, there is a very strong correlation between these values (range of correlation coefficients, $r = .92$ to .98). Within this range of values, pulse oximetry accurately reflects *functional* hemoglobin saturation. Most current manufacturers report a bias of 2%, which indicates that the actual value of saturation may be 2% higher or lower than the actual value. However, when oxygen saturation values are less than 70%, pulse oximetry may provide a falsely high value because of the calculation algorithm used (Nitzan et al., 2014). This is due to the development and testing of these instruments in healthy adults only; ethical considerations precluded developers from reducing oxygen saturation in healthy volunteers to levels developed by acutely and critically ill patients. SpO_2 may be a clinically useful indirect indicator of oxygen transport; however, both the clinician and the researcher must remember that the use of a functional measurement of oxygen saturation does not reflect tissue oxygen delivery.

Accuracy of Pulse Oximetry

Certain clinical and technical phenomena may reduce the accuracy of saturation values obtained by pulse oximetry (Shamir et al., 2012; Table 13.2).

Bias for pulse-oximetry values vary depending on the degree of hypoxemia; so, as oxygen saturation decreases, bias increases. Bias for pulse-oximetry measures ranges from less than 0.5% to as much as 10%. Thus, the measured values could be seriously inaccurate, particularly at critical values. Pulse-oximetry values in general are reported to have a margin of error or bias of $\pm$ 2% of the actual SaO_2 value. This degree of error provides a wide range of potential values if SpO_2 values are normally distributed. Clinicians and investigators must determine whether measures with this degree of potential error provide sufficiently accurate data to address the clinical and research objectives.

Precision and Reliability of Oxygen Saturation by Pulse Oximetry

Pulse oximetry can detect a 1% change in oxygen saturation. However, the speed of response by the pulse oximeter decreases as actual SaO_2 values decreases. A statistical measure of the reproducibility of pulse-oximetry measures is precision. This value is obtained by calculating the standard deviation of the bias measurement. The precision measure is analogous to the scatter of data points in measures made over time. Precision measures for pulse oximetry are reported to range from 2% to 4% (Perkins et al., 2003; Wilson et al., 2010). Pulse-oximetry measures are generally consistent over time (Nitzan et al., 2014); a majority of reliability evaluation studies evaluated consistency of measurement over time using different probe types (reusable or disposable, finger,

TABLE 13.2 Clinical and Technical Factors That Reduce the Accuracy of SpO$_2$ Values

CATEGORY	FACTOR	CLINICAL SITUATION
Individual	Weak arterial pulsation	Shock states, hypothermia with shunting of blood flow from the periphery, or increased systemic vascular resistance may result in significantly reduced or absent light absorption detection by the sensor
	Venous pulsation	Right ventricular failure or a partial obstruction to venous outflow. In the presence of both arterial and venous pulsatile flow, the SpO$_2$ value is a composite value and will be lower than the actual arterial saturation
	Anemia	May be secondary to the scattering of light in the plasma, which produces a shift in the degree of red light absorbed (Nitzan et al., 2014)
	Presence of significant portion of hemoglobin unavailable for oxygen binding (HbCO, Hbmet)	At a CO partial pressure of only 0.1 mmHg, hemoglobin is 50% saturated with CO, but a functional measurement of saturation by the pulse oximeter may indicate very high oxygen saturation, as the remaining 50% of hemoglobin may be fully saturated with oxygen. High levels of HbCO increases the affinity of hemoglobin for oxygen and reduces oxygen unloading from hemoglobin at the tissues
	Hyperbilirubinemia and highly pigmented skin	The majority of studies that compare SaO$_2$ with SpO$_2$ in the presence of hyperbilirubinemia (bilirubin up to 46.3 mg/dL) suggested that high bilirubin levels do not interfere with the accuracy of SpO$_2$ when saturation is above 90% (Nitzan et al., 2014) Reduced at low saturations in individuals with highly pigmented skin, with errors up to 10% (Feiner et al., 2007)
	Use of systemic dyes	Indigo carmine, indocyanine green, and methylene blue absorb light at wavelengths similar to those used by the pulse oximeter (660 nm) and alter the accuracy of SpO$_2$ values
	Hyperlipidemia	From endogenous lipids or administration of exogenous lipid solutions, in conjunction with total parenteral nutrition, may produce an artificially lower SpO$_2$ value
	Artificial nails	Fingernail polish does not influence the accuracy of SpO$_2$. Use of artificial nails may reduce the transmission of light and influence the measures made (Rodden et al., 2007)
Technical factors	Motion artifact	May be interpreted by the photodetector as arterial pulsation
	Ambient light	High-intensity, high-quantity ambient light like heat lamps, surgical lights, and fluorescent lights may reduce the accuracy of SpO$_2$ values, as ambient light may be detected by the pulse-oximetry photodetector. Photodetector receives information from both the LEDs and the ambient light source; SpO$_2$ value is then a composite value and is likely inaccurate
	Optical shunt	Some of the light from the LEDs is transmitted to the photodetector without passing through a pulsatile vascular bed; degree of red and infrared light received by the photodetector is again a composite of light exposed to hemoglobin and light not exposed to pulsatile blood

(continued)

TABLE 13.2 Clinical and Technical Factors That Reduce the Accuracy of SpO$_2$ Values (*continued*)

CATEGORY	FACTOR	CLINICAL SITUATION
	Optical cross-talk	Sensor placed in proximity to another instrument also using red and/or infrared light; light emitted by the secondary instrument received by the pulse-oximetry photodetector will result in a composite value for the SpO$_2$
	Excessive signal noise/electrical interference	Impedes signal acquisition; signal processing may be disrupted with resultant delayed values that may be inaccurate

ear, and nose). The development of motion artifact appears to be the primary influence on the reliability of pulse-oximetry measures. However, other threats to accuracy also influence the reliability of this type of measurement.

Guidelines to Increase the Utility of Pulse Oximetry for Research Purposes

If SpO$_2$ values are used as research data, the investigator must ensure that these data are valid, precise, and reliable. Milner and Mathews (2012) evaluated 847 pulse-oximeter sensors used in 27 hospitals, and found that 11% of these contained electrical malfunctions that reduced accuracy, 23% of the oximeters emitted light spectra different from that reported by the manufacturer, and 31% of the oximeters were not functioning as expected. None of the inpatient facilities had a procedure or the equipment available for evaluation and calibration of these oximeters. Dugani et al. (2011) found that the use of an oximeter tester could identify faulty electronics and demonstrate the degree of error in SpO$_2$ measurements, but only 65% of biomedical engineers responding to a survey self-reported accuracy testing of pulse oximeters in their facility. These data indicate that the accuracy of clinical values of SpO$_2$ may be questionable in many facilities. The following guidelines improve the likelihood that the acquired SpO$_2$ data will be useful.

- Select a pulse oximeter with indicators of pulsatile signal strength and ability to observe a pulse waveform to ensure that adequate, appropriate signal quality is available.

- Ensure that probe type, size, and position are optimal to detect arterial pulsation without technical interference from ambient light, optical shunt, or cross-talk.

- Assess the association between the apical heart rate and the heart rate detected by the pulse oximeter. These values should be the same.

- Evaluate the individual for the presence of dysfunctional hemoglobin, hyperbilirubinemia, hyperlipidemia, and anemia prior to data collection to ensure that these factors do not influence SpO$_2$.

- Stabilize the probe so that motion artifact is not a significant confounding factor.

- Analyze the relationship between SpO$_2$ and SaO$_2$ obtained by CO-oximetry regularly. These values should be highly correlated with minimal bias and precision. Calculate the bias and precision to evaluate the accuracy and repeatability of the data.

- Perform instrument calibration and accuracy testing prior to each experimental use of the biomedical instrument, and evaluate the equipment using a known standard concentration.

Physiologic Measurement in Community Settings Used for Research

Until recently the use of biomedical instruments for clinical care and research were confined to clinical and laboratory settings. Currently, biomedical activity monitoring devices are widely marketed to individuals in the community as a strategy to improve overall health through regular measurement of daily activity and fitness. These devices are one component of self-care and a support for behavior change, as they provide rapid feedback to the user, and may be useful in evaluation of specific goals. These are easy to use, interface with smartphones or other electronic devices, and readily track activity and other measures like heart rate, oxygen saturation and sleep using technology. This technology may provide useful data for clinicians and researchers. However, as with all biomedical devices, it is necessary to evaluate the appropriateness, validity, accuracy, and reliability of these devices before collection of data.

Activity monitoring devices may measure a number of variables that include heart rate, steps taken, distance traveled, minutes of activity, activity level (light, moderate, vigorous), expected calories expended during activity, oxygen saturation, and estimates of sleep time. More advanced activity models may be global positioning system (GPS)-enabled for precise tracking of location and distance, and may evaluate activity by the hour, calculation of sedentary time for a specified period, and provision of reminders to move if sedentary time reaches a set threshold. Many activity monitors contain a three-way accelerometer, an altimeter, and a gyroscope. An accelerometer measures the magnitude of individual acceleration in one to three planes of movement; the altimeter measures the altitude of the individual and changes in altitude over time; while the gyroscope measures orientation and rotation of the individual during activity. Algorithms that use data from each of these technologies calculate activity frequency, extent of time of activity, estimate of the intensity of the activity and subsequent patterns of activity over time (Broderick et al., 2014). For activity devices that provide sleep measures, an actigraph is one component of the device. An actigraph detects movement and may provide an estimate of sleep time in individuals with normal sleep patterns. However, these devices do not evaluate sleep stages or quality of sleep, and sleep time is based only on lack of movement during a designated sleep period.

As with any biomedical device, demographic and clinical characteristics of the study participants will influence the choice of equipment. For example, a study of patients with heart failure may require cross-sectional measurement of heart rate, body weight, and activity level during the 24-hour period and could use a device that would evaluate activity frequency and degree of intensity, measure heart rate, and connect wirelessly to a smart bathroom scale to upload body weight data.

There are a number of activity devices that use photoplethysmography to measure heart rate. This technique requires an optical emitter that projects a minimum of two wavelengths of light into the skin, a digital signal processor that captures refracted light, an accelerometer to detect motion, and specific algorithms to take the data from the processor and the accelerometer and calculate a motion-tolerant heart rate measurement (Carpenter & Frontera, 2016). The inclusion of activity detected by the accelerometer is vital to the accuracy of these algorithms, as activity increases motion artifact in the signal, which reduces the accuracy of the measure. There are a number of clinical and device characteristics that may reduce the accuracy of the heart rate data captured; these include skin pigmentation, presence of tattoos or the use of henna, skin temperature, severe peripheral vascular disease, hypotension, dysrhythmias, and variations in skin pressure where the sensor is placed. These characteristics may result in inaccurate heart rate calculations. Poor adherence to self-monitoring behaviors may also result in extended periods of missing data (Chung et al., 2017).

Before the data collected by these devices is included in research studies or used to guide clinical care, it is vital to evaluate the validity, accuracy, and reliability of these devices. Heart rate measures with these devices have demonstrated fair to poor accuracy when compared to gold standard measures with mean absolute percentage of error of 9.17% ± 10.9% for an activity monitor compared with a gold standard measure (Lee et al., 2016). In older adults, the pace and speed of ambulation is often slower and may require the use of assistive devices. Unfortunately, most activity detection devices are not able to sense this, which results in increased error in calculations of movement and distance. Floegel et al. (2017) evaluated accuracy of four activity monitors in impaired and non-impaired older adults, and found that the number of directly observed steps taken were underestimated by 2.6% to 26.9%, and in impaired older adults, steps were underestimated by 1.7% to 16.3%. In those older adults using a cane or walker, directly observed steps were underestimated by 1.3% to more than 11.5%. Leininger et al. (2016) compared one commercial activity monitor to a research grade actigraph and found that the commercial device significantly overestimated the number of steps taken, and did not accurately discriminate between light and vigorous physical activity. Byun et al. (2016) identified a mean absolute percentage of error of 9.2% for sedentary time, 70.1% for moderate to vigorous activity, and 14.5% for total physical activity for an activity monitor compared with a research grade actigraph in healthy preschoolers. Thus, a high degree of error is common currently in many of these commercial devices.

Although commercial activity monitors have become ubiquitous over the past decade, their accuracy, precision, and reliability have not been clearly demonstrated by rigorous study. These evaluations are required before the data from these devices can be useful in research and clinical care. However, early research findings supported the use of consumer-based activity monitors because of their positive effects on self-monitoring behaviors, and their utility to support lifestyle changes and improve health (Chung et al., 2017). With improved technology and rigorous evaluation of the accuracy, precision, and reliability, these devices may provide important data for investigators in the future, and they clearly may be useful adjuncts to interventions to support behavior changes.

▪ SUMMARY

When evaluating and critiquing the appropriateness of research studies to implement EBP in the clinical setting, knowledge about biomedical instrumentation is essential to determine the validity, accuracy, and reliability of the physiological data acquired for those studies and to determine the degree of certainty about the findings. Consideration must be given to the ability of any biomedical instrument to provide valid, precise, and reliable data to ensure that the conclusions derived from research studies are from rigorous measures, and are meaningful and useful.

▪ PSYCHOSOCIAL DATA COLLECTION METHODS

Psychosocial measures are instruments that researchers and advanced practice registered nurses (APRNs) use to measure variables related to psychological, emotional, behavioral, and related areas in a study. In general, instruments focus on certain topics or content domains such as depression or anxiety. Psychosocial data collection methods are important to guide the use of evidence in nursing practice. They are often used for approved research studies; however, increasingly, these tools are used to evaluate patients clinically or to assess treatment response.

Where do the instruments exist, and how does a researcher or APRN locate them? One place to start is with other established researchers in the field. Another source is relevant articles located and reviewed in preparation for the study. An examination of the methods and instruments section of earlier studies often gives a detailed account of which measures were used and some of their key characteristics. Since most published manuscripts do not include the actual scales, the reference list should contain a citation for the original instrument. Permission to use a new or original scale may have to be requested from the author(s). Libraries and internet sources also contain compilations of standardized instruments that can be obtained by searching for key words that reflect the concept under study. Finally, databases and websites such as the Patient Reported Outcome Measurement Information System (PROMIS; www.nia.nih.gov/research/resource/patient-reported-outcomes-measurement-information-system-promis) can be accessed for potential instruments for clinical practice and research on patient reported outcomes (PROs).

There are also books that include primarily tools for measuring concepts (Frank-Stromborg & Olsen, 2004). Some instruments are copyrighted and can be purchased for a fee. The fee may be a one-time purchase fee or a per-copy or per-use fee. To purchase some instruments, one may need to have certain credentials, such as a PhD. A variety of well-established scales of different types exist to measure concepts such as depression and anxiety and to answer different research questions. These concepts may be measured using interviews, whether structured or semi-structured, or questionnaires that are administered by the researcher and/or completed by the participant. Other methods, such as observation and checklists, may be used along with standardized tests to collect data on behaviors in order to validate observations. For example, a study that examines the sleep of hospitalized cancer patients may include nursing observations and an established patient self-report scale.

■ SELECTION OF INSTRUMENTS

The selection of a measurement tool for psychosocial variables depends upon the research question, variables of interest, ages of participants, and other factors. A general rule is that the research question dictates the broader method to be used, whether qualitative, quantitative, or mixed method. Having a research question and key variables that are well defined helps to direct the selection of a method. Before considering various established instruments, the researcher should think about several important questions, including the study purpose, characteristics of the sample, the concept or content to be measured, and practical considerations. In order for the measure to be suitable, it should have established *reliability* and *validity* (Box 13.1).

■ INSTRUMENT DEVELOPMENT

Occasionally, an investigator who is interested in a certain concept or area of study may find that there are no available scales or instruments that reflect that specific research problem. Creating new scales or questionnaires can be tempting; however, their development requires a deliberate and systematic approach. Beginning researchers may think it is a simple process to create a new scale for psychosocial variables; however, there are several steps involved. An initial step is often to bring together a group of experts in the field; these may be patients who experience a certain

---

BOX 13.1 Factors to Consider When Selecting an Instrument

Does the instrument measure the concept being examined?
What are the psychometric properties of the instrument?
Reliability
    Stability
    Equivalence
    Homogeneity
Validity
    Content validity
    Criterion-related validity
    Construct validity
Is the instrument feasible?
    Instrument availability
    Costs of data-collection tools
    Nature of the study sample

Source: From Mateo, M. A., & Kirchhoff, K. T. (1999). *Using and conducting nursing research in the clinical setting* (p. 263). W. B. Saunders.

---

diagnosis or response to a problem, or experienced nurses who know the topic well and can serve as content experts. For example, a nurse researcher interested in immigrant mothers' health practices with their children may bring together six or eight representative mothers to generate potential items for a questionnaire during a meeting that lasts from 1 to 2 hours. Next, content experts should review the draft questions, which should also be pretested, revised, and tested for validity and reliability. Overall, the creation of a new instrument requires extensive time and effort, but is appropriate when existing measures are unavailable or inadequate for the purpose. It is generally more feasible to use existing scales. Then results can be compared across samples.

Reliability and Validity

Reliability and *validity* are two important and essential concepts that relate to each potential instrument that the investigator is considering. They have specific definitions in research and can be easily confused. *Validity* refers to whether the instrument actually measures what it is supposed to measure. For example, if the nurse is interested in measuring acute stress, the instrument should measure the concept of stress and not related ones, such as anxiety or depression. There are different types of validity, detailed later in this chapter. *Reliability* refers to whether the tool conveys consistent and reproducible data, for example, from one participant to another or from one point in time to another. Several types of reliabilities exist as well. For a scale to be valid, it must be reliable.

Validity

Validity is the degree to which a tool measures what it is supposed to measure (Mateo & Kirchhoff, 1999). There are three types of validity: content, criterion-related, and construct.

Content validity relates to an instrument's adequacy in covering all concepts pertaining to the phenomenon being studied. If the purpose of the tool is to learn whether the patient is anxious before taking an examination, the questions should include a list of behaviors that anxious people report when they are experiencing anxiety. Content experts are vital in the development of valid and reliable tools (Mateo & Kirchhoff, 1999). Generally, "content experts," colleagues with expertise and experience in the area, are identified. Ways to identify experts include publications in refereed journals, research in the phenomenon of interest, clinical expertise, and familiarity with the dimensions being measured. It is important that an instrument be reviewed for content by persons who possess characteristics and experiences similar to those of the participants in a study.

Criterion-related validity, which can be either predictive or concurrent, measures the extent to which a tool is related to other criteria (Mateo & Kirchhoff, 1999). Predictive validity is the adequacy of the tool to estimate the individual performance or behavior in the future. For example, if a tool is developed to measure clinical competence of nurses, persons who respond to the tool can be followed over time to see if this score correlates with other measures of competence, such as performance appraisals, commendations, or other indications of competence. If results indicate that there is a high coefficient correlation (0.90), it means that the clinical competence scale can be used to predict future performance appraisals. Concurrent validity is the ability of a tool to compare the respondent's status at a given time to a criterion (Mateo & Kirchhoff, 1999). For example, when a patient is asked to complete a questionnaire to determine the presence of anxiety, results of the test can be compared to the same patient's ratings on an established measure of anxiety administered at the same time.

Construct validity is concerned with the ability of the instrument to adequately measure the underlying concept (Mateo & Kirchhoff, 1999). With this type of validity, the researcher's concern relates to whether the scores represent the degree to which a person possesses a trait. Since construct validity is a judgment based on a number of studies, it takes time to establish this type of validity. These studies compare results in groups that should be similar (convergent validity) or different (divergent validity). Scores on the anxiety tool should be lower among those who are receiving a massage and higher among those taking a final exam.

Reliability

Reliability is a basic characteristic of an instrument when it is used for collecting accurate, stable, and usable research data (Mateo & Kirchhoff, 1999). The reliability of a tool is the degree of consistency in scores achieved by subjects across repeated measurements. The comparison is usually reported as a *reliability coefficient*. The reliability coefficient is determined by the proportion of true variability (attributed to true differences among respondents) to the total obtained variability (attributed to the result of true differences among respondents and differences related to other factors). Reliability coefficients normally range between 0 and 1.00; the higher the value, the greater the reliability. In general, coefficients greater than 0.70 are considered appropriate; however, in some circumstances this will vary. The researcher takes a chance that data across repeated administrations will not be consistent when instruments with reliability estimates of 0.60 or lower are used (Mateo & Kirchhoff, 1999).

Three aspects should be considered when determining the reliability of instruments: (a) stability, (b) equivalence, and (c) homogeneity (Gray et al., 2017; Mateo & Kirchhoff, 1999). The *stability* of a tool refers to its ability to consistently measure the phenomenon being studied; this is determined through test–retest reliability. The tool is administered to the same persons on two separate occasions. Scores of the two sets of data are then compared, and the correlation is derived. The recommended interval between testing times is 2 to 4 weeks (Gray et al., 2017; Mateo & Kirchhoff, 1999). The time that must lapse between the two points of measurements is important; it should be long enough so that respondents do not remember their answers on the first test, yet not so long that change in the respondents can take place. Interpretation of the test–retest correlation coefficient should be done with caution, because it might not represent the stability of the instrument; rather, it might indicate that change has occurred in those being assessed. For example, change can occur among nurses being evaluated with regard to their attitudes toward work schedules; for instance, persons who responded to the first test may since have gained seniority and may now be working their preferred shifts. In this case, the second test might yield a more positive result, and the correlation coefficient obtained when the two sets of scores are compared would represent a change in the respondents rather than being an accurate measure of the stability of the tool (Mateo & Kirchhoff, 1999).

Equivalence should be determined when two versions of the same tool are used to measure a concept (alternative forms) or when two or more persons are asked to rate the same event or the behavior of another person (interrater reliability; Mateo & Kirchhoff, 1999). In alternative form reliability, two versions of the same instrument are developed and administered. The scores obtained from the two tools should be similar. It is helpful for the researcher to know whether a published instrument has alternate forms; when there are, a decision must be made about which form to use. For example, the Beck Depression Inventory (BDI) has a long and a short form (Beck & Steer, 1993). The researcher might decide to use the short form to test patients with short attention spans or low energy levels. Establishing interrater reliability is important when two or more observers are used for collecting data. Considerations relating to this type of reliability have already been discussed.

The *homogeneity* of an instrument is determined most commonly by calculating a Cronbach's α coefficient. This test is found in a number of statistical packages. This test is a way of determining whether each item on an instrument measures the same thing. Internal consistency reliability estimates are also calculated by using the Kuder–Richardson formula, described in measurement textbooks. When more than one concept is measured in an instrument, the Cronbach's α is computed on the subscales, rather than the whole scale. If the scale does not attempt to measure a single concept or has subscales that measure several concepts, this test is not useful.

▣ TYPES AND CHARACTERISTICS OF INSTRUMENTS

In general, there are several common types of measures or instruments available to measure the selected concept under investigation. Researchers use *semi-structured* or *structured* interviews with detailed questions that either guide (semi-structured) the interviewer or outline a specific set of questions. The principal investigator or study staff follows the order of questions during an interview with the participant. Another option is *self-report scales* that are given to the research subject to complete; examples include scales such as the BDI. Self-report instruments differ from clinician- and nurse-rated ones on the basis of who actually completes them. Other scales may contain *open-ended* or *closed questions*. Open-ended questions allow more exploration and the opportunity for freer responses, without restraint or limitation. For example, in qualitative research, the researcher frequently asks open-ended questions, such as "What is your experience with . . ." or "Tell me about. . . ." Open-ended responses allow participants to answer in their own words. Closed questions, while more common, direct respondents to choose an answer from a predetermined list of possible alternatives. As a result, the participants may be pointed in certain directions that may not be appropriate or that lack uniqueness. Many of the scales used in psychosocial research have *ordinal items*, with numbers assigned to different categories that reflect increasing order, such as 0 = none, 1 = slight, 2 = mild, 3 = moderate, 4 = severe.

Visual Analog Scales

The visual analog scale (VAS) uses a 100-mm line with "anchors" at either end to explore the participant's opinion about a specific concept along a continuum. Respondents place an X on the line to mark where they stand on the continuum. For example, questions on pain prompt the respondents to describe their experience of pain at the corresponding point on the line, which has anchors of "none" and "very much"; a mark made 80 mm from the end signifies that the person rates his or her pain as quite severe. Convenient and simple, a VAS is an attractive means of rating continuous measurement.

Whether structured, detailed, or open-ended, every scale has advantages as well as limitations. There are several things to consider for psychosocial tools. Many of the instruments result in a certain rating (e.g., a numerical score that indicates a moderate level of depression). These rating scales attempt to measure the underlying concept (depression) efficiently and comprehensively and to attach to it a number that then is interpreted to represent a certain range (a given score indicates a given level of depression). The researcher cannot assume that a certain score or level of score on an established scale indicates the presence of a disorder. For example, the researcher cannot assume that a total score on a depression scale means that the participant actually should be diagnosed with depression. Some people assume, incorrectly, that a scale score that results in a certain degree or severity of symptoms produces a diagnosis. These instruments are in reality only part of an evaluation for a disorder.

There are several general types of instruments that measure psychological symptoms or overall functioning. Each uses either *continuous* or *categorical* responses. Continuous variables or items usually have quantifiable intervals or values, such as weight or blood pressure. In general, categorical items contain forced and mutually exclusive choices, such as *strongly agree, agree, disagree, strongly disagree*, in contrast to continuous items, which literally contain a blended continuum of responses without specific choices. When there are two possible choices or values, such as gender, the categorical variable is termed *dichotomous*. For psychological or psychosocial ratings, the focus is generally on self-report (or parent report for children) or clinician-rated symptoms. While these scales are most typically used for research purposes, they can also be used in clinical situations to aid in diagnostic evaluation or to help to monitor treatment response or symptoms over time. The instruments focus on particular symptoms or concepts such as anxiety, depression, suicide ideation, mania, suicide risk, or attention problems. Examples of commonly used instruments, along with their purpose and a general overview of their characteristics, are described.

Clinical Global Impressions Scale

Clinical Global Impressions (CGI) is a categorical scale used for rating change from baseline over the duration of a clinical trial (Guy, 1976). The CGI consists of three global scales formatted for use with similar scoring. The scales assess global improvement, severity of illness, and efficacy index. Clinical Global Impressions-Improvement (CGI-I) is a clinician-administered scale commonly used in studies of adults and children to assess posttreatment ratings at the discretion of the researcher.

The CGI-I consists of one item ranked 0 to 7 that compares patient condition at admission to the project to the patient's condition at a later time (Guy, 1976). The seven levels of improvement include 0 = not assessed, 1 = very much improved, 2 = much improved, 3 = minimally improved, 4 = no change, 5 = minimally worse, 6 = much worse, and 7 = very much worse. They are most commonly rated by the clinician and the patient. Investigators looking for at least moderate improvement on a global generic scale usually expect an improvement score of 50% or more (Bobes, 1998).

Mini-Mental State Examination

Several versions of the Mini-Mental State Examination (MMSE) have been developed and used since its original development (Folstein et al., 1975). Widely used as a screening instrument for cognitive impairment, the MMSE is an easy tool to assess changes in cognitive function, often with older adults, and as a screening for dementia. This is a common instrument that nurses use to identify changes in mental status such as orientation, registration, attention and calculation, word recall, and language and visuospatial ability. It contains 11 questions and takes about 10 minutes to administer. The maximum score is 30; scores less than 24 may indicate cognitive impairment, while scores between 10 and 19 may reflect moderate levels of cognitive impairment. Educational level, age, and other factors may also influence the score. Similar to other available instruments, the MMSE is not a diagnostic tool for Alzheimer's disease or other forms of dementia and does not substitute for a mental status exam. Since its creation in 1975, the MMSE has been validated and extensively used in both clinical practice and research (Crum et al., 1993).

Since its introduction, the MMSE has been revised to address problematic items and adjust tasks to difficulty level. While raw scores remain the same, the most recent version, the MMSE-2: Standard Version, has comparable scores to the MMSE. In addition, there are two other versions: the MMSE-2: Brief Version, used for quick clinical or research screening, and the MMSE-2: Expanded Version that includes additional tasks related to memory and processing. The MMSE-2: Expanded Version is more sensitive to different dementia symptoms and aging effects. Versions are available in many different languages for application to different patient populations. The original MMSE is free; however, the current official versions are copyrighted and are purchased through Psychological Assessment Resources (PAR; www.parinc.com).

Brief Psychiatric Rating Scale

The Brief Psychiatric Rating Scale (BPRS) is one of the most frequently used clinician-rated measures. It has existed for more than 40 years (Overall & Gorham, 1962, 1976). It consists of 18 items rated on a 7-point severity scale and is used for general overall assessment of broad psychiatric symptoms. The BPRS takes about 20 minutes to complete. Its scoring results in an overall total score as well as scores on five major factors: anxious depression, thinking disturbance, withdrawal-retardation, hostile suspiciousness, and tension-excitement. More specific yet similar scales that measure positive and negative symptoms of major mental illnesses (such as the Positive and Negative Symptoms Scale [PANSS]) are derived partly from the BPRS and have well-established validity and reliability. Validity of the items and subscales separated three homogeneous psychiatric diagnoses in patients (Lachar et al., 2001). The ratings of each individual item were compared for different raters. Using large samples of psychiatric patients in multiple studies, individual BPRS item interrater reliability estimates ranged from 0.54 to 0.92 (median 0.785), with the majority of values (10–18) demonstrating very good agreement (greater than 0.74; Lachar et al., 2001). Interrater reliability rater agreement was $r = 0.57$ for total scores and ranged from $r = 0.60$ to 0.84 for the factor subscales.

CAGE Questionnaire

Alcohol and substance abuse are increasingly prevalent in traditional nursing settings and with younger populations, including college students. Screening for potential alcohol problems is important in all settings, particularly medical settings. Alcohol abuse and alcoholism may be hidden for years and thus nurses are in a prime position to detect potentially serious situations. A variety of instruments are available, but the CAGE is one short, simple, easy-to-use tool to assess patients upon admission or during treatment (Ewing, 1984). The CAGE detects alcohol problems over the course of a person's lifetime. It is easy to remember and has been shown to be effective in detecting a range of alcohol problems (Ewing, 1984). It includes four simple questions:

C   Have you ever felt you should cut down on your drinking?
A   Have people annoyed you by criticizing your drinking?
G   Have you ever felt bad or guilty about your drinking?
E   Eye opener: Have you ever had a drink first thing in the morning to steady your nerves or to get rid of a hangover?

Two positive answers indicate a positive test. Once detected on a screening tool such as this, a more complete evaluation is frequently recommended. Several hundred instruments also exist that delve into more information and can detect serious alcohol abuse or dependence, and can be found at www.niaaa.nih.gov/publications/protraining.htm.

Drug Abuse Screening Test

Abuse of illicit and prescription drugs is on the rise, with a concomitant increase in the prevalence of misuse and substance abuse disorders. Another salient issue is the rise of opioid and heroin abuse, leading to more stringent oversight measures in the prescription of controlled drugs (Dart et al., 2015). A key element to prevent and mitigate substance use is the assessment and identification of individuals at risk for substance abuse and dependence. There are many options available for screening and evaluation; one of the most common is the Drug Abuse Screening Test (DAST; Skinner, 1982), which has undergone various iterations, revision, and shortening. Condensed versions include the 20-item DAST and 10-item DAST, available at www.drugabuse.gov/sites/default/files/files/DAST-10.pdf.

The DAST-20 or DAST-10 may be used as either a self-report or in an interview format to provide a quick assessment of drug abuse problems. It should not be used if the APRN suspects that the patient is currently under the influence of or withdrawing from drugs. Typically, an introduction is used for administration of either test: "The following questions concern information about your potential involvement with drugs, not including alcoholic beverages" (Skinner, 1982). When using the DAST, "drug abuse" refers to either excess use of prescribed or over-the-counter medications, or nonmedical use of illicit drugs such as cannabis, solvents/glue, anxiolytics, cocaine, stimulants, hallucinogens, or narcotics.

There is both an adult and adolescent version of the DAST-20. The instrument contains questions that elicit information about using drugs for nonmedical reasons, the ability to stop use, withdrawal symptoms, blackouts, and other related behaviors such as feeling guilty about drug use. Scoring instructions are available at http://cde.drugabuse.gov/ instruments, and the total score is calculated. A score of 0 indicates no reported evidence of drug abuse. Increasing scores generally indicate higher levels of drug problems, with the maximum score (20 and 10, respectively, for DAST-20 and DAST-10) revealing significant problems. The authors suggest tentative guidelines for interpreting total scores on each of the DAST instruments, from low and intermediate, to substantial or severe. A DAST score over 5 suggests further evaluation and intervention, on an outpatient basis for patients at intermediate risk, or inpatient hospitalization or intensive treatment for those at substantial or severe risk.

Originally the DAST was modeled after the screening tool used for alcohol use/abuse, the MAST. Its psychometric properties were first explored with over 250 patients with drug/alcohol abuse (Skinner, 1982). Internal consistency revealed very good reliability estimates; $r = 0.92$. Similarly, a factor analysis of the 28 items revealed intercorrelations among the items and one dimension emerged. Variables associated with substance abuse such as frequency of drug use and psychopathology revealed concurrent validity, especially related to more frequent use of cannabis, barbiturates, and nonheroin opioids. Revision of the DAST led to shortening the instrument to 20 and 10 items (DAST-20, DAST-10). The 20-item DAST demonstrated very high reliability ($r = 0.99$) with the 28-item scale, as well as very high internal consistency ($\alpha = 0.95$). The 10-item DAST also demonstrated high correlations ($r = 0.98$) and internal consistency reliability ($\alpha = 0.92$ [total sample]; 74 [drug abuse subsample]) with the DAST-20. Thus, both brief screening instruments are valid and reliable tools for use in daily practice to evaluate and screen for substance misuse and abuse (Staley & el-Guebaly, 1990; Yudko et al., 2007). Including evaluation for drug use and potential abuse is important for holistic clinical care, and the DAST can be used for early identification as well as evaluating treatment efficacy.

Child Behavior Checklist

The Child Behavior Checklist (CBCL) is a 118-item standardized measure that rates general behavior for children ages 4 to 18 years, drawing on hundreds of studies of children (Achenbach, 1991). Parents (and/or guardians) complete questions about the child's social competence and behavioral or emotional problems, reflecting either the child's current behavior or behaviors that have occurred over the past 6 months. Items are rated from 0 to 2, with 0 = not true; 1 = somewhat or sometimes true; 2 = very true or often true. The 20 social competence items reflect the child's amount and quality of participation in sports, hobbies, games, activities, organizations, jobs and chores, friendships; how well the child gets along with others and plays and works by themself; and school performance (Achenbach, 1991). Two open-ended questions are included as well.

The CBCL has well-established reliability and construct validity. Intraclass correlations for individual items equal 0.90 "between item scores obtained from mothers filling out the CBCL at 1-week intervals, mothers and fathers filling out the CBCL on their clinically-referred children, and three different interviewers obtaining CBCLs from parents of demographically matched triads of children" (Achenbach, 1991). Good stability of the scale exists for both behavior problems and social competencies over time, with correlations of 0.84 and 0.97, respectively. Test–retest reliability of mothers' ratings is generally 0.89.

Modified Checklist for Autism in Toddlers, Revised

Autism and related developmental disorders are on the rise, estimated to affect more than 1% of children (Autism and Developmental Disabilities Monitoring Network Surveillance Year 2008 Principal Investigators; Centers for Disease Control and Prevention, 2012). Symptoms frequently begin early in childhood and persist into adulthood, leading to significant functional impairment. Thus, early identification is important to begin diagnostic assessment of young children who may have autism and begin early intensive intervention (Gura et al., 2011).

There are several instruments available to evaluate risk for Autism Spectrum Disorder (ASD). The M-CHAT-R is a screening tool that assesses risk for ASD in toddlers 16 and 30 months of age (Robins, Fein, & Barton, 1999). This 20-item tool takes only a few minutes to complete and asks the rater to indicate observations (yes or no) related to eye contact, unusual movements, play, and other age- and developmentally related behaviors. One item for example is, does the child point with one finger to ask for something or to show you something interesting? It can be administered by either APRNs, for example, during a well-child visit, or by parents to assess risk for ASD, and takes about 2 minutes to score. Scoring guidelines are available at mchatscreen.com, and children's scores fall into three categories of risk: low, medium, or high. The instrument tends to overestimate risk for autism-related conditions, leading to false positives. Since it is designed to assess potential risk, further follow-up is needed to make a diagnosis of ASD. Similar to other screening instruments, it is not used for diagnosis, but indicates the need for diagnostic evaluation and further follow-up, particularly for children who score in the high-risk category. It is designed to be used with the Modified Checklist for Autism in Toddlers, Revised, with Follow-Up (M-CHAT-R/F; Robins et al., 2009), a copyrighted tool, also available by download. Both instruments may be administered for clinical, research, or educational reasons, at no cost. If the tool is to be incorporated into the electronic medical record, permission needs to be requested from DianaLRobins@gmail.com. The format follows the questions of the first screening instrument, and only those items that the child failed need further evaluation with the M-CHAT-R/F.

Validity of the instrument was recently documented evaluating over 16,000 toddlers whose parents completed the M-CHAT-R during their well-childcare appointments (Robins et al., 2014). Those toddlers identified to be at risk then completed the follow-up M-CHAT-R/F. Children scoring over 2 initially and over 1 after follow-up had a 48% risk of being diagnosed with ASD (confidence interval [95% CI] 0.41–0.54) and a 95% risk of any developmental delay or concern (95% CI 0.92–0.98). Of clinical significance, earlier detection was evident; children who were identified in the study to be at risk were diagnosed 2 years younger than the national median age of diagnosis (Robins et al., 2014).

Hamilton Depression Rating Scale

For depression, there are several commonly used rating scales to measure symptoms and severity of depression. The Hamilton Depression Rating Scale (HDRS) consists of 17 or 21 items (Hamilton, 1967). It is the most widely used continuous measure to determine severity of depressive symptoms in adults and adolescents because of its comprehensive coverage of depressive symptoms. The HDRS is the standard depression outcome measure used in clinical trials presented to the U.S. Food and Drug Administration by pharmaceutical companies seeking approval of new drug applications and is the standard by which all other depression scales are measured. Although other depressive scales exist, including some developed and used for adults, the HDRS remains the most reliable and valid. The scale takes approximately 30 minutes to complete and score.

The scale contains items defined by anchor point descriptions that increase in intensity. The rater is instructed to begin each query with the first recommended depression symptom question. Raters consider intensity and frequency of symptoms when assigning values. Total possible scores range from 0 to 63. Ten of the 21 items are rated on a scale from 0 to 4, nine items are rated from 0 to 2, and two are rated from 0 to 3. Each item score is summed to calculate total HDRS scores. Since the test's development in the 1950s, total HDRS scores have demonstrated reliability and a high degree of concurrent and discriminant validity (Carroll et al., 1973).

Beck Depression Inventory

The Beck Depression Inventory (BDI; Beck & Steer, 1993; Beck et al., 1988) is a self-report depression severity scale, designed for individuals 13 years and older, that consists of 21 multiple-choice questions. It is one of the most commonly used scales in both the clinical and the research arenas. Participants are asked to rate their depressive symptoms and behaviors during the past week. The BDI assesses common symptoms of depression such as hopelessness, irritability, guilt, and self-harm, as well as physical symptoms such as fatigue, weight loss, and lack of interest in sex, with four possible forced-choice answers that range in intensity, such as:

(0) I do not feel sad.
(1) I feel sad.
(2) I am sad all the time and I can't snap out of it.
(3) I am so sad or unhappy that I can't stand it.

Values are assigned to each question and then totaled, and the total score is compared to validated scores to determine the severity of depression. Total scores between 0 and 9 indicate few to no depressive symptoms; between 10 and 18 indicate mild to moderate depression; between 19 and 29 indicate moderate to severe depression; and between 30 and 63 indicate severe depression (Beck & Steer, 1993; Beck et al., 1988). The BDI is a copyrighted scale. Therefore, the researcher needs to request permission and actually purchase the instrument for use.

Conners Rating Scale-Revised

The Conners Rating Scale-Revised (CRS-R) consists of several versions, with differing numbers of items, aimed specifically at parents, teachers, or adolescents, that allows them to rate childhood behaviors (Conners et al., 1998). The CRS-R is a means of standardized evaluation in children and adolescents ages 3 to 17 years for emotional, behavioral, and attentional symptoms, particularly Attention Deficit Hyperactivity Disorder. It takes up to 20 minutes to complete, depending on the version. A 10-item short version may be used to assess baseline severity of behavioral problems and to assess treatment response over time.

Short and long versions of the Conners Parent Rating Scales (CPRS), Conners Teacher Rating Scales (CTRS), and Conners Adolescent Self-Report Scales (CASS) exist; the longer versions are more comprehensive and provide a more thorough psychosocial evaluation. The parent version consists of either 80 or 27 items that focus on inattention, opposition, and hyperactive behaviors. The teacher versions, consisting of 87 or 27 items, cover similar domains. Age- and gender-based norms are available for comparison for each of the subscales and overall score.

Instruments for Measurement of Anxiety

For anxiety, there are several rating scales available. The most common tool is the Beck Anxiety Inventory (Beck, Epstein, et al., 1988) where 21 items are rated by the clinician. For children ages 6 to 19 years, the revised Children's Manifest Anxiety Scale consists of 37 items completed by the child (Reynolds & Richmond, 1994). Obsession symptoms or those that reflect Obsessive-Compulsive Disorder can be measured by the Yale-Brown Obsessive Compulsive Scale (Y-BOCS; Goodman et al., 1989). The adult version contains about 20 items rated by the clinician, while the child version (CY-BOCS), targeted at children aged 14 years, contains approximately 40 items (Scahill et al., 1997).

Pittsburgh Sleep Quality Index

Sleep is an important and essential life function and the effects of sleep deprivation and sleep disorders can have devastating consequences for individuals and society. Sleep plays a critical role in immune function, metabolism, attention, memory, learning, and other key health functions. The Pittsburgh Sleep Quality Index (PSQI) is a 19-item self-report instrument that evaluates sleep quality and disturbance over a 1-month period (Buysse et al., 1989). Simple and easy to use, the PSQI takes about 10 minutes to complete. These 19 items lead to 7 components including subjective sleep quality, sleep latency (or time to fall asleep), sleep duration, sleep efficiency, sleep disturbances, use of medication to sleep, and daytime dysfunction (Buysse et al., 1989). The tool includes questions about time to fall asleep, night-time waking, breathing/snoring, nightmares, daytime sleepiness, and fatigue. The tool also includes a section for the patient's bed partner or roommate to report on snoring, apneic events, and leg movements or restlessness. Total scores range from 0 to 21 points and include only the self-rated items. Scores range from 0 to 3 on each of the seven component scores. The global score is derived from the sum of the seven component items, ranging from 0 (no reported sleep difficulty) to 21, indicating severe sleep disturbance in all areas. Detailed scoring guidelines can be found in the original article (Buysse et al., 1989).

The PSQI is used for screening sleep problems and is also used to describe the nature of the sleep disturbance. The results may suggest the need for further evaluation of sleep dysfunction, including specific areas of disturbance, such as difficulty falling asleep or daytime somnolence. It can also be used for research purposes, to monitor the course of sleep disruption, or to assess the effects of treatment over time.

This instrument is copyrighted and owned by the University of Pittsburgh and may be reprinted without charge only for noncommercial research and educational purposes. The psychometric properties of the PSQI were assessed over 18 months with healthy controls, "good sleepers," and depressed and sleep-disordered patients, who were identified as poor sleepers. The seven component scores demonstrated a high degree of internal consistency, with an overall reliability coefficient (Cronbach's $\alpha = 0.83$), suggesting that they all reflected one measurement, sleep quality (Buysse et al., 1989). Similarly, individual items were strongly correlated with one another, and demonstrated the identical reliability coefficient ($\alpha = 0.83$). Validity was established comparing group differences in total scores by subject groups, with sleep and depressed subjects showing significantly higher scores, as predicted. Further evidence for the validity of this tool resulted from comparing PSQI estimates of sleep with polysomnography, especially on the component of sleep latency. Total scores on the PSQI over 5 led to diagnostic sensitivity of 90% and specificity of 87% ($\kappa = 0.75, p < .001$) in differentiating good versus poor sleepers (Buysse et al., 1989).

■ SUMMARY

Much of what nurses do as part of daily practice can be based on systematic research. Once the research question(s) are identified and the design elucidated, APRNs can focus on specific existing instruments that are valid and reliable to measure the concept of interest. Psychosocial data collection tools commonly address mood (e.g., depression, anxiety), behavior, general psychiatric or psychological symptoms, and measures of global impression. The APRN or researcher may complete some instruments, and the participant may complete others. Using appropriate tools to elicit psychological or behavioral content helps quantify and answer the question under investigation. Data derived using these methods can provide documentation to answer relevant clinical questions or test an intervention. As a result, the APRN can use evidence to direct and guide practice and contribute to knowledge development in a given domain.

SUGGESTED LEARNING ACTIVITIES

Physiological Measures

1. Select a research article in which biomedical instrumentation was used to collect physiological data. Review and critique the article. Evaluate whether the data collected using the instrumentation were valid, accurate, and reliable. Determine whether the results of the reviewed study are rigorous and appropriate to apply to further research studies and clinical practice.

2. Select a physiological variable, such as carbon dioxide. Search the literature to determine different methods to measure carbon dioxide, including measurement from blood (blood gases in vitro) or in vivo measures of tissue carbon dioxide ($TcPCO_2$) or exhaled carbon dioxide ($ETCO_2$). Design a study to measure carbon dioxide in a human research subject and provide the rationale for the choice on the basis of the method of measurement and human subject concerns (direct vs. indirect method and in vivo vs. in vitro method). Compare and contrast the validity, reliability, and accuracy of these methods.

Psychological Measures

1. Find a recent newspaper or internet article of interest that reports the results of a study. Go to the original source (peer-reviewed article) and examine which instruments were used. For example, did the authors develop a survey, or did they use an existing measurement tool? What was the underlying concept that was being measured?

2. Next, read the description of the instrument in the journal article. What key characteristics are outlined about the instrument? What types of reliability and validity were used, and what is your interpretation of them?

3. Select a concept related to your practice as a nurse/APRN. Using established procedures and references, find at least two relevant instruments that reflect the concept. If your search results in no appropriate tool, detail the next three steps to consider instrument development.

REFERENCES

Achenbach, T. M. (1991). *Integrative guide for the 1991 CBCL/4–18, YSR, and TRF profiles*. University of Vermont, Department of Psychiatry.

Autism and Developmental Disabilities Monitoring Network Surveillance Year 2008 Principal Investigators; Centers for Disease Control and Prevention. (2012). Prevalence of autism spectrum disorders—Autism and Developmental Disabilities Monitoring Network, 14 sites, United States, 2008. *MMWR Surveillance Summary, 61*(3), 1–19.

Avellan, S., Uhr, I., McKelvey, D., & Sondergaard, S. (2017). Identifying the position of the right atrium to align pressure transducer for CVP: Spirit level or 3D electromagnetic positioning? *Journal of Clinical Monitoring and Computing, 31*(5), 943–949. https://doi.org/10.1007/s10877-016-9918-5

Beck, A. T., Epstein, N., Brown, G., & Steer, R. A. (1988). An inventory for measuring clinical anxiety: Psychometric properties. *Journal of Consulting and Clinical Psychology, 56*(6), 893–897. https://doi.org/10.1037/0022-006X.56.6.893

Beck, A. T., & Steer, R. A. (1993). *Manual for the Beck Depression Inventory.* Psychological Corporation.

Beck, A. T., Steer, R. A., & Garbing, M. G. (1988). Psychometric properties of the Beck Depression Inventory: Twenty-five years of evaluation. *Clinical Psychology Review, 8,* 77–100. https://doi.org/10.1016/0272-7358(88)90050-5

Bobes, J. (1998). How is recovery from social anxiety disorder defined? *Journal of Clinical Psychiatry, 59*(Suppl. 17), 12–19.

Broderick, J. M., Ryan, J., O'Donnell, D. M., & Hussey, J. (2014). A guide to assessing physical activity using accelerometry in cancer patients. *Supportive Care in Cancer, 22*(4), 1121–1130. https://doi.org/10.1007/s00520-013-2102-2

Buysse, D. J., Reynolds, C. F., Monk, T. H., Berman, S. R., & Kupfer, D. J. (1989). The Pittsburgh Sleep Quality Index: A new instrument for psychiatric practice and research. *Psychiatry Research, 28*(2), 193–213. https://doi.org/10.1016/0165-1781(89)90047-4

Byun, W., Barry, A., & Lee, J. M. (2016). Accuracy of the Fitbit for measuring preschoolers' physical activity. *Medicine & Science in Sports & Exercise, 48*(5, Suppl. 1), 778. https://doi.org/10.1249/01.mss.0000487337.24755.a2

Carpenter, A., & Frontera, A. (2016). Smart-watches: A potential challenger to the implantable loop recorder? *Europace: European Pacing, Arrhythmias, and Cardiac Electrophysiology, 18*(6), 791–793. https://doi.org/10.1093/europace/euv427

Carroll, B. J., Fielding, J. M., & Blashki, T. G. (1973). Depression rating scales: A critical review. *Archives of General Psychiatry, 28*(3), 361–366. https://doi.org/10.1001/archpsyc.1973.01750330049009

Chung, A. E., Skinner, A. C., Hasty, S. E., & Perrin, E. M. (2017). Tweeting to health: A novel mHealth intervention using Fitbits and Twitter to foster healthy lifestyles. *Clinical Pediatrics, 56*(1), 26–32. https://doi.org/10.1177/0009922816653385

Conners, C. K., Sitarenios, G., Parker, J. D., & Epstein, J. N. (1998). The revised Conners' Parent Rating Scale (CPRS-R): Factor structure, reliability, and criterion validity. *Journal of Abnormal Child Psychology, 26*(4), 257–268. https://doi.org/10.1023/A:1022602400621

Crum, R. M., Anthony, J. C., Bassett, S. S., & Folstein, M. F. (1993). Population-based norms for the Mini-Mental State Examination by age and educational level. *Journal of the American Medical Association, 269*(18), 2386–2391. https://doi.org/10.1001/jama.1993.03500180078038

Dart, R. C., Surratt, H. L., Cicero, T. J., Parrino, M. W., Severtson, S. G., Bucher-Bartelson, B., & Green, J. L. (2015). Trends in opioid analgesic abuse and mortality in the United States. *New England Journal of Medicine, 372*(3), 241–248. https://doi.org/10.1056/NEJMsa1406143

Dugani, S., Hodzovic, I., Sindhakar, S., Nadra, A., Dunstan, C., Wilkes, A. R., & Mecklenburgh, J. (2011). Evaluation of a pulse oximeter sensor tester. *Journal of Clinical Monitoring and Computing, 25*(3), 163–170. https://doi.org/10.1007/s10877-011-9283-3

Enderle, J., & Bronzino, J. (2012). *Introduction to biomedical engineering* (3rd ed.). Elsevier.

Feiner, J. R., Severinghaus, J. W., & Bickler, P. E. (2007). Dark skin decreases the accuracy of pulse oximeters at low oxygen saturation: The effects of oximeter probe type and gender. *Anesthesia and Analgesia, 105*(6, Suppl.), S18–S23. https://doi.org/10.1213/01.ane.0000285988.35174.d9

Ewing, J. A. (1984). Detecting alcoholism. The CAGE questionnaire. *Journal of the American Medical Association, 252*(14), 1905–1907. https://doi.org/10.1001/jama.1984.03350140051025

Floegel, T. A., Florez-Pregonero, A., Hekler, E. B., & Buman, M. P. (2017). Validation of consumer-based hip and wrist activity monitors in older adults with varied ambulatory abilities. *The Journals of Gerontology, 72*(2), 229–236. https://doi.org/10.1093/gerona/glw098

Folstein, M. F., Folstein, S. E., & McHugh, P. R. (1975). "Mini-mental state." A practical method for grading the cognitive state of patients for the clinician. *Journal of Psychiatric Research, 12*(3), 189–198. https://doi.org/10.1016/0022-3956(75)90026-6

Frank-Stromborg, M., & Olsen, S. J. (2004). *Instruments for clinical health-care research* (3rd ed.). Jones & Bartlett.

Goodman, W. K., Price, L. H., Rasmussen, S. A., Mazure, C., Fleischmann, R. L., Hill, C. L., Heninger, G. R., & Charney, D. S. (1989). The Yale-Brown Obsessive Compulsive Scale. I. Development, use, and reliability. *Archives of General Psychiatry, 46*(11), 1006–1011. https://doi.org/10.1001/archpsyc.1989.01810110048007

Gray, J. R., Grove, S. K., & Sutherland, S. (2017). *The practice of nursing research: Appraisal, synthesis, and generation of evidence* (8th ed.). Elsevier.

Gura, G. F., Champagne, M. T., & Blood-Siegfried, J. E. (2011). Autism spectrum disorder screening in primary care. *Journal of Developmental and Behavioral Pediatrics, 32*(1), 48–51. https://doi.org/10.1097/DBP.0b013e3182040aea

Guy, W. (1976). *Clinical global impression: ECDEU assessment manual for psychopharmacology, revised.* National Institute of Mental Health.

Hamilton, M. (1967). Development of a rating scale for primary depressive illness. *British Journal of Social and Clinical Psychology, 6*(4), 278–296. https://doi.org/10.1111/j.2044-8260.1967.tb00530.x

Jacq, G., Gritti, K., Carré, C., Fleury, N., Lang, A., Courau-Courtois, J., Bedos, J-P., & Legriel, S. (2015). Modalities of invasive arterial pressure monitoring in critically ill patients: A prospective observational study. *Medicine, 94*(39), e1557. https://doi.org/10.1097/MD.0000000000001557

Kennedy, A., Finlay, D. D., Guldenring, D., Bond, R., Moran, K., & McLaughlin, J. (2016). The cardiac conduction system: Generation and conduction of the cardiac impulse. *Critical Care Nursing Clinics of North America, 28*(3), 269–279. https://doi.org/10.1016/j.cnc.2016.04.001

Lachar, D., Bailley, S. E., Rhoades, H. M., Espadas, A., Aponte, M., Cowan, K. A., Gummattira, P., Kopecky, C. P., & Wassef, A. (2001). New subscales for an anchored version of the Brief Psychiatric Rating Scale: Construction, reliability, and validity in acute psychiatric admissions. *Psychological Assessment, 13*(3), 384–395. https://doi.org/10.1037/1040-3590.13.3.384

Lee, J. M., An, H., Kang, S. K., Kim, Y., & Dinkel, D. (2016). Examining the validity of Fitbit Charge HR for measuring heart rate in free-living conditions. *Medicine & Science in Sports & Exercise, 48*(5, Suppl. 1), 786–787. https://doi.org/10.1249/01.mss.0000487361.48518.aa

Leininger, L. J., Cook, B. J., Jones, V., Bellumori, M., & Adams, K. I. (2016). Validation and accuracy of Fitbit Charge: A pilot study in a university worksite walking program. *Medicine & Science in Sports & Exercise, 48*(5, Suppl. 1), 96. https://doi.org/10.1249/01.mss.0000485293.86436.f1

Mateo, M. A., & Kirchhoff, K. T. (1999). *Using and conducting nursing research in the clinical setting* (p. 263). W. B. Saunders.

Milner, Q. J., & Mathews, G. R. (2012). An assessment of the accuracy of pulse oximeters. *Anaesthesia, 67*(4), 396–401. https://doi.org/10.1111/j.1365-2044.2011.07021.x

Muntner, P., Shimbo, D., Carey, R. M., Charleston, J. B., Gaillard, T., Misra, S., Myers, M. G., Ogedegbe, G., Schwartz, J. E., Townsend, R. R., Urbina, E. M., Viera, A. J., White, W. B., & Wright Jr, J. T. (2019). Measurement of blood pressure in humans: a scientific statement from the American Heart Association. *Hypertension, 73*(5), e35–e66. https://doi.org/10.1161/HYP.0000000000000087

Nitzan, M., Romem, A., & Koppel, R. (2014). Pulse oximetry: Fundamentals and technology update. *Medical Devices, 7*, 231–239. https://doi.org/10.2147/MDER.S47319

O'Brien, E. (2000). Replacing the mercury sphygmomanometer. Requires clinicians to demand better automated devices. *British Medical Journal (Clinical Research Edition), 320*(7238), 815–816. https://doi.org/10.1136/bmj.320.7238.815

Overall, J. L., & Gorham, D. R. (1962). The brief psychiatric rating scale. *Psychological Reports, 10*, 799–812. https://doi.org/10.2466/pr0.1962.10.3.799

Overall, J. L., & Gorham, D. R. (1976). The Brief Psychiatric Rating Scale. In W. Guy (Ed.), *ECDEU assessment manual for psychopharmacology* (pp. 157–160). U.S. Department of Health, Education and Welfare.

Ozone, S., Shaku, F., Sato, M., Takayashiki, A., Tsutsumi, M., & Maeno, T. (2016). Comparison of blood pressure measurements on the bare arm, over a sleeve and over a rolled-up sleeve in the elderly. *Family Practice, 33*(5), 517–522. https://doi.org/10.1093/fampra/cmw053

Perkins, G. D., McAuley, D. F., Giles, S., Routledge, H., & Gao, F. (2003). Do changes in pulse oximeter oxygen saturation predict equivalent changes in arterial oxygen saturation? *Critical Care, 7*(4), R67. https://doi.org/10.1186/cc2339

Pinar, R., Ataalkin, S., & Watson, R. (2010). The effect of clothes on sphygmomanometric blood pressure measurement in hypertensive patients. *Journal of Clinical Nursing, 19*(13–14), 1861–1864. https://doi.org/10.1111/j.1365-2702.2010.03224.x

Polit, D. F., & Hungler, B. P. (1987). *Nursing research: Principles and methods* (3rd ed.). Lippincott.

Reynolds, C. R., & Richmond, B. O. (1994). *Revised children's Manifest Anxiety Scale*. Western Psychological Services.

Robins, D. L., Casagrande, K., Barton, M., Chen, C. M., Dumont-Mathieu, T., & Fein, D. (2014). Validation of the Modified Checklist for Autism in Toddlers, Revised with Follow-up (M-CHAT-R/F). *Pediatrics, 133*(1), 37–45. https://doi.org/10.1542/peds.2013-1813

Robins, D. L., Fein, D., & Barton, M. L. (1999). *Modified Checklist for Autism in Toddlers (M-CHAT) follow-up interview.* Self-published.

Robins, D. L., Fein, D., & Barton, M. (2009). *The Modified Checklist for Autism in Toddlers (M-CHAT).* Self-published.

Rodden, A. M., Spicer, L., Diaz, V. A., & Steyer, T. E. (2007). Does fingernail polish affect pulse oximeter readings? *Intensive & Critical Care Nursing, 23*(1), 51–55. https://doi.org/10.1016/j.iccn.2006.08.006

Scahill, L., Riddle, M. A., McSwiggin-Hardin, M., Ort, S. I., King, R. A., Goodman, W. K., Cicchetti, D., & Leckman, J. F. (1997). Children's Yale-Brown Obsessive Compulsive Scale: Reliability and validity. *Journal of the American Academy of Child and Adolescent Psychiatry, 36*(6), 844–852. https://doi.org/10.1097/00004583-199706000-00023

Shamir, M. Y., Avramovich, A., & Smaka, T. (2012). The current status of continuous noninvasive measurement of total, carboxy, and methemoglobin concentration. *Anesthesia and Analgesia, 114*(5), 972–978. https://doi.org/10.1213/ANE.0b013e318233041a

Skinner, H. A. (1982). The Drug Abuse Screening Test. *Addictive Behaviors, 7*(4), 363–371. https://doi.org/10.1016/0306-4603(82)90005-3

Song, I. K., Park, H. S., Lee, J. H., Kim, E. H., Kim, H. S., Bahk, J. H., & Kim, J. T. (2016). Optimal level of the reference transducer for central venous pressure and pulmonary artery occlusion pressure monitoring in supine, prone and sitting position. *Journal of Clinical Monitoring and Computing, 31*(2), 381–386. https://doi.org/10.1007/s10877-016-9864-2

Staley, D., & el-Guebaly, N. (1990). Psychometric properties of the Drug Abuse Screening Test in a psychiatric patient population. *Addictive Behaviors, 15*(3), 257–264. https://doi.org/10.1016/0306-4603(90)90068-9

Thompson, H. J. (2011). *Care of the patient undergoing intracranial pressure monitoring/external ventricular drainage or lumbar drainage.* AACN.

Wilson, B. J., Cowan, H. J., Lord, J. A., Zuege, D. J., & Zygun, D. A. (2010). The accuracy of pulse oximetry in emergency department patients with severe sepsis and septic shock: A retrospective cohort study. *BMC Emergency Medicine, 10*, 9. https://doi.org/10.1186/1471-227X-10-9

Wohlfahrt, P., Cikova, R., Krajcoviechova, A., Sulc, P., Bruthans, J., Linhart, A., Filipovsky, J., Mayer, O., & Widimsky, J. (2019). Comparison of three office blood pressure measurement techniques and their effect on hypertension prevalence in the general population. *Journal of Hypertension, 38*(4), 656–662. https://doi.org/10.1097/HJH.0000000000002322

Yudko, E., Lozhkina, O., & Fouts, A. (2007). A comprehensive review of the psychometric properties of the Drug Abuse Screening Test. *Journal of Substance Abuse Treatment, 32*(2), 189–198. https://doi.org/10.1016/j.jsat.2006.08.002

Zaouter, C., & Zavorsky, G. S. (2012). The measurement of carboxyhemoglobin and methemoglobin using a non-invasive pulse CO-oximeter. *Respiratory Physiology & Neurobiology, 182*(2–3), 88–92. https://doi.org/10.1016/j.resp.2012.05.010

III

USING AVAILABLE EVIDENCE

14

LITERATURE REVIEWS

KATHLEEN R. STEVENS

▪ INTRODUCTION

Science is largely composed of two types of research: (a) primary research—original studies based on observation or experimentation; and (b) secondary research—reviews of published research that draw together the findings of two or more primary studies.

Once a number of studies on the same topic accumulate, the challenge becomes determining implications for clinical decision-making. In response to this challenge, health professionals and scientists have worked together to develop approaches that summarize research results into a single, clinically useful knowledge form, often called "*reviews.*" With the introduction of the *systematic review* in the mid 1990s by the Cochrane Collaboration, the general concept of a review has expanded and the terminology has grown broader and sometimes confounding. The shared goal of all reviews is similar to the traditional *review of literature*, meant to provide the scientific foundation for the "next step" in the use of the research evidence, either toward application in clinical practice or as the basis upon which to build the next research study. This chapter provides an overview of a number of types of *evidence summaries*, pointing to similarities in purpose, rigor, and clinical usefulness while providing examples.

The discussion explores the following types of reviews: systematic review, integrative review, qualitative review, scoping review, and narrative review. The discussion proceeds from those that produce the strongest level of evidence to guide clinical decisions to those that are less rigorous or are done for a different purpose.

▪ SYSTEMATIC REVIEWS

Systematic reviews (SRs) are widely accepted as the most reliable source of knowledge from research. The SR is regarded as the most rigorous and scientific way to summarize research evidence in evaluating healthcare interventions intended to prevent and treat illness. SRs can distinguish interventions that work from those that are ineffective, harmful, or wasteful and give reliable estimates about how well various care options work. SRs also identify gaps in knowledge requiring further research.

SRs are a type of research design within the larger field of the science of *research synthesis*. SRs emerged as an integral part of the evolution of evidence-based practice (EBP), and are considered foundational not only to effective clinical practice but also to further research. When done well, SRs are considered the highest level of evidence for clinical decision-making; that is, the SR indicates the likelihood that the clinical intervention will produce the intended clinical outcome. Systematic reviews of quantitative research results are central to the clinical decisions of those providing healthcare services. Systematically derived answers address questions such as: (a) Does this intervention work? (b) How accurate is this screening approach? SRs bring together all evidence to answer a specific review topic.

A primary value of SRs is that they generate new knowledge that is not otherwise apparent from examining the set of primary research studies. This summary is accomplished through the use of rigorous scientific methods, for example, meta-analysis. As in other research designs, the application of systematic research methods is central in constructing accurate, valid, and unbiased results.

The purpose of this section is to highlight the need for SRs in research; to introduce the methodology necessary to produce rigorous, credible conclusions; and to discuss who produces SRs, where SRs may be found, and the importance of critically appraising SRs.

■ DEFINITIONS OF SYSTEMATIC REVIEWS

The Cochrane Collaboration uses the following definition for SRs: "SRs are concise summaries of the best available evidence that seek to collate evidence that fits pre-specified eligibility criteria in order to answer a specific research question, and minimize bias, with systematic methods that are documented in advance" (Chandler et al., 2019, n.p.). SRs are further described as a "review of a clearly formulated question that uses systematic and explicit methods to identify, select, and critically appraise relevant research and to collect and analyze data from the studies that are included in the review; statistical methods (meta-analysis) may or may not be used to analyze and summarize the results of the included studies" (Higgins et al., 2019, n.p.).

In short, the SR is a type of evidence summary that uses a rigorous scientific approach to combine results from a body of primary research studies into a clinically meaningful whole (Stevens, 2015). It is essential to evaluate the methodological quality of the SR prior to moving the new evidence into clinical decision-making; reporting guidelines for such appraisals are discussed in this chapter.

As a scientific investigation, the SR focuses on a specific type of research question and uses explicit, transparent methods through each step of identifying, selecting, assessing, and summarizing individual research studies (Haynes et al., 2006; West et al., 2002). Essential aspects of each of these steps in the SR methodology are discussed in this chapter. It is crucial that SR investigative methods be preplanned, transparent, and replicable, as is true in other research designs. Reviews may or may not include a quantitative analysis of the results of selected studies to develop inferences (conclusions) about the population of interest (Institute of Medicine [IOM], 2008, 2011).

■ HIGHLIGHTS OF THE EVOLUTION OF SYSTEMATIC REVIEWS

Because of the relative nascence of SRs as a research design, the health science field uses multiple terms to refer to similar, sometimes overlapping, sometimes less rigorous approaches to summarizing the science on a given topic. These terms include *review* (used in the medical literature), *state-of-the-science review* (used in the nursing literature), and *review of literature* (traditionally used in research methods textbooks). There are, however, important distinctions to be made. Today, the SR is considered to be the most reliable information from research on the benefits and harms of specific interventions, actions, or strategies. All review types other than the SR are considered to be weaker forms of evidence and likely to provide biased conclusions about what works in clinical care. Even the traditional review of literature, performed to demonstrate a gap in knowledge, and therefore a need for a research study, has come under scrutiny for lack of rigor (IOM, 2011). Indeed, experts agree that two forms of knowledge point to "what works in healthcare," that is, systematic reviews and credible clinical practice guidelines (IOM, 2008, 2011).

A high level of scientific rigor in research synthesis is not yet reflected in all published SRs. In seminal research, Mulrow (1987) created a strong case for moving from the then loosely performed "review" in medicine to the more scientifically performed SR. Mulrow's assessment of 50 "reviews" published in the medical literature showed that the rigor of the reviews was woefully lacking and that, therefore, the conclusions were not trustworthy.

The distinction between SRs, traditional literature reviews, and other types of reviews discussed in this chapter is the strict scientific design that is employed in SRs. As in other research designs, if strict methods are not employed, then the conclusion is called into question for bias and accuracy. That is, the conclusion could be wrong about the efficacy of the intervention, either missing the impact or overestimating the impact on the health outcome. Because clinicians rely on SRs to summarize what is known about a clinical intervention, it is crucial that the results of reviews be highly reliable (IOM, 2011) before application in clinical decision-making. It is equally important to understand what is known before investing additional resources to conduct additional primary research—perhaps over questions for which the answers are already known.

Since Mulrow (1987), several other studies have appraised the quality of reviews in the medical literature. Kelly et al. (2001) conducted a study in which they assessed the quality of SRs in the emergency medicine literature. Likewise, Choi et al. (2001) conducted a critical appraisal of SRs in the anesthesia literature. Dixon et al. (2005) completed a critical appraisal study in which they evaluated meta-analyses in the surgical literature. In each case, the rigor of the published SRs was found to be lacking.

Stevens (2006) demonstrated that SRs published in the nursing literature also reflected a lack of rigor. In a study similar to that of Mulrow's (1987), SRs were located in nursing journals. Randomly selected articles classified in the Cumulative Index to Nursing and Allied Health Literature (CINAHL) of the publication type "systematic review" were evaluated using the Overview Quality Assessment Questionnaire (OQAQ; Oxman & Guyatt, 1991), a widely used critical appraisal instrument. This study showed that SRs are overclassified in CINAHL, with classification as SR occurring when the article did not specify that the SR methods were used. In addition, 90% of the SRs fell short of the expected level of rigor.

The poignant caution of an early EBP leader drives home the point of the need for rigorous SRs:

> More than a decade has passed since it was first shown that patients have been harmed by failure to prepare scientifically defensible reviews of existing research evidence. There are now many examples of the dangers of this continuing scientific sloppiness. Organizations and individuals concerned about improving the effectiveness and safety of healthcare now look to systematic reviews of research—not individual studies—to inform their judgments. (Chalmers, 2005)

Recognizing the poor state of rigor of SRs and the significance of "getting the evidence straight," the IOM (2008) assessed what is needed to move the synthesis of science forward. Their report acknowledged the great strides made in the new science of SRs. However, it called for more methodological research to produce better SRs. The report suggested that investing in the science of research synthesis will increase the quality and value of evidence in SRs. The IOM committee recommended establishment of EBPs for SRs (IOM, 2008, 2011).

A primary mover in the field of SRs, the Cochrane Collaboration (Clarke & Chalmers, 2018; Higgins et al., 2019) methodology workgroup continues to evolve methods for conducting SRs. Likewise, the IOM strongly urges continued development of methodological foundations and rigorous standards for SRs.

THE NEED FOR SYSTEMATIC REVIEWS

SRs are critical in assisting clinicians, patients, and policy makers to be able to keep up with the hundreds of thousands of new and often conflicting studies published every year. SRs offer a number of advantages to practice and in planning the next primary study. An SR distills a volume of data into a manageable form, clearly identifies cause-and-effect relationships, increases generalizability across settings and populations, reduces bias, resolves complexity and incongruence across single studies, increases rate of adoption of research into care, and offers a basis for ease of update as new evidence emerges (Mulrow, 1994). With such enduring advantages, the need for rigorous execution of SRs is clear.

SRs are a type of secondary research that follows highly rigorous and prescribed methods to produce an unbiased summary of what is known on a particular topic. In science, there is general agreement about a hierarchy of knowledge produced through various methods. In this hierarchy, the SR is considered the most robust, producing the most accurate view of objective truth. That is, SRs are deemed the most reliable form of research that provides conclusions about "what works" in healthcare to produce intended patient outcomes (IOM, 2008, 2011).

Moreover, given their value in determining the state of the science and the rigorous scientific standards now supporting the conduct of SRs, these reviews are considered a research design worthy of specific funding and support. This point was demonstrated in a study of the relative citation impact of study designs in the health sciences (Patsopoulos et al., 2005). The investigators compared the frequency of citation across a variety of research designs (SR, true experiment, cohort, case–control, case report, nonsystematic review, and decision analysis). Meta-analyses were cited significantly more often than all other designs after adjusting for year of publication, journal impact factor, and country of origin. When limited to studies that addressed treatment effects, meta-analyses received more citations than randomized trials (Patsopoulos et al., 2005).

The purpose of an SR is twofold: (a) to indicate what we know about the clinical effectiveness of a particular healthcare process; and (b) to identify gaps in what is known, pointing to a need for further research. So valuable is the SR in setting the stage for further research that leaders have recommended denial of funding of proposals that are not preceded by a SR on the topic (Chalmers, 2005).

Three of the most important reasons for conducting SRs are (a) to reduce the volume of literature that must guide clinical decisions, (b) to reduce bias arising from several sources, and (c) to provide a resolution among single primary studies that draw conflicting conclusions about whether an intervention is effective.

Reducing the Volume of Literature

An oft-cited benefit of a SR is that it reduces a number of single research studies into one, harmonious statement reflecting the state of the science on a given topic. Literally thousands of new health research studies are published weekly. In 2019, MEDLINE alone had 956,390 new citations (National Institutes of Health [NIH] National Library of Medicine [NLM], 2020); this represents over 2,600 new articles per day. Others suggest the doubling of global scientific output roughly every 9 years (Van Noorden, 2014). Individual readers are daunted by the challenge of reading and staying abreast of the published literature. The SR offers a solution in that it reduces the world's scientific literature to a readable summary of synthesized knowledge, ready for use in clinical care.

For example, to demonstrate the value of SRs in informing care, suppose a nursing practice council sets out to improve care with the goal of preventing falls in the elderly. The council chooses to develop an evidence-based approach and searches the literature. A CINAHL search on "falls prevention" yields 5,639 articles. Limiting the search to "research publications" reduces the list to 2,092 articles. Narrowing the search further to "systematic reviews" yields 168 articles and adding the population "elderly" produces one SR. The SRs range in rigor; however, one article on the subject (Gillespie et al., 2009) was published in the Cochrane Database of Systematic Reviews, ensuring that the synthesis was conducted in a highly systematic (scientific) way. This SR report notes that, after searching multiple bibliography databases and screening studies for relevance and quality, the authors included 62 trials involving 21,668 people in the SR (Gillespie et al., 2009). Upon synthesizing effects using meta-analysis, the researchers drew conclusions about interventions that are likely to be beneficial in reducing falls and interventions for which the effectiveness is unknown. Results are expressed in terms of relative risk and confidence intervals. An example of a beneficial intervention is expressed as follows. A significant pooled relative risk (0.86 with a 95% confidence interval of 0.76–0.98) from five studies representing 1,176 participants, suggests the clinical effectiveness of a multidisciplinary multifactorial risk screening and an intervention program for elders with a history of falling or those at high risk to reduce falls (Gillespie et al., 2009).

SRs consolidate research results from multiple studies on a given topic to increase the power of what we know about cause and effect, making an excellent foundation for clinical decision-making.

Avoiding Bias

The term *bias* refers to a deviation in accuracy of the conclusion of the summarized studies (Higgins et al., 2019). A SR reduces bias and provides a true representation of the scientifically produced knowledge. Common sources of bias in SRs are (a) an incomplete literature search, (b) biased selection of literature, and (c) exclusion of nonpublished literature. Conducting SRs according to a structured scientific approach ensures that a true representation of knowledge is presented.

Resolving Conflicting Results

Rapid growth in the number of healthcare studies has sharpened the need for SRs to assist clinicians, patients, and policy makers in sorting through the confusing and sometimes conflicting array of available evidence. Although one study may conclude that an intervention is effective, a second study may conclude that the intervention offers no advantage over the comparison. Nurses are cautioned that the simplistic approach of comparing the number of studies that favor an intervention to the number that does not will most likely lead to an erroneous conclusion about intervention efficacy. Instead, rigorous methods, such as SRs, are a superior approach to combining results across all studies to come to this conclusion of efficacy. Some studies have larger sample sizes or higher quality methodologies and therefore carry more weight. Some studies of poor quality may be excluded by using preset criteria.

The growth and maturation of methods and expertise for conducting and using SRs have increased the reliability of evidence for use in making healthcare decisions. It is crucial that nurses apply the accepted principles to conduct rigorous SRs and critically appraise those that are presented in the literature.

■ FUNDAMENTALS OF SYSTEMATIC REVIEWS

Whether they are serving as the lead investigator or as a member of an interprofessional team, nurses should have knowledge and skills related to SRs. Essential competencies for nurses include locating, critically appraising, and conducting SRs (Stevens, 2009).

Two of the primary organizations that have established guidelines for conducting SRs, include the Agency for Healthcare Research and Quality (AHRQ) and the Cochrane Collaboration. The process has been adapted and renamed by other organizations; however, there are commonly accepted principles for conducting a SR.

A rigorous SR includes a detailed description of the approach and parameters used to ensure completeness in identifying the available data, the rationale for study selection, the method of critical appraisal of the primary studies (evidence), and the method of analysis and interpretation. Documentation of each step is requisite and provides the necessary transparency so that the SR may be replicated. It is strongly suggested that persons well versed in SR methods be part of the research team for all SR studies.

The five basic steps listed here should be followed, and the key decisions that constitute each step of the review should be clearly documented (IOM, 2011):

Step 1: Formulate the research question.

Step 2: Construct an analytic (or logic) framework.

Step 3: Conduct a comprehensive search for evidence.

Step 4: Critically appraise the evidence.

Step 5: Synthesize the body of evidence.

Methodologically sound SRs are understood to include a clear basic and clinical hypothesis, a predefined protocol, designation of search strategies and bibliographic resources, a thorough search (regardless of publication status), transparent selection criteria, qualification of studies selected, synthesis of study data and information, relevant summary, and conclusion.

Step 1: Formulate the Research Question

Like other research designs, SRs use specific methods of inquiry to yield new and valid knowledge. The aim of an SR is to create a summary of scientific evidence related to the effects (outcome) produced by a specific action (intervention). Therefore, the research question used in a SR is designed in a very specific way. A well-formulated, clearly defined question lays the foundation for a rigorous SR. The question guides the analytic framework; the overall research design, including the search for evidence; decisions about types of evidence to be included; and critical appraisal of the relevant evidence from single research studies.

The SR research question must define a precise, unambiguous, answerable research question. The mnemonic PICO was devised (Richardson et al., 1995) to reflect the four key elements of the SR question:

1. Patient population
2. Intervention
3. Comparison
4. Outcome(s) of interest

The following is an example of a well-stated SR question used to guide a SR on the topic of "Interventions for Substance Use Disorders in Adolescents" (Steele et al., 2020):

> What are the effects of behavioral, pharmacologic, and combined interventions (I) compared with placebo (C) or no active treatment (C) for substance use disorders and problematic substance use in adolescents (P) to achieve abstinence, reduce quantity and frequency of use, improve functional outcomes, and reduce substance-related harms (O)? (Steele et al., 2020)

A second question on promoting smoking cessation during pregnancy, in which the comparison condition is implied, is as follows:

> What are the effects of smoking cessation programs (I) implemented during pregnancy on the health (O) of the fetus, infant, mother, and family (P)? (Lumley et al., 2004)

Note that, in this example, the implied comparison is the absence of smoking-cessation programs.

The population characteristics, such as age, gender, and comorbidities, usually vary across studies and are likely to be factors in the effect of an intervention. In addition, a given intervention may produce a number of outcomes of interest. The SR question is formulated so that it includes beneficial *and* adverse outcomes. For example, although prostate cancer treatment reduces mortality, the SR should also examine harmful effects of treatment such as urinary incontinence (IOM, 2008, 2011).

Depending on the specific SR question, different types of primary studies will be of interest. For example, questions about effectiveness of prescription drugs will generate searches for randomized controlled trials (RCTs). On the other hand, a question about the effects of illicit drug use will find no trials that assign one group to such drug use; in this case, the question will generate a search for observational studies that compare the health of otherwise similar groups of users and nonusers.

The SR question is typically formulated during initial literature searches and evolves as the SR team examines background literature. In addition, a broader group of stakeholders is often involved in question formulation. These may include policy makers, managers, health professionals, and consumers (AHRQ, 2005).

Step 2: Construct an Analytic (or Logic) Framework

After stating the SR question, the research team then constructs a framework. This framework maps the relations between the intervention and the outcomes of interest. In the case of the relations between screening and various outcomes as depicted in Figure 14.1, the analytic framework was developed by the U.S. Preventive Services Task Force (USPSTF) to depict causal pathways (USPSTF, 2020).

The analytic framework (Figure 14.1) demonstrates which factors are intermediate to the outcomes of interest and guides the construction of the search.

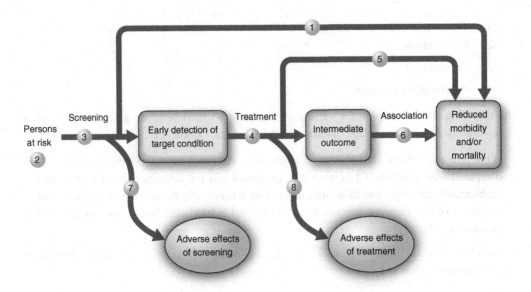

FIGURE 14.1 Generic analytic framework used by the U.S. Preventive Services Task Force for topics about health screening.

Source: From U.S. Preventive Service Task Force. (2020). *Procedure Manual.* https://www.uspreventiveservicestaskforce.org/uspstf/procedure-manual

Step 3: Conduct a Comprehensive Search for Evidence

The comprehensive search for evidence is the most important—and time-consuming—step in conducting a reliable and valid SR (Higgins et al., 2019). The search is crucial to identifying *all* relevant studies; in addition, search details must be documented so that the search can be replicated. The comprehensiveness of the search is what distinguishes a SR from a traditional narrative review (Moynihan, 2004). The question asked generates the specific search for evidence from original studies.

Constructing an adequate search strategy requires the skills of a librarian knowledgeable about EBP. The expert search strategy may consist of more than three pages of search terms, limited, for example, to human research, RCTs, the specific intervention, outcomes of interest, and multiple bibliographic databases. The world's literature is searched across databases such as CINAHL, MEDLINE, EMBASE, and others. Often, the initial search may yield 2,000 to 3,000 articles. In addition to these databases, other sources are searched, including review group registers (e.g., Cochrane Central Register of Controlled Trials Database), and hand searches of textbook bibliographies, citation indexes, and website resources are also conducted.

The inclusion of unpublished studies reduces publication bias. Because studies that find no effect are less likely to be published (Dickersin, 2005), reliance on published studies produces an overestimate of the effects of interventions. To minimize publication bias, it is important to find "fugitive" or "grey" literature—for example, conference proceedings and unpublished studies. Researchers often contact experts directly to locate research results and data sources that were not found in the literature.

Step 4: Critically Appraise the Evidence

Once located, studies are screened to ensure methodologic quality and to guard against selection bias. Studies are judged according to explicit criteria for design quality, strength of findings, and consistency with other studies in the set. Each study is examined to determine its applicability to the population and outcomes of interest and internal and external validity (AHRQ, 2005; Higgins et al., 2019; IOM, 2011).

Using specifically designed data collection forms, the research team extracts data from the studies that meet the quality criteria for inclusion. This abstraction process treats each study as a "subject" of the SR. The data extracted includes the effect size of the intervention on the outcome. To maintain rigor and reduce bias, at least two investigators independently extract data; if opinions about either quality or data extraction diverge, consensus is gained through discussion and/or third-party adjudication (Higgins et al., 2019).

Step 5: Synthesize the Body of Evidence

Summarizing Across Studies

SRs originally were developed to summarize quantitative research using statistical techniques. Summary approaches in synthesizing nonexperimental and qualitative research are also used. To synthesize a body of quantitative evidence, many SRs use meta-analyses. This is an approach that statistically combines results of separate original studies into a single result, originated by Glass (1976) and advanced by the Cochrane Collaboration and AHRQ as useful in SRs. The meta-analytic method provides a more precise estimate of the effect of the intervention than other methods such as vote counting, in which the number of positive studies is compared to the number of negative studies. Meta-analysis takes into account the weight of the effect of each individual study.

The results of a meta-analysis can be displayed in a forest plot (Figure 14.2). The plot provides a simple visual representation of the information from the individual studies that went into the meta-analysis. The graphical display conveys the strength of evidence in quantitative studies.

Forest plots are usually presented in two columns. The left column lists studies, and the right column is a plot of the measure of effect for each study. Effect estimates and confidence intervals for both individual studies and meta-analyses are displayed (Lewis & Clarke, 2001). Single-study estimates are represented by a square, the size of which reflects its weight in the meta-analysis. The confidence interval for that study is represented by a horizontal line extending on either side of the block. The length of the line is an indication of the width of the confidence interval around the result; the longer the line, the wider the confidence interval and the less precise the estimate of effect size. The meta-analyzed measure of effect (pooled result across all the included studies) is plotted as a diamond, with the lateral points reflecting the synthesized confidence interval (Higgins et al., 2019).

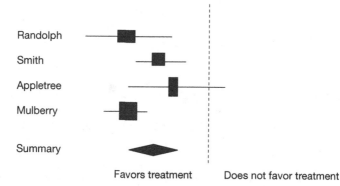

FIGURE 14.2 Example of a forest plot with four fictitious studies.

A vertical line is also plotted, representing "no effect." If the confidence interval line crosses the vertical line, it cannot be said that the result was different from no effect—that is, there was no statistically significant difference between intervention and comparison conditions. The same applies for the meta-analyzed measure of effect.

Analyzing Bias

Two primary types of bias can occur: bias in the individual studies that are incorporated into the SR and biases resulting from the selection of studies into the SR. To examine bias of individual studies, researchers use traditional design critique. Bias in study selection is examined using approaches that detect publication bias (studies that show an effect are more likely to be published), citation bias (studies that show an intervention effect are more often cited), language bias (large studies are typically published in English-language journals), and multiple publication bias (the same study results are sometimes published multiple times). All of these biases are in the same direction, indicating that the intervention was effective.

The funnel plot is the primary analytic technique employed to assess bias. The funnel plot detects publication bias by examining the range of effect sizes represented in the set of studies. If small studies are represented, then the funnel plot is asymmetric (AHRQ, 2005; Higgins et al., 2019). In the absence of bias, the funnel plot is symmetric, as represented in Figure 14.3. Note that the points in the figure form an upside-down funnel. Figure 14.4 depicts a funnel plot reflecting bias, probably arising from publication bias.

■ EVALUATING THE SYSTEMATIC REVIEW AS THE BASIS FOR CLINICAL DECISION-MAKING

SRs are critical in helping clinical and policy decision-makers interpret the state of knowledge from the large collection of studies around a topic. While an increasing number of SRs are being conducted, the usefulness of SRs is limited if the methodology is less than rigorous or flawed and if the reporting is incomplete. Examination of the current rigor of SRs to date shows that, while SRs are increasingly sought after, the quality of both the conduct and the reporting varies widely (Page et al., 2016). This provides misleading results that will misinform clinical decisions. If this

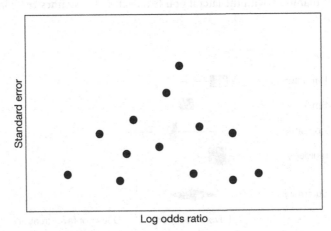

FIGURE 14.3 Funnel plot representing no bias.

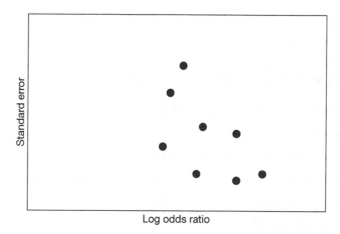

FIGURE 14.4 Funnel plot representing bias.

were the case, then clinicians should not accept the findings of SRs without critically appraising the rigor.

One solution is to use checklists to assess SRs found in the literature. Over the course of the past decade, specific evaluation approaches have been developed, such as the Preferred Reporting Items for Systematic Reviews and Meta-Analyses (PRISMA; Moher et al., 2009). PRISMA was developed on previous checklists and is the most widely used approach to ensuring adequate development of SR reports.

Another appraisal approach is especially useful when considering applying the synthesized evidence in clinical practice: This is the checklist produced by the Critical Appraisal Skills Programme (CASP, 2020; Exhibit 14.1). The CASP tool addresses three broad issues important in appraisal of SR: (a) Are the results valid? (b) What are the results? (c) Will the results benefit local care? This checklist will help distinguish among narrative reviews and SRs and will assess the quality and rigor of the SR methodology.

■ BEYOND THE SYSTEMATIC REVIEW

The variety of knowledge generated from primary research is valuable to clinical decision-making. SRs remain the "gold standard" for summarizing RCTs about intervention studies to inform clinical decisions about what works. However, other forms of evidence summaries have emerged to serve other purposes. Popular approaches to non-RCT bodies of evidence include the scoping review, narrative review, integrative review, and qualitative review (IOM, 2008). The underlying rationale for using one approach over the other largely depends on the nature of the body of literature and to some degree, the purpose of the review. Table 14.1 presents the definition and purpose, and an example for each of these types of reviews: Qualitative Review, Integrative Review, Scoping Review, and Narrative Review.

Because of their importance, the qualitative review and scoping review are further discussed below.

Qualitative Review. Nursing is rich with qualitative evidence; in tandem, approaches to synthesizing this type of evidence have emerged (e.g., Barnett-Page & Thomas, 2009). Although not a cause-and-effect conclusion, evidence summaries of qualitative research offer insights into the meaning of healthcare and patient preferences that are valuable in guiding clinical decisions. On a

---

EXHIBIT 14.1

CHECKLIST TO MAKE SENSE OF SYSTEMATIC REVIEWS

1. Did the review ask a clearly focused question?
2. Did the authors include the right type of papers?
3. Are all the important, relevant studies included?
4. Was enough done to assess the quality of the studies that were included?
5. If results were combined, was it reasonable to do so?
6. What are the overall results?
7. How precise are the results?
8. Can the results be applied to the local population?
9. Were all important outcomes considered?
10. Are benefits worth the harms and costs?

Sources: From Critical Appraisal Skills Programme. (2020). *CASP Checklists: 10 questions to help you make sense of a review*. Author. http://www.casp-uk.net

---

specific topic, a number of qualitative studies may provide a valuable array of evidence that could be summarized to inform practice (Sandelowski et al., 2007). The particular nature of a clinical question may lend itself to a systematic review that includes qualitative summaries.

Scoping Review. Another evidence summary approach is the scoping study. The scoping review is deemed most appropriate when there is a need to determine the gaps in science with

TABLE 14.1 Other Types of Reviews

REVIEW/KEY RESOURCE	DEFINITION/PURPOSE	EXAMPLE
Qualitative Review Sandelowski, M., Barroso, J., & Voils, C. I. (2007). Using qualitative metasummary to synthesize qualitative and quantitative descriptive findings. *Research in Nursing & Health, 30*(1), 99–111. https://doi.org/10.1002/nur.20176 Noyes, J., Booth, A., Cargo, M., Flemming, K., Harden, A., Harris, J., Garside, R., Hannes, K., Pantoja, T., & Thomas, J. (2019). Qualitative evidence. *Cochrane Handbook for Systematic Reviews of Interventions, 23*, 525–545. https://doi.org/10.1002/9781119536604.ch21	A qualitative metasummary is an approach to combine findings of qualitative studies. Qualitative findings are systematically collected and synthesized from topical or thematic surveys in the relevant literature.	Experiences of elderly patients regarding participation in their hospital discharge: A qualitative metasummary (Lilleheie et al., 2019)

(continued)

TABLE 14.1 Other Types of Reviews (*continued*)

REVIEW/KEY RESOURCE	DEFINITION/PURPOSE	EXAMPLE
Integrative Review Whittemore, R., & Knafl, K. (2005). The integrative review: Updated methodology. *Journal of Advanced Nursing, 52*(5), 546–553. https://doi.org/10.1111/j.1365-2648.2005.03621.x	A broad type of research review, allowing for simultaneous inclusion of experimental and non-experimental research. Integrative reviews have the potential to build nursing science, informing research, practice, and policy initiatives.	Respite care and stress among caregivers of children with autism spectrum disorder: An integrative review (Whitmore, 2016) TeamSTEPPS®: An evidence-based approach to reduce clinical errors threatening safety in outpatient settings: An integrative review (Parker et al., 2019)
Scoping Review Arksey, H., & O'Malley, L. (2005). Scoping studies: Towards a methodological framework. *International Journal of Social Research Methodology: Theory and Practice, 8*(1), 19–32. https://doi.org/10.1080/1364557032000119616 Munn, Z., Peters, M. D., Stern, C., Tufanaru, C., McArthur, A., & Aromataris, E. (2018). Systematic review or scoping review? Guidance for authors when choosing between a systematic or scoping review approach. *BMC Medical Research Methodology, 18*(1), 143. https://doi.org/10.1186/s12874-018-0611-x	Using a scoping framework, this review identifies the types of existing evidence on a topic, clarifies key concepts and definitions, and surveys designs used in the research topic. The purpose is to identify knowledge gaps on the particular topic.	Epidemiology, causes, clinical manifestation and diagnosis, prevention and control of coronavirus disease (COVID-19) during the early outbreak period: A scoping review. (Adhikari et al., 2020)
Narrative Review Ferrari, R. (2015). Writing narrative style literature reviews. *Medical Writing, 24*(4), 230–235. https://doi.org/10.1179/2047480615z.000000000329	Also called the traditional literature review, this is a non-systematic overview of current knowledge on a topic. Traditionally used to set the background discussion and context or establish a theoretical framework for a primary study. Because these reviews lack systematic rigor, the results are prone to bias. Narrative reviews are useful as novices become familiar with a problem of interest. However, contemporary thinking is that narrative reviews are always insufficient to identify knowledge for clinical decisions and to identify gaps for research studies. Rather research should be preceded with a systematic review to clearly point to gaps in knowledge. Narrative reviews are inappropriate to guide clinical decision-making.	Compassion fatigue in palliative care nursing: A concept analysis (Cross, 2019)

regard to setting a research agenda (Arksey & O'Malley, 2005). Scoping reviews play an important role in identifying what has already been discovered through other primary research and can provide a strong rationale for obtaining funding and resources to fill the knowledge gap. The use of scoping reviews has surged, and accompanying methods further developed (Munn et al., 2018).

■ SUMMARY

All systematically derived evidence has value for advancing the scientific foundations of nursing care. Evidence summaries transform the multitude of studies on a topic into a usable form for clinical decision-making. SRs put the "science" into reviews of literature. The rigorous approach used in producing SRs ensures that the synthesis of studies is valid, representing accuracy and truth. The IOM notes:

> Systematic reviews of evidence on the effectiveness of healthcare services provide a central link between the generation of research and clinical decision making. SR is itself a science and, in fact, is a new and dynamic science with evolving methods. (IOM, 2008, p. 108)

If nursing care is to be effective in producing intended outcomes, it must be based on rigorously conducted SRs. Clinicians must systematically appraise the rigor with which the evidence was summarized through a SR prior to applying the results. Nurse scientists make significant contributions to the evolution of methodologies that match the science of nursing. High priority is given to conducting quantitative and qualitative SRs and carefully employing the methodologies that guide these processes (Higgins et al., 2019; IOM, 2008, 2011) to transform research evidence into a useable form of knowledge. Nurse scientists, clinical scholars, and clinical experts are called on to engage in the conduct of SRs to guide clinical decision-making in nursing and healthcare.

SUGGESTED LEARNING ACTIVITIES

1. Visit the Cochrane Collaboration website at www.cochrane.org. Read the introduction.
   a. Search for "logo" in the website search box and read the explanation of the Cochrane Collaboration logo. The direct link is www.cochrane.org/about-us/difference-we-make#:~:text=We%20call%20this%20representation%20a,life%20of%20the%20newborn%20child. Does it represent a "count" or a meta-analysis?
   b. View the short video entitled, "What are Systematic Reviews" under "What We Do, Goal 1." What does the diamond in the logo represent?
2. Locate an SR in your topic of interest; use the CASP checklist to critically appraise the rigor and validity of the methodology available from www.casp-uk.net; summarize the practice implications for your local population of interest. Is the SR a convincing foundation for making practice change?
3. Visit the website for the AHRQ at www.ahrq.gov
   Go to effectivehealthcare.ahrq.gov/sites/default/files/pdf/health-careassociated-infections_research.pdf and read about Prevention of Healthcare Associated Infections. Read the structured abstract.
   a. What four infections were studied?
   b. What was shown to be effective and to what strength of evidence?

REFERENCES

Adhikari, S. P., Meng, S., Wu, Y. J., Mao, Y. P., Ye, R. X., Wang, Q. Z., Sun, C., Sylvia, S., Rozelle, S., Raat, H., & Zhou, H. (2020). Epidemiology, causes, clinical manifestation and diagnosis, prevention and control of coronavirus disease (COVID-19) during the early outbreak period: A scoping review. *Infectious Diseases of Poverty, 9*(1), 1–12. https://doi.org/10.1186/s40249-020-00646-x

Agency for Healthcare Research and Quality. (2005). *Evidence-based practice centers partner's guide.* Author.

Arksey, H., & O'Malley, L. (2005). Scoping studies: Towards a methodological framework. *International Journal of Social Research Methodology: Theory and Practice, 8*(1), 19–32. https://doi.org/10.1080/1364557032000119616

Barnett-Page, E., & Thomas, J. (2009). Methods for the synthesis of qualitative research: A critical review. *BMC Medical Research Methodology, 9*, 59. https://doi.org/10.1186/1471-2288-9-59

Chalmers, I. (2005). Academia's failure to support systematic reviews. *Lancet, 365*(9458), 469. https://doi.org/10.1016/S0140-6736(05)17854-4

Chandler, J., Cumpston, M., Thomas, J., Higgins, J. P. T., Deeks, J. J., & Clarke, M. J. (2019). Chapter I: Introduction. In: J. P. T. Higgins, J. Thomas, J. Chandler, M. Cumpston, T. Li, M. J. Page, & V. A. Welch (Eds.), *Cochrane handbook for systematic reviews of interventions* version 6.0. Cochrane, 2019. www.training.cochrane.org/handbook

Choi, P. T., Halpern, S. H., Malik, N., Jadad, A. R., Tramèr, M. R., & Walder, B. (2001). Examining the evidence in anesthesia literature: A critical appraisal of systematic reviews. *Anesthesia and Analgesia, 92*(3), 700–709. https://doi.org/10.1213/00000539-200103000-00029

Clarke, M., & Chalmers, I. (2018). Reflections on the history of systematic reviews. *BMJ Evidence-Based Medicine, 23*, 121–122. https://doi.org/10.1136/bmjebm-2018-110968

Critical Appraisal Skills Programme. (2020). *CASP Checklists: 10 questions to help you make sense of a review.* Author. http://www.casp-uk.net

Cross, L. A. (2019). Compassion fatigue in palliative care nursing: A concept analysis. *Journal of Hospice and Palliative Nursing, 21*(1), 21. https://doi.org/10.1097/NJH.0000000000000477

Dickersin, K. (2005). Publication bias: Recognizing the problem, understanding its origins and scope, and preventing harm. In H. Rothstein, A. Sutton, & M. Borenstein (Eds.), *Publication bias in meta-analysis: Prevention, assessment, and adjustments.* John Wiley.

Dixon, E., Hameed, M., Sutherland, F., Cook, D. J., & Doig, C. (2005). Evaluating meta-analyses in the general surgical literature: A critical appraisal. *Annals of Surgery, 241*(3), 450–459. https://doi.org/10.1097/01.sla.0000154258.30305.df

Ferrari, R. (2015). Writing narrative style literature reviews. *Medical Writing, 24*(4), 230–235. https://doi.org/10.1179/2047480615z.000000000329

Gillespie, L. D., Gillespie, W. J., Robertson, M. C., Lamb, S. E., Cumming, R. G., & Rowe, B. H. (2009). Interventions for preventing falls in elderly people. *Cochrane Database of Systematic Reviews, 4*, CD000340. https://doi.org/10.1002/14651858.CD007146.pub2

Glass, G. V. (1976). Primary, secondary and meta-analysis. *Educational Researcher, 5*(10), 3–8. https://doi.org/10.3102/0013189X005010003

Haynes, R. B., Sackett, D. L., Guyatt, G. H., & Tugwell, P. (2006). *Clinical epidemiology: How to do clinical practice research* (3rd ed.). Lippincott Williams & Wilkins.

Higgins, J. P., Thomas, J., Chandler, J., Cumpston, M., Li, T., Page, M. J., & Welch, V. A. (Eds.). (2019). *Cochrane handbook for systematic reviews of interventions.* John Wiley & Sons.

Institute of Medicine. (2008). *Knowing what works in health care.* National Academies of Science.

Institute of Medicine. (2011). *Finding what works in health care: Standards for systematic reviews.* National Academies Press (Committee on Standards for Systematic Reviews of Comparative Effective Research; Board on Health Care Services).

Kelly, K. D., Travers, A., Dorgan, M., Slater, L., & Rowe, B. H. (2001). Evaluating the quality of systematic reviews in the emergency medicine literature. *Annals of Emergency Medicine, 38*(5), 518–526. https://doi.org/10.1067/mem.2001.115881

Lewis, S., & Clarke, M. (2001). Forest plots: Trying to see the wood and the trees. *British Medical Journal (Clinical Research Edition), 322*(7300), 1479–1480. https://doi.org/10.1136/bmj.322.7300.1479

Lilleheie, I., Debesay, J., Bye, A., & Bergland, A. (2019). Experiences of elderly patients regarding partici-pation in their hospital discharge: a qualitative metasummary. *BMJ Open, 9*(11), e025789. https://doi.org/10.1136/bmjopen-2018-025789

Lumley, J., Oliver, S. S., Chamberlain, C., & Oakley, L. (2004). Interventions for promoting smok-ing cessation during pregnancy. *Cochrane Database of Systematic Reviews, 4*, CD001055. https://doi.org/10.1002/14651858.CD001055.pub2

Moher, D., Liberati, A., Tetzlaff, J., & Altman, D. G.; PRISMA Group. (2009). Preferred reporting items for systematic reviews and meta-analyses: The PRISMA statement. *Annals of Internal Medicine, 151*(4), 264–269, W64. https://doi.org/10.7326/0003-4819-151-4-200908180-00135

Moynihan, R. (2004). *Evaluating health services: A reporter covers the science of research synthesis.* Milbank Memorial Fund.

Mulrow, C. D. (1987). The medical review article: State of the science. *Annals of Internal Medicine, 106*(3), 485–488. https://doi.org/10.7326/0003-4819-106-3-485

Mulrow, C. D. (1994). Rationale for systematic reviews. *British Medical Journal (Clinical Research Edition), 309*(6954), 597–599. https://doi.org/10.1136/bmj.309.6954.597

Munn, Z., Peters, M. D., Stern, C., Tufanaru, C., McArthur, A., & Aromataris, E. (2018). Systematic review or scoping review? Guidance for authors when choosing between a systematic or scoping review approach. *BMC Medical Research Methodology, 18*(1), 143. https://doi.org/10.1186/s12874-018-0611-x

National Institutes of Health National Library of Medicine. (2020). *Citations added to Medline by Fiscal Year.* National Library of Medicine. https://www.nlm.nih.gov/bsd/stats/cit_added.html

Noyes, J., Booth, A., Cargo, M., Flemming, K., Harden, A., Harris, J., Garside, R., Hannes, K., Pantoja, T., & Thomas, J. (2019). Qualitative evidence. *Cochrane Handbook for Systematic Reviews of Interventions, 23*, 525–545. https://doi.org/10.1002/9781119536604.ch21

Oxman, A. D., & Guyatt, G. H. (1991). Validation of an index of the quality of review articles. *Journal of Clinical Epidemiology, 44*(11), 1271–1278. https://doi.org/10.1016/0895-4356(91)90160-B

Page, M. J., Shamseer, L., Altman, D. G., Tetzlaff, J., Sampson, M., Tricco, A. C., Catalá-López, F., Li, L., Reid, E. K., Sarkis-Onofre, R., & Moher, D. (2016). Epidemiology and reporting characteristics of systematic reviews of biomedical research: A cross-sectional study. *PLOS Medicine, 13*(5), e1002028. https://doi.org/10.1371/journal.pmed.1002028

Parker, A. L., Forsythe, L. L., & Kohlmorgen, I. K. (2019). TeamSTEPPS®: An evidence-based approach to reduce clinical errors threatening safety in outpatient settings: An integrative review. *Journal of Healthcare Risk Management, 38*(4), 19–31. https://doi.org/10.1002/jhrm.21352

Patsopoulos, N. A., Analatos, A. A., & Ioannidis, J. P. (2005). Relative citation impact of various study designs in the health sciences. *Journal of the American Medical Association, 293*(19), 2362–2366. https://doi.org/10.1001/jama.293.19.2362

Richardson, W. S., Wilson, M. C., Nishikawa, J., & Hayward, R. S. (1995). The well-built clinical question: A key to evidence-based decisions. *ACP Journal Club, 123*(3), A12–A13.

Sandelowski, M., Barroso, J., & Voils, C. I. (2007). Using qualitative metasummary to synthesize qual-itative and quantitative descriptive findings. *Research in Nursing & Health, 30*(1), 99–111. https://doi.org/10.1002/nur.20176

Steele, D. W., Becker, S. J., Danko, K. J., Balk, E. M., Saldanha, I. J., Adam, G. P., Bagley, S. M., Friedman, C., Spirito, A., Scott, K., Ntzani, E. E., Saeed, I., Smith, B., Popp, J., & Trikalinos, T. A. (2020). *Interventions for Substance Use Disorders in Adolescents: A Systematic Review. Review No. 225.* AHRQ Publication No. 20-EHC014. Agency for Healthcare Research and Quality.

Stevens, K. R. (2006). *Evaluation of systematic reviews in nursing literature. Proceedings of the Summer Institute on Evidence-Based Practice.* University of Texas Health Science Center.

Stevens, K. R. (2009). *Essential competencies for evidence-based practice in nursing* (2nd ed.). University of Texas Health Science Center.

Stevens, K. R. (2015). *Stevens star model of knowledge transformation.* The University of Texas Health Science Center at San Antonio. https://www.uthscsa.edu/academics/nursing/star-model

U.S. Preventive Service Task Force. (2020). *Procedure Manual.* https://www.uspreventiveservicestaskforce.org/uspstf/procedure-manual

Van Noorden, R. (2014). Global scientific output doubles every nine years. Blog. *Nature.* http://blogs.nature.com/news/2014/05/global-scientific-output-doubles-every-nine-years.html

West, S., King, V., Carey, T. S., Lohr, K. N., McKoy, N., Sutton, S. F., & Lux, L. (2002). Systems to rate the strength of scientific evidence. *Evidence Report/Technology Assessment, 47*, 1–11.

Whitmore, K. E. (2016). Respite care and stress among caregivers of children with autism spectrum disorder: An integrative review. *Journal of Pediatric Nursing, 31*(6), 630–652. https://doi.org/10.1016/j.pedn.2016.07.009

Whittemore, R., & Knafl, K. (2005). The integrative review: updated methodology. *Journal of Advanced Nursing, 52*(5), 546–553. https://doi.org/10.1111/j.1365-2648.2005.03621.x

PROGRAM EVALUATION

KAREN J. SAEWERT

▣ INTRODUCTION

This chapter provides basic knowledge about the process, principles, and steps of program evaluation and their application to healthcare practice, education, and research. Meaningful use of program evaluation to healthcare remains essential as economic resources for new clinical programs shrink and the viability and impact of existing programs are challenged. Program evaluation serves many purposes including program improvement; accountability and decision-making; judgments of merit, worth, and significance; and ultimately social welfare promotion and measurement of success, relevance, and sustainability (Ardisson et al., 2015; Gargani & Miller, 2016). Program evaluation studies use various frameworks and methods, but commonly share goals to analyze new or existing programs within a specific social context, produce information for evaluating the program's effectiveness, and use information to make decisions about program refinement, revision, and/or continuation.

▣ OVERVIEW AND PRINCIPLES OF PROGRAM EVALUATION

Program evaluation is defined as the systematic collection, analysis, and reporting of descriptive and judgmental information about the merit and worth of a program's goals, design, process, and outcomes in an effort to address improvement, accountability, and understanding of the phenomenon (Posavac & Carey, 2010; Stufflebeam & Shinkfield, 2007). As a broad concept, program evaluation includes a range of approaches (e.g., formative, summative) with similarities to continuous quality improvement viewed by some within a continuum of approaches to support organizations and program delivery, yet distinguished by the ultimate goal of determining program merit and worth (Donnelly et al., 2016). A distinctive feature of program evaluation is that it examines programs—a set of specific activities designed for an intended purpose that has quantitatively and/or qualitatively measurable goals and objectives. Because programs come in a variety of shapes and sizes, the models and methods for evaluating them are also varied (Stufflebeam & Shinkfield, 2007).

There is no clear consensus or agreement about the use of any one model in program evaluation. The choice of an approach to program evaluation is not so much a hunt for the perfect model as it is a reflective exercise through which the evaluator recognizes a model's inherent biases and decides on an appropriate combination of available approaches to supplement and ensure that all of the relevant elements of the evaluation are captured (Haji et al., 2013). Understanding the program that is being evaluated is an overriding principle in model selection. This encompasses the program context and history, the purpose of undertaking a program evaluation, and the time, expertise, and resources required for conducting a program evaluation (Billings, 2000;

Hackbarth & Gall, 2005; Posavac & Carey, 2010; Shadish et al., 1991; Spaulding, 2008; Stufflebeam & Shinkfield, 2007). Selection of an evaluation model should also consider the needs and interests of, and yield the most useful and organized information for, various stakeholders (Hackbarth & Gall, 2005). Table 15.1 provides an overview of eight program evaluation models.

TABLE 15.1 Selected Overview of Program Evaluation Models

MODEL	DESCRIPTION AND CONSIDERATIONS
Objective-based	• The predominant model used for program evaluation. Uses objectives written by the creators of the program and the evaluator. The emphasis of this approach is on the stated program goals and objectives that guide the evaluation data to be collected.
	• Focus on the goals and objectives should not neglect an examination of reasons the program succeeds or fails, additional desirable or untoward program effects, or whether the selected goals and objectives were best-suited for the key stakeholder audiences.
Goal-free	• Assumes that evaluators work more effectively if they do not know the goals of the program. Considerable effort is spent studying the program as administered (e.g., staff, clients, setting, records, etc.) to identify all program impacts (positive and negative). Program staff and funders decide whether evaluation findings demonstrate that the program meets the needs of the clients. • An expensive approach. Its open-ended nature may be perceived as threatening. Problematic for projects that receive funding and are required to conduct data collection and analysis for specific outcomes based on goals and objectives, that if excluded, may not be considered.
Expert-oriented	• Focus on the evaluator as a content expert who carefully examines a program to render a judgment about its quality. The evaluator judges a program or service on the basis of an established set of criteria as well as their own expertise. Decisions are based on quantitative as well as qualitative data.
	• This approach is frequently used when the entity being evaluated is large, complex, and unique. Involves program evaluator sent to the site by agencies that grant accreditation to institutions, programs, or services. Issues may include the specificity of criteria, interpretation of criteria by various experts, and the level of content expertise of the evaluator.
Naturalistic	• The evaluator becomes the data gatherer using a variety of direct observation and qualitative techniques to develop a deep, rich, and thorough understanding of the program (e.g., clients, social environment, setting, etc.). Direct observations by the evaluator are thought to be an advantage to construct the meaning of numerical information. • This approach generates lengthy reports because of the detail included.
Participative-oriented	• The evaluator invites stakeholders to participate actively in the program evaluation and gain skills from the experience (e.g., instrument development, data analysis, report findings). • This approach requires close contact with the stakeholders. Benefits may include a potential increase in the likelihood of stakeholders enacting recommendations and subsequently reducing the amount of time the process for improvement may take. Some argue that this approach compromises the validity of the evaluation.

(continued)

TABLE 15.1 Selected Overview of Program Evaluation Models (*continued*)

MODEL	DESCRIPTION AND CONSIDERATIONS
Improvement-focused	• Assumes an explicit assumption that program improvement is the focus of the evaluation. The evaluator helps program staff discover discrepancies between program objectives and the needs of the target population, between program implementation and program plans, and between expectations of the target population and the services actually delivered. • This approach tends to lead to an integrated understanding of the program and its effects. Quantitative and qualitative data are used to identify strengths of the program (merit and worth) and, conversely, the ways that the program may fall short of its goals and benefit from improvement.
Success case	• Detailed information is obtained from those who benefit most from the program. • This approach can lead program managers to tailor programs to those most likely to succeed rather than those most in need of the program when naively applied.
Theory-driven	• The evaluation is based on a careful description of the services to be offered in the program to participants, the way the program is expected to change the participants, and the specific outcomes to be achieved. Analysis consists of discovering the relationships among the participant characteristics and services, services and the immediate changes, and the immediate changes and outcome variables. • Qualitative understanding of the program that requires resources and expertise not available or funded may go unaddressed.

Standards of Program Evaluation

Program evaluations are expected to meet specific standards based on five fundamental concepts: *utility*, *feasibility*, *propriety*, *accuracy*, and *accountability*. Concepts and related standards of the original four categories of evaluation quality recommended by The Joint Committee on Standards for Educational Evaluation are central to the Centers for Disease Control and Prevention (CDC) framework (Stufflebeam & Shinkfield, 2007).

In brief, *utility* refers to the usefulness of an evaluation for those persons or groups involved with or responsible for implementing the program. Evaluators should ascertain the users' information needs and report the findings in a clear, concise, and timely manner. The general underlying principle of utility is that program evaluations should effectively address the information needs of clients and other audiences with a right to know and inform program improvement processes. If there is no prospect that the findings of a contemplated evaluation will be used, the evaluation should not be done.

Program evaluation should employ procedures that are *feasible*, parsimonious, and operable in the program's environment without disrupting or impairing the program. Feasibility also addresses the control of political forces that may impede or corrupt the evaluation. Feasibility standards require evaluations to be realistic, prudent, diplomatic, politically viable, frugal, and cost-effective.

Evaluations should meet conditions of *propriety*. They should be grounded in clear, written agreements that define the obligations of the evaluator and program client with regard to supporting and executing the evaluation and protecting the rights and dignity of all involved. In general, the propriety standards require that evaluations be conducted legally, ethically, and with due regard for the welfare of those involved in the evaluation and those affected by the results.

Accuracy includes standards that require evaluators to describe the program as it was planned and executed, present the program background and setting, and report valid and reliable findings. This fundamental concept and related standards require that evaluators obtain sound information, analyze it correctly, report justifiable conclusions, and note any pertinent caveats (Stufflebeam & Shinkfield, 2007).

Accountability includes standards that encourage adequate documentation and an internal and external meta-evaluative (evaluation of the evaluation) perspective focused on improvement and accountability for evaluation processes and products (Yarbrough et al., 2011).

Guiding Principles

In addition to these fundamental concepts and related standards of evaluation, the American Evaluation Association has set forth guiding principles for evaluators intended to guide the professional practice of evaluators and to inform evaluation clients and the general public about the principles they can expect to be upheld by professional evaluators (American Evaluation Association, n.d.). These principles—*systematic inquiry, competence, integrity and honesty, respect for people,* and *responsibilities for general and public welfare*—focus on the following areas and are fully detailed at the Association's website (www.eval.org/p/cm/ld/fid=51).

■ FORMATIVE AND SUMMATIVE EVALUATIONS

Formative and *summative* evaluations are common components of program evaluation. Experts note that the role of formative evaluation is to assist in developing and implementing programs, whereas summative evaluation is used to judge the value of the program. It is not the nature of the collected data that determines whether an evaluation is formative or summative but the purpose for which the data are used (Stufflebeam & Shinkfield, 2007). Data for summative and formative evaluations can be *qualitative* and/or *quantitative* in nature; the former is a nonnumerical (e.g., narrative and observation) approach (quality), whereas the latter is a numerical or statistical approach (quantity).

Formative Evaluation

Formative evaluations are used to assess, monitor, and report on the development and progress of implementing a program (Stetler et al., 2006; Stufflebeam & Shinkfield, 2007; Wyatt et al., 2008). This type of evaluation is directed at continuously improving operations and offers guidance to those who are responsible for ensuring the program's quality. A well-planned and executed formative evaluation helps ensure that the purpose of the program is well defined, its goals are realistic, and its variables of interest are measurable. In addition, a formative evaluation may focus on the proper training of staff who will be involved in the program implementation. During this evaluation phase, data are collected that serve to monitor the project's activities. The evaluator should interact closely with program staff, and the evaluation plan needs to be flexible and responsive to the development and implementation of the program.

Summative Evaluation

In contrast, a summative evaluation focuses on measuring the general effectiveness or success of the program by examining its outcomes. A summative evaluation addresses whether the program reached its intended goals, upheld its purpose, and produced unanticipated outcomes; it may also compare the effectiveness of the program with that of other, similar interventions (Posavac & Carey, 2010). This type of evaluation is meant to assess a program at its completion. Summative evaluation might be used to compare the effectiveness of the different treatment programs if more than one is implemented, or to make comparisons among members of the "treatment" group (e.g., those enrolled in a pulmonary rehabilitation program) and a natural comparison group (e.g., those not enrolled in a pulmonary rehabilitation program). Longitudinal comparisons may also be examined to determine the relative influence of the program at different stages. In other words, the summative evaluation seeks to determine the long-term and lasting effects on clients of having participated in the program (Posavac & Carey, 2010; Stufflebeam & Shinkfield, 2007).

▨ USE OF PROCESS AND OUTCOME DATA

Formative and summative evaluations can be further understood in terms of *process* (program implementation and progress) and *outcome* (program success). Process refers to *how* the program is run or *how* the program reaches its desired results. A formative evaluation is process focused and requires a detailed description of the operating structure required for a successful program. Outcome refers to the success of a program and the effects, including, but not limited to, cost and quality. Outcomes can be individualized to show the effects and determine the impact of the program on each program participant. Outcomes can also be program based to examine the success and determine the impact of the program on an organizational level. Program-based outcomes are often analyzed in terms of their fiscal impact or success through a comparison with similar programs.

▨ USE OF QUALITATIVE AND QUANTITATIVE DATA

Both *qualitative* and *quantitative* data are useful for program evaluation. Qualitative data, with a rich and narrative quality, provide an understanding of the impact of the program on individuals enrolled in the program. The descriptive nature of qualitative data allows one to understand the operating structure of a program and the individualized outcomes of a program. On the other hand, quantitative data, with their strictly numerical nature, allow a mathematical understanding of the factors involved in a program (e.g., statistical significance and power analysis). In addition, quantitative data provide descriptive analysis (e.g., frequency counts, means or averages) of the variables of interest. The statistical nature of quantitative data facilitates understanding of overall programmatic outcomes and makes possible direct comparisons among program participants and, if applicable, between program groups. Frequently, only one of these data types is used, neglecting the often beneficial and complementary provisions of the other. For qualitative data, direct observation and description are emphasized, as these lead to a form of discovery or an understanding of individual level impact of program factors. Qualitative methods may also provide insight into the context in which the program is delivered. Quantitative data tend to rely on standardized instrumentation and variable control and provide numerical figures that depict level of program success.

Triangulation is one way that both qualitative and quantitative data can be incorporated into a program evaluation to enhance the validity of program evaluation findings. Denzin (1978) described four forms of triangulation: data, investigator, theory, and methodology focused on a technological solution for ensuring validity (Mathison, 1988). These forms, applied in the context of program evaluation, are outlined in the following:

1. *Data triangulation:* Use of multiple data sources to conduct program evaluation that may include time and setting variations.

2. *Investigator triangulation:* Involvement of more than one evaluator in the program evaluation process.

3. *Theory triangulation:* Use of various perspectives to interpret evaluation results.

4. *Methodological triangulation:* Application of different methods to different understandings related to program evaluation.

Mathison (1988) proposed an alternative conceptualization of triangulation strategies useful to consider: convergence, inconsistency, and contradiction. This alternative perspective takes into account that triangulation results in convergent, inconsistent, and contradictory evidence that must be rendered sensible by the evaluator. This belief shifts the responsibility for constructing and making sense of program evaluation findings to the program evaluator and suggests that triangulation as a strategy provides evidence for the evaluator to consider, but the triangulation strategy does not, in and of itself, do this. This viewpoint, applied to program evaluation, is extrapolated as follows:

1. *Convergence:* Occurs when program evaluation data collected from different sources, investigators, perspectives, and/or methods *agree.*

2. *Inconsistency:* Occurs when program evaluation data collected from different sources, investigators, perspectives, and/or methods are *inconsistent but not confirmatory or contradictory.*

3. *Contradiction:* Occurs when program evaluation data collected from different sources, investigators, perspectives, and/or methods are *not simply inconsistent, but contradictory.*

Triangulation strategies explicate existing, often unarticulated problems realistically—rarely in agreement and frequently inconsistent and/or contradictory—challenging evaluators to make sense of evaluation finds within a holistic context and understanding (Mathison, 1988).

■ STEPS IN PROGRAM EVALUATION

Overview

Program evaluation should not focus solely on *proving* whether a program or initiative works. Historically, emphasis on the positivist scientific approach and on proving that programs work has created an imbalance in human service evaluation work—with a heavy emphasis on proving that programs work through the use of quantitative, impact designs and not enough attention to more naturalistic, qualitative designs aimed at improving programs (W. K. Kellogg Foundation, 2017). Program evaluation should consider a more pluralistic approach that includes a variety of perspectives. Questions to consider include:

■ Does the program work? Why does it work or not work?

■ What factors impact the implementation and effectiveness of the program?

■ What are program strengths?

■ What opportunities exist for program improvement?

Internal and External Evaluators

Evaluators can relate to an organization seeking program evaluation in two primary ways: internally or externally. Internal evaluators work for the organization seeking program evaluation and may do a variety of evaluations in that setting on an episodic or ongoing basis. External evaluators may be independent consultants or work for a research firm, university, or a government agency contracted to conduct a specific program evaluation. An evaluator's affiliation has implications for program evaluations and should be considered along with competence, personal qualities, and the purpose of the evaluation (Posavac & Carey, 2010).

Competence factors include methodological and knowledge expertise needed to conduct the program evaluation. Internal evaluators often have knowledge and access advantages consistent with an internal alliance with the program, its participants, and staff. The methodological expertise of an evaluator must also be considered; this includes the extent to which an evaluator has access to resources and individuals to bridge any knowledge and/or methodological disparities. Although not absolute, external evaluators frequently have access to a wider range of resources and methodological experts than are often available to an internal evaluator. Selecting an evaluator with the program content expertise and experience may enhance the evaluator's insight into crucial issues; conversely, an evaluator with limited expertise and experience may contribute avoidable interpretive errors.

A program evaluator's trustworthiness, objectivity, sensitivity, and commitment to program improvement are critical to a program evaluation effort. The perception of these attributes by others may vary depending on whether the evaluator is internal or external to the organization. For example, an internal evaluator might be expected to have a higher degree of commitment to improving the program and may be readily trusted by program participants, staff, and administrators. The internal evaluator's institutional credibility should be anticipated to influence their ability to conduct the evaluation. In contrast, an external evaluator may be perceived as more objective and may find it easier to elicit sensitive information. Developing a reputation for tackling sensitive issues is often made easier when evaluators consistently emphasize that the majority of program improvement opportunities are associated with system issues versus the performance of individuals. Regardless of internal or external organizational affiliation, individual qualities remain an important consideration in selecting a program evaluator.

Finally, the purpose of the evaluation can provide additional guidance to those charged with making an evaluator selection decision. The internal evaluator may have the advantage in performing formative evaluations and leveraging existing relationships with program participants, staff, and administrators and maximize the effectiveness of communication and adoption of program improvement recommendations. In contrast, if the primary purpose of the evaluation is summative in nature and is intended to decide whether a program is continued, expanded, or discontinued, an external evaluator may be a preferable choice (Posavac & Carey, 2010).

Initial Communication

When an evaluation is being conducted it is imperative that communication between the evaluator and program representatives be clear and agreements and expectations made explicit. Evaluators must acknowledge, be flexible, and be willing to accommodate the competing demands of program administrators. Agreements, if written, advisably serve as both a reminder and record of decision-making. Seeing evolving evaluation plans described in writing can draw attention to implications that neither evaluators nor administrators have previously considered.

PLANNING AND CONDUCTING THE EVALUATION: ESSENTIAL STEPS

Ideally, program evaluation should begin when programs are planned and implemented. Formative evaluation, described earlier in this chapter, is a technique often used during program planning and implementation. However, some programs may already be underway and may never have undergone a formal evaluation process. Evaluation of such programs requires that the evaluator understand the program and how it is being implemented as part of the evaluation process. The Centers for Disease Control and Prevention (CDC) framework for evaluation (see Figure 15.1) will be used as the guide in describing the program evaluation steps (CDC, 2012).

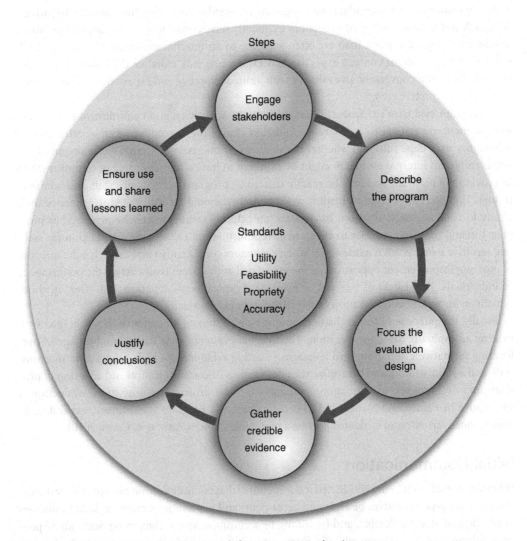

FIGURE 15.1 Recommended framework for program evaluation.

Source: From Centers for Disease Control and Prevention. (2012). *A framework for program evaluation.* https://www.cdc.gov/mmwr/PDF/rr/rr4811.pdf

Step 1: Engaging Stakeholders

The evaluation cycle begins by engaging stakeholders—the persons or organizations that have an investment in what will be learned from an evaluation and what will be done with the knowledge. Stakeholders include program staff, those who derive some of their revenue or income from the program (e.g., program administrators), sponsors of the program (e.g., CEO of an organization, foundations, and government agencies), and clients or potential participants in the program. Understanding the needs of intended program recipients is necessary because it is for their welfare that the program has been developed. This may require undertaking a needs assessment and gathering information on the demographics and health status indicators of the target populations. These data may reside in existing data sources (e.g., health statistics from local or state health departments) or may be collected from key informants through surveys, focus groups, or observations (Hackbarth & Gall, 2005; Laryea et al., 1999). Stakeholders must be engaged in the inquiry to ensure that their perspectives are understood. When stakeholders are not engaged, an evaluation may fail to address important elements of a program's objectives, operations, and outcomes (Hackbarth & Gall, 2005; Posavac & Carey, 2010).

Step 2: Describing the Program

Program descriptions convey the mission and objectives of the program being evaluated. Descriptions should be sufficiently detailed to ensure understanding of (a) program goals and strategies, (b) the program's capacity to effect change, (c) its stage of development, and (d) how it fits into the larger organization and community. Program descriptions set the frame of reference for all subsequent decisions in an evaluation. The description enables the evaluator to compare the program with similar programs and facilitates attempts to connect program components to their effects. Moreover, different stakeholders may have different ideas regarding the program's goals and purposes. Working with stakeholders to formulate a clear and logical program description will bring benefits even before data are available to evaluate the program's effectiveness. Aspects to include in a program description are need (nature and magnitude of the problem or opportunity addressed by the program, target populations, and changing needs); expected effects (what the program must accomplish to be considered successful, immediate and long-term effects, and potential unintended consequences); activities (what activities the program undertakes to effect change, how these activities are related, and who does them); resources (time, talent, technology, equipment, information, money, and other assets available to conduct program activities; congruence between desired activities and resources); stage of development (newly implemented or mature); and context (setting and environmental influences within which the program operates). An understanding of environmental influences such as the program's history, the politics involved, and the social and economic conditions within which the program operates is required to design a context-sensitive evaluation and to aid in interpreting findings accurately (Barkauskas et al., 2004; Jacobson Vann, 2006; Menix, 2007).

Questions to facilitate program descriptions include: (a) Who wants the evaluation? (b) What is the focus of the evaluation? (c) Why is the evaluation wanted? (d) When is the evaluation needed? and (e) What resources are available to support the evaluation? Addressing these questions will assist in helping individuals understand the goals of the program evaluation, arrive at an overall consensus on the purpose of evaluations, and determine the time and resources available to carry out the evaluation. These questions also assist in uncovering the assumptions and conceptual basis of the program. For example, diabetes care programs may be based on the chronic care model, a disease management model, or a health belief model, and it is important that the evaluator understand the program's conceptual basis to understand essential information to include in the program evaluation (Berg & Wadhwa, 2007).

Development of a logic model is part of the work of describing the program. A logic model sequences the events for bringing about change by synthesizing the main program elements into a picture of how the program is supposed to work. Often, this model is displayed in a flowchart, map, or table to portray the sequence of steps that will lead to the desired results. One of the virtues of a logic model is its ability to summarize the program's overall mechanism of change by linking processes (e.g., exercise) to eventual effects (e.g., improved quality of life, decreased coronary risk). A logic model can also display the infrastructure needed to support program operations. Elements that are connected within a logic model generally include inputs (e.g., trained staff, exercise equipment, space); activities (e.g., supervised exercise three times per week, education about exercise at home); outputs (e.g., increased distance walked); and results, whether immediate (e.g., decreased dyspnea with activities of daily living), intermediate (e.g., ability to participate in desired activities of life, improved social interactions), or long term (e.g., improved quality of life). Creating a logic model allows stakeholders to clarify a program's strategies and reveal assumptions about the conditions necessary for the program to be effective. The accuracy of a program description can be confirmed by consulting with diverse stakeholders and comparing reported program descriptions with direct observation of the program activities (CDC Evaluation Working Group, 2008; Dykeman et al., 2003; Ganley & Ward, 2001; Hulton, 2007).

Step 3: Focusing the Evaluation Plan

On the basis of the information gained in steps 1 and 2, the evaluator needs to set forth a focused evaluation plan (Table 15.2). A systematic and comprehensive plan anticipates the program's intended uses and creates an evaluation strategy with the greatest chance of being useful, feasible, ethical, and accurate. Although the components of the plan may differ somewhat depending on the information and understanding of the program gained in steps 1 and 2, essential elements of the evaluation plan are discussed here.

Purpose

Articulating an evaluation's purpose (i.e., intent) prevents premature decision-making regarding how the evaluation should be conducted. Characteristics of the program, particularly its stage of development and context, influence the evaluation's purpose. The purpose may include gaining insight into program operations that affect program outcomes so that knowledge can be put to use in designing future program modifications; describing program processes and outcomes for the purpose of improving the quality, effectiveness, or efficiency of the program; and assessing the program's effects by examining the relationships between program activities and observed consequences. It is essential that an evaluation purpose be set forth and agreed on, as this will guide the types and sources of information to be collected and analyzed.

Selecting and Defining Variables of Interest

Defining the *independent* (process and context) and *dependent* (outcome) variables to be measured carefully and accurately is an essential part of focusing the evaluation plan. This step is likely to be the most daunting, as well as the most important. Selection and definition of the variables must be precise enough so as not to generate unwieldy data management and analysis, yet

TABLE 15.2 Examples of Steps 3, 4, and 5 for Formative and Summative Evaluations

COMPONENTS	FORMATIVE EVALUATION	SUMMATIVE EVALUATION
Selecting and defining variables of interest	Focus on process variables that determine how well the program is running. • Are clients being recruited? • Has staff been properly trained in the program protocol? • Are staff members following program protocol? • Are clients adhering to program requirements?	Focus on outcome variables that determine the effectiveness of the program. • Were clients and staff satisfied with the program? • Did client health improve significantly? • Were medical resources reduced as a result of the program? • Are clients continuing the program on their own once the program is completed?
Measuring variables of interest	Focus on ways to measure how well the program is being run. Use: • Focus groups to discuss problem areas and ways to improve the program. • Direct observation to measure how the staff is following the protocol. • Staff diary data to measure problems that occur on a daily basis. • Interviews of clients to determine how well they are adhering to the program requirements.	Focus on ways to measure the impact the program has had. Use: • Self-reports of clients and staff to report on the progress of clients in terms of health status, functioning, and symptomatology. • Collateral reports to get a second rating on the clients' improvements. • Biomedical data to determine changes in biological parameters of functioning. • Chart abstractions to measure healthcare resource use.
Selecting a program evaluation design	Use descriptive designs or narrative accounts. • Allow for a narrative account of how well the program is being run. • Provide feedback from clients and staff on areas in need of improvement. • Document client adherence levels to the program requirements. • Track process variables over the implementation of the program.	Use experimental, quasi-experimental, or sequential designs (when possible). • Allow for a comparison among groups of clients that were assigned to groups that received the program or did not receive the program. • Use random assignment to program groups whenever possible. • Use over time examinations, if resources permit. • Allow for determination of impact that the program has had on clients' lives.

(continued)

TABLE 15.2 Examples of Steps 3, 4, and 5 for Formative and Summative Evaluations (continued)

COMPONENTS	FORMATIVE EVALUATION	SUMMATIVE EVALUATION
Collecting data	Use uniform collection procedures that do not disrupt the program implementation. • Collected data must be coded according to a uniform system that translates narrative data into meaningful groupings. For example, focus group comments can be grouped into comments about staff-related problems, patient-related problems, recruitment difficulties, adherence difficulties, and so on. • Program evaluators should not bias data collection strategies by holding preconceptions about how well the program is being run.	Use systematic procedures for collecting data across groups (if more than one) and across time. • Collected data must be coded with a uniform system that translates the data into numerical values so that data analysis can be conducted. For example, responses to a question about health status that includes responses such as *poor, fair, good, and excellent* need to be coded as 0, 1, 2, or 3. • Across-time data collection must follow the same procedures. For example, all patients receive self-reports either in the mail or from the program site. The procedures must not vary.
Evaluating data analysis	Use both qualitative and quantitative approaches. • Qualitative approaches provide a narrative description of the process variables and allow for descriptive understanding of how well the program is running. • Quantitative approaches provide frequency counts and means or averages for some of the variables of interest. • Allows evaluators to make recommendations based on data.	Use both qualitative and quantitative approaches. • Qualitative approaches provide a narrative description of the impact that the program has had on individual clients. • Quantitative approaches provide a statistical comparison between groups (if more than one) or across time. Can determine whether the program was effective in improving clients' health status, increasing staff and client satisfaction, and reducing healthcare resources utilized. • Quantitative approaches can also be used to make comparisons with other similar clinical programs. • Enables evaluators to make recommendations based on data.

Source: From Centers for Disease Control and Prevention. (1999). Framework for program evaluation. *Morbidity and Mortality Weekly Report, 48*(RR 11). https://www.cdc.gov/mmwr/PDF/rr/rr4811.pdf

retain variables that are both meaningful and measurable. During formative evaluations, *process* variables are of primary interest, whereas during summative evaluations both *process* and *outcome* variables are of interest.

Independent or Process Variables

An example of an important independent or process variable is the level of adherence to any treatments or self-care regimens prescribed by a program. More than 25 years of research indicates that, on average, 40% of clients fail to adhere to the recommendations prescribed to them to treat their acute or chronic conditions (DiMatteo & DiNicola, 1982). How well participants adhere to program requirements, a focus of formative evaluation, is intimately linked to a program's overall effectiveness. Nonadherence has been found to be a causal factor in the time and money wasted in healthcare visits (Haynes et al., 1979) and must not be overlooked in determining how well a program is being implemented. As an illustration, if a program introduces barriers to adherence (e.g., by requiring time-intensive self-care routines, by introducing complex treatments with numerous factors to remember, by making it difficult to get questions answered, or by having uninformed or untrained staff), program client adherence will likely be diminished. An accompaniment to adherence is the issue of how well the program staff maintains or adheres to the program's protocol. The integrity of an intervention or program is not upheld unless the staff members assigned to carry it out are diligent in following procedures and protocol (Kirchhoff & Dille, 1994). In addition to assessing adherence, program evaluators need to ascertain the level at which staff members are adhering to the program protocols.

Process variables include how participants are recruited into the program, how well trained and informed the staff members are about the program's purpose and importance, how staff members identified barriers (if any) to the implementation of the program, the level at which the program site is conducive to conducting a well-run program, and the perceptions held by program staff and participants related to the usefulness of the program. These factors generally are easier to realign than are issues of participant and staff adherence. For this reason, evaluators need to spend a considerable amount of time formatively assessing and adjusting program procedures and protocols to maximize participant and staff adherence.

All programs are situated within a community or organization. This context exerts some degree of influence on how the program works and on its effectiveness. The need to examine which contextual factors have the greatest impact on program success and which factors may help or hinder the optimization of the program's goals and objectives is likely to arise in program evaluation. Variables such as leadership style, cultural competence, organizational culture, and collaboration are all examples of contextual factors that the evaluator should consider. Gathering this type of information through either quantitative or qualitative techniques will help the evaluator understand why components of the program worked or did not work (Greenhalgh et al., 2005; Stetler et al., 2008). Other areas worthy of examination include the federal and state climates, the impact of these climates on program processes and effectiveness, and how these climates have changed over time (Randell & Delekto, 1999).

Dependent or Outcome Variables

Examples of dependent or outcome variables (Fitzgerald & Illback, 1993) that are measured by social scientists and healthcare services evaluators in determining the effectiveness of healthcare programs include:

■   Participant health status and daily functioning.

■   Client satisfaction with program providers and care received.

■   Program provider satisfaction.

■   Cost containment.

Evaluators and nurses alike should consider each of these variables as outcomes of a clinical program. The evaluator who conducts a program evaluation and who attempts to determine the effectiveness or success of a program should pay particular attention to these four outcomes.

The first important outcome variable defines and measures whether the program has facilitated the client's ability to improve his or her health and/or functional status. The outcome of importance is whether the program has improved quality of life and whether health goals have been achieved. If the program does not increase these outcome variables and the protocol or intervention has been followed (i.e., client and staff have adhered to the program), then the program's effectiveness is questionable. Although expectations for health improvements may not be a focus of the program, client health status is an important outcome variable that needs to be examined. For this reason, health status measurements taken multiple times and in multiple ways using triangulation techniques over the course of the program and even after the program is completed must be considered.

An important outcome of the healthcare delivery and program evaluation is client satisfaction. Research suggests that an intervention that decreases satisfaction with healthcare may lead to poorer health (Kaplan et al., 1989), poorer adherence to treatments (Ong et al., 1995), poorer attendance at follow-up appointments (DiMatteo et al., 1986), and greater interest in obtaining healthcare elsewhere (Ross & Duff, 1982) than is the case among those whose satisfaction has increased. Evaluators need to take into account changes in client satisfaction with the program in particular, and with their healthcare in general, because any decrease in satisfaction can point to problems in the program's purpose, scope, and execution.

Another outcome that is often overlooked is that of staff satisfaction. Slevin et al. (1996) measured staff satisfaction during the evaluation of a quality improvement initiative and found that satisfaction was related to better interpersonal care of clients. Level of satisfaction can pertain directly to the process and implementation of the intervention or can be more generally defined and include professional satisfaction. Any program that introduces frustrations for its staff may risk contributing to it being conducted in the manner other than intended, serve to diminish the quality of care delivered, and perhaps negatively influence client satisfaction and health status. The satisfaction of program staff who implement the intervention on a daily basis and interact and negotiate with clients must be addressed. Evaluation of programs must attend to the impact that the program has on the staff involved, and not simply the impact that it has on the client (Slevin et al., 1996).

Finally, of considerable importance to program evaluation is the outcome variable of cost containment and/or reduction. An effective program is one that improves the quality and delivery of care outcomes, while maintaining and perhaps even reducing costs to both the organization and the client. This evaluation outcome, however, is generally long-term in nature and requires multiple follow-ups; this can pose a considerable burden for programs with limited resources. Data that may be available to assist in this aspect of outcome evaluation include information about any program clients' hospitalizations and related lengths of stay, emergency department visits, regular healthcare provider office visits, supplies and equipment costs, and personnel time. It is beneficial for program evaluators to work collaboratively with financial management personnel to obtain this important information.

Measuring Variables

The next step is to select the way in which each variable of interest will be measured. In making this decision, it is important to consider, first, the many ways in which variables can be assessed and measured (e.g., self-reports, biomedical instrumentation, direct observation, or chart abstraction) and, second, the source from which the data will be collected (e.g., program client, program staff, healthcare records, or other written documents). Measurement is an important element of program evaluation, for without rigorous, reliable, and valid information, the data obtained and subsequent recommendations are questionable.

Program evaluators need to consider, if possible, the use of valid and reliable instruments, rather than develop new instruments to measure the variable of interest. Exhibit 15.1 outlines potential benefits of this approach. Many forms of instrumentation exist that have been used for purposes of program evaluation.

Several reference books are available that have compiled a multitude of research instruments and normative data for measures (Frank-Stromberg & Olsen, 2004; Robinson et al., 1991; Stewart & Shamdasani, 1990).

Fitzgerald and Illback (1993) delineate the various methods of obtaining information and corresponding data sources to consider in program evaluation. Data sources and collection methods to consider are outlined in Exhibit 15.2. *Self-reports* from program clients and staff are likely the most widely used technique for acquiring information about the process and effects of a program intervention. These measures, completed by program participants and staff, can often be completed at the individual's leisure. The main advantages of self-reports include ease of use, cost-efficiency, limited coding and data-entry requirements, and reduced need for highly trained staff to implement their use. The main disadvantage is the prevalent belief that self-report instruments elicit self-presentation tendencies (i.e., the tendency of individuals to present themselves in a socially desirable manner or in a positive light). This view is often unfounded, as many measurement experts now hold the view that most of the people, most of the time, are accurate in their self-reported responses (Stewart & Ware, 1992; Ware et al., 1978).

In addition to self-report inventories completed by the program participant, *collateral reports* can be obtained. Collateral reports are completed by an individual closely related to the program

---

EXHIBIT 15.1

POTENTIAL BENEFITS OF USING PUBLISHED INSTRUMENTS TO GATHER SELF-REPORT INFORMATION

- Gathered information has a greater chance of being reliable and valid; that is, the instrument measures what it intends to measure and has internal consistency.

- The program evaluator has a normative group by which to compare ranges, means, and standard deviations on the instrument to the sample being evaluated.

- The instrument is composed of items or questions that are understandable by the majority of respondents.

- The instrument has a response format that both fits with the stem of the question and is responded to with relative ease.

EXHIBIT 15.2

WAYS TO MEASURE VARIABLES

Data Collection Methods and Sources

Self-reports obtained from program clients or staff.

Collateral reports obtained from family members.

Structured or unstructured interviews conducted by a trained interviewer.

Direct observation of the program implementation mechanisms.

Focus groups on program benefits and problems.

Biomedical information to substantiate program client progress.

Health care record or other written document abstractions.

Diary data obtained from program clients or staff.

---

participant. These reports rely on the same instruments as those used for self-reports, with slight modifications in wording, and can provide additional information about the program client. These types of reports have not been used to a great extent in nursing research, though they have been used extensively in psychological research. Collateral measures have been found to be highly correlated with the self-report data and can serve as either a validity check on the self-report data or an additional source of variant information to be used in the program evaluation.

Use of *structured* and *unstructured interviews* is another method for acquiring information. The practice of interviewing program participants provides benefits beyond those of self-report questionnaires but also introduces a few drawbacks. The benefits of interviews include the ability to clarify any confusing questions or items, increase response rates, obtain more complete information (individuals are often more likely to leave questions blank on questionnaires), and obtain narrative accounts unrestricted by standardized questions and response formats. The main drawback to interviews, however, is the need for interviewers trained to avoid leading questions and introducing bias. Another drawback includes the reduced ability to acquire vast amounts of information more easily achieved with self-report questionnaires.

Direct observation is an alternative method of measurement that does not rely on the reports of the program participants in the project. Observations, like interviews, require highly trained observers. To effectively obtain data, observers must record very specific and narrow pieces of information, often limiting the amount of time a particular action is observed. For instance, a program client may be observed through the use of time-sampling techniques in which only the first 5 minutes or last 5 minutes of every hour is observed and recorded. In addition, direct observations can provide information only about observable behaviors and do not allow insight into program participant perceptions or attitudes.

A variation on interviews and direct observations is the use of *focus groups* (Becker et al., 2007; Laryea et al., 1999; Packer et al., 1994; Wyatt et al., 2008). The qualitative information obtained from focus groups helps evaluators performing formative and summative evaluations to assess areas that need to be further refined, changed altogether, or even eliminated. Focus groups were first used by market researchers and have been a favored method by which to obtain information about consumer preferences (Stewart & Shamdasani, 1990). The use of focus groups, however, is becoming more widespread among program evaluators seeking to understand program client preferences and expectations. For example, a focus group can be used to gather pertinent information about a group of clients participating in a program or to obtain process feedback about how the program is proceeding. Focus groups can also be used to learn about how clients talk about a program or its directive and to ascertain perceptions about program effectiveness and utility (Morgan, 1988; Stewart & Shamdasani, 1990).

Stewart and Shamdasani (1990) discuss the role of focus groups in program evaluation and define the focus group technique as the collective interview of usually eight to 12 individuals who are brought together to discuss a particular topic for an hour or two. The group is generally facilitated by a trained moderator who keeps the discussion focused on the topic of interest, enhances group interaction, and probes for necessary details. Morgan (1988) points out that information acquired from group discussions is often more readily accessible than it would be for individual interviews, as individual members are cued or primed to give information that they might not give in an interview. The topic of interest can vary depending on whether this technique is used for the purpose of formative or summative program evaluation.

Biomedical data include laboratory tests; blood pressure, heart and respiratory rates; and other types of data that require the use of a bioinstrument for collection (e.g., use of blood pressure monitor, heart rate monitor, or stress test). Because of the expense of some medical tests, their use as the sole means of data collection in program evaluation may not be practical. If the program requires use of biomedical data collection as part of its protocol, however, the evaluator might be able to acquire this information. The type of biomedical information collected for program evaluation must provide information relevant to the program and its evaluation and must hold meaning outside basic medical parameters. In other words, biomedical information is useless unless it can be translated into information that is directly meaningful in the determination of a program's effectiveness (e.g., if the program's goal is to reduce hypertension, then the bioinstrumentation must demonstrate that blood pressure has been lowered among the program's participants).

Healthcare record reviews or *written document abstractions* are another source of data to consider when conducting a program evaluation. Use of healthcare records as a data source requires development of a standardized evaluation form and coding scheme to use in abstracting data. These types of reviews need trained abstractors who are clear about the information to be gathered and the need to be systematic in the review process. These types of reviews often allow for the gathering of information that cannot be found in any other manner. The main drawback to this data collection method is associated with document completeness, readability, and accuracy. The primary advantage of this method is the evaluator's ability to rely on existing data.

Diary data (self-report) are another source of data that can be used to measure variables of interest. Diary data can be completed by either the healthcare provider or the client and provide information that is immediate and time relevant. Data can be collected once a day (e.g., a nightly count of food consumed for that day), several times a day (e.g., when every prescription medication is taken), or even randomly (prompted by some form of an alert). The main disadvantage of using diary data is that individuals may not always take the necessary time to complete the forms completely or accurately. Diary data, however, represent an advance in data collection methods when used in combination with other forms of data previously discussed.

Selecting the Design

The next step is to select the method that will provide the information necessary to determine a program's effectiveness. Numerous evaluation methods are available that can serve as both practical and efficient means to determine the effectiveness of programs. A brief review of evaluation methods or designs that an evaluator can consider in selecting a technique for program evaluation is outlined by Rossi et al. (2004) and includes the amount of time and financial expense required to implement it, the type of analysis plan necessary, the level of control it offers the evaluator over the variables of interest, and the level of associated statistical power.

True randomized controlled trials (RCTs) involve a comparison between one or more experimental groups that have an intervention group and a control group that does not receive the intervention. Participants in the experimental group(s) participate in the program that is intended to affect a measurable outcome, whereas those in the control group serve as a comparison (Chan et al., 2000). The key component to true experiments is the random assignment of subjects to either the experimental or the control group. This assignment theoretically eliminates any individual differences among the groups before the implementation of the program.

According to program evaluation experts, this type of design is difficult to implement in the dynamic, real-world setting where programs reside. Furthermore, this design requires withholding ongoing feedback regarding information related to program improvement during the experiment (Stufflebeam & Shinkfield, 2007). Opportunities to meet the requirements of randomized experiments in program evaluation, particularly in service fields such as healthcare and social service, are quite limited. The expectation of federal agencies and government mandates—that program evaluations employ RCTs—has had a crippling and wasteful influence on the practice of program evaluations (Stufflebeam & Shinkfield, 2007).

Quasi-experiments involve the same intervention and comparison component as true experiments, except that quasi-experiments differ in one critical way: Random assignment of subjects or participants to a "treatment" group is not feasible. The evaluation process for quasi-experiments is similar to that for true experiments. The main difference, however, occurs during the summative evaluation. Since random assignment to treatment groups is not feasible, it is not possible to be certain that changes in outcome variables are the result of the intervention or program. Differences among the individuals in the assigned groups or other factors cannot be ruled out as the cause for observed changes in the outcome variable(s) of interest.

One drawback to both experiments and quasi-experiments is the need for a control or a natural comparison group. This need for an additional group can pose a limitation for sites where client participation is limited, recruitment takes a great deal of time, or there is no natural comparison group readily available. In addition, some have argued the ethical implications of providing some clients with care or experimental care and not providing equivalent care to others. For these reasons, a *cross-sequential design* might be the most practical. In the cross-sequential design, the program evaluator observes or assesses several different groups of clients over several time periods, but each group is observed initially in the same period, for example, 6 weeks after admission to the program (Rosenthal & Rosnow, 1991). This type of design allows the time of measurement and the client group to serve as the basis for comparison, eliminating the need for a control group. In essence, a cross-sequential design simultaneously compares several different groups of clients on a set of variables observed during a single designated time period. The evaluator is able to assess for possible variations in how the program is conducted. If clients observed during the beginning of the program have different outcomes from those recruited later in the program, the evaluator can attempt to determine whether these differences are due to individual differences among the clients or to differences in program implementation.

Finally, *descriptive designs* are also useful to employ in program evaluations. These designs serve to track and describe key outcome variables over time and examine data for patterns and trends. Descriptive designs can be employed that use a cross-sectional examination of the reports of program clients and staff or a longitudinal examination of trends in relationships among variables of interest and provide narrative descriptions of the component parts of the program as viewed by clients and staff. These designs are particularly relevant for formative evaluations, because this phase of evaluation is focused on the process of planning and implementing the program as well as on *how* the program is being executed. Descriptions of the program can help to illuminate problems in program execution, especially in program client and staff adherence.

Sample Size in Program Evaluations

When selecting a design for program evaluation, the evaluator must consider effective sampling and representation as an important aspect of meaningful evaluation. Sample size depends on several factors. Among these are the expected effect size of the intervention (i.e., whether the intervention will produce a small amount or a large amount of change), type of design used, plan for data analysis, and budgetary constraints. For a further explanation of sample size and its related statistical power to detect significant effects, please refer to Chapter 11 on sampling.

Step 4: Gathering Credible Evidence: Data Collection

The collection of valid, reliable, and systematic data serves as the foundation of an effective program evaluation and requires establishing the conditions and systematic procedures for data collection. Clear and consistent procedures must be used to collect data to enhance the utility, accuracy, and trustworthiness of the evaluation findings.

Data Collection Quality

Once the evaluator has identified the sources of information and data collection strategies, quality control mechanisms must be established to protect data integrity. These quality control mechanisms should include monitoring the quality of information obtained and taking practical steps to improve the quality of data and/or data collection procedures if indicated. Similar problems may become evident with all forms of data. Data collection procedures and data analysis are highly sensitive to variations. Goals of the evaluator include ensuring uniformity across the program, maintaining systematic procedures, and eliminating sources of potential bias.

Data Coding

One of the most tedious components of the evaluation process is the coding and entering of all relevant data (Coffey & Atkinson, 1996; Keppel & Zedeck, 1989; Lipsey, 1994). The protocol for coding data needs to be well developed early in program planning and, whenever possible, to follow a standardized and published method. Because data collected during an evaluation may be narrative, the coding scheme for analyzing the accounts must be succinct, time efficient, and meaningful. The accounts are usually sorted through and divided into a manageable number of conceptual or programmatic categories. Often, not all of these categories will be used in the evaluation of the program, but nonetheless, a systematic coding scheme needs to be followed. Additionally, all self-report data, biomedical data, and document-based data need to be coded into numerical values that can be used in the computations for the final evaluations. Again, these coding procedures need to be uniform across all participants (participant and staff reports) and across all forms of data.

The evaluator must also keep track of the manner in which items are phrased or data from written documents and bioinstruments are abstracted so that these can be accurately recoded. Items may be phrased in an alternate manner to reduce acquiescent and response biases that may require recoding. Multiple items that measure the same variable should be analyzed only when they are all directionally coded for consistency.

Step 5: Justifying Conclusions: Data Analysis, Interpretation, and Recommendations

Techniques for analyzing, interpreting, and synthesizing findings should be agreed on before data collection begins and guide this phase of program evaluation. Once all data are accurately coded and entered into a database, the evaluator can move forward with data analysis. The reader is referred to Chapter 13 for a thorough discussion of how to conduct an appropriate analysis. Analysis and synthesis of an evaluation's findings may detect patterns in the evidence, either by isolating important findings (analysis) or by combining sources of information to reach a broader understanding (synthesis). Mixed-method evaluations require the separate analysis of each evidence element and a synthesis of all sources to allow for an examination of patterns of agreement, convergence, or complexity.

The program evaluator must be cautious in interpreting the results of an evaluation once it has been completed. Interpretation is the process of determining the significance of results before determining what the findings mean and is part of the overall effort to understand the evidence gathered in an evaluation. The uncovering of facts regarding a program's performance is not a sufficient basis on which to draw evaluative conclusions. Evaluation evidence must be interpreted to determine the practical significance of what has been learned. Interpretations draw on information and perspectives that stakeholders bring to the evaluation inquiry.

The results of data analysis can sometimes be confusing but are often unassuming. Effect size refers to the magnitude of the relationship between two variables; the smaller the related coefficient, the smaller the effect. The evaluator must keep in mind that the effect size coefficient is meaningful only in a statistical sense and does not mean that the effect it has on the lives of individuals is small (Cohen, 1988; Rosenthal & Rosnow, 1991). The determination, based on quantitative data analysis, that a program has a small effect may be predominant; however, a small effect does not mean that the effect is unimportant. To interpret qualitative data, the evaluator should employ qualitative analysis techniques, using quotations and stories to illustrate themes and concepts. Qualitative information is important to include; it illustrates the basis for recommendations derived from the data, particularly for components that address program implementation.

Judgments about the program are made on the basis of data analysis and interpretation. Statements about the program are set forth, and they focus on the merit, worth, or significance of the program and are based on the agreed-upon values or standards set by the stakeholders in the planning stages of program evaluation. They are formed by comparing the findings and interpretations regarding the program against one or more of the selected standards. Because multiple standards can be applied to a given program, some evaluative statements may be incongruent. However, one of the unique features of program evaluation is that the evaluator makes judgment statements based on standards that are set a priori and reflect the perspectives of various stakeholder groups. For example, a 10% increase in pulmonary rehabilitation program annual enrollment may be viewed as positive by the program manager, whereas potential participants in the program may view this figure differently and argue that a critical threshold for access to this service has not been reached. Conflicting statements regarding a program's quality, value, or importance may suggest that stakeholders are using different standards on which to base their judgment. In the context of an evaluation, such disagreement can be a catalyst for clarifying relevant values and the worth of the program (CDC, 2012).

Recommendations

Recommendations are proposed actions for consideration that grow out of the evaluation. Forming recommendations is a distinct element of program evaluation that requires information beyond what is necessary to form judgments regarding program performance (CDC, 2012). Knowing that a program is able to reduce the risk of disease does not necessarily translate into a recommendation to continue the effort, particularly when competing priorities or other effective alternatives exist. Thus, summative evaluation recommendations related to continuing, expanding, redesigning, or terminating a program are separate from judgments regarding a program's effectiveness. Making recommendations requires information concerning the context, particularly the organizational context, in which programmatic decisions will be made. Recommendations that lack sufficient evidence or those that are not aligned with stakeholders' values can undermine an evaluation's credibility. By contrast, an evaluation can be strengthened by recommendations that anticipate the political sensitivities of intended users and that highlight areas that users can control or influence. Sharing draft recommendations, soliciting feedback from multiple stakeholders, and presenting alternative options instead of directive advice increase the likelihood that recommendations will be relevant and well received.

Conclusions and recommendations are strengthened by (a) summarizing the plausible mechanisms of change, (b) delineating the temporal sequence between activities and effects, (c) searching for alternative explanations and showing why they are unsupported by the evidence, and (d) showing that the effects can be repeated (CDC, 2012). When different but equally well-supported conclusions exist, each can be presented with a summary of its strengths and weaknesses.

Step 6: Ensure Use and Share Lessons Learned: The Written Report and Follow-Up

Lessons learned in the course of an evaluation do not automatically translate into informed decision-making and appropriate action. Deliberate effort is needed to ensure that the evaluation processes and findings are used and disseminated appropriately (CDC, 2012).

Writing an Evaluation Plan and Report

Writing an evaluation report and disseminating the report to key stakeholders are essential final steps in program evaluation (see also Chapter 21 on reporting results through publication). The checklist in Exhibit 15.3 is a helpful tool to ensure effective reports.

A report that addresses these elements and is supported by evidence contributes to the usefulness, the primary purpose, of the program evaluation. An *executive summary* is beneficial for administrators and those individuals with program decision-making responsibilities. It is critical that the executive summary clearly documents the association between the program and the outcomes of interest and demonstrates program benefits, cost savings, and the number of program participants served. The executive summary is usually written after the evaluator has completed the final report designed to be a more comprehensive report of the program evaluation. The executive summary needs to succinctly address the outcomes of the program evaluation linked to the evidence gathered and be consistent with the agreed-upon standards of the stakeholders. A well-written final report and the subsequent executive summary for a new or continuing program may seem like a daunting task, but it can serve as a useful template for subsequent program reviews.

EXHIBIT 15.3

CHECKLIST FOR ENSURING EFFECTIVE EVALUATION REPORTS

Provide interim and final reports to intended users in time for use.

- Tailor the report content, format, and style for the audience(s) by involving audience members.
- Include an executive summary.
- Summarize the description of the stakeholders and how they were engaged.
- Describe essential features of the program (e.g., in appendices).
- Explain the focus of the evaluation and its limitations.
- Include an adequate summary of the evaluation plan and procedures.
- Provide all necessary technical information (e.g., in appendices).
- Specify the standards and criteria for evaluative judgments.
- Explain the evaluative judgments and how they are supported by the evidence.
- List both strengths and weaknesses of the evaluation.
- Discuss recommendations for action with their advantages, disadvantages, and resource implications.
- Ensure protection for program clients and other stakeholders.
- Anticipate how people or organizations might be affected by the findings.
- Present minority opinions or rejoinders where necessary.
- Verify that the report is accurate and unbiased.
- Organize the report logically and include appropriate details.
- Remove technical jargon.
- Use examples, illustrations, graphics, and stories.

Source: Adapted from Worthen, B. R., Sanders, J. R., & Fitzpatrick, J. L. (1997). *Program evaluation: Alternative approaches and practical guidelines* (2nd ed.). Addison Wesley Longman.

Follow-Up

Follow-up refers to the support provided to users to enable them to disseminate and enact the program evaluation findings as appropriate (CDC, 2012). Active follow-up might be necessary to remind intended users of the planned use of the report. Follow-up might also be required to ensure that lessons learned are not lost or ignored in the process of making complex or politically sensitive decisions. To guard against such oversights, someone involved in the evaluation process should serve as an advocate for the evaluation's findings during the decision-making phase. This type of advocacy increases appreciation of what was discovered and what actions are consistent with the findings.

Facilitating use of evaluation findings also carries with it the responsibility for preventing misuse. Evaluation results are always bound by the context in which the evaluation was conducted. However, some results may be interpreted or taken out of context and used for purposes other than those agreed on. For example, individuals who seek to undermine a program might misuse results by overemphasizing negative findings without regard to the program's positive attributes. Active follow-up can help prevent these and other forms of misuse by ensuring that evidence is not misinterpreted and is not applied to situations, time periods, persons, contexts, and purposes other than those for which the findings are applicable and that were the central focus of the evaluation (CDC, 2012).

■ SUMMARY

The evolution of program evaluation as a discipline links questions being asked and program elements that must be evaluated to answer them, and highlights relationships among program interventions and desired outcomes (to address not only the fundamental question of *whether* a program worked, but also *how* and *why* it worked, and *what else* happened) within the *context* in which the program is operating (Haji et al., 2013). The process of planning, conducting, and analyzing a well-designed and comprehensive program evaluation is time-consuming, creative, and challenging. The effort put forth can be rewarded with fiscal reinforcement, community recognition, and a sound future for the program. Programs that are found to be effective in terms of increasing participant and staff satisfaction, improving health status, and increasing cost savings are likely the ones that will be considered for continued or increased funding. Ultimately, the program evaluator needs to examine and protect the program's integrity at all levels, because, if integrity is not maintained, the outcomes of the program are questionable.

SUGGESTED LEARNING ACTIVITIES

1. You have been asked by the chief nursing officer to evaluate the cardiovascular case management program at your community hospital. Describe how you will proceed in developing an evaluation plan for this program. Include a purpose statement for the evaluation, a list of the key stakeholders you will need to communicate with, and the program evaluation methods you will use to gather information to include in the evaluation.

2. Contrast the use of an internal evaluator and an external evaluator for program evaluation. Examine the advantages and disadvantages of having an individual employed by the institution conduct the evaluation versus contracting with an external program evaluator.

REFERENCES

American Evaluation Association. (n.d.). *Guiding principles for evaluators.* https://www.eval.org/p/cm/ld/fid=51

Ardisson, M., Smallheer, B., Moore, G., & Christenbery, T. (2015). Meta-evaluation: Experiences in an accelerated graduate nurse education program. *Journal of Professional Nursing, 31*(6), 508–515. https://doi.org/10.1016/j.profnurs.2015.04.009

Barkauskas, V. H., Pohl, J., Breer, L., Tanner, C., Bostrom, A. C., Benkert, R., & Vonderheid, S. (2004). Academic nurse-managed centers: Approaches to evaluation. *Outcomes Management, 8*(1), 57–66.

Becker, K. L., Dang, D., Jordan, E., Kub, J., Welch, A., Smith, C. A., & White, K. M. (2007). An evaluation framework for faculty practice. *Nursing Outlook, 55*(1), 44–54. https://doi.org/10.1016/j.outlook.2006.10.001

Berg, G. D., & Wadhwa, S. (2007). Health services outcomes for a diabetes disease management program for the elderly. *Disease Management, 10*(4), 226–234. https://doi.org/10.1089/dis.2007.104704

Billings, J. R. (2000). Community development: A critical review of approaches to evaluation. *Journal of Advanced Nursing, 31*(2), 472–480. https://doi.org/10.1046/j.1365-2648.2000.01278.x

Centers for Disease Control and Prevention. (1999). Framework for program evaluation. *Morbidity and Mortality Weekly Report, 48*(RR 11). https://www.cdc.gov/mmwr/PDF/rr/rr4811.pdf

Centers for Disease Control and Prevention. (2012). *A framework for program evaluation.* https://www.cdc.gov/mmwr/PDF/rr/rr4811.pdf

Centers for Disease Control and Prevention Evaluation Working Group. (2008). *Framework for program evaluation in public health.* Author. https://www.cdc.gov/mmwr/preview/mmwrhtml/rr4811a1.htm

Chan, S., MacKenzie, A., Ng, D. T., & Leung, J. K. (2000). An evaluation of the implementation of case management in the community psychiatric nursing service. *Journal of Advanced Nursing, 31*(1), 144–156. https://doi.org/10.1046/j.1365-2648.2000.01250.x

Coffey, A., & Atkinson, P. (1996). *Making sense of qualitative data: Complementing research strategies.* SAGE.

Cohen, J. (1988). *Statistical power analysis for the behavioral sciences* (2nd ed.). Erlbaum.

Denzin, N. K. (1978). *The research act.* McGraw-Hill.

DiMatteo, M. R., & DiNicola, D. D. (1982). *Achieving patient compliance: The psychology of the medical practitioner's role.* Pergamon Press.

DiMatteo, M. R., Hays, R. D., & Prince, L. M. (1986). Relationship of physicians' nonverbal communication skill to patient satisfaction, appointment noncompliance, and physician workload. *Health Psychology, 5*(6), 581–594. https://doi.org/10.1037/0278-6133.5.6.581

Donnelly, C., Shulha, L., Klinger, D., & Letts, L. (2016). Using program evaluation to support knowledge translation in an interprofessional primary care team: A case study. *BMC Family Practice, 17*(1), 142. https://doi.org/10.1186/s12875-016-0538-4

Dykeman, M., MacIntosh, J., Seaman, P., & Davidson, P. (2003). Development of a program logic model to measure the processes and outcomes of a nurse-managed community health clinic. *Journal of Professional Nursing, 19*(4), 197–203. https://doi.org/10.1016/S8755-7223(03)00070-X

Fitzgerald, E., & Illback, R. J. (1993). Program planning and evaluation: Principles and procedures for nurse managers. *Orthopedic Nursing, 12*(5), 39–44, 70. https://doi.org/10.1097/00006416-199309000-00009

Frank-Stromberg, M., & Olsen, S. J. (2004). *Instruments for clinical health care research.* Jones & Bartlett.

Ganley, H. E., & Ward, M. (2001). Program logic: A planning and evaluation method. *Journal of Nursing Administration, 31*(1), 4, 39. https://doi.org/10.1097/00005110-200101000-00001

Gargani, J., & Miller, R. L. (2016). What is program evaluation? *American Journal of Public Health, 106*(6), e13. https://doi.org/10.2105/AJPH.2016.303159

Greenhalgh, T., Robert, G., Bate, P., Macfarlane, F., & Kyriakidou, O. (2005). *Diffusion of innovations in health service organisations: A systematic literature review.* Blackwell.

Hackbarth, D., & Gall, G. B. (2005). Evaluation of school-based health center programs and services: The whys and hows of demonstrating program effectiveness. *The Nursing Clinics of North America, 40*(4), 711–724, x. https://doi.org/10.1016/j.cnur.2005.07.008

Haji, F., Morin, M. P., & Parker, K. (2013). Rethinking programme evaluation in health professions education: Beyond "did it work?" *Medical Education, 47*(4), 342–351. https://doi.org/10.1111/medu.12091

Haynes, R. B., Taylor, D. W., & Sackett, D. L. (1979). *Compliance in health care.* Johns Hopkins University Press.

Hulton, L. J. (2007). An evaluation of a school-based teenage pregnancy prevention program using a logic model framework. *Journal of School Nursing, 23*(2), 104–110. https://doi.org/10.1177/10598405070230020801

Jacobson Vann, J. C. (2006). Measuring community-based case management performance: Strategies for evaluation. *Lippincott's Case Management, 11*(3), 147–159. https://doi.org/10.1097/00129234-200605000-00006

Kaplan, S. H., Greenfield, S., & Ware, J. E. (1989). Assessing the effects of physician-patient interactions on the outcomes of chronic disease. *Medical Care, 27*(3, Suppl.), S110–S127. https://doi.org/10.1097/00005650-198903001-00010

Keppel, G., & Zedeck, S. (1989). *Data analysis for research designs: Analysis of variance and multiple regression correlation approaches.* W. H. Freeman.

Kirchhoff, K. T., & Dille, C. A. (1994). Issues in intervention research: Maintaining integrity. *Applied Nursing Research, 7*(1), 32–38. https://doi.org/10.1016/0897-1897(94)90018-3

Laryea, M., Sen, P., Glen, L., Kozma, A., & Palaclo, T. (1999). Using focus groups to evaluate an education program. *The International Journal of Psychiatric Nursing Research, 4*(3), 482–488.

Lipsey, M. W. (1994). Identifying potentially interesting variables and analysis opportunities. In H. Cooper & L. V. Hedges (Eds.), *The handbook of research synthesis* (pp. 111–123). Russell Sage Foundation.

Mathison, S. (1988). Why triangulate. *Educational Researcher, 17*(2), 13–17. https://doi.org/10.3102/0013189X017002013

Menix, K. D. (2007). Evaluation of learning and program effectiveness. *Journal of Continuing Education in Nursing, 38*(5), 201–208; quiz 209. https://doi.org/10.3928/00220124-20070901-05

Morgan, D. L. (1988). *Focus groups as qualitative research.* SAGE University paper series on qualitative research methods (Vol. 16). SAGE.

Ong, L. M., de Haes, J. C., Hoos, A. M., & Lammes, F. B. (1995). Doctor-patient communication: A review of the literature. *Social Science & Medicine (1982), 40*(7), 903–918. https://doi.org/10.1016/0277-9536(94)00155-M

Packer, T., Race, K. E. H., & Hotch, D. F. (1994). Focus groups: A tool for consumer-based program evaluation in rehabilitation agency settings. *Journal of Rehabilitation, 60*(3), 30–33.

Posavac, E. J., & Carey, R. G. (2010). *Program evaluation: Methods and case studies* (8th ed.). Pearson.

Randell, C. L., & Delekto, M. (1999). Telehealth technology evaluations process. *Journal of Healthcare Information Management, 13*(4), 101–110.

Robinson, J. P., Shaver, P. R., & Wrightsman, L. S. (Eds.). (1991). *Measures of personality and social psychological attitudes* (Vol. 1). Academic Press.

Rosenthal, R., & Rosnow, R. L. (1991). *Essentials of behavioral research: Methods and data analysis.* McGraw-Hill.

Ross, C. E., & Duff, R. S. (1982). Returning to the doctor: The effect of client characteristics, type of practice, and experiences with care. *Journal of Health and Social Behavior, 23*(2), 119–131. https://doi.org/10.2307/2136509

Rossi, P., Lipsey, M. W., & Freeman, H. E. (2004). *Evaluation: A systematic approach* (7th ed.). SAGE.

Shadish, W. R., Jr., Cook, T. D., & Leviton, L. C. (1991). *Foundations of program evaluation: Theories of practice.* SAGE.

Slevin, E., Somerville, H., & McKenna, H. (1996). The implementation and evaluation of a quality improvement initiative at Oaklands. *Journal of Nursing Management, 4*(1), 27–34. https://doi.org/10.1111/j.1365-2834.1996.tb00024.x

Spaulding, D. T. (2008). *Program evaluation in practice: Core concepts and examples for discussion and analysis.* Jossey-Bass.

Stetler, C. B., Legro, M. W., Wallace, C. M., Bowman, C., Guihan, M., Hagedorn, H., Kimmel, B., Sharp, N. D., & Smith, J. L. (2006). The role of formative evaluation in implementation research and the QUERI experience. *Journal of General Internal Medicine, 21*(Suppl. 2), S1–S8. https://doi.org/10.1007/s11606-006-0267-9

Stetler, C. B., McQueen, L., Demakis, J., & Mittman, B. S. (2008). An organizational framework and strategic implementation for system-level change to enhance research-based practice: QUERI series. *Implementation Science, 3*, 30. https://doi.org/10.1186/1748-5908-3-30

Stewart, A. L., & Ware, J. E., Jr. (Eds.). (1992). *Measuring functioning and well-being: The medical outcomes study approach.* Duke University Press.

Stewart, D. W., & Shamdasani, P. M. (1990). *Focus groups: Theory and practice.* Applied social research methods series (Vol. 20). SAGE.

Stufflebeam, D. L., & Shinkfield, A. J. (2007). *Evaluation theory, models and applications.* Jossey-Bass.

Ware, J. E., Jr., Davies-Avery, A., & Donald, C. A. (1978). *Conceptualization and measurement of health for adults in the health insurance study: Vol. V, General health perceptions.* RAND Corporation.

W. K. Kellogg Foundation. (2017, November). *W. K. Kellogg Foundation step-by-step guide to evaluation: How to become savvy evaluation consumers.* https://www.wkkf.org/resource-directory/resources/2017/11/the-step-by-step-guide-to-evaluation--how-to-become-savvy-evaluation-consumers

Worthen, B. R., Sanders, J. R., & Fitzpatrick, J. L. (1997). *Program evaluation: Alternative approaches and practical guidelines* (2nd ed.). Addison Wesley Longman.

Wyatt, T. H., Krauskopf, P. B., & Davidson, R. (2008). Using focus groups for program planning and evaluation. *Journal of School Nursing, 24*(2), 71–77. https://doi.org/10.1177/10598405080240020401

Yarbrough, D. B., Shulha, L. M., Hopson, R. K., & Caruthers, F. A. (2011). *The program evaluation standards: A guide for evaluations and evaluation users* (3rd ed.). SAGE.

ADDITIONAL RESOURCES

American Evaluation Association. (n.d.). *American Evaluation Association: Guiding principles for evaluators.* http://www.eval.org

Centers for Disease Control and Prevention. (2012, December 11). *CDC evaluation framework* [Video]. YouTube. https://www.youtube.com/watch?v=tOjieBh1ce0

Holden, D. J., & Zimmerman, M. A. (Eds.). (2009). *A practical guide to program evaluation planning: Theory and case examples.* SAGE.

Western Michigan University. (n.d.). *The evaluation center.* https://www.wmich.edu/evaluation

IMPLEMENTING EVIDENCE-BASED PRACTICE

LISA J. HOPP

▓ INTRODUCTION

The use of evidence-based practice (EBP) has become the expected standard in healthcare; yet, in spite of decades of high-quality health care research and a growing evidence base, its impact at the point of care remains inconsistent. Fragmented care, health inequities, and regional variability in healthcare practices and outcomes coupled with a recognition of the highest care and mediocre outcomes have created a demand for using evidence to improve health and healthcare (Dzau et al., 2017; see also Institute of Medicine [IOM], 2008). In the United States, health and healthcare disparities persist while spending and estimated waste both increase. In 2015, total spending on healthcare was estimated at $3.2 trillion with 30% of it committed to waste or excess including unnecessary treatment, inefficiencies, missed prevention, and even fraud (Dzau et al., 2017). Clearly, despite high-quality research availability this overall health picture persists. In 2006, Graham et al. reported that in both the United States and the Netherlands, 30% to 40% of patients do not receive evidence-based care, and 20% to 25% of patients receive unneeded or potentially harmful care. Similarly, Sanchez et al. (2020) cited a near doubling in the use of statins in one area of Spain despite the limited primary prevention value for cardiovascular disease in low-risk patients. Foy et al. (2015) emphasized that the lack of uptake of what we know from research produces research waste and an "invisible ceiling on the potential for research to enhance population outcomes" (p. 2).

In an effort to improve patient care, government bodies and individual organizations have focused time, attention, and resources on compiling and evaluating research findings, as shown by the increase in published systematic reviews. The Cochrane Database of Systematic Reviews (CDSR) alone has published 7,500 reviews with plain language summaries in 14 languages and the organization has 11,000 members, 68,000 supporters from more than 130 countries (Cochrane, 2020). Other organizations contribute to the growing volume of systematic reviews through their libraries and evolving methodologies to conduct systematic reviews such as the Joanna Briggs Institute (JBI). The findings from these reviews on topics relevant to preventive, acute, and chronic healthcare have been used to develop behavioral interventions, evidence-based healthcare programs, and evidence-based guidelines and protocols. However, despite these efforts, use of EBPs at the point of care remains inconsistent (Campbell et al., 2015; Foy et al., 2015).

There is a need for focused research to identify effective strategies to increase the use of evidence-based programs, guidelines, and protocols and how to incorporate the evidence into health systems with the goal of better outcomes and patient experiences at a better value (Whicher et al., 2018). Some questions that point to how to improve the way we use evidence for better health and healthcare are: What strategies are effective in increasing the use of EBP? Are these strategies effective in all settings (e.g., acute care, long-term care, school health, and primary care)? Who should provide the interventions through what channels? Are they effective with all end users (e.g., nurses, physicians, pharmacists, housekeeping staff)? Are they effective with different evidence-based healthcare practices (prescribing drugs, handwashing, fall prevention)? What strategies work to de-implement or undo ineffective practices? In summary, we need to know what strategies to use and in what setting and by and with whom for varying topics when implementing EBPs in an organization.

This chapter describes the field of implementation science, a relatively new area of study that is addressing these questions through research. Included are emerging definitions, an overview of promising models, and the current state of the science, and concludes with suggestions for future research needed to move the field forward.

■ DEFINITION OF TERMS

Based on the National Institutes of Health program announcement, *implementation* is "the process of putting to use or integrating evidence-based interventions within a setting" (Rabin et al., 2008, p. 118). According to the editors of the periodical *Implementation Science*, *implementation research* is:

> the scientific study of methods to promote the systematic uptake of evidence-based interventions into practice and policy and hence to improve health. In this context, it includes the study of influences on professional, patient and organizational behavior in healthcare, community or population contexts. (Foy et al., 2015, p. 2)

In the "about" section of the journal pages, the editors include "de-implementation" as part of implementation science. This relates to the study of how to remove interventions of low or no benefit from routine practice (*Implementation Science*, 2020; Norton & Chambers, 2020). It includes research that helps us understand how to move knowledge of the evidence-based healthcare practices into routine use (Brownson et al., 2012). It includes research to (a) understand context variables that influence adoption of EBPs, and (b) test the effectiveness of interventions to promote and sustain use of evidence-based healthcare practices. *Implementation science* then relates to both the systematic investigation of methods, interventions, and variables that influence adoption of evidence-based healthcare practices and the organized body of knowledge gained through such research (Foy et al., 2015).

Implementation research is a young science, so standardized definitions of commonly used terms are emerging (Canadian Institutes of Health Research [CHIR], 2020; Graham et al., 2006; McKibbon et al., 2010). This is evidenced by differing definitions and the interchanging of terms that, in fact, may represent different concepts to different people. Adding to the confusion, terminology may vary depending on the country in which the research was conducted. Graham et al. (2006) reported identifying 29 terms in nine countries that refer to some aspect of translating research findings into practice. For example, researchers in Canada may use the terms *research utilization, knowledge-to-action, integrated knowledge translation, knowledge transfer,* or *knowledge translation* interchangeably, whereas researchers in the United States, the United Kingdom, and Europe may be more likely to use the terms *dissemination research, implementation,* or *research translation* to express similar concepts (Canadian Institutes of Health Research, 2020; Colquhoun et al., 2014; U.S. Department of Health and Human Services, 2018). McKibbon et al.

(2010) collected terms across a broad but purposeful set of literature sources during 1 year (2006). They found more than 100 terms that they regarded as equivalent or closely related to knowledge translation. They further analyzed the terms to try to find words that more likely differentiated knowledge translation literature from nonknowledge translation literature. Table 16.1 provides examples of currently used definitions of common terms describing concepts related to implementation science. Although these definitions provide an explanation of terms used in articles about implementation science, terms such as *implementation, dissemination, research translation,*

TABLE 16.1 Definitions Associated With Implementing Evidence in Practice

	DEFINITION	SOURCE
Diffusion	"The process by which an innovation is communicated through certain channels over time among members of a social system."	Rogers (2003)
Dissemination	"An active approach of spreading evidence-based interventions to the target audience via determined channels using planned strategies."	Rabin et al. (2008)
Dissemination research	"The scientific study of targeted distribution of information and intervention materials to a specific public health or clinical practice audience. The intent is to understand how best to spread and sustain knowledge and the associated evidence-based interventions."	U.S. Department of Health and Human Services (2018), background
Implementation research	"The scientific study of methods to promote the systematic uptake of clinical research findings and other evidence-based practices into routine practice" in order to improve the quality and effectiveness of health care.	Graham et al. (2006)
Implementation science	"The investigation of methods, interventions, and variables that influence adoption of evidence-based health care practices by individuals and organizations to improve clinical and operational decision making and includes testing the effectiveness of interventions to promote and sustain use of evidence-based healthcare practices."	Titler, Everett, & Adams (2007)
	"All aspects of research relevant to the scientific study of methods to promote the uptake of research findings into routine health care in both clinical and policy contexts."	Graham et al. (2006)
Integrated knowledge translation	"A way of doing research that involves decision makers/knowledge-users—usually as members of the research team— in all stages of the research process."	Canadian Institutes of Health Research (2020)
Knowledge broker	"An intermediary who facilitates and fosters the interactive process between producers (i.e., researchers) and users (i.e., practitioners, policymakers) of knowledge through a broad range of activities."	Rabin & Brownson (2012)

(continued)

TABLE 16.1 Definitions Associated With Implementing Evidence in Practice (*continued*)

	DEFINITION	SOURCE
Knowledge to action	A broad concept that encompasses both the transfer of knowledge and the *use* of knowledge by practitioners, policy makers, patients, and the public, including use of knowledge in practice and/or the decision-making process. The term is often used interchangeably with knowledge transfer or knowledge translation.	Straus et al. (2013)
Knowledge transfer	"Knowledge transfer is used to mean the process of getting knowledge used by stakeholders." "The traditional view of 'knowledge transfer' is a unidirectional flow of knowledge from researchers to users."	Graham et al. (2006)
Knowledge translation	"Knowledge translation is the exchange, synthesis and ethicallysound application of knowledge within a complex system of interactions among researchers and users to accelerate the capture of the benefits of research for Canadians through improved health, more effective services and products, and a strengthened health care system."	Canadian Institutes of Health Research (2016)
Knowledge user	"An individual who is likely to be able to use research results to make informed decisions about health policies, programs and/or practices. A knowledge user's level of engagement in the research process may vary in intensity and complexity depending on the nature of the research and on his/her information needs. A knowledge user can be, but is not limited to, a practitioner, a policy maker, an educator, a decision maker, a health care administrator, a community leader or an individual in a health charity, patient group, private sector organization or media outlet."	Canadian Institutes of Health Research (2020)
Research utilization	"That process by which specific research-based knowledge (science) is implemented in practice."	Estabrooks et al. (2003)
Translation research	The process of turning observations in the laboratory, clinic, and community into interventions that improve the health of individuals and the public—from diagnostics and therapeutics to medical procedures and behavioral changes.	National Center for Advancing Translational Sciences (2018)

and *knowledge transfer* may be used interchangeably, and the reader must determine the exact meaning from the content of the article. As implementation science progresses, there is increased emphasis on the dynamic nature of knowledge translation and that it involves reciprocal, bidirectional interaction among knowledge creators, translators, and users.

The interchange of terms leads to confusion about how implementation research fits into the broader picture of conduct and use of research. One way to understand this relationship is to compare implementation research and the commonly used scientific terms for the steps of scientific discovery: basic research, methods development, efficacy trials, effectiveness trials, and dissemination trials (Sussman et al., 2006). For example, the term *translation* denotes the idea of moving something from one form to another. The National Institutes of Health (NIH) used this term to describe the process of moving basic research knowledge that may be directly or indirectly relevant to health behavior changes into a form that eventually has impact on patient outcomes (National Center for Advancing Translational Sciences [NCATS], 2018). The NIH built a "roadmap" that identified two gaps in translation. The first exists between discovery of biochemical and physiological mechanisms learned at the bench and the second between the bench and development of better diagnostic and treatment solutions (Zerhouni, 2003). Westfall et al. (2007) suggested that the gap between bench and human trials be identified as "T1" and that the research designs that best fit discovery would be phase 1 and phase 2 clinical trials as well as case series. They named the gap between human clinical research and clinical practice "T2" and recommended that this type of translational research needs to go beyond traditional effectiveness trials (phase 3) to more pragmatic approaches or "practice-based research." They further identified T3 as the next gap requiring effective dissemination and uptake through synthesis, guideline development, and implementation research in order to achieve the goal of moving knowledge into routine practices, systems, and policies. Finally, T4 research has emerged to evaluate the impact of implementing discovery in populations (Brownson et al., 2012). Since this ground-breaking work, the movement and translation knowledge from research is thought of being highly dynamic, with multiple opportunities for data gathering and analysis, dissemination, and interactions among phases (IOM, 2013; NCATS, 2018). As we learn more about the complexities of moving and bridging the "know–do" gap, undoubtedly the science and underpinning language and theory will grow. Rabin and Brownson (2012) provided a summary of terms used in what they call "dissemination and implementation" activities as one reference guide to emerging terminology. Building a common taxonomy of terms in implementation science is of primary importance to this field and must involve input from a variety of stakeholders and researchers from various disciplines (e.g., healthcare, organizational science, psychology, and health services research; IOM, 2007b).

■ IMPLEMENTATION MODELS

EBP models began to emerge in the nursing literature as focus shifted from research utilization to broader concepts. These earlier models guided the overall process of EBP (Rosswurm & Larrabee, 1999; Stetler, 2001; Titler et al., 2001). They include implementation as a concept and the process reflected a problem-solving process much like the nursing process, including identifying clinical problems, collecting and analyzing evidence, making the decision to use the evidence to change practice, and evaluating the change after implementation. But little detail and/or guidance was provided regarding the actual process or "how" of implementation. Users of these models were told to simply "implement," a directive that fails to take into account the complexity of the process of implementation. Implementing and sustaining change is a complex and multifaceted process, requiring attention to both individual and organizational factors (Grimshaw et al., 2012).

Many experts believe that using a model specifically focused on implementation provides a framework or mental map for identifying factors that may be pertinent in different settings or circumstances, and allows for testing and comparing tailored strategies for individual settings. The hope is this will allow for some generalization of results (Esmail et al., 2020; Kirk et al., 2016). Although no single model may apply to all situations, an effective model must be sufficiently specific to guide both implementation research and implementation at the point of care but general enough to cross various populations. Birken et al. (2017) surveyed implementation scientists to determine what factors influenced their choice of theory to guide their implementation studies. Two hundred twenty-three implementation scientists from 12 countries responded to the survey. The investigators found that this group used 100 different theories. The factors that most influenced their choice were: analytic level (i.e., individual, organization, system); logical consistency and plausibility (e.g., relationships that reflected face-validity); empirical support; and description of a change process. They concluded that implementation scientists vary greatly in the way they make decisions on how to select a theoretical approach and that investigators often use theories rather superficially, not at all, or even misuse them. Therefore, they recommended that implementation scientists represent their reasons for their selection of theory more transparently. In 2018, Birken et al. developed a tool called T-CaST (Implementation Theory Comparison and Selection Tool) to guide selection using 16 specific criteria in four domains: applicability, usability, testability and acceptability (online access is available at impsci.tracs.unc.edu/tcast).

Several attempts have been made to search for and organize the multitude of theories, models, and frameworks that are used to promote changes in practice or behavior. Just as the terms for implementation science are often used interchangeably, although technically they are not the same, the terms *conceptual frameworks/models* and *theoretical frameworks/models* are often used interchangeably, although they differ in their level of abstraction (Nilsen, 2015; Titler, 2018). In this discussion, the term *model* will be used as a general term, unless the model is specifically identified as a theory or conceptual framework by its creator. A model, then, for our purposes, is a set of general concepts and propositions that are integrated into a meaningful configuration to represent how a particular theorist views the phenomena of interest, in this case the implementation of evidence into practice (Fawcett, 2005).

Although an extensive review of all models suggested for possible use in implementation science is beyond the scope of this chapter, several promising models are discussed in some detail. For a summary of additional models, see the review by Grol et al. (2007) who reviewed a wide variety of models relevant to quality improvement and the implementation of change in healthcare. Bucknall and Rycroft-Malone's (2010) monograph focused on models highly relevant to nursing practice. Tabak et al. (2012) reviewed 61 different models and most recently Nilsen (2015) analyzed and categorized existing implementation theories, models, and frameworks according to their purposes and aims and proposed a taxonomy to allow analysis and differentiation of models, frameworks and theories relevant to implementation science.

In this chapter, one theory and two frameworks will be reviewed. The first, Rogers's Diffusion of Innovation Theory, is ubiquitously present across disciplines and incorporated in many other models and frameworks. The second, the Promoting Action on Research Implementation in Health Services (PARIHS) and its successor, the Integrated PARIHS (i-PARIHS) was selected because of its usability and ease of adaptation to nursing practice. Finally, the Consolidated Framework for Implementation Research (CFIR) was chosen as it is a meta-synthesis of many models and structures the what, where, who, and how of implementation while pointing its users to specific implementation strategies. All three of these approaches recognize that implementation is complex, nonlinear and ultimately messy.

■ DIFFUSION OF INNOVATIONS

Probably the most well-known and frequently used theory for guiding change in practice is Everett Rogers's (2003) Diffusion of Innovations Theory. In the theory, he proposed that the rate of adoption of an innovation is influenced by the nature of the innovation, the manner in which the innovation is communicated, and the characteristics of the users and the social system into which the innovation is introduced. Rogers's theory has undergone empirical testing in a variety of different disciplines (Barta, 1995; Feldman & McDonald, 2004; Greenhalgh et al., 2004; Lia-Hoagberg et al., 1999; Michel & Sneed, 1995; Rogers, 2003; Wiecha et al., 2004).

According to Rogers (2003), an innovation can be used to describe any idea or practice that is perceived as new by an individual or organization; evidence-based healthcare practices are considered an innovation according to this theory. Rogers acknowledges the complex, nonlinear interrelationships among organizational and individual factors as people move through five stages when adopting an innovation: knowledge/awareness, persuasion, decision, implementation, and evaluation, and focuses on characteristics of the innovation such as relative advantage, compatibility, complexity, trialability, and observability that influence the probability of change. These elements are incorporated in many other models and frameworks, including i-PARIHS and the CFIR among many others.

The PARIHS/i-PARIHS Framework

The PARIHS framework is a promising model proposed to help practitioners understand and guide the implementation process. The originating authors began to develop the framework inductively in 1998 as a result of work with clinicians to improve practice. Subsequently, the framework has undergone concept analysis and has been used as a guide for structuring research and implementation projects at the point of care (Ellis et al., 2005; Wallin et al., 2005, 2006), evaluation (Kitson et al., 2008), and further development of the role of facilitation (Harvey & Kitson, 2015). This framework proposes that implementation is a function of the relationship among the nature and strength of the evidence, the contextual factors of the setting, and the method of facilitation used to introduce the change. Kitson and colleagues suggested that the model may be best used as part of a two-stage process: First, the practitioner uses the model to perform a preliminary evaluation measure of the elements of the evidence and the context, and, second, the practitioner uses the data from the analysis to determine the best method to facilitate change. In 2008, Kitson et al. evaluated the progress of the framework's development and recognized that while evidence supported the conceptual integrity, face, and content validity, further work remained. Subsequently, Helfrich et al. (2010) synthesized 24 published papers; they identified that investigators most commonly used the framework as a heuristic guide and recommended more prospective implementation studies that would clarify the relationship among the major subconcepts and implementation strategies. Since their synthesis, 40 papers on the model have been published but few included prospective application.

Based on this evaluative work, Harvey and Kitson (2015) developed a guide for facilitation that revisits the model based on the prior evaluative findings. They call the revised framework "i-PARIHS" with a shift in focus on innovation and its characteristics (see Rogers's attributes) where available research evidence informs the innovation. They have expanded upon the notion of context to include inner (the immediate setting such as the unit or clinic) and outer (the wider health system including the policies and regulatory systems) settings. The revision also refocuses on facilitation as the "active ingredient" rather than one of the elements of implementation. In addition, successful implementation is conceptualized more broadly to include achievement of the goals, the uptake, and the embedding of the innovation in practice; stakeholders are engaged and motivated to own the innovation, and variation across settings is minimized (Harvey & Kitson, 2015). Thus, they have revised the formula: $SI = Fac^n (I + R+ C)$ where SI is successful implementation, Fac^n is facilitation, I is innovation, R is recipients, and C is context. They include Rogers's characteristics of the innovation as part of what needs to be considered in implementation. They added the construct of recipients, the targets of the implementation after feedback from the model's users and reviewers, and define characteristics such as the motivation, values and beliefs, skills, knowledge, and so forth. Finally, the active ingredient—facilitation—includes both role and strategies. See Harvey and Kitson (2015) for a complete explanation of the framework as well as application cases. Since the updated framework's publication in 2015, there have been 68 citations in the database Scopus identifying the use of PARIHS or i-PARIHS, but most referred to the original model.

Strengths of the model include an explicit recognition that implementation is nonlinear and complex; the framework provides a pragmatic map to make sense of the inherent complexity and the design of tools and methods to diagnose and design interventions. In addition, users can flex the facilitation process to the level of evidence and the level of context support available, making it adaptable to various situations.

Consolidated Framework for Implementation Research (CFIR)

In 2009, Damshroder et al. recognized that the plethora of models, frameworks, and theories was potentially hindering development of a coherent approach to conducting implementation research and the use of this knowledge. They conducted a broad review of theories used to guide implementation. The outcome was a meta-theoretical synthesis from 19 commonly cited implementation models to net a structure of constructs from existing theories. While they organized these constructs into a schema, they did not attempt to depict interrelationships or generate hypotheses. Instead, they aimed to produce a common language and comprehensive set of constructs that researchers use as "building blocks" to generate testable models and hypotheses using this common structure.

The CFIR is composed of five domains that include the intervention, inner and outer settings, the people involved, and the process of implementation (Damschroder et al., 2009). Taking some liberty to simplify, the framework is organized by the "what" (intervention and its characteristics), "where" (inner and outer settings or context), "who" (individuals involved and their characteristics), and the "how" (the process of implementation). Within these domains, they further defined constructs (Table 16.2). (The definitions of each in construct can be found in the electronic supplements to Damschroder et al's original article.)

A decade after the CFIR was published, Kirk et al. (2016) conducted a systematic review of studies that used the CFIR to determine how it has been used and its impact on implementation science. They found that investigators cited the framework in 429 publications but they excluded nearly 83% of them because the researchers did not use the model in a meaningful manner (incorporating the framework in the methods and reporting of the findings). The remaining 26 studies used the framework to varying degrees of depth with the majority using it to guide data analysis.

■ IMPLEMENTATION STRATEGIES

When implementing EBP, as previously stated, it is helpful to use a model to provide structure and guidance in targeting interventions to increase the rate of adoption. Fundamentally, the questions that any implementation model or framework must address is: What is to be implemented? To and by whom should the knowledge be translated? Where should it be translated? How should it

TABLE 16.2 Consolidated Framework for Implementation Research Elements

DOMAIN	CONSTRUCTS
Intervention characteristics	• Intervention source, evidence strength, and quality • Relative advantage • Adaptability • Trialability • Complexity • Design quality and packaging • Cost
Outer setting	• Patient needs and resources • Cosmopolitanism • Peer pressure • External policy and incentives

Inner setting	• Structural characteristics
	• Networks and communication
	• Culture
	• Implementation climate
	  ◦ Tension for change
	  ◦ Compatibility
	  ◦ Relative priority
	  ◦ Organizational incentives and rewards
	  ◦ Goals and feedback
	  ◦ Learning climate
	• Readiness for implementation
	  ◦ Leadership engagement
	  ◦ Available resources
	  ◦ Access to knowledge and information

Characteristics of the individual	• Knowledge and beliefs about the intervention • Self-efficacy • Individual stage of change • Individual identification with the organization • Other personal attributes

Process	• Planning
	• Engaging
	  ◦ Opinion leaders
	  ◦ Formally appointed internal implementation leaders
	  ◦ Champions
	  ◦ External change agents
	• Executing
	• Reflecting and evaluating

Source: Adapted from Damschroder, L. J., Aron, D. C., Keith, R. E., Kirsh, S. R., Alexander, J. A., & Lowery, J. C. (2009). Fostering implementation of health services research findings into practice: A consolidated framework for advancing implementation science. *Implementation Science, 4*, 50. https://doi.org/10.1186/1748-5908-4-50

be translated? To what effect? (Damschroder et al., 2009; Grimshaw et al., 2012; Harvey & Kitson, 2015). As recently as 2011, the IOM (now the National Academy of Medicine) recommended using multifaceted strategies (IOM, 2011). However, Squires et al. (2014) conducted an overview of 25 systematic reviews that compared a single component to multi-faceted (two or more) components and they failed to find that multifaceted strategies were superior to single strategies. Nonetheless, multiple factors (e.g., the context, individuals, the intervention, types of barriers and facilitators) may necessitate selecting more than one strategy.

Innovation: The "What"

If an innovation is to be "evidence-based," it should be based on the best available evidence. "Available" implies that an exhaustive search has revealed all the evidence that exists and "best" implies that someone has appraised the evidence and judiciously selected it as the most valid and reliable information. Grimshaw et al. (2012) wrote, "the basic unit of knowledge translation should be up-to-date systematic reviews or other syntheses of global evidence" (p. 3). They based their argument on the work of Ioannidis and colleagues who found that studies of particular treatments or associations showed larger, sometimes extravagant effect size in the initial trials that diminished with replications (Grimshaw et al., 2012).

Even when ideal evidence exists, the nature or characteristics of the EBP influence the rate of adoption. However, the attributes of an evidence-based healthcare practice as perceived by the users and stakeholders are not stable but change depending on the interaction between the users and the context of practice (Damschroder et al., 2009; Harvey & Kitson, 2015). For example, an identical guideline for improving pain management may be viewed as pertinent and not complex by users in one setting (e.g., labor and delivery) but as less of a priority and as difficult to implement by staff in another unit (e.g., geropsychiatry). Although a positive perception of the EBP alone is not sufficient to ensure adoption, it is important that the information be perceived as pertinent and presented in a way that is credible and easy to understand (Greenhalgh et al., 2004, 2005; Harvey & Kitson, 2015). Some characteristics of the innovation known to influence the rate of adoption are the complexity or simplicity of the evidence-based healthcare practice, the credibility and pertinence of the evidence-based healthcare practice to the user, and the ease or difficulty of assimilating the change into existing behavior (Harvey & Kitson, 2015; Rogers, 2003). However, although these characteristics are important, the adopter's decision to use and sustain an EBP is complex. This is evident in the continued failure to achieve a consistent high rate of adherence to handwashing recommendations in spite of the relative simplicity of the process and the knowledge of its pertinence to optimal patient outcomes. EBP guidelines are one tested method of presenting information (Flodgren et al., 2016; Grimshaw et al., 2004; Guihan et al., 2004; IOM, 2011). EBP guidelines are designed to assimilate large, complex amounts of research information into a usable format (Grimshaw et al., 2004; Lia-Hoagberg et al., 1999) and are ideally based on a synthesis of systematic reviews (Grimshaw et al., 2012; IOM, 2008). Appropriately designed guidelines are adaptable and easy to assimilate into the local setting. Empirically tested methods of adapting guidelines and protocols to the local practice setting include practice prompts, quick reference guides, decision-making algorithms, computer-based decision support systems, and patient-mediated interventions (Eccles & Grimshaw, 2004; Feldman et al., 2005; Fønhus et al., 2018; Grimshaw, Eccles, Thomas, et al., 2006; Wensing et al., 2006). Flodgren et al. (2016) conducted a systematic review of the effect of tools developed and disseminated to accompany a practice guideline. While this science is young and the studies were too heterogeneous to conduct a meta-analysis, tools such as paper-based education targeting barriers to uptake, reminders, and order forms improved adherence to the guideline.

Communication: To Whom and By Whom and How?

The method and the channels used to communicate with potential users about an innovation influence the speed and extent of adoption of the innovation (Manojlovich et al., 2015; Rogers, 2003). Communication channels include both formal methods of communication that are established in the hierarchical system and informal communication networks that occur spontaneously throughout the system. Communication networks are interconnected individuals who are linked by patterned flows of information (Rogers, 2003). Manojlovich et al. (2015) make the argument that communication should be viewed as transformational and able to cause change in the context of implementation rather than viewed simply as transactional.

Mass media communication methods are effective in raising awareness at the population or community level; for example, of public health issues such as the need for immunizations and screenings and include the use of television, radio, newspapers, pamphlets, posters, and leaflets (Bala et al., 2017; Carson-Chahhoud et al., 2017; see also Grilli et al., 2002; Rogers, 2003). Many acute care EBP implementation projects also use awareness campaigns in the early stages that may include similar strategies (e.g., bulletin boards, flyers, posters, and newsletters). Although research has been done on the effectiveness of mass media campaigns at the population level to guide message content and delivery to the general public (Bala et al., 2017; Carson-Chahhoud et al., 2017; Grilli et al., 2002; Randolph & Viswanath, 2004), less evidence is available to guide the message content or delivery methods needed to affect the rate of adoption of EBP among healthcare workers and in varying levels of wealth world-wide.

Rogers (2003) would predict that interpersonal communication is more effective than mass media communication in persuading people to change practice. Communication strategies tested in healthcare systems that use interpersonal communication channels include education (Forsetlund et al., 2009; see also Davis et al., 1995); opinion leaders (Anderson & Titler, 2014; Flodgren et al., 2019; see also Locock et al., 2001); change champions (Guihan et al., 2004; Kaasalainen et al., 2015); facilitators (Harvey & Kitson, 2015; Kitson et al., 1998; Stetler et al., 2006); audit and feedback (Grimshaw et al., 2004; Hysong et al., 2006; Ivers et al., 2012; Landis-Lewis et al., 2020); and outreach consultation and education by experts (Bero et al., 1998; Davis et al., 1995; Feldman & McDonald, 2004; Hysong et al., 2006; O'Brien et al., 2007).

The literature indicates that education using didactic teaching strategies or traditional dispersion of printed educational material and formal conference presentations may increase awareness but has little impact on changing practice (Giguère et al., 2012). Interactive teaching methods, especially when combined with other methods, are generally more effective (Bero et al., 1998; Forsetlund et al., 2009; O'Brien et al., 2007). Educational strategies that lead to improvement in EBP adherence include educational meetings with an interactive component, small-group educational meetings (which are more effective than large-group meetings), and educational meetings that include an opportunity to practice skills (Forsetlund et al., 2009).

Local opinion leaders are informal leaders from the local peer group who are viewed as respected sources of information and judgment regarding the appropriateness of the innovation (Anderson & Titler, 2014; Effective Practice and Organisation of Care [EPOC], 2015). They are trusted to evaluate new information and to determine the appropriateness of the innovation for the setting. Opinion leaders have been effective in promoting the practitioner uptake of an EBP (Flodgren et al., 2019) alone or in combination with other strategies such as outreach and performance feedback (Flodgren et al., 2019; see also Dopson et al., 2002; Forsetlund et al., 2009; Locock et al., 2001). However, the impact on patient outcomes remains unclear (Flodgren et al., 2019). In addition, while the effects of opinion leaders in natural settings have been well documented, selecting and engaging opinion leaders for specific projects is complex (Flodgren et al., 2019; Greenhalgh et al., 2004; Grimshaw, Eccles, Greener, et al., 2006). For changes in practice that involve multiple disciplines, opinion leaders should be selected from each of the various disciplines involved. These opinion leaders must be respected members of their group—competent, knowledgeable, and enthusiastic about the innovation, and able to understand how the new practice fits with the group norms (Collins et al., 2000; Grimshaw et al., 2012). Opinion leaders thought of as change champions are expert practitioners from the local peer group who promote the use of the innovation (Rogers, 2003). Change champions can be nurses who provide information and encouragement, are persistent, and have positive working relationships with their colleagues. Advanced practice nurses (nurse practitioners and clinical nurse specialists) have been effective while using a variety of implementation strategies such as audit and feedback, educational outreach, reminders, and a variety of interpersonal communication techniques to improve uptake of pain management guidelines (Kaasalainen et al., 2015). The use of change champions has been shown to be effective in other settings (Estabrooks et al., 2003; Rycroft-Malone et al., 2004). Research suggests that nurses prefer interpersonal communication with peers rather than other sources of information, so the presence of a change champion may be crucial in facilitating the adoption of the innovation (Adams & Barron, 2009; Estabrooks et al., 2005; Estabrooks, O'Leary, et al., 2003).

Using a core group or team that has the same goal of promoting EBP, along with the change champion, increases the likelihood of obtaining the critical mass of users necessary to promote and sustain the adoption of the practice change (Dopson et al., 2002; Nelson et al., 2002; Rogers, 2003; Titler, 2006). Practical advice includes having members of the core group represent the various shifts and days of the week to assume responsibility for providing information, daily reinforcement of the change, and positive feedback to their peers.

Educational outreach, also called academic detailing, is one-on-one communication between an external topic expert and healthcare practitioners in their practice setting to provide information on the practice change. The expert should be knowledgeable about the research base for the EBP change and able to respond to questions and concerns that arise during implementation. Feedback on performance and/or education may be provided at that time. When used alone or in combination with other strategies, outreach has impact on the adoption of EBP (Feldman & McDonald, 2004; Nkansah et al., 2010; O'Brien et al., 2007).

A related concept is the facilitator role identified as an essential component in the original PARiHS model of translation of EBP (Harvey et al., 2002) and reenvisioned as the "active ingredient" in the i-PARIHS model. The facilitator role is flexible and fluid and adaptive to the context. It may range from task-focused activities (e.g., outreach and academic detailing) to holistic interactions designed to enable individuals, teams, and organizations to change practice (Harvey et al., 2002; Kitson et al., 1998; Stetler et al., 2006). The facilitator may be internal to the organization or external to the organization, and facilitation may encompass more than one individual (both internal and external), in contrast to outreach, which is typically external to the organization (Greenhalgh et al., 2005; Stetler et al., 2006). A full discussion of facilitation as an active ingredient in i-PARIHS is beyond the scope of this chapter; see Harvey and Kitson's publication (2015) to learn more about building the knowledge and skills for effective facilitation.

Knowledge brokers are another type of agent of change that share many of the roles of a facilitator or linker. Bornbaum et al. (2015) conducted a systematic review to classify the function of knowledge brokers and to examine their effectiveness in translating knowledge into practice. While they found 29 studies, only two examine effectiveness, so they were unable to determine the impact of knowledge brokers. However, they identified 10 categories of activities across three domains: knowledge management, linkage and exchange, and capacity building. Future research will focus on the effectiveness of knowledge broker roles and activities.

Several studies have analyzed attitudes and characteristics that influence adoption of EBP by individual users (Estabrooks et al., 2003; Jun et al., 2015; Milner et al., 2006; Squires et al., 2011). Characteristics such as favorable attitude toward research and previous involvement in research studies are consistently associated with use of research findings in practice (Squires et al., 2011; see also Estabrooks, Floyd, et al., 2003). Additional characteristics such as educational level, professional role (e.g., management vs. staff nurse), autonomy, conference attendance, cooperativeness and self-efficacy, job satisfaction, professional association membership, and time spent reading professional journals may influence a user's readiness to adopt EBP, but the findings are not consistent across various studies (Estabrooks, 1999; Hutchinson & Johnston, 2004; Jun et al., 2015; McKenna et al., 2004; Milner et al., 2006; Squires et al., 2014).

Implementation strategies targeted at the individual user include audit and feedback and gap analysis. Gap analysis and audit and feedback have consistently shown positive affects on changing the practice behavior of providers (Hysong et al., 2006; Ivers et al., 2012). An audit and analysis of practice gaps provide *baseline* performance data specific to the EBPs being implemented (e.g., pain assessment and fall rates) prior to the implementation process (Ivers et al., 2012), accompanied by a discussion about the gap between current practices and the desired EBPs. For example, investigators who were testing the effectiveness of a translating-research-into-practice intervention for acute pain management in older adults met with physicians and nurses at each experimental site at the beginning of the implementation process to review indicators of acute pain management (e.g., avoid meperidine prescription) specific to their setting and to discuss gaps between current practices and recommended EBPs in areas such as frequency of pain assessment, dosing of opioids, and around-the-clock administration of analgesics (Titler et al., 2009). Audit and feedback follow and consist of ongoing audit of performance indicators specific to the EBP being implemented (e.g., pain assessment practices or fall prevention practices and fall rates), followed by presentation and discussion of the data with key stakeholders. Although these strategies show a consistently positive effect on adoption of EBPs, the effect size varies among studies. Greater effectiveness is associated with additional factors such as low baseline compliance and increased intensity of the feedback (Bero et al., 1998; Davis et al., 1995; Grimshaw et al., 2004; Hysong et al., 2006; Ivers et al., 2012). Organizations with a successful record of EBP guideline adherence provide nonpunitive, individualized feedback in a timely manner throughout the implementation process (Hysong et al., 2006). Feedback is more effective when it comes from a supervisor or colleague, is offered more than once in both verbal and written formats, and includes an action plan aimed at particular targets and offered at least monthly (Hysong et al., 2006; Ivers et al., 2012). Providing individual feedback, as opposed to unit or facility-level feedback, is also associated with better adherence to EBP guidelines. Offering positive feedback, in addition to pointing out areas where the practitioner can improve performance, provides better results than providing feedback only when staff members fall short of optimal performance (Hysong et al., 2006). Recently, Landis-Lewis et al. (2020) described a three-stage approach to designing feedback while engaging the user in an iterative process to maximize the usability and impact of the feedback. Their work emphasizes that recipients' and users' need to be part of the implementation process. They developed prototypical feedback displays first with paper designs and then in electronic displays. Further research is indicated to determine the return on the investment of the time and resources required to develop this type of feedback system but it holds the promise of integrating the needs of the users with the process of implementation.

Settings and Context

The social system or context of care delivery influences adoption of an innovation (Damschroder et al., 2009; Duffy et al., 2015; Fraser, 2004a, 2004b; Harvey & Kitson, 2015; IOM, 2001; Kirk et al., 2015; Rogers, 2003). However, multiple definitions and conceptualizations of social setting or context create a lack of clarity in how to address this element of the implementation puzzle.

To date, much of implementation research has focused on acute and primary care. However, healthcare is delivered in a wide variety of healthcare delivery systems, including occupational settings, school settings, long-term care and assisted-living facilities, and homes and community settings through public health and home healthcare agencies. These settings have obvious differences because of their unique nature, but, even within similar settings, each organization has its own culture that may or may not support EBP. This is a result of the interaction of individuals through communication channels and social networks within the organizational structure and hierarchy, as well as interaction with the larger community as a whole. It is important to remember that the resulting social system is unique to each setting and is complex and dynamic (Damschroder et al., 2009; Garside, 1998; Greenhalgh et al., 2005; Scott et al., 2003a, 2003b).

When choosing strategies to increase adoption of EBP, it is necessary to focus on both the organizational structures, the individual adopters within the social system, and their interactions. For example, requiring a change in pain assessment frequency by individual caregivers but not providing the accompanying organizational changes (appropriate forms, changes in the electronic charting system, and inclusion of the new standards in performance evaluations) is shortsighted and reduces the likelihood that the change will be sustained in practice.

There are several structural characteristics that are consistently associated with increased use of EBP, such as size, slack resources, and urbanicity. Organizations that are larger in size and divided into differentiated and specialized semiautonomous units are associated with innovativeness. Slack resources (i.e., uncommitted resources) are associated with larger organizations and may be partially responsible for the impact of organization size on adoption rates. Larger organizations may have more resources available, both financial and human, to support EBP in practice. Clinical agencies that partner with academic institutions who lend an embedded expert may have improved knowledge of frontline nurses and may improve uptake over time if these relationships can be sustained (Duffy et al., 2016). Urbanicity provides organizations with access to more interpersonal and mass media channels, access to resources and education opportunities, exposure to new ideas, and contact with other innovative organizations (Damschroder et al., 2009; Greenhalgh et al., 2005; Rogers, 2003).

There is no question that leadership at all levels in the organization is critical to adoption of EBP. The leader defines and communicates the organization's goals and vision (Harvey et al., 2019; IOM, 2001; Warren et al., 2016). Most early studies focused on measurable characteristics such as educational background and tenure of individuals holding key leadership positions (Greenhalgh et al., 2005). Melnyk et al. (2016) surveyed chief nurse executives in the United States. While they valued EBP as important to achieve high-quality care, one quarter of them were unsure of the steps of the process, three fourths reported committing only 0% to 10% of their annual operating budgets to growing and sustaining EBP in their institutions, and 60% reported that EBP was practiced not at all or very little in their organizations. Yet their top priorities were quality and safety. Clearly, this represents a disconnect between how nurse executives linked quality and safety to EBP, and how they resourced the endeavor.

The wider contribution of leadership is harder to explicitly measure but includes efforts in areas such as promoting a climate that facilitates adoption, which can include communication style, providing a nonpunitive environment for risk taking, providing resources for EBP projects, providing time for research activities, and promoting a learning environment (Greenhalgh et al., 2005; Melnyk et al., 2016). Frontline managers can serve as the linker between the organizational level support for uptake of evidence and individual nurses through facilitating roles such as mentoring, collaborating, translating, role modeling, and providing a learning environment (Harvey et al., 2019; Matthew-Maich et al., 2014). Other influences of leadership include setting role expectations that include the use of research in practice, providing role clarity, and supporting democratic and inclusive decision-making processes (Bradley, Webster et al., 2004; IOM, 2001; McCormack et al., 2002; Meijers et al., 2006). Based on a scoping review, some of the science is ready for synthesis but other areas need further development to understand what strategies enhance nurses' knowledge, skills, and attitudes for using evidence in their decision-making in tertiary settings (Yost et al., 2014). However, more targeted research needs to be done on specific leadership strategies at the unit manager level that may impact the adoption of EBP.

Additional strategies are (a) the use of multidisciplinary teams, especially in the care of chronic illnesses, and (b) the revising of professional roles. Both strategies have been effective in improving patient outcomes through better adherence to recommended EBP guidelines and also have resulted in reduced healthcare costs (Wensing et al., 2006). The use of multidisciplinary teams seeks to improve communication and cooperation between professional groups (e.g., physicians and nurses) and also to streamline services (Zwarenstein & Reeves, 2006). However, all teams are not created equal, and measuring the characteristics of teams that improve patient outcomes is difficult. Some characteristics of high-functioning teams that show positive impact on patient care include team composition; stability; collaboration; time allotted for the various tasks; explicit, appropriate task and role definitions; and having a team leader (Schouten et al., 2008). A related strategy, revision of professional roles (e.g., reassigning prevention interventions to nonphysician staff, such as nurses), has also resulted in improved patient outcomes through better adherence to EBP guidelines (Zwarenstein & Reeves, 2006). Since these groundbreaking studies were completed, Reeves et al. (2017) completed a systematic review to understand the impact of different types of interventions designed to increase interprofessional collaboration on patient outcomes, efficiencies, and collaborative behaviors. They found that in nine studies with 6,540 participants, there were slight improvements in patient functional status, healthcare professionals' adherence to recommended practices and use of healthcare resources with externally facilitated interprofessional activities. However, there is too much uncertainty to determine how these techniques affected patient-assessed quality of care, continuity of care, or collaborative working behaviors. Interprofessional rounds and checklists had a slight impact to improve use of resources and interprofessional meetings may improve adherence to recommended practices and use of resources. The reviewers recommended further research focused on scaled-up interventions effectiveness, a wider range of interventions, and more focus on circumstances of the interventions.

Documentation systems for effective data recording aid in the implementation and sustainability of guidelines and protocols by providing appropriate forms for outcome measurement and information for quality-improvement programs (Garside, 1998; Greenhalgh et al., 2004; Wensing et al., 2006). In addition, access to computer technology can improve professional performance and client outcomes in two ways. First, use of data recording, patient record keeping, computer prompts, and reminders may increase adherence to EBP (Rappolt et al., 2005; Wensing & Grol, 1994; Wensing et al., 2006), even if the computer-generated reminders are delivered to the provider on paper (Arditi et al., 2017). Second, information systems, including computer technology, hold promise for better knowledge acquisition and management (Bradley, Holmboe, et al., 2004; Wensing et al., 2006). The IOM's 2001 report, *Crossing the Quality Chasm: A New Health System for the 21st Century*, stresses the importance of computerized information technology systems, but in order to take advantage of these systems, healthcare workers need not only access to the systems but the skills to use them (IOM, 2001). Organizations that provide needed resources and access to support for EBP, such as technology and sufficient training to allow staff to become proficient, libraries, research findings, computer databases, journals, time, and financial support for continuing education, and time for research participation and implementation, are more likely to implement and sustain EBP in practice (Bryar et al., 2003; Dopson et al., 2001; Duffy et al., 2015; Estabrooks, 2003; Estabrooks, O'Leary, et al., 2003; Meijers et al., 2006; Melnyk et al., 2016; Pravikoff et al., 2005).

Undoing or De-Implementation

Most of the discussion to date relates to improving the uptake of evidence and how best to improve outcomes through this uptake. Recently, the EBP community has begun to focus on how to undo or de-implement practices that hold no value, increase the cost of care or indeed may cause harm (Norton & Chambers, 2020; Prasad & Ioannidis, 2014). Similar to the implementation work, lack of consistency and clarity of definitions plagues this early field. In fact, Norton and Chambers (2020) identified 43 different terms for de-adoption, de-implementation, and another set of models. Like implementation, de-implementation is complex and multi-layered with similar "who" (providers, patients, etc.), "what" (intervention), "where" (context), "why" (impacts and outcomes) but perhaps different "how" (strategies) implications. These authors describe four different approaches to de-implementation: removing, replacing, reducing, or restricting the practice. The methods for accomplishing one of these modes of de-implementation may be similar or unique to what works for implementation. For example, in the past several years, efforts have been aimed at "reducing" when healthcare teams determined that indwelling catheters should only be used in a narrow set of circumstances (Gould et al., 2019). Norton and Chambers advise that, like implementation strategies, de-implementation strategies should be multi-level (aimed at leaders, stakeholders, systems, etc.) and tailored to specific contextual barriers and facilitators. Undoubtedly, research will progress this work as research protocols have begun to appear in the literature (Aron et al., 2014; Hasson et al., 2018; Sanchez et al., 2020) and some emerging reports (Voorn et al., 2017).

■ DESIGNING IMPLEMENTATION STUDIES

Non-governmental and governmental agencies have sponsored a variety of workshops with proceedings meant to guide the implementation research. For example, the IOM Forum on the Science of Quality Improvement and Implementation Research held several workshops on implementation science in which researchers have addressed various perspectives in conducting studies in this field (www.nap.edu). Given the complexity of implementation science and associated types of research questions, its methods vary from qualitative, phenomenological studies to randomized controlled trials (RCTs) and systematic reviews of the primary research. Links between generalizable scientific evidence for a given healthcare topic and specific contexts create opportunities for experiential learning in implementation science (IOM, 2007a). Given this perspective, qualitative methods may be used to better understand why specific implementation strategies work in some settings and not in others. For example, an investigator might ask why Centers for Medicare & Medicaid Services (CMS)-regulated EBPs for heart failure patients are adhered to in some hospitals and not others. A study designed to understand these differences might use qualitative approaches such as interviews with front-line staff, observation of clinical care delivery, and practitioner focus groups (Tripp-Reimer & Doebbeling, 2004). This qualitative study might generate hypotheses for future investigations as well as provide deep knowledge related to the subjective nature of decision-making choices. Such studies provide a sound basis for empirical studies on the effectiveness of implementation interventions.

Rigorous evaluations of implementation interventions provide a solid base of research that can be built upon. Much can be learned from empirical evaluation of naturally occurring adoption efforts such as the implementation of rapid-response teams in acute-care settings. Implementation studies that investigate natural experiments provide several benefits, including testing the relationships among various individual and system factors and the level of practice adoption. Understanding these factors and their relationships is important as one designs studies to test the effectiveness of implementation interventions. For example, Colquhoun et al. (2017) conducted a systematic review of methods used in studies designed to change individual providers behavior. They learned that there are four key "tasks" when anyone designs an intervention to change individual behaviors: identify barriers, select intervention components, use theory, and engage the end user. They were unable to find any definitive conclusions related to system-level intervention methods.

At the IOM workshops, Grimshaw discussed the disagreement in the field of implementation science regarding the use of RCTs to evaluate the effectiveness of implementation interventions (IOM, 2007a, 2007b). Debate continues as to the role of RCTs in complex social contexts such as the process of implementation of EBPs, although others believe RCTs to be an extremely valuable method of evaluating these interventions. Randomized trials of implementation interventions tend to be pragmatic and focus on effectiveness in order to elucidate whether an intervention will be effective in a real-world setting. Such RCTs, unlike RCTs that focus on efficacy (e.g., drug trials), have broad inclusion criteria and are designed to improve our understanding of both the influence of context on the effectiveness of the intervention and why changes occurred. One method of achieving this understanding is to use observational approaches in conjunction with data from the RCT to test multilevel hypotheses about which interventions work and which do not. RCTs build on the knowledge generated by observational studies and case studies (IOM, 2007a). The best method to evaluate a given intervention depends on the research question(s), hypotheses, and the specifics of the implementation intervention. One should always attempt to choose a mixture of the best possible methods, given the individual circumstances.

Building this body of research knowledge will require development in many areas. Theoretical developments are needed to provide frameworks and predictive theories that will lead to generalizable research such as studies on how to change individual and organizational behavior. Methodological developments are also required, as are exploratory studies aimed at improving our understanding of the experiential and organizational learning that accompanies implementation. Rigorous evaluations are needed to evaluate the effectiveness and efficiency of implementation interventions, and partnerships are needed to encourage communication among researchers, theorists, and implementers and to help researchers understand what types of knowledge are needed and how that knowledge can best be developed (Damschroder et al., 2009; Dawson, 2004; Proctor et al., 2013; Titler, 2004a, 2004b; Tripp-Reimer & Doebbeling, 2004). Finally, synthesis methodologies need to be further developed to accommodate complex interventions. But primary researchers need to specify their interventions using standardized language and deep description of the process in order for systematic reviewers to determine appropriateness of pooling data.

■ FUTURE DIRECTIONS

Although the evidence base for implementation strategies is growing, there is much work to be done. In 2003, the U.S. Invitational Conference "Advancing Quality Care Through Translation Research" convened, funded in part by the Agency for Healthcare Research and Quality's (1 R13

HS014141–01). The objective was to set forth a future research agenda for translation (or implementation) science. Seventy-seven participants representing 25 states and all geographic regions of the United States were selected to attend on the basis of their knowledge and skills in research, education, practice, and public policy; the goal was to advance a translation science agenda. The conference set forth an agenda that remains relevant today.

Conference participants recommended giving high priority to testing multifaceted, interdisciplinary implementation interventions in a variety of settings, and to designing multisite studies that increase understanding about what interventions work in similar types of settings (e.g., acute care) with different contextual factors. Priority was also given to comparing the effectiveness of implementation interventions in different types of clinical settings (e.g., acute vs. home health) to foster understanding of the components of the intervention that need modification depending on the type of setting. These implementation priorities are congruent with recommendations of others (Dopson et al., 2002; Greenhalgh et al., 2004; Grimshaw et al., 2004; Proctor et al., 2013).

A unique finding of the U.S. Invitational Conference was the call to prioritize research on (a) methods for engaging stakeholders to increase their support and (b) implementation of clinical topics for nursing practice based on existing guidelines and synthesis reports.

The conference attendees identified these recommended research priorities for implementation science:

- Test implementation strategies across different types and contexts of care delivery to determine which strategies are most effective for which type of healthcare setting and context.

- Test interdisciplinary approaches (e.g., physicians, nurses, and physical therapists) to implementation.

- Test combined or multiple implementation strategies such as education plus use of opinion leaders plus audit and feedback.

- Test various dissemination methods and implementation strategies such as electronic information technology, communication strategies, and facilitator roles.

- Determine best methods for engaging stakeholders to promote the use of evidence in practice.

- Focus on measurement and methodological issues encountered in translation science regarding process measures, outcome measures, intervention dose, core dependent measures (e.g., process vs. outcome measures), organizational context, nested designs, and qualitative methods.

- Investigate leadership and organizational context variables and measures that promote EBPs.

- Develop and test measures of organizational readiness for EBP.

- Determine ways to create practice cultures that facilitate change.

- Test organizational-level interventions that promote EBPs.

■ SUMMARY

The use of EBP remains sporadic in spite of a growing evidence base and the increasing availability of systematic reviews and predeveloped EBP guidelines. Implementation science provides a research focus for identifying effective strategies to increase the use of evidence-based programs, guidelines, and protocols in different settings and among different end users. Because this is a young science, standardized definitions have not been established. Commonly used terms were identified in this chapter, along with promising models to guide implementation at the point of care. The current evidence base for implementation strategies is growing and, although additional research is needed, there is sufficient evidence to warrant use of evidence-based strategies when implementing a change in practice.

SUGGESTED LEARNING ACTIVITIES

1. You are the nurse manager of an adult surgical inpatient unit (30 beds) at a 500-bed community hospital. Staff members are changing practice for assessment of bowel mobility following abdominal surgery. The practice change includes "giving up" listening for bowel sounds. Describe a de-implementation plan with specific strategies for making this change in practice.

2. You are the school nurse supervising other school nurses in a rural consolidated school district. This school district includes three high schools, five elementary schools, and four middle schools. There are nine school nurses: Two covering the high schools, two covering the middle schools, and five covering the elementary schools.

   a. Select a topic of interest to school nurses to promote the health of the population of students with a rationale for why this topic was selected.

   b. Identify evidence sources for each topic.

   c. Describe implementation strategies for the selected topics.

REFERENCES

Adams, S., & Barron, S. (2009). Use of evidence-based practice in school nursing: Prevalence, associated variables and perceived needs. *Worldviews on Evidence-Based Nursing, 6*(1), 16–26. https://doi.org/10.1111/j.1741-6787.2008.00141.x

Anderson, C. A., & Titler, M. (2014). Development and verification of an agent-based model of opinion leadership. *Implementation Science, 9,* Article 136 (2014). https://doi.org/10.1186/s13012-014-0136-6

Arditi, C., Rege-Walther, M., Durieux, P., & Burnand, B. (2017). Computer-generated reminders delivered on paper to healthcare professionals? Effects on professional practice and healthcare outcomes. *Cochrane Database of Systematic Reviews.* https://doi.org/10.1002/14651858.CD001175.pub4

Aron, D. C., Lowery, J., Tseng, C., Conlin, P., & Kahwati, L. (2014). De-implementation of inappropriately tight control (of hypoglycemia) for health protocol with an example of a research grant application. *Implementation Science, 9,* Article 58 (2004). https://doi.org/10.1186/1748-5908-9-58

Bala, M. M., Stzeszynski, L. & Topor-Madry, R. (2017). Mass media interventions for smoking cessation in adults. *Cochrane Database of Systematic Reviews.* https://doi.org/10.1002/14651858.CD004704.pub4

Barta, K. M. (1995). Information-seeking, research utilization, and barriers to research utilization of pediatric nurse educators. *Journal of Professional Nursing, 11*(1), 49–57. https://doi.org/10.1016/S8755-7223(95)80073-5

Bero, L. A., Grilli, R., Grimshaw, J. M., Harvey, E., Oxman, A. D., & Thomson, M. A. (1998). Closing the gap between research and practice: An overview of systematic reviews of interventions to promote the implementation of research findings. *British Medical Journal (Clinical Research Edition), 317*(7156), 465–468. https://doi.org/10.1136/bmj.317.7156.465

Birken, S. A., Powell, B. J., Shea, C. M., Haines, E. R., Kirk, M. A., Leeman, J., Rohweder, C., Damshroder, L., & Presseau, J. (2017). Criteria for selecting implementation science theories and frameworks: results from an international study. *Implementation Science, 12,* 124. https://doi.org/10.1186/s13012-017-0656-y

Birken, S., Rohweder, C. L., Powell, B. J., Shea, C. M., Scott, J., Leeman, J., Grewe, M. E., Kirk, M. A., Damschroder, L., Aldridge, W. A., Haines, E. R., Straus, S., & Presseau, J. (2018). T-CaST: An implementation theory comparison and selection tool. *Implementation Science, 13*, 143. https://doi.org/10.1186/s13012-018-0836-4

Bornbaum, C. C., Kornas, K., Peirson, L., & Rosella, L. C. (2015). Exploring the function and effectiveness of knowledge brokers as facilitators of knowledge translation in health-related settings: A systematic review and thematic analysis. *Implementation Science, 10*, 162. https://doi.org/10.1186/s13012-015-0351-9

Bradley, E. H., Holmboe, E. S., Mattera, J. A., Roumanis, S. A., Radford, M. J., & Krumholz, H. M. (2004). Data feedback efforts in quality improvement: Lessons learned from U.S. hospitals. *Quality & Safety in Health Care, 13*(1), 26–31. https://doi.org/10.1136/qhc.13.1.26

Bradley, E. H., Webster, T. R., Baker, D., Schlesinger, M., Inouye, S. K., Barth, M. C., Lapane, K. L., Lipson, D., Stone, R., & Koren, M. J. (2004). Translating research into practice: Speeding the adoption of innovative health care programs. *Issue Brief (Commonwealth Fund), 724*, 1–12.

Brownson, R. C., Colditz, G. A., & Proctor, E. K. (Eds.). (2012). *Dissemination and implementation research in health: Translating science to practice.* Oxford University Press.

Bryar, R. M., Closs, S. J., Baum, G., Cooke, J., Griffiths, J., Hostick, T., Kelly, S., Knight, S., Marshall, K., &.Thompson, D. R.; Yorkshire BARRIERS project. (2003). The Yorkshire BARRIERS project: Diagnostic analysis of barriers to research utilisation. *International Journal of Nursing Studies, 40*(1), 73–84. https://doi.org/10.1016/S0020-7489(02)00039-1

Campbell, J. M., Umapathysivam, K., Xue, Y., & Lockwood, C. (2015). Evidence-based practice point-of-care resources: A quantitative evaluation of quality, rigor, and content. *Worldviews on Evidence-Based Nursing, 12*(6), 313–327. https://doi.org/10.1111/wvn.12114

Canadian Institutes of Health Research. (2020). *Glossary of funding-related terms.* https://cihr-irsc.gc.ca/e/34190.html#k

Carson-Chahhoud, K. V., Ameer, F., Sayehmiri, K., Hnin, K., van Agteren, J. E. M., Sayehmiri, F., Brinn, M. P., Esterman, A. J., Chang, A. B., & Smith, B. J. (2017). Mass media interventions for preventing smoking in young people. *Cochrane Database of Systematic Reviews.* https://doi.org/10.1002/14651858.CD001006.pub3

Cochrane. (2020). *About us.* https://www-cochrane-org.pnw.idm.oclc.org/about-us

Collins, B. A., Hawks, J. W., & Davis, R. (2000). From theory to practice: Identifying authentic opinion leaders to improve care. *Managed Care (Langhorne, Pa.), 9*(7), 56–58, 61.

Colquhoun, H., Leeman, J., Michie, S., Lokker, C., Bragge, P., Hempel, S., McKibbon, A., Gjalt-Jorn, P., Stevens, K., Wilson, M. J., & Grimshaw, G. (2014). Towards a common terminology: A simplified framework of interventions to promote and integrate evidence into health practices, systems and policies. *Implementation Science, 9*, Article 781 (2014). https://doi.org/10.1186/1748-5908-9-51

Colquhoun, H. L., Squires, J. E., Kolehmainen, N., Fraser, C., & Grimshaw, J. (2017). Methods for designing interventions to change healthcare professionals' behavior: A systematic review. *Implementation Science, 12*, Article 30 (2017). https://doi.org/10.1186/s13012-017-0560-5

Damschroder, L. J., Aron, D. C., Keith, R. E., Kirsh, S. R., Alexander, J. A., & Lowery, J. C. (2009). Fostering implementation of health services research findings into practice: A consolidated framework for advancing implementation science. *Implementation Science, 4*, 50. https://doi.org/10.1186/1748-5908-4-50

Davis, D. A., Thomson, M. A., Oxman, A. D., & Haynes, R. B. (1995). Changing physician performance: A systematic review of the effect of continuing medical education strategies. *Journal of the American Medical Association, 274*(9), 700–705. https://doi.org/10.1001/jama.1995.03530090032018

Dawson, J. D. (2004). Quantitative analytical methods in translation research. *Worldviews on Evidence-Based Nursing, 1*(Suppl. 1), S60–S64. https://doi.org/10.1111/j.1524-475X.2004.04040.x

Dzau, V. J., McClellan, M., McGinnis, J. M. & Finkelman, E. (Eds). (2017). *Vital directions for health & health care: An initiative of the National Academy of Medicine.* National Academy of Medicine.

Department of Health and Human Services. (2018). *Dissemination and implementation research in health (R01).* Funding Opportunity Announcement. https://grants.nih.gov/grants/guide/pa-files/par-16-238.html

Dopson, S., FitzGerald, L., Ferlie, E., Gabbay, J., & Locock, L. (2002). No magic targets! Changing clinical practice to become more evidence based. *Health Care Management Review, 27*(3), 35–47. https://doi.org/10.1097/00004010-200207000-00005

Dopson, S., Locock, L., Chambers, D., & Gabbay, J. (2001). Implementation of evidence-based medicine: Evaluation of the Promoting Action on Clinical Effectiveness programme. *Journal of Health Services Research & Policy, 6*(1), 23–31. https://doi.org/10.1258/1355819011927161

Duffy, J. R., Culp, S., Sand-Jecklin, K., Stroupe, L., & Lucke-Wold, N. (2016). Nurses' research capacity, use of evidence, and research productivity in acute care. *Journal of Nursing Administration, 46,* 12–17. https://doi.org/10.1097/NNA.0000000000000287

Duffy, J. R., Culp, S., Yarberry, C., Stroupe, L., Sand-Jeckline, K., & Coburn, A. S. (2015). Nurses' research capacity and use of evidence in acute care: Baseline findings from a partnership study. *Journal of Nursing Administration, 45,* 158–164. https://doi.org/10.1097/NNA.0000000000000176

Eccles, M. P., & Grimshaw, J. M. (2004). Selecting, presenting and delivering clinical guidelines: Are there any "magic bullets"? *The Medical journal of Australia, 180*(6 Suppl), S52–S54. https://doi.org/10.5694/j.1326-5377.2004.tb05946.x

Effective Practice and Organisation of Care. (2015). *EPOC Taxonomy.* https://epoc.cochrane.org/epoc-taxonomy

Ellis, I., Howard, P., Larson, A., & Robertson, J. (2005). From workshop to work practice: An exploration of context and facilitation in the development of evidence-based practice. *Worldviews on Evidence-Based Nursing, 2*(2), 84–93. https://doi.org/10.1111/j.1741-6787.2005.04088.x

Esmail, R., Hanson, H. M., Holroyd-Leduc, J., Brown, S., Stifler, L., Straus, S. E., Niven, D. J., & Clement, F. M. (2020). A scoping review of full-spectrum knowledge translation theories, models and frameworks. *Implementation Science, 15,* Article 11 (2020). https://doi.org/10.1186/s13012-020-0964-5

Estabrooks, C. A. (1999). Modeling the individual determinants of research utilization. *Western Journal of Nursing Research, 21*(6), 758–772. https://doi.org/10.1177/01939459922044171

Estabrooks, C. A. (2003). Translating research into practice: Implications for organizations and administrators. *The Canadian Journal of Nursing Research, 35*(3), 53–68.

Estabrooks, C. A., Chong, H., Brigidear, K., & Profetto-McGrath, J. (2005). Profiling Canadian nurses' preferred knowledge sources for clinical practice. *The Canadian Journal of Nursing Research, 37*(2), 118–140.

Estabrooks, C. A., Floyd, J. A., Scott-Findlay, S., O'Leary, K. A., & Gushta, M. (2003). Individual determinants of research utilization: A systematic review. *Journal of Advanced Nursing, 43*(5), 506–520. https://doi.org/10.1046/j.1365-2648.2003.02748.x

Estabrooks, C. A., O'Leary, K. A., Ricker, K. L., & Humphrey, C. K. (2003). The Internet and access to evidence: How are nurses positioned? *Journal of Advanced Nursing, 42*(1), 73–81. https://doi.org/10.1046/j.1365-2648.2003.02581.x

Estabrooks, C. A., Wallin, L., & Milner, M. (2003). Measuring knowledge utilization in health care. *International Journal of Policy Analysis & Evaluation, 1,* 3–36.

Fawcett, J. (2005). *Contemporary nursing knowledge: Analysis and evaluation of nursing models and theories* (2nd ed.). F. A. Davis.

Feldman, P. H., & McDonald, M. V. (2004). Conducting translation research in the home care setting: Lessons from a just-in-time reminder study. *Worldviews on Evidence-Based Nursing, 1*(1), 49–59. https://doi.org/10.1111/j.1741-6787.2004.04007.x

Feldman, P. H., Murtaugh, C. M., Pezzin, L. E., McDonald, M. V., & Peng, T. R. (2005). Just-in-time evidence-based e-mail "reminders" in home health care: Impact on patient outcomes. *Health Services Research, 40*(3), 865–885. https://doi.org/10.1111/j.1475-6773.2005.00389.x

Flodgren, G., Hall A. M., Goulding, L., Eccles, M. P., Grimshaw, J. M., Leng, G. C., & Shepperd S. (2016). Tools developed and disseminated by guideline producers to promote the uptake of their guidelines. *Cochrane Database of Systematic Reviews.* https://doi.org/10.1002/14651858.CD010669.pub2

Flodgren, G., O'Brien, M. A., Parmelli, E., & Grimshaw, J. M. (2019). Local opinion leaders: Effects on professional practice and health care outcomes. *Cochrane Database of Systematic Reviews, 6.* https://doi.org/10.1002/14651858.CD000125.pub5

Fønhus, M. S., Dalsbø, T. K., Johansen, M., Fretheim, A., Skirbekk, H., & Flottorp, S. A. (2018). Patient-mediated interventions to improve professional practice. *Cochrane Database of Systematic Reviews.* https://doi.org/10.1002/14651858.CD012472.pub2

Forsetlund, L., Bjørndal, A., Rashidian, A., Jamtvedt, G., O'Brien, M. A, Wolf, F., Davis, D., Odgaard-Jensen, J., & Oxman, A. D. (2009). Continuing education meetings and workshops: Effects on professional practice and health care outcomes. *Cochrane Database of Systematic Reviews.* https://doi.org/10.1002/14651858.CD003030.pub2

Foy, R., Sales, A., Wensing, M., Aarons, G. A., Flottrop, S., Kent, B., Michie, S., O'Connor, D., Rogers, A., Sevdalis, N., Straus, S., & Wilson, P. (2015). Implementation Science: A reappraisal of our journal mission and scope. *Implementation Science, 10*(51). https://doi.org/10.1186/s13012-015-0240-2

Fraser, I. (2004a). Organizational research with impact: Working backwards. *Worldviews on Evidence-Based Nursing, 1*(Suppl. 1), S52–S59. https://doi.org/10.1111/j.1524-475X.2004.04044.x

Fraser, I. (2004b). Translation research: Where do we go from here? *Worldviews on Evidence-Based Nursing, 1(Suppl. 1)*, S78–S83. https://doi.org/10.1111/j.1524-475X.2004.04046.x

Garside, P. (1998). Organisational context for quality: Lessons from the fields of organisational development and change management. *Quality in Health Care, 7*(Suppl.), S8–S15.

Graham, I. D., Logan, J., Harrison, M. B., Straus, S. E., Tetroe, J., Caswell, W., & Robinson, N. (2006). Lost in knowledge translation: Time for a map? *The Journal of Continuing Education in the Health Professions, 26*(1), 13–24. https://doi.org/10.1002/chp.7

Greenhalgh, T., Robert, G., Bate, P., Macfarlane, F., & Kyriakidou, O. (2005). *Diffusion of innovations in health service organisations: A systematic literature review.* Blackwell.

Greenhalgh, T., Robert, G., Macfarlane, F., Bate, P., & Kyriakidou, O. (2004). Diffusion of innovations in service organizations: Systematic review and recommendations. *The Milbank Quarterly, 82*(4), 581–629. https://doi.org/10.1111/j.0887-378X.2004.00325.x

Giguère, A., Légaré, F., Grimshaw, J., Turcotte, S., Fiander, M., Grudniewicz, A., Makosso-Kallyth, S., Wolf, F. M., Farmer, A. P., & Gagnon, M. P. (2012). Printed educational materials: effects on professional practice and healthcare outcomes. *Cochrane Database of Systematic Reviews, 10.* https://doi.org/10.1002/14651858 .CD004398.pub3

Gould, C. V., Umscheid, C. A., Agarwal, R., Kuntz, G., Pegues, D. A., & the Healthcare Infection Control Practices Advisory Committee. (2019). *Guideline for prevention of catheter-associated urinary tract infections 2009.* Centers for Disease Control and Prevention. https://www.cdc.gov/infectioncontrol/guidelines/cauti

Grilli, R., Ramsay, C., & Minozzi, S. (2002). Mass media interventions: Effects on health services utilisation. *Cochrane Database of Systematic Reviews, 1,* CD000389. https://doi.org/10.1002/14651858.CD000389

Grimshaw, J. M., Eccles, M. P., Greener, J., Maclennan, G., Ibbotson, T., Kahan, J. P., & Sullivan, F. (2006). Is the involvement of opinion leaders in the implementation of research findings a feasible strategy? *Implementation Science, 1,* 3. https://doi.org/10.1186/1748-5908-1-3

Grimshaw, J. M., Eccles, M. P, Lavis, J. N., Hill, S. J., & Squires, J. E. (2012). Knowledge translation of research findings. *Implementation Science, 7,* 50. https://doi.org/10.1186/1748-5908-7-5

Grimshaw, J., Eccles, M., Thomas, R., MacLennan, G., Ramsay, C., Fraser, C., & Vale, L. (2006). Toward evidence-based quality improvement. Evidence (and its limitations) of the effectiveness of guideline dissemination and implementation strategies 1966-1998. *Journal of General Internal Medicine, 21*(Suppl. 2), S14–S20. https://doi.org/10.1007/s11606-006-0269-7

Grimshaw, J. M., Thomas, R. E., MacLennan, G., Fraser, C., Ramsay, C. R., Vale, L., Whitty, P., Eccles, M. P., Matowe, L., Shirran, L., Wensing, M., Dijkstra, R., & Donaldson, C. (2004). Effectiveness and efficiency of guideline dissemination and implementation strategies. *Health Technology Assessment (Winchester, England), 8*(6), iii–iv, 1. https://doi.org/10.3310/hta8060

Grol, R. P., Bosch, M. C., Hulscher, M. E., Eccles, M. P., & Wensing, M. (2007). Planning and studying improvement in patient care: The use of theoretical perspectives. *The Milbank Quarterly, 85*(1), 93–138. https://doi.org/10.1111/j.1468-0009.2007.00478.x

Guihan, M., Bosshart, H. T., & Nelson, A. (2004). Lessons learned in implementing SCI clinical practice guidelines. *SCI Nursing, 21*(3), 136–142.

Harvey, G., & Kitson, A. (2015). *Implementing evidence-based practice in healthcare: A facilitation guide.* Routledge.

Harvey, G., Loftus-Hills, A., Rycroft-Malone, J., Titchen, A., Kitson, A., McCormack, B., & Seers, K. (2002). Getting evidence into practice: The role and function of facilitation. *Journal of Advanced Nursing, 37*(6), 577–588. https://doi.org/10.1046/j.1365-2648.2002.02126.x

Harvey, G., Gifford, W., Cummings, G., Kelly, J., Kislov, R., Kitson, A., Pettersson, L., Wallin, L, Wilson, P., & Ehrenberg, A. (2019). Mobilising evidence to improve nursing practice: A qualitative study of leadership roles and process in four countries. *International Journal of Nursing Studies, 80,* 21–30. https://doi .org/10.1016/j.ijnurstu.2018.09.017

Hasson, H., Nilsen, P., Augustsson, H., & Schwarz, U. (2018). Empirical and conceptual investigation of de-implementation of low-value care from professional and health care system perspectives: A study protocol. *Implementation Science, 13,* 67. https://doi.org/10.1186/s13012-018-0760-7

Helfrich, C. D., Damschroder, H. J., Hagedorn, H. J., Daggertt, G. S., Sahay, A., T., Ritchie, M., Damush, T., Guihan, M., Ullrich, P., & Stetler, C. B. (2010). A critical synthesis of literature on the promoting action on research implementation in health services (PARIHS) framework. *Implementation Science, 5,* 82. https://doi.org/10.1186/1748-5908-5-82

Hutchinson, A. M., & Johnston, L. (2004). Bridging the divide: A survey of nurses' opinions regarding barriers to, and facilitators of, research utilization in the practice setting. *Journal of Clinical Nursing, 13*(3), 304–315. https://doi.org/10.1046/j.1365-2702.2003.00865.x

Hysong, S. J., Best, R. G., & Pugh, J. A. (2006). Audit and feedback and clinical practice guideline adherence: Making feedback actionable. *Implementation Science, 1,* Article 9 (2006). https://doi.org/10.1186/1748-5908-1-9

Implementation Science. (2020). *About, Aims and Scope.* https://implementationscience.biomedcentral.com/about

Institute of Medicine. (2001). *Crossing the quality chasm: A new health system for the 21st century.* National Academies Press.

Institute of Medicine. (2007a). *Advancing quality improvement research: Challenges and opportunities.* Workshop summary. National Academies Press.

Institute of Medicine. (2007b). *The state of quality improvement and implementation research: Expert reviews.* Workshop summary. National Academies Press.

Institute of Medicine. (2008). *Knowing what works in health care: A roadmap for the nation.* Committee on reviewing evidence to identify highly effective clinical services. National Academies Press.

Institute of Medicine. (2011). *Clinical Practice Guidelines We Can Trust.* The National Academies Press.

Institute of Medicine. (2013). *The CTSA Program at NIH: Opportunities for advancing clinical and translational research.* The National Academies Press.

Ivers, N., Jamtvedt, G., Flottorp, S., Young, J. M., Odgaard-Jensen, J., French, S. D., O'Brien, M. A., Johansen, M., Grimshaw, J., & Oxman, A. D. (2012). Audit and feedback: Effects on professional practice and healthcare outcomes. *Cochrane Database of Systematic Reviews, 2012*(6), Art. No. CD000259. https://doi.org/10.1002/14651858.CD000259.pub3

Jun, J., Kovner, C. T., & Stimpfel, A. W. (2015). Barriers and facilitators of nurses' use of clinical practice guidelines: An integrative review. *International Journal of Nursing Studies, 60,* 54–68. https://doi.org/10.1016/j.ijnurstu.2016.03.006

Kaasalainen, S., Ploeg, J., Donald, F., Coker, E., Brazil, K., Martin-Misener, R., Dicenso, A., & Hadjistavropoulos, T. (2015). Positioning clinical nurse specialists and nurse practitioners as change champions to implement a pain protocol in long-term care. *Pain Management Nursing, 16,* 78–88. https://doi.org/10.1016/j.pmn.2014.04.002

Kirk, M.A., Kelley, C., Yankey, N., Birken, N., Abadie, B., & Damschroder, L. (2016). A systematic review of the use of the Consolidated Framework for Implementation Research. *Implementation Science, 11,* Article 72 (2015). https://doi.org/10.1186/s13012-016-0437-z

Kitson, A., Harvey, G., & McCormack, B. (1998). Enabling the implementation of evidence based practice: A conceptual framework. *Quality in Health Care, 7*(3), 149–158. https://doi.org/10.1136/qshc.7.3.149

Kitson, A., Rycroft-Malone, J., Harvey, G., McCormack, B., Seers, K., & Titchen, A. (2008). Evaluating the successful implementation of evidence into practice using the PARiHS framework: Theoretical and practical challenges. *Implementation Science, 3*(1). http://www.implementationscience.com

Landis-Lewis, Z., Kononowech, J., Scott, W. J., Hogikyan, R. V., Carpenter, J. G., Periyakoil, V. S., Miller, S. C., Levy, C., Ersek, M., & Sales, A. (2020). Designing clinical practice feedback reports: Three steps illustrated in Veterans Health Affairs long-term care facilities and programs. *Implementation Science, 15,* 7. https://doi.org/10.1186/s13012-019-0950-y

Lia-Hoagberg, B., Schaffer, M., & Strohschein, S. (1999). Public health nursing practice guidelines: An evaluation of dissemination and use. *Public Health Nursing, 16*(6), 397–404. https://doi.org/10.1046/j.1525-1446.1999.00397.x

Locock, L., Dopson, S., Chambers, D., & Gabbay, J. (2001). Understanding the role of opinion leaders in improving clinical effectiveness. *Social Science & Medicine (1982), 53*(6), 745–757. https://doi.org/10.1016/S0277-9536(00)00387-7

Matthew-Maich, N., Ploeg, J., Dobbins, M., & Jack, S. (2014). Supporting the uptake of nursing guidelines: What you really need to know to move nursing guidelines into practice. *Worldviews on Evidence Based Nursing, 10,* 104–115. https://doi.org/10.1111/j.1741-6787.2012.00259.x

Manojlovich, M., Squires, J. E., Davies, B., & Graham, I. (2015). Hiding in plain sight: Communication theory in implementation science. *Implementation Science, 10*, 58. https://doi.org/10.1186/s13012-015-0244-y

McCormack, B., Kitson, A., Harvey, G., Rycroft-Malone, J., Titchen, A., & Seers, K. (2002). Getting evidence into practice: The meaning of "context." *Journal of Advanced Nursing, 38*(1), 94–104. https://doi.org/10.1046/j.1365-2648.2002.02150.x

McKenna, H., Ashton, S., & Keeney, S. (2004). Barriers to evidence based practice in primary care: A review of the literature. *International Journal of Nursing Studies, 41*(4), 369–378. https://doi.org/10.1016/j.ijnurstu.2003.10.008

McKibbon, K. A., Lokker, C., Wilczynski, N. L., Ciliska, D., Dobbins, M., Davis, D. A., Haynes, B., & Straus, S. E. (2010). A cross-sectional study of the number and frequency of terms used to refer to knowledge translation in a body of health literature in 2006: A Tower of Babel? *Implementation Science, 5*, 16. https://doi.org/10.1186/1748-5908-5-16

Meijers, J. M., Janssen, M. A., Cummings, G. G., Wallin, L., Estabrooks, C. A., & Halfens, R. (2006). Assessing the relationships between contextual factors and research utilization in nursing: Systematic literature review. *Journal of Advanced Nursing, 55*(5), 622–635. https://doi.org/10.1111/j.1365-2648.2006.03954.x

Melnyk, B. M., Gallagher-Ford, L., Thomas, B. K., Troseth, M., Wyngarden, K., & Szalacha, L. (2016). A Study of chief nurse executives indicates low prioritization of evidence-based practice and shortcomings in hospital performance metrics across the United States. *Worldviews on Evidence-Based Nursing, 13*(1), 6–14. https://doi.org/10.1111/wvn.12133

Michel, Y., & Sneed, N. V. (1995). Dissemination and use of research findings in nursing practice. *Journal of Professional Nursing, 11*(5), 306–311. https://doi.org/10.1016/S8755-7223(05)80012-2

Milner, M., Estabrooks, C. A., & Myrick, F. (2006). Research utilization and clinical nurse educators: A systematic review. *Journal of Evaluation in Clinical Practice, 12*(6), 639–655. https://doi.org/10.1111/j.1365-2753.2006.00632.x

National Center for Advancing Translational Science. (2018). *Translation science spectrum*. https://ncats.nih.gov/translation/spectrum

Nelson, E. C., Batalden, P. B., Huber, T. P., Mohr, J. J., Godfrey, M. M., Headrick, L. A., & Wasson, J. H. (2002). Microsystems in health care: Part 1. Learning from high-performing front-line clinical units. *The Joint Commission Journal on Quality Improvement, 28*(9), 472–493. https://doi.org/10.1016/S1070-3241(02)28051-7

Nilsen, P. (2015). Making sense of theories, models and frameworks. *Implementation Science, 10*, Article 53 (2015). https://doi.org/10.1186/s13012-015-0242-0

Nkansah, N., Mostovetsky, O., Yu, C., Chheng, T., Beney, J., Bond, C. M., & Bero, L. (2010). Effect of outpatient pharmacists' non-dispensing roles on patient outcomes and prescribing patterns. *Cochrane Database of Systematic Reviews, 7*. https://doi.org/10.1002/14651858.CD000336.pub2

Norton, W. E., & Chambers, D. A. (2020). Unpacking the complexities of de-implementing inappropriate health interventions. *Implementation Science, 15*, 2. https://doi.org/10.1186/s13012-019-0960-9

O'Brien, M. A., Rogers, S., Jamtvedt, G., Oxman, A. D., Odgaard-Jensen, J., Kristoffersen, D. T., Forsetland, L., Bainbridge, D., Freemantle, N., Davis, D., Haynes, R. B., & Harvey, E. C. (2007). Educational outreach visits: Effects on professional practice and health care outcomes. *Cochrane Database of Systematic Reviews, 4*. https://doi.org/10.1002/14651858.CD000409.pub2

Prasad, V., & Ioannidis, J. P. A. (2014). Evidence-based de-implementation for contradicted, unproven, and aspiring healthcare processes. *Implementation Science, 9*, Article 1 (2014). https://doi.org/10.1186/1748-5908-9-1

Pravikoff, D. S., Tanner, A. B., & Pierce, S. T. (2005). Readiness of U.S. nurses for evidence-based practice. *The American Journal of Nursing, 105*(9), 40–51; quiz 52. https://doi.org/10.1097/00000446-200509000-00025

Proctor, E. K., Powell, B. J., & McMillen, J. C. (2013). Implementation strategies: Recommendations for specifying and reporting. *Implementation Science, 8*, Article 139 (2013). https://doi.org/10.1186/1748-5908-8-139

Rabin, B. A., & Brownson, R. C. (2012). Developing the terminology for dissemination and implementation research. In R. C. Brownson, G. A. Colditz, & E. K. Proctor (Eds.), *Dissemination and implementation research in health* (pp. 23–51). Oxford University Press.

Rabin, B. A., Brownson, R. C., Haire-Joshu, D., Kreuter, M. W., & Weaver, N. L. (2008). A glossary for dissemination and implementation research in health. *Journal of Public Health Management and Practice, 14*(2), 117–123. https://doi.org/10.1097/01.PHH.0000311888.06252.bb

Randolph, W., & Viswanath, K. (2004). Lessons learned from public health mass media campaigns: Marketing health in a crowded media world. *Annual Review of Public Health, 25*, 419–437. https://doi.org/10.1146/annurev.publhealth.25.101802.123046

Rappolt, S., Pearce, K., McEwen, S., & Polatajko, H. J. (2005). Exploring organizational characteristics associated with practice changes following a mentored online educational module. *The Journal of Continuing Education in the Health Professions, 25*(2), 116–124. https://doi.org/10.1002/chp.16

Reeves, S., Pelone, F., Harrison, R., Golman, J., & Zwarenstein, M. (2017). Interprofessional collaboration to improve professional practice and healthcare outcomes. *Cochrane Database of Systematic Reviews, 6.* https://doi.org/10.1002/14651858.CD000072.pub3

Rogers, E. (Ed.). (2003). *Diffusion of innovations* (5th ed.). Simon & Schuster.

Rosswurm, M. A., & Larrabee, J. H. (1999). A model for change to evidence-based practice. *Image—The Journal of Nursing Scholarship, 31*(4), 317–322. https://doi.org/10.1111/j.1547-5069.1999.tb00510.x

Rycroft-Malone, J., & Bucknall, T. (Eds). (2010). *Models and frameworks for implementing evidence-based practice: Linking evidence to action.* Wiley-Blackwell.

Rycroft-Malone, J., Harvey, G., Seers, K., Kitson, A., McCormack, B., & Titchen, A. (2004). An exploration of the factors that influence the implementation of evidence into practice. *Journal of Clinical Nursing, 13*(8), 913–924. https://doi.org/10.1111/j.1365-2702.2004.01007.x

Sanchez, A., Pijoan, J. I., Pablo, S., Mediavilla, M., Sainz de Rosa, R., Lekue, I., Gonzalez-Larragan, S., Lantaron, G., Argote, J., Garcia-Alvarez, A, Latorre, P. M., Helfrich, C. D., & Grandes, G. (2020). Addressing low-value pharmacologic prescribing in primary prevention of CVD through a structured evidence-based and theory-informed process for the design and testing of de-implementation strategies: The De-imFAR study. *Implementation Science, 15*, 8. https://doi.org/10.1186/s13012-020-0966-3

Schouten, L. M., Hulscher, M. E., Akkermans, R., van Everdingen, J. J., Grol, R. P., & Huijsman, R. (2008). Factors that influence the stroke care team's effectiveness in reducing the length of hospital stay. *Stroke: A Journal of Cerebral Circulation, 39*(9), 2515–2521. https://doi.org/10.1161/STROKEAHA.107.510537

Scott, T., Mannion, R., Davies, H. T., & Marshall, M. N. (2003a). The quantitative measurement of organizational culture in health care: A review of the available instruments. *Health Services Research, 38*(3), 923–945. https://doi.org/10.1111/1475-6773.00154

Scott, T., Mannion, R., Davies, H. T., & Marshall, M. N. (2003b). Implementing culture change in health care: Theory and practice. *International Journal for Quality in Health Care, 15*(2), 111–118. https://doi.org/10.1093/intqhc/mzg021

Squires, J. E., Estabrooks, C. A., Gustavsson, P., & Wallin, L. (2011). Individual determinants of research utilization by nurses: A systematic review update. *Implementation Science, 6*, Article 1 (2011). https://doi.org/10.1186/1748-5908-6-1

Squires, J. E., Sullivan, K., Eccles, M. P., Worswick, J., & Grimshaw, J. M. (2014). Are multifaceted interventions more effective than single-component interventions in changing health-care professionals' behaviours? An overview of systematic reviews. *Implementation Science, 9*, Article 152 (2014). https://doi.org/10.1186/s13012-014-0152-6

Stetler, C. B. (2001). Updating the Stetler model of research utilization to facilitate evidence-based practice. *Nursing Outlook, 49*(6), 272–279. https://doi.org/10.1067/mno.2001.120517

Stetler, C. B., Legro, M. W., Rycroft-Malone, J., Bowman, C., Curran, G., Guihan, M., Hagedorn, H., Pineros, S., & Wallace, C. M. (2006). Role of "external facilitation" in implementation of research findings: A qualitative evaluation of facilitation experiences in the Veterans Health Administration. *Implementation Science, 1*, 23. https://doi.org/10.1186/1748-5908-1-23

Straus, S. E., Tetroe, J., & Graham, I. (2013). *Knowledge translation in health care: Moving from evidence to practice.* Wiley.

Sussman, S., Valente, T. W., Rohrbach, L. A., Skara, S., & Pentz, M. A. (2006). Translation in the health professions: Converting science into action. *Evaluation & the Health Professions, 29*(1), 7–32. https://doi.org/10.1177/0163278705284441

Tabak, R. G., Khoong, E. C., Chambers, D. A., & Brownson, R. C. (2012). Bridging research and practice. *American Journal of Preventative Medicine, 43*, 337–350. https://doi.org/10.1016/j.amepre.2012.05.024

Titler, M. G. (2004a). Methods in translation science. *Worldviews on Evidence-Based Nursing, 1*(1), 38–48. https://doi.org/10.1111/j.1741-6787.2004.04008.x

Titler, M. G. (2004b). Translation science: Quality, methods and issues. *Communicating Nursing Research, 37*(15), 17–34.

Titler, M. G. (2006). Developing an evidence-based practice. In G. LoBiondo-Wood & J. Haber (Eds.), *Nursing research: Methods and critical appraisal for evidence-based practice* (6th ed.). Mosby.

Titler, M. G. (2018). Translation research in practice: An introduction. *Online Journal of Issues in Nursing, 23(2)*, manuscript 1.

Titler, M. G., Everett, L. Q., & Adams, S. (2007). Implications for implementation science. *Nursing Research, 56*(4 Suppl.), S53–S59. https://doi.org/10.1097/01.NNR.0000280636.78901.7f

Titler, M., Herr, K., Brooks, J., Xie, X., Ardery, G., Schilling, M. L., Marsh, J. L., Everett, L. Q., & Clarke, W. R. (2009). Translating research into practice intervention improves management of acute pain in older hip fracture patients. *Health Services Research, 44*(1), 264–287. https://doi.org/10.1111/j.1475-6773.2008 .00913.x

Titler, M. G., Kleiber, C., Steelman, V. J., Rakel, B. A., Budreau, G., Everett, L. Q., Buckwalter, K. C., Tripp-Reimer, T., & Goode, C. J. (2001). The Iowa model of evidence-based practice to promote quality care. *Critical Care Nursing Clinics of North America, 13*(4), 497–509. https://doi.org/10.1016/ S0899-5885(18)30017-0

Tripp-Reimer, T., & Doebbeling, B. (2004). Qualitative perspectives in translational research. *Worldviews on Evidence-Based Nursing, 1*, S65–S72. https://doi.org/10.1111/j.1524-475X.2004.04041.x

Voorn, V. M. A., Marang-van de Mheen, P. J., van der Hout, A., Hofstede, S. N., So-Osman, C., Elske van den Akker-van Marle, M., Kaptein, A. A., Stijnen, T., Koopman-van Gemert, A. W. M. M., Vliet Vlieland, T. P. M. M., Nelissen, R. G. H. H., & van Bodegom-Vos, L. (2017). The effectiveness of a de-implementation strategy to reduce low-value blood management techniques in primary hip and knew arthroplasty: A pragmatic cluster-randomized controlled trial. *Implementation Science, 12*, 72. https://doi.org/10.1186/ s13012-017-0601-0

Wallin, L., Ewald, U., Wikblad, K., Scott-Findlay, S., & Arnetz, B. B. (2006). Understanding work contextual factors: A short-cut to evidence-based practice? *Worldviews on Evidence-Based Nursing, 3*(4), 153–164. https://doi.org/10.1111/j.1741-6787.2006.00067.x

Wallin, L., Rudberg, A., & Gunningberg, L. (2005). Staff experiences in implementing guidelines for kangaroo mother care—A qualitative study. *International Journal of Nursing Studies, 42*(1), 61–73. https://doi .org/10.1016/j.ijnurstu.2004.05.016

Warren, J. I., McLaughlin, M., Bardsley, J., Eich, J., Esche, C. A., Kropkowski, L., & Risch, S. (2016). The strengths and challenges of implementing EBP in healthcare systems. *Worldviews on Evidence-Based Nursing, 13*, 15–24. https://doi.org/10.1111/wvn.12149

Wensing, M., & Grol, R. (1994). Single and combined strategies for implementing changes in primary care: A literature review. *International Journal for Quality in Health Care, 6*(2), 115–132. https://doi.org/10.1093/ intqhc/6.2.115

Wensing, M., Wollersheim, H., & Grol, R. (2006). Organizational interventions to implement improvements in patient care: A structured review of reviews. *Implementation Science, 1*, Article 2 (2006). https://doi .org/10.1186/1748-5908-1-2

Westfall, J. M., Mold, J. M., & Fagman, L. (2007). Practice-based research—"Blue Highways" on the NIH roadmap. *Journal of American Medical Association, 297*, 403–406. https://doi.org/10.1001/jama.297.4.403

Wiecha, J. L., El Ayadi, A. M., Fuemmeler, B. F., Carter, J. E., Handler, S., Johnson, S., Strunk, N., Korzec-Ramirez, D., & Gortmaker, S. L. (2004). Diffusion of an integrated health education program in an urban school system: Planet health. *Journal of Pediatric Psychology, 29*(6), 467–474. https://doi.org/10.1093/ jpepsy/jsh050

Whicher, D., Rosengren, K., Siddiqi, S. & Simpson, L. (Eds.). (2018). *The future of health services research: Advancing health systems research and practice in the United States*. National Academy of Medicine.

Yost, J., Thompson, D., Ganann, R., Aloweni, F., Newman, K., McKibbon, A., Dobbins, M., & Ciliska, D. (2014). Knowledge translation strategies for enhancing nurses' evidence-informed decision making: A scoping review. *Worldviews on Evidence-Based Nursing, 11*, 156–167. https://doi.org/10.1111/wvn.12043

Zerhouni, E. (2003). The NIH roadmap. *Science, 302*(72), 63–64. https://doi.org/10.1126/science.1091867

Zwarenstein, M., & Reeves, S. (2006). Knowledge translation and interprofessional collaboration: Where the rubber of evidence-based care hits the road of teamwork. *Journal of Continuing Education in the Health Professions, 26*(1), 46–54. https://doi.org/10.1002/chp.50

IV

EVALUATING THE IMPACT OF
EVIDENCE-BASED PRACTICE,
ETHICAL ASPECTS OF A STUDY,
AND COMMUNICATING RESULTS

COST AS A DIMENSION OF EVIDENCE-BASED PRACTICE

BRIANA J. JEGIER AND TRICIA J. JOHNSON

INTRODUCTION

The healthcare industry is facing increasing pressure to improve value through the provision of higher quality and/or more efficient care. Value is the balance between the quality of care a patient receives and the cost of the care. The cost component of value has received increased attention because healthcare spending represents roughly 17.7% of the gross domestic product of the United States and is one of the single most expensive budget items that businesses face today (Centers for Medicare & Medicaid Services [CMS], 2018; Congressional Budget Office [CBO], 2019). For example, the cost to the U.S. federal government for the Medicare, Medicaid, and State Children's Health Insurance Program (CHIP) accounts for 28% of the federal budget, with future projections estimating that spending on these programs could reach as high as 41% of the budget by 2049 (CBO, 2019; CMS, 2018). Thus, it is important for healthcare researchers and practitioners to be conscious of the cost implications of their research and practice by including cost measurement in addition to quality-of-care measurement. The purpose of this chapter is to introduce the concept of cost, to describe how to incorporate cost methodology into research and practice, and to improve the critical evaluation of cost findings published in research and practice publications.

THE DEFINITION OF COST

Before integrating cost into research and practice, the definition and perspective must be clearly defined. Most people outside the field of economics refer to cost as the monetary value paid by a purchaser (e.g., a consumer, a provider, a payer, a government, a society) for goods or services. The monetary value, referred to in economics literature as the price, is certainly one aspect of cost, but is not the only aspect. Cost is more accurately defined as the resources that are expended for goods or services. These resources may or may not have an associated or measurable monetary value (Drummond et al., 2005; Gold et al., 1996). By defining cost in this broader sense of resource expenditure, it allows us to consider the fact that the acquisition of goods or services occurs within a complex, multifaceted environment where the resources that must be expended involve multiple parties. It also allows us to consider that not all goods and services include a price that is paid, in part or in full, by the individual or group receiving the goods or services. For example, a patient rarely pays the full price of their medical care services, yet the patient is the one who benefits from those services.

A single good from a healthcare situation illustrates this complex relationship: What is the cost of 1 hour of nursing care for a hospitalized patient? To answer this question, you might start by asking yourself the cost to whom? One hour of nursing care could involve the participation of five different parties: the nurse, the hospital, the patient, the patient's family, and the insurance carrier. Table 17.1 demonstrates the resources that each party would expend for 1 hour of nursing care. These resources can be conceptualized into two primary categories: time (e.g., nurse, other healthcare professionals and staff, patient, patient's family, insurance carrier employee) and resources (e.g., supplies, utilities, space).

Definition: Cost

Cost is defined as the resources that are expended for goods or a service. The resources may or may not have an associated monetary value.

■ TYPES OF COST

The Cost of Time

The cost of time is usually characterized as opportunity cost. Opportunity cost is the resource trade-off a person faces when deciding how to allocate their time. People face resource trade-off decisions to determine how to allocate their time every day. For example, a person chooses between watching a favorite television program and going to the gym, or chooses to work overtime instead of having dinner with a friend. In each instance, the person weighs the resources that would need to be expended for each choice. Perhaps the favorite television show is selected over the gym because the gym requires that the person drive 30 minutes, whereas the television program only requires that they walk to the den. Working overtime may be selected over dinner with a friend, because working overtime right now allows them to spend the whole weekend with the friend later. Each decision about how to allocate time incorporates the process of measuring and valuing the opportunity cost of each choice. The selected choice will have the most favorable opportunity cost to the individual making the decision.

Opportunity cost can present a measurement challenge given that every person has a complex decision-making process for how they spend time. In research and practice, researchers and providers also need to systematically measure opportunity cost using a standard unit of measure, and this is ideally reported in monetary terms. Therefore, economists define the measurement of opportunity cost as the monetary value of the next best alternative choice. Thus, in the "1 hour of nursing care" example, the nurse's opportunity cost was the nurse's decision to spend time at work versus some other activity they might enjoy (Table 17.1). The monetary value of that opportunity cost is the compensation they received for the additional hour spent at work instead of pursuing another paid or unpaid activity.

The Cost of Resources

The cost of resources is characterized as the cost of equipment, supplies, and other "objects" expended to provide the good or service. Using our example, the cost to provide the bed that a hospital uses for a patient is the monetary value the hospital paid to purchase, install, maintain, and replace the bed so that it would be available for the patient for their 1 hour of nursing care. The cost of a resource is generally allocated over the life span of that object. Using the bed as an example, the cost for that 1 hour of the bed would be the total cost of purchase, installation, and

TABLE 17.1 Resources and Associated Monetary Value for the Delivery of 1 Hour of Nursing Care to a Hospitalized Patient

PERSPECTIVE	NURSE DELIVERING CARE	HOSPITAL WHERE THE CARE IS DELIVERED	HOSPITALIZED PATIENT	PATIENT'S FAMILY	INSURANCE CARRIER
Resources used	The nurse provides their time, knowledge, and expertise to the patient.	The institution provides the environment for the care to be delivered (e.g., bed, supplies, electricity, nursing administration time).	The patient provides their time and presence during the care episode.	The patient's family members may also provide time during the care episode (e.g., waiting for patient).	The insurance carrier provides staff time to approve the hospitalization, process the payment for the hospital, and answer any benefits questions the patient or family members have.
Monetary value	Measured monetarily as the compensation (salary and benefits) the nurse accepts from the hospital for the time they spend with the patient. If the nurse had not accepted this compensation, they could have done something else (e.g., spend time with friends/family, read a book, watch a movie).	Compensation paid to the nurse as well as the amount paid for supplies, maintenance, utilities, and the space.	Wages and the monetary value of unpaid work (e.g., household work) forgone by the patient because of the hospitalization as well as other out-of-pocket expenses incurred as a result of that hospitalization.	Wages and the monetary value of unpaid work (e.g., household work) forgone by other family members because of the hospitalization and other out-of-pocket expenses incurred as a result of that hospitalization.	Compensation paid to the employee(s) who handle the claim, what the insurance carrier pays to operate their business, and what they pay to the hospital on behalf of their patient.

maintenance for the bed divided by the number of hours the bed is expected to be in use. Thus if the bed cost $500 to purchase, $300 to install, and $400 to maintain over its life span, then the total cost of the bed would be $1,200. If the bed was expected to be in use for 10,000 hours, then the cost of the bed for that 1 hour of care would be $1,200/10,000 or $0.12 per hour of use.

Direct and Indirect Cost

Once the time and resources used to provide a good or service are identified, then you can further classify each resource based on how they contribute to the delivery of that good or service. Costs can be classified as direct, indirect, or intangible costs. If the resource is absolutely integral to the delivery of the good or service, then that resource would be considered a direct cost. Using the example of 1 hour of nursing care, the cost of the bed would be a direct cost for a hospitalized patient because the bed is absolutely necessary for the delivery of care to the hospitalized patient. If the resource is needed but not an integral part of the delivery of the good or service, then that resource would be considered an indirect cost. Using the example of 1 hour of nursing care, the cost of the hospital maintenance worker would be an indirect cost for a hospitalized patient. It is considered indirect because all patients must use the service of the maintenance worker in some way because they ensure that the beds are available; however, this work is not absolutely necessary for the delivery of care to any one individual hospitalized patient. Another indication of an indirect cost is if the cost is distributed equally regardless of the actual use by any given individual. For example, if a bed breaks during the care of one patient, that patient might use more maintenance resources than a patient whose bed continues to function properly. Both patients are allocated the same amount of maintenance worker resources when the final costs of their respective stays are calculated. Another example is a hospital finance specialist who processes the patient's insurance claim. The time the finance specialist spends processing the claim does not change substantively based on the insurance provider. Thus, each patient receives the same charge for a finance specialist. Indirect costs in healthcare are sometimes called overhead costs.

Intangible Cost

The last type of cost is the intangible cost. An intangible cost is the cost for resources that do not have a clear and direct value, monetary or otherwise. Some examples of intangible costs include the cost of lost life due to a medical error and the cost of pain and suffering the patient experiences during care. It is clear that patients can experience pain and suffering during care, but there is not a uniform, straightforward way of placing value on that experience. For most intangible costs, there are standardized approaches to assign monetary values. These systems are most often developed by actuaries, but can also be products of process (such as the legal system) or by other types of professionals. For example, in legal cases the value of lost life due to a medical error might be valued at the lost wages estimated over one's life span.

◼ MEASURING COST

In the nursing care example, time and resources from five different perspectives all contributed to the cost of 1 hour of nursing care. However, before measuring the monetary value of these costs, the decision concerning which perspective to use must be made. That decision is often dictated by who commissioned the measurement activity. The perspectives that might be used in any given cost analysis are the individual consumer; the program, corporation, or business (e.g., hospital, healthcare provider, health insurer); the government; and society as a whole. The societal perspective as a whole is the most encompassing view of cost because it considers all of the potential perspectives. In the United States, a consensus was developed in the late 1990s by the Cost Evaluation Taskforce to use the societal viewpoint for all healthcare cost studies to maximize the ability to compare costs across studies (Weinstein et al., 1996) and is the "gold standard" for economic evaluations. Thus, unless the cost measurement is commissioned from a distinct perspective (e.g., the provider), the societal perspective should be used when measuring costs or should be reported in conjunction with other perspectives. Once you have identified the perspective of the costs, all of the individual personnel time and resources are identified. The exact process of identification and measurement is determined by the type of cost analysis performed.

■ TYPES OF COST ANALYSIS

Drummond et al. (2005) identify eight types of cost analyses: (a) cost description, (b) cost–outcome description, (c) cost, (d) cost minimization, (e) cost consequence, (f) cost-effectiveness, (g) cost–utility, and (h) cost–benefit analysis. The type of cost analysis that should be used depends on two factors: (a) whether a single activity or multiple alternative activities will be compared, and (b) whether costs alone or costs and their associated outcomes or consequences (e.g., improved health and reduced length of hospitalization) will be measured. Figure 17.1 presents a

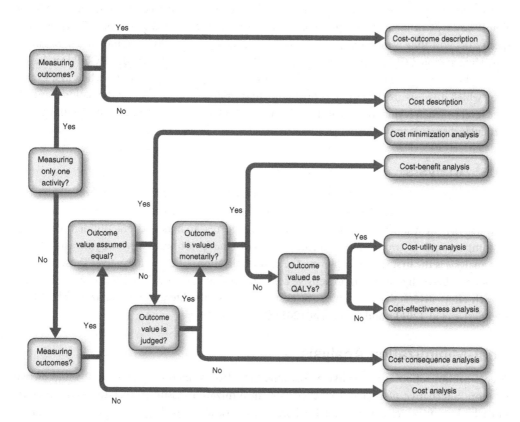

FIGURE 17.1 Flow diagram to select type of cost analysis.
QALYs, quality-adjusted life years.

flow diagram for selecting the type of cost analysis. The next section explores each of the eight types of analyses in further detail.

Cost Description and Cost–Outcome Description

The cost description and the cost–outcome description analyses measure the cost of a single activity. The cost description solely measures the cost of the activity, whereas the cost–outcome measures both the cost and the outcome that results from the activity. The outcome of an activity is also referred to as the consequence, effect, or benefit. The cost and the cost–outcome descriptions are useful tools for researchers and practitioners, because they help quantify the cost implications of a single type of activity. Both are used widely in healthcare to examine the economic magnitude of disease because they can be used to answer questions such as: "How much does hospitalization for a heart transplant cost?" or "What is the hospital cost for stroke treatment and how long will I be hospitalized if I experience it?" The initial example of the cost of 1 hour of nursing care would be considered a cost description because it measured a single activity—an hour of nursing care—and did not seek to identify any outcomes that might result from that activity (e.g., the patient living 1 day longer than they would without the care). Some examples of cost description and cost–outcome description from the published literature are Johnson et al. (2013), American Diabetes Association (2013), and Gross et al. (2013).

Further, the cost and cost–outcome description analyses are so prevalent in healthcare that the Agency for Healthcare Research and Quality (AHRQ) has a free online tool, HCUPnet, that researchers and practitioners can use to identify the mean and median cost and length of stay for almost any type of inpatient hospitalization (HCUP Databases, 2012). The tool allows users to specify the cost they want by a specific diagnosis-related group (DRG), an individual diagnosis code (International Classification of Diseases [ICD]-9), or a procedure code (HCUP Databases, 2012). This is a particularly useful tool for researchers and practitioners to use when first examining which diseases are the largest contributors to overall healthcare costs at the national and/or state level or when trying to present the "big picture" case for why developing interventions for a particular disease is important.

Cost Analysis

A cost analysis is an analysis that solely measures the monetary cost of two or more alternative activities. A cost analysis does not consider any consequences or benefits that may result from each activity. Cost analysis can be especially useful to researchers and practitioners when the cost implications of two or more alternative activities have not been previously measured. The cost analysis is the first step in exploring the cost implications of each alternative. These analyses are often followed by more comprehensive cost studies that compare the costs and consequences of each alternative activity. Examples of cost analyses in the literature are Jegier et al. (2010), Leendertse et al. (2011), and Chan et al. (2014).

Cost-Minimization Analysis

A cost-minimization analysis, like a cost analysis, also compares the monetary value of two or more alternative activities. However, cost minimization assumes that the consequences of each alternative activity are equal, whereas the cost analysis does not measure the consequences or formulate any assumptions about them. Cost-minimization analyses are particularly useful when comparing two different treatment modalities for delivering the exact same treatment, for example, intravenous compared to oral delivery of a specific pain medication. In this example, the consequence of the pain medication (e.g., pain relief) should theoretically be equal; however, the cost to administer a drug orally versus intravenously would drastically differ. A cost-minimization analysis is also useful when effectiveness studies have already been completed to demonstrate that the outcomes are equal. This type of analysis identifies the lowest cost alternative, and it would be the recommended alternative. Some examples of cost-minimization analyses in the published literature are Dasta et al. (2010), Schuurman et al. (2009), and Behera et al. (2012).

Cost-Consequence Analysis

A cost-consequence analysis also compares the costs and the consequences of two or more alternative activities. The cost-consequence analysis, however, does not assume that the consequences all have equal worth. Instead, the cost and each consequence are presented to the reader or audience. The audience or reader must then decide which alternative to choose using their own judgment regarding the balance between the cost and the consequences for each alternative activity. A cost-consequence analysis would be presented as follows—cost activity 1: consequences of activity 1. Cost consequence can be particularly helpful if there are multiple possible consequences and/or if there is disagreement over the value of any consequence. The reader is allowed to weigh the relationship between the costs and consequences and consider that multiple consequences are possible. Examples of a cost-consequence analysis in the published literature are Kroese et al. (2011) and Jegier et al. (2016).

Cost-Effectiveness Analysis

A cost-effectiveness analysis compares the monetary costs with the consequence of two or more alternative activities. The cost-effectiveness analysis measures the consequences of each alternative using a clinical outcome as the unit of measure. For example, if a new program claims to reduce the length of hospital stay, a cost-effectiveness analysis would compare the costs and outcomes of the new program to other existing programs. Cost-effectiveness analysis is particularly useful for clinical providers because it breaks down the costs to a cost per clinical outcome, and this clinical outcome is usually the most important outcome from a clinical or practice perspective. For example, a cost-effectiveness analysis might identify the cost per day of hospitalization saved. This can be quite powerful when presenting a business case for a new clinical program because it ties the cost and clinical outcomes together. Some examples of cost-effectiveness analyses in the literature are Behl et al. (2012), Petrou et al. (2011), and Patel et al. (2013).

Cost–Utility Analysis

A cost–utility analysis builds on the framework of a cost-effectiveness analysis. Specifically, cost–utility incorporates a standardized measure of quality of life as the consequence being measured. Thus, the typical consequence that is measured in cost–utility analysis is the quality-adjusted life year (QALY; pronounced KW-ALL-EE) or the disability-adjusted life year (DALY; pronounced DA-LEE). There are many different techniques for quantifying QALYs and DALYs; however, there are three scales that are typically used in clinical research. They are the Quality of Well-Being (QWB) Scale (Kaplan & Anderson, 1988; Kaplan et al., 1996); the EuroQol 5-D (EuroQol Group, 1990; available at www.eurolqol.org); or the Short Form 36 (SF-36; Brazier et al., 2002). The use of QALY and DALY in the cost–utility analysis can be very helpful to healthcare providers,

---

EXHIBIT 17.1

PATIENT REPORTED OUTCOMES MEASUREMENT INFORMATION SYSTEM (PROMIS): THE FUTURE OF QUALITY ADJUSTED LIFE YEARS (QALY) AND DISABILITY ADJUSTED LIFE YEARS (DALY) MEASUREMENT

PROMIS is a U.S. federal initiative funded through the National Institutes of Health that provides standardized tools for measuring quality of life from the patient's perspective (Cella et al., 2007; Revicki et al., 2009). The tools are free for research use and provide researchers with a way to capture physical, mental, and social well-being using a series of validated and standardized questionnaires. These tools offer a unique opportunity to incorporate greater quality measures into research particularly because they include an electronic data collection system.

More information about PROMIS is available at www.nihpromis.org/default.

---

particularly when counseling patients, because it allows the provider to present the quality of life added by a treatment rather than just the raw time alone. This also allows comparison of the cost-effectiveness across different types of programs or interventions. Some examples of cost–utility analyses in the literature are Kaimal et al. (2011), Smith et al. (2012), and Leung et al. (2016). See also Exhibit 17.1.

Cost–Benefit Analysis

A cost–benefit analysis compares the cost and consequence of two or more alternative activities using monetary value for both the costs and the consequence. Cost–benefit analyses are helpful because the cost and the consequences are measured using the same unit of measurement, which allows the reader to quantify the absolute monetary value of the activity. There is often controversy when consequences are measured in monetary value. If the consequence of an activity is that you live a year longer, how much is that additional year of life worth? Cost–benefit analysis requires assigning a monetary value to consequences, even if the consequence comes with an intangible cost. In addition to some of the standard approaches previously mentioned from certain professions (e.g., actuaries), there is a plethora of economic literature that explores how to apply monetary valuation to costs and consequences that typically are not measured monetarily. Some resources for monetary valuation are Viscusi and Zeckhauser (1994) and Viscusi and Aldy (2003). Further, some examples of cost–benefit analyses in the literature are Puzniak et al. (2004) and Kang et al. (2012).

■ CONDUCTING THE COST ANALYSIS

Once the type of cost analysis planned is identified then measurement and analysis begin. There are five general steps for cost analyses: (a) defining the analysis assumptions, (b) measuring the resources used for each cost, (c) measuring the outcomes or consequences associated with each cost, (d) conducting a sensitivity analysis, and (e) comparing the cost and consequences of each alternative activity. Each of these steps is explored further in the following.

Defining the Analysis Assumptions

The first step of any type of cost analysis is to define the assumptions that will guide the analysis. Assumptions are a set of rules that the researcher will follow when conducting the analysis and in considering the costs and consequences of each activity. Assumptions typically fall into two categories: analysis standards and analysis scope. The analysis standards are the researcher's rules for the perspective that will be used (individual, business, and society) and how costs and consequences will be standardized. As previously described, the perspective is most often dictated by who commissioned the study. Standardization assumptions entail describing the way in which the researcher will measure all costs and consequences. Standardization involves the selection of a single year (e.g., 2017) to measure all costs and consequences. By selecting this year, the researcher is stating that all costs and consequences will be measured using the monetary value from 2017. If the study spans multiple years, then the researcher would inflate or deflate the costs from other years to match the value of money in 2017. It is important to standardize to a single year so that the costs and the consequences can be accurately compared. If the researcher does not standardize the costs and consequences, then any differences in costs and/or consequences may not be real, but rather reflect the fact that a dollar today is worth more than a dollar tomorrow (and a dollar yesterday is worth more than a dollar today). In the United States, a common method of standardizing the costs and consequences to a single year is to use the rate of inflation from the U.S. consumer price index for all goods or the consumer price index specifically for medical care (Bureau of Labor Statistics, 2012). Cost analysis in other countries may use those countries' comparable price indices.

The analysis scope assumptions generally include items that are similar to inclusion and exclusion criteria in a traditional research study. They are similar because analysis scope assumptions frame the types of costs and consequences that will be measured. To illustrate an analysis scope assumption, let us examine a cost analysis that compares whether mothers/parents who pump breast milk for their premature infants have lower healthcare costs than mothers/parents who do not pump. In this analysis, one resource that the researcher might consider is travel time to bring the human milk to the neonatal intensive care unit (NICU). In this analysis, the researcher might assume that the travel time to bring the human milk to the NICU is zero because bringing the human milk typically occurs as a part of the mother's/parent's usual visit to the NICU. The researcher might support this assumption by providing data that demonstrates mothers/parents who breastfeed visit their infants the same number of times as mothers/parents who do not breastfeed.

Measuring the Resources Used for Each Cost

Once the assumptions have been identified, the researcher must identify all of the resources that will be used to create the total cost for each alternative that will be measured. These resources should include all time and resources expended, and ideally information about these resources is collected at the time that other data are collected during the study. During this step, it is often helpful to create a table that captures the name of each resource, how it is defined, how it is measured, how much it costs, what year the costs are measured, and where the cost data are obtained (Table 17.2). After all of the resources have been identified and the monetary value has been measured, the monetary value of all the resources used is summed to create a total cost for each activity in the analysis.

TABLE 17.2 A Guide to Measuring the Resources Used for Each Cost Using Selected Resources From the Example of 1 Hour of Nursing Care

RESOURCE NAME	DEFINITION OF RESOURCE	RESOURCE MEASUREMENT	TOTAL COST	COST YEAR	SOURCE(S) OF COST DATA
Nurse time	Nurse time reflects the time spent by the nurse directly with the patient and completing activities related to care for that patient (e.g., charting the activities that occurred and submitting a patient's blood sample to the lab).	This resource was measured through direct observation of the nurse before, during, and after interaction with the patient by a research assistant (RA). The RA noted on a standardized time log the name and the total time in minutes for each distinct activity (e.g., interacting with patient and entering documentation into the health record). RAs followed the nurse for 2 weeks. The total cost per hour of care was measured as the nurse's hourly wage plus the hourly cost of the benefits the hospital provides. (Hourly wage = $25; hourly benefit cost = $1)	$27	2019	Research Assistant (RA) standardized time log; hospital human resource department
Supplies	Supplies reflect the actual supplies that were used during the care of the patient during a 1-hour time period.	This resource was measured through direct observation of the encounter with the patient by an RA. The RA noted each individual supply that was used and/or present in the room using a standardized supply log. These observations were cross-checked against the hospital supply system, which requires that a code unique to the patient room is entered before the supply can be sent to the room or is taken from the local supply system machine on the unit. The cost for each item was obtained from the hospital purchasing department. The total cost was the sum of the individual costs of each item.	$158	2019	RA standardized supply log; hospital supply system; hospital purchasing department
Space	Space reflects the total square footage of the room that the patient occupies during a 1-hour time period.	This resource was measured as the total square feet of the room. This measure was obtained from the hospital planning department. The total cost of the room for 1 hour was calculated by multiplying the total square feet of the room by the total hourly cost per square foot. (Total square feet = 100; total hourly cost = $1)	$106	2019	Hospital planning department

Measuring the Outcomes or Consequences Associated With Each Cost

After measuring the total cost of each activity, the same process is repeated to measure the outcomes or consequences associated with each activity. The outcomes or consequences can be measured for each individual resource used within the activity or for the activity as a whole. The monetary value of each outcome or consequence can be measured at the same time or immediately after each is identified, if the monetary value is required for the type of cost analysis selected. For most analyses, a single outcome or consequence is used to compare activities or programs. If multiple consequences/outcomes are needed, consider using a cost-consequence analysis.

Conducting a Sensitivity Analysis

Before comparing the costs and consequences of each alternative activity, it is important to determine which resources contribute the most to total costs. A sensitivity analysis is a technique that examines what happens to the total cost of each activity if the underlying costs of the resources that are used change. Therefore, a sensitivity analysis is the process of recalculating the total costs by changing the underlying resource costs one at a time (i.e., "univariate" sensitivity analysis). Costs can be changed using a percentage method (e.g., changing each cost by 10%) or using a replacement method (e.g., replacing the actual hourly wage with a standard wage like the minimum wage for the location). As the cost of each resource is changed, the raw change in total cost and the percentage change in total cost are measured. The process of changing the cost of each resource is usually repeated until the total cost of the activity is doubled or tripled. The resource or resources that represent the largest or fastest change in total cost are the resources that a researcher would say the total cost of the activity is sensitive to or that drive the total cost of the activity. Knowing which resources drive the total cost of an activity allows the researcher to portray the potential cost range for the activity. Other more advanced methods of sensitivity analysis include multivariate sensitivity approaches that use bootstrapping, Monte Carlo, and/or Markov modeling methods. To account for the nonnormal distribution of the ratio of costs and outcomes, bootstrapping methods can be used to calculate 95% confidence intervals for evaluating uncertainty in cost-effectiveness ratios (Briggs et al., 1997; Polsky et al., 1997; Tambour & Zethraeus, 1988). Monte Carlo and Markov approaches are used to evaluate uncertainty in analyses that examine costs and consequences over time. These more advanced methods should be performed in consultation with an expert in health economics as they require knowledge of advanced econometric modeling.

Comparing the Costs and Consequences of Each Alternative Activity

The final step in a cost analysis is to compare the costs and consequences of each alternative activity that was measured. The way in which the comparison of the cost and consequences is presented depends on the type of cost analysis used. Table 17.3 provides the presentation style for each type of cost analysis. Generally, the activity with the lowest cost and the best consequence is the activity that would be selected by the cost analysis as the optimal outcome.

TABLE 17.3 Presentation of the Comparison of Costs and Consequences by Type of Cost Analysis

TYPE OF COST ANALYSIS	PRESENTATION	FICTITIOUS EXAMPLES
Cost description	Total cost of single activity	A heart disease prevention program costs $50,000.
Cost–outcome description	Total cost of single activity per unit of the outcome	Lung cancer hospitalization costs $10,000 per hospitalization and each hospitalization is an average of 5 days in the hospital.
Cost analysis	Total cost of each individual activity	Heart disease program A costs $50,000. Heart disease program B costs $60,000.
Cost minimization	Total cost of each activity assuming constant consequence	Drug A and Drug B cure a bacterial infection in 5 treatment days. Drug A costs $1 per day of treatment; Drug B costs $2 per day of treatment.
Cost consequence	Total cost of each activity and total consequence of each activity	Heart disease program A costs $50,000. Heart disease program B costs $60,000 dollars. Heart disease program A saves $100,000 in hospital costs and reduces readmission by 10%. Heart disease program B saves $150,000 in hospital costs and reduces readmission by 10%.
Cost–benefit	Cost/savings of the unit of the outcome per total cost of each activity	Mammography screening saves $3 in cancer expenditure per $1 spent on screening. Teaching self-breast exam techniques saves $5 in cancer expenditure per $1 spent on teaching.
Cost-effectiveness	Total cost of each activity per unit of the outcome	Smoking-cessation program A saves $1,000 in annual primary care visits per patient who quits smoking. Smoking-cessation program B saves $1,500 in annual primary care visits per patient who quits smoking.
Cost–utility	Total cost of each activity per quality-adjusted unit of the outcome	Intramuscular injection flu immunization costs $10 per disability-adjusted life year gained. Nasal mist flu immunization costs $11 per disability-adjusted life year gained.

■ SPECIAL CONSIDERATIONS

This section examines some considerations for common situations and scenarios that researchers and practitioners may encounter when conducting a cost analysis. These considerations include selecting the standardization year, discounting, depreciation, and a brief description of some of the software programs that can assist with cost analysis.

Selecting the Standardization Year

Selecting to what year to standardize all costs can be a difficult decision, particularly when conducting the cost analysis long after the actual data were collected or when using a historical data set where considerable time has lapsed. There are two good options for selecting the standardization year: Use the final year in which data were collected or use the present year. Using the final year the data were collected can be attractive because the costs are tied most closely to the time period the data were collected, and this limits the assumptions and decisions about the rate of inflation to use. The downside to using the final year is that the data may not reflect the costs of the present day, making interpretation for the reader more difficult. Using the present year can be attractive, because it ensures that the data are most relevant to the time period when the findings will actually be used. The downside to using the present year is that the researcher may have to make a number of assumptions regarding how to inflate the cost values to present-day dollars. Although the inflation can be complex, using the present year is preferable to the final study year, because the results will be most relevant to the present.

Discounting

Discounting is another topic that must be considered when conducting a cost analysis (Attema et al., 2018). Discounting is the process by which we standardize the value of any future costs, savings, or outcomes/consequences (Krahn & Gafni, 1993). Similar to inflation, discounting allows the researcher to ensure comparability of outcomes as well as avoid overstating the potential future implications. Typically a 3% discount rate per year is applied to the value of future costs, savings, or outcomes/consequences when comparing each alternative. However, the U.S. Federal Reserve in 2019 reaffirmed its 2012 policies and target inflation rates of 2%; this suggests that perhaps a 2% discount rate is sufficient (Board of Governors of the Federal Reserve System, 2019). Researchers should clearly articulate what rate they used and may want to consult the governing body in the country/locality where their research occurs for monetary policy (e.g., Federal Reserve, Department of Treasury) to identify the best discount rate for their work. Attema et al. (2018) summarize national guidelines for discounting for a number of countries. Additionally, a range of results using different assumptions for the discount rate can be reported.

Depreciation

Depreciation is an important consideration for cost analyses that examine resources that can be used for multiple years with substantial capital investments, such as expensive equipment. Depreciation allows the researcher to allocate the cost of that resource equally over the years of use that the resource will have rather than simply applying the total cost of the resource in the first year of its life. Depreciation is also a way to account for the cost of replacement for the resource at the end of its useful life. Typically, depreciation is allocated by equally dividing the total cost of the item over the expected total years of use. Sometimes a replacement investment percentage can be added to the total cost of the item to allow for the measurement of future resource expenses. To determine what depreciation, if any, should be included in your analysis, it is best to discuss how depreciation is accounted for with the organization that is commissioning the analysis. If the societal perspective is used, depreciation may not be specifically measured.

Programs That Assist With Cost Analysis

There are many software programs that can be used for cost analysis. Any basic or advanced spreadsheet program (e.g., Microsoft Excel) can be used to capture costs and outcomes data. These programs also have formulas that will assist the researcher in standardizing costs and discounting to present value. These types of programs are likely all that is required for cost description, cost–outcome description, cost, and cost-minimization and cost-consequence analyses. However, if you are pursuing cost-effectiveness, cost–utility, and cost–benefit analyses, a more sophisticated software package may be helpful. Software packages that are designed to allow decision tree construction and Monte Carlo Markov Chain modeling allow easy execution of cost-effectiveness, cost–utility, and cost–benefit analyses. One of the most user-friendly programs is TreeAge (Williamstown, MA). SPSS (Chicago, IL) and SAS (Cary, NC) can also be used to build more complex cost-analysis models.

Other Costing Tools

There are a growing number of online costing tools that have been made publicly available to researchers, policymakers, and others for the purpose of providing economic evidence to support policies, interventions, and practices (Stuebe et al., 2017; Trogdon et al., 2015; Walters et al., 2019). These tools enable individuals to explore the cost of different health outcomes and the interventions that can be used to change their incidence or prevalence. These tools generally explore modification of a specific risk factor or set of risk factors. These tools can be simple math-based models that use probabilities and costs, or they can be complex simulations that incorporate a wide variety of mathematical, probability, and predictive modeling techniques. Researchers should explore what tools are available to them to determine what may be useful in their work or what may inform their own cost studies.

◼ ADVANCED TECHNIQUE: MONTE CARLO

This section examines the advanced cost-analysis technique, the Monte Carlo Model (MCM). The MCM was first published in 1949 (Metropolis & Ulam, 1949) and has been used in a wide variety of sectors including financial/insurance firms, manufacturing, and government. MCM is an umbrella term for a series of related modeling techniques (e.g., Simple, Markov Chain) that use mathematical approaches to model various size systems/problems with inputs (e.g., risk factors/interventions) and outputs (e.g., outcomes) that we can reasonably estimate. The use of MCM models is growing in healthcare because, while we have many systems that have estimable inputs and outputs, our ability to conduct large, population size studies is limited. For example, MCM can be used to estimate the number of expected breast cancer cases in the U.S. population accounting for the impact of exposure to protective and/or harmful risk factors. Because the MCM uses mathematical approaches, it allows researchers to build uncertainty around the magnitude of impact of modeled risk factors. This is important because it recognizes that the actual impact of any given risk factor might vary. For example, the impact of breastfeeding on reducing breast cancer cases varies based on breastfeeding duration and the estimate of this impact includes both a point estimate and a 95% confidence interval (Collaborative Group on Hormonal Factors in Breast Cancer, 2002). Thus, using the MCM approach, we can model population outcomes (breast cancer cases) that account for exposure differences (breastfeeding duration) and the impact variance (95% confidence interval for breastfeeding impact). This ability to model a large population and to model uncertainty has great potential for a variety of healthcare outcomes. Researchers should be cautioned to only undertake a MCM approach in partnership with experts in econometrics and/or computer programming. An example of a study that utilizes MCM is Bartick et al. (2016).

◼ SUMMARY

Throughout this chapter, we discussed the definition of costs, cost measurement, types of cost analysis, the process of conducting a cost analysis, and special considerations that should be taken into account when working with costs and undertaking a cost analysis. It is important that, as researchers and practitioners, you apply the practices described in this chapter to critically evaluate the cost literature. This critical evaluation is important because cost analyses are another tool that can be used to support evidence-based practice. To integrate cost analyses, we must apply the same rigorous standards used to evaluate efficacy, effectiveness, and other clinical research. Cost analyses that do not clearly describe the resources they measured, the assumptions they made, or the year that their costs represent can lead the reader to erroneous conclusions that may hinder the implementation of valuable programs.

SUGGESTED LEARNING ACTIVITIES

1. For each for the scenarios that follow identify what would be the appropriate type of cost analysis.

    a. A study that compares the cost of four different types of chemotherapy treatment for patients with lung cancer

    b. A study that measures the cost of a new enhanced discharge planning program

    c. A study that compares the cost and incidence of back injury among nurses following the implementation of new patient lift assist devices

    d. A study that measures the cost and health outcomes at 5 years of life for infants born preterm and term

    e. A study that compares the cost and quality of life for community health workers who undergo an academic training program versus an on-the-job program

    f. A study that compares the costs and lengths of stay for patients who receive open versus minimally invasive spinal surgery

2. For each of the scenarios in Question 1, what point of view would this study most likely use (individual, institution/corporation, government, society)?

3. Using a peer-reviewed article of your choosing or one of the exemplars listed in the chapter, review the article and identify the following:

    a. What is the main purpose of the article?

    b. What type of economic/cost analysis did they perform?

    c. What type of point of view did they use? Were they consistent in limiting their discussion to that point of view?

    d. How did they define costs and, if appropriate, outcomes/benefits?

    e. Was the analysis comprehensive? Is there anything you think they should have added? Did they address any comprehensiveness issues in their limitations?

    f. What were the main conclusions from the article?

    g. Would you use the findings in the article to influence your practice? Why or why not?

REFERENCES

American Diabetes Association. (2013). Economic costs of diabetes in the U.S. in 2012. *Diabetes Care, 36*(4), 1033–1046. https://doi.org/10.2337/dc12-2625

Attema, A. E., Brouwer, W. B. F., Claxton, K. (2018). Discounting in economic evaluations. *Pharmacoeconomics, 36*, 745–775. https://doi.org/10.1007/s40273-018-0672-z

Bartick, M. C., Schwarz, E. B., Green, B. D., Jegier, B. J., Reinhold, A. G., Colaizy, T. T., Bogen, D. L., Schaefer, A. J., & Stuebe, A. M. (2017). Suboptimal breastfeeding in the United States: Maternal and pediatric health outcomes and costs. *Maternal & Child Nutrition, 13*, e12366. https://doi.org/10.1111/mcn.12366

Behera, M. A., Likes, C. E., Judd, J. P., Barnett, J. C., Havrilesky, L. J., & Wu, J. M. (2012). Cost analysis of abdominal, laparoscopic, and robotic-assisted myomectomies. *Journal of Minimally Invasive Gynecology, 19*(1), 52–57. https://doi.org/10.1016/j.jmig.2011.09.007

Behl, A. S., Goddard, K. A., Flottemesch, T. J., Veenstra, D., Meenan, R. T., Lin, J. S., & Maciosek, M. V. (2012). Cost-effectiveness analysis of screening for *KRAS* and *BRAF* mutations in metastatic colorectal cancer. *Journal of the National Cancer Institute, 104*(23), 1785–1795. https://doi.org/10.1093/jnci/djs433

Board of Governors of the Federal Reserve System. (2019). *Statement on Longer-Run Goals and Monetary Policy Strategy.* https://www.federalreserve.gov/faqs/statement-on-longer-run-goals-monetary-policy-strategy-FOMC.htm

Brazier, J., Roberts, J., & Deverill, M. (2002). The estimation of a preference-based measure of health from the SF-36. *Journal of Health Economics, 21*(2), 271–292. https://doi.org/10.1016/S0167-6296(01)00130-8

Briggs, A. H., Wonderling, D. E., & Mooney, C. Z. (1997). Pulling cost-effectiveness analysis up by its bootstraps: A non-parametric approach to confidence interval estimation. *Health Economics, 6*(4), 327–340. https://doi.org/10.1002/(SICI)1099-1050(199707)6:4<327::AID-HEC282>3.0.CO;2-W

Bureau of Labor Statistics. (2012). *Consumer price index for all urban consumers and all items.* http://www.bls.gov/cpi/#tables

Cella, D., Yount, S., Rothrock, N., Gershon, R., Cook, K., Reeve, B., Ader, D., Fries, J. F., Bruce, B., & Rose, M.; PROMIS Cooperative Group. (2007). The Patient-Reported Outcomes Measurement Information System (PROMIS): Progress of an NIH Roadmap cooperative group during its first two years. *Medical Care, 45*(5, Suppl. 1), S3–S11. https://doi.org/10.1097/01.mlr.0000258615.42478.55

Centers for Medicare & Medicaid Services. (2018). *National health expenditure data.* https://www.cms.gov/Research-Statistics-Data-and-Systems/Statistics-Trends-and-Reports/NationalHealthExpendData/NHE-Fact-Sheet

Chan, K., Hernandez, L., Yang, H., & Bidwell Goetz, M. (2014). Comparative cost analysis of clinical reminder for HIV testing at the Veterans Affairs Healthcare System. *Value in Health, 17*(4), 334–339. https://doi.org/10.1016/j.jval.2014.03.001

Collaborative Group on Hormonal Factors in Breast Cancer. (2002). Breast cancer and breastfeeding: Collaborative reanalysis of individual data from 47 epidemiological studies in 30 countries, including 50,302 women with breast cancer and 96,973 women without the disease. *Lancet, 360*, 187–195. https://doi.org/10.1016/S0140-6736(02)09454-0

Congressional Budget Office. (2019). *The 2019 long-term budget outlook* (CBO Publication No. 55331). U.S. Government Printing Office. https://www.cbo.gov/publication/55331

Dasta, J. F., Kane-Gill, S. L., Pencina, M., Shehabi, Y., Bokesch, P. M., Wisemandle, W., & Riker, R. R. (2010). A cost-minimization analysis of dexmedetomidine compared with midazolam for long-term sedation in the intensive care unit. *Critical Care Medicine, 38*(2), 497–503. https://doi.org/10.1097/CCM.0b013e3181bc81c9

Drummond, M. F., Sculpher, M. J., Torrance, G. W., O'Brien, B. J., & Stoddart, G. L. (2005). *Methods for the economic evaluation of health care programmes* (3rd ed.). Oxford University Press.

EuroQol Group. (1990). EuroQol—A new facility for the measurement of health-related quality of life. *Health Policy, 16*, 199–208. https://doi.org/10.1016/0168-8510(90)90421-9

Gold, M. R., Siegel, J. E., Russell, L. B., & Weinstein, M. C. (1996). *Cost-effectiveness in health and medicine.* Oxford University Press.

Gross, C. P., Long, J. B., Ross, J. S., Abu-Khalaf, M. M., Wang, R., Killelea, B. K., Gold, H. T., Chagpar, A. B., & Ma, X. (2013). The cost of breast cancer screening in the Medicare population. *JAMA Internal Medicine, 173*(3), 220–226. https://doi.org/10.1001/jamainternmed.2013.1397

HCUP Databases. (2012). *Healthcare cost and utilization project (HCUP): 2006–2011.* Agency for Healthcare Research and Quality. www.hcup-us.ahrq.gov/databases.jsp

Jegier, B. J., Meier, P., Engstrom, J. L., & McBride, T. (2010). The initial maternal cost of providing 100 mL of human milk for very low birth weight infants in the neonatal intensive care unit. *Breastfeeding Medicine, 5*(2), 71–77.

Jegier, B. J., O'Mahony, S., Johnson, J., Flaska, R., Perry, A., Runge, M., & Sommerfeld, T. (2016). Impact of a centralized inpatient hospice unit in an academic medical center. *American Journal of Hospice & Palliative Care, 33*(8), 755–759. https://doi.org/10.1089/bfm.2009.0063

Johnson, T. J., Patel, A. L., Jegier, B. J., Meier, P. P., & Engstrom, J. L. (2013). The cost of morbidities in very low birth weight infants. *Journal of Pediatrics, 162*(2), 243–249. https://doi.org/10.1016/j.jpeds.2012.07.013

Kaimal, A. J., Little, S. E., Odibo, A. O., Stamilio, D. M., Grobman, W. A., Long, E. F., Owens, D. K., & Caughey, A. B. (2011). Cost-effectiveness of elective induction of labor at 41 weeks in nulliparous women. *American Journal of Obstetrics and Gynecology, 204*(2), 137.e1–137.e9. https://doi.org/10.1016/j.ajog.2010.08.012

Kang, J., Mandsager, P., Biddle, A. K., & Weber, D. J. (2012). Cost-effectiveness analysis of active surveillance screening for methicillin-resistant *Staphylococcus aureus* in an academic hospital setting. *Infection Control and Hospital Epidemiology, 33*(5), 477–486. https://doi.org/10.1086/665315

Kaplan, R. M., & Anderson, J. P. (1988). A general health policy model: Update and applications. *Health Services Research, 23*(2), 203–235.

Kaplan, R. M., Alcaraz, J. E., Anderson, J. P., & Weisman, M. (1996). Quality-adjusted life years lost to arthritis: Effects of gender, race, and social class. *Arthritis Care and Research, 9*(6), 473–482. https://doi.org/10.1002/art.1790090609

Krahn, M., & Gafni, A. (1993). Discounting in the economic evaluation of health care interventions. *Medical Care, 31*(5), 403–418. https://doi.org/10.1097/00005650-199305000-00003

Kroese, M. E., Severens, J. L., Schulpen, G. J., Bessems, M. C., Nijhuis, F. J., & Landewé, R. B. (2011). Specialized rheumatology nurse substitutes for rheumatologists in the diagnostic process of fibromyalgia: A cost-consequence analysis and a randomized controlled trial. *Journal of Rheumatology, 38*(7), 1413–1422. https://doi.org/10.3899/jrheum.100753

Leendertse, A. J., Van Den Bemt, P. M., Poolman, J. B., Stoker, L. J., Egberts, A. C., & Postma, M. J. (2011). Preventable hospital admissions related to medication (HARM): Cost analysis of the HARM study. *Value in Health, 14*(1), 34–40. https://doi.org/10.1016/j.jval.2010.10.024

Leung, W., Kvizhinadze, G., Nair, N., & Blakely, T. (2016). Adjuvant trastuzumab in HER2-positive early breast cancer by age and hormone receptor status: A cost-utility analysis. *PLOS Med, 13*(8), e1002067. https://doi.org/10.1371/journal.pmed.1002067

Metropolis, N., & Ulam, S. (1949). The Monte Carlo method. *Journal of the American Statistical Association, 44*(247), 335–341. https://doi.org/10.2307/2280232

Patel, A. L., Johnson, T. J., Engstrom, J. L., Fogg, L. F., Jegier, B. J., Bigger, H. R., & Meier, P. P. (2013). Impact of early human milk on sepsis and health-care costs in very low birth weight infants. *Journal of Perinatology, 33*(7), 514–519. https://doi.org/10.1038/jp.2013.2

Petrou, S., Taher, S., Abangma, G., Eddama, O., & Bennett, P. (2011). Cost-effectiveness analysis of prostaglandin E2 gel for the induction of labour at term. *BJOG: An International Journal of Obstetrics and Gynaecology, 118*(6), 726–734. https://doi.org/10.1111/j.1471-0528.2011.02902.x

Polsky, D., Glick, H. A., Willke, R., & Schulman, K. (1997). Confidence intervals for cost-effectiveness ratios: A comparison of four methods. *Health Economics, 6*(3), 243–252. https://doi.org/10.1002/(SICI)1099-1050(199705)6:3<243::AID-HEC269>3.0.CO;2-Z

Puzniak, L. A., Gillespie, K. N., Leet, T., Kollef, M., & Mundy, L. M. (2004). A cost-benefit analysis of gown use in controlling vancomycin-resistant *Enterococcus* transmission: Is it worth the price? *Infection Control and Hospital Epidemiology, 25*(5), 418–424. https://doi.org/10.1086/502416

Revicki, D. A., Kawata, A. K., Harnam, N., Chen, W. H., Hays, R. D., & Cella, D. (2009). Predicting EuroQol (EQ-5D) scores from the patient-reported outcomes measurement information system (PROMIS) global items and domain item banks in a United States sample. *Quality of Life Research, 18*(6), 783–791. https://doi.org/10.1007/s11136-009-9489-8

Schuurman, J. P., Schoonhoven, L., Defloor, T., van Engelshoven, I., van Ramshorst, B., & Buskens, E. (2009). Economic evaluation of pressure ulcer care: A cost minimization analysis of preventive strategies. *Nursing Economics, 27*(6), 390–400, 415.

Smith, K. J., Wateska, A. R., Nowalk, M. P., Raymund, M., Nuorti, J. P., & Zimmerman, R. K. (2012). Cost-effectiveness of adult vaccination strategies using pneumococcal conjugate vaccine compared with pneumococcal polysaccharide vaccine. *Journal of the American Medical Association, 307*(8), 804–812. https://doi.org/10.1001/jama.2012.169

Stuebe, A. M., Jegier, B. J., Schwarz, E. B., Green, B. D., Reinhold, A. D., Colaizy, T. T., Bogen, D. L., Schaefer, A. J., Jegier, J. T., Green, N. A., & Bartick, M. C. (2017). An online calculator to estimate the impact of changes in breastfeeding rates on population health and costs. *Breastfeeding Medicine, 12*(10), 645–658. https://doi.org/10.1089/bfm.2017.0083

Tambour, M., & Zethraeus, N. (1998). Bootstrap confidence intervals for cost-effectiveness ratios: Some simulation results. *Health Economics, 7*(2), 143–147. https://doi.org/10.1002/(SICI)1099-1050(199803)7:2<143::AID-HEC322>3.0.CO;2-Q

Trogdon, J. G., Murphy, L. B., Khavjou, O. A., Li, R., Maylahn, C. M., Tangka, F. K., Nurmagambetov, T. A., Ekwueme, D. U., Nwaise, I., Chapman, D. P., & Orenstein, D. (2015). Costs of chronic diseases at the state level: The chronic disease cost calculator. *Prev Chronic Dis, 12*, 150131. https://doi.org/10.5888/pcd12.150131

Viscusi, W. K., & Aldy, J. E. (2003). *The value of a statistical life: A critical review of market estimates throughout the world*. National Bureau of Economic Research (Working Paper 9487). http://www.nber.org/papers/w9487

Viscusi, W. K., & Zeckhauser, R. J. (1994). The fatality and injury costs of expenditures. *Journal of Risk and Uncertainty, 8*(1), 19–41. https://doi.org/10.1007/BF01064084

Walters, D. D., Phan, L. T. H., & Mathisen, R. (2019).The cost of not breastfeeding: global results from a new tool. *Health Policy and Planning, 34*(6), 407–417, https://doi.org/10.1093/heapol/czz050

Weinstein, M. C., Siegel, J. E., Gold, M. R., Kamlet, M. S., & Russell, L. B. (1996). Recommendations of the panel on cost-effectiveness in health and medicine. *Journal of the American Medical Association, 276*(15), 1253–1258. https://doi.org/10.1001/jama.1996.03540150055031

EVALUATION OF OUTCOMES

ANNE W. ALEXANDROV

■ INTRODUCTION

Knowing the results of healthcare services is key to demonstrating value; likewise, measurement of results or *outcomes* is critical to stimulating improvement in healthcare structures and processes. Today, outcome measurement has become not only necessary, but also an expectation among all healthcare service stakeholders, yet methods supporting measurement alongside program improvement remain complex, especially in comparison to the ease of structure and process measurement.

A number of measures constitute health outcomes, including traditional measures such as those focused on disease morbidity and mortality, as well as health economic measures, quality of life, functional status, and stakeholder satisfaction with healthcare services. Some of the earliest attempts to measure outcomes were made by Florence Nightingale in the 1850s when she monitored the impact of interventions aimed at improving survival rates during the Crimean War (Nightingale, 1863). Attempts to evaluate healthcare can increasingly be seen in the literature since that time, but the work of Donabedian (1966) describing structure, process, and outcome as the three key monitoring areas supporting health systems improvement significantly advanced the field of quality management.

Definitions for what constitutes healthcare quality likely differ depending on the stakeholder, but most would probably identify quality healthcare as that which provides safe, accessible evidence-based health services that have been shown to ensure optimal health, functional status and wellness, and can be delivered at an acceptable cost. Regardless of how it is defined, the evaluation of quality always starts with identification of an *outcome target*; methods are then proposed and developed, and systems built or augmented in a manner that supports achievement of the outcome. The implementation, and ultimately the evaluation of these processes and structural systems, support completion of a *quality loop*. Whether the outcome is advanced practice registered nurse (APRN)–role specific (e.g., position turnover; role satisfaction) or associated with a medical diagnosis (e.g., complication rate; disease severity), the process remains the same, providing healthcare practitioners with an ability to not only understand their impact, but also to clarify the contribution of implemented processes and systems of care, including the need for further improvement. APRNs must embrace outcome measurement alongside evaluation of process and structural system components, using it as a potent method to demonstrate the value of their services and to provide ongoing feedback that incentivizes improvement in both systems of care and the processes used.

◼ DEFINITION AND INTRODUCTION OF TERMS

Health Outcomes Research

Health outcomes research evaluates the results of specific healthcare treatments or interventions (Agency for Healthcare Research and Quality [AHRQ], 2020). The conduct of health outcomes research requires use of experimental or mixed methods designs with the intent to understand differences between two clinical approaches to a problem. Interventions tested may include a broad range of items, from new structures providing a similar standard of care process in a new setting, to new roles, or to use of a variety of different processes that aim to improve outcomes.

Efficacy and Effectiveness Research

Randomized controlled trials (RCTs) test either *efficacy* or *effectiveness* of an intervention. Classically, patients are randomized to either receive an intervention, or to become part of the control group that is managed in the currently acceptable manner. Differences in the targeted outcome are then analyzed to determine whether the intervention is efficacious or effective depending on the phase of intervention testing. *Efficacy* testing is conducted within the context of what is commonly referred to as a *phase 3* RCT, where the *potential* benefits of an intervention are studied under ideal, highly controlled conditions (Piantadosi, 2017; U.S. Food and Drug Administration [FDA], 2020). In comparison, *effectiveness* testing or *phase 4* research refers to testing the intervention in a real-world, less controlled setting, often using what is referred to as an *historical control group* from a previous efficacy RCT (Hulley et al., 2013; Piantadosi, 2017; FDA, 2020). The rationale for use of an historical control group is that if an intervention has been found to be efficacious in previous phase 3 research, it may be unethical to withhold its use in a phase 4 effectiveness trial; therefore, the historical control serves as the group for comparison instead of randomizing patients to a control arm where they may be significantly and unethically disadvantaged (Piantadosi, 2017). The findings from effectiveness research are much more generalizable to a variety of patients, practitioners, and clinical settings because of its implementation within less strictly controlled circumstances (Piantadosi, 2017). As more and more nurse researchers are being prepared as clinical trialists, the future will likely hold findings from numerous efficacy and effectiveness RCTs led by APRN investigators.

Comparative Effectiveness Research

Comparative effectiveness research is conducted to test use of an intervention that has already been found to be effective, but now will be delivered in a new manner (Piantadosi, 2017). For example, treatment with intravenous tissue plasminogen activator (tPA) has been found to be both efficacious and effective in the treatment of acute ischemic stroke patients within 4.5 hours of symptom onset. Treatment with tPA is classically given within the walls of an acute care hospital and has been studied extensively in these settings. The emergence of mobile stroke units (ambulances with computed tomography scanning capabilities) provides the opportunity for a comparative effectiveness study of tPA treatment in the field compared to that provided in the hospital. Similarly, tPA treatment is classically provided by physicians after clinical examination and review of neuroimaging; however, use of APRNs to diagnose stroke and prescribe/administer tPA is increasing dramatically due a shortage of vascular neurologists. Therefore. a comparison of APRN-prescribed to physician-prescribed tPA provides another example of a comparative effectiveness research project. While these examples pertain strictly to acute stroke, APRNs are encouraged to think of how they might design comparative effectiveness research that could support role expansion and the discovery of better methods to support optimal patient outcomes.

Risk and/or Severity Adjustment

Risk adjustment refers to accounting or controlling for patient-specific factors that may impact outcomes (Alexandrov et al., 2019; Duncan, 2018). Risk adjustment "levels the playing field," so to speak, in an effort to determine the efficacy or effectiveness of an intervention in patients that may inherently carry differences in risk, for example a young otherwise healthy athlete being treated for a sports-related extremity fracture, versus an elderly patient with multiple comorbidities and disabilities who is being treated similarly for the same extremity fracture. Without risk adjustment inaccurate conclusions might be made if treatment outcomes are poor, when in reality the cause might be inherent patient factors. There are varying methods of risk adjustment and using the most appropriate method depends on which outcomes are being evaluated, the time period under study, the study population, and the purpose of the evaluation (Duncan, 2018). The most common variables used for risk adjustment include age, severity of illness, and comorbid conditions (Alexandrov et al., 2019; Duncan, 2018).

■ EVALUATING OUTCOMES

Evolution of Outcome Evaluation

As briefly described, Florence Nightingale (1863) is credited with much of the early work in medicine that was tied to outcome evaluation, with scrutiny of processes and structures when results were determined to be unacceptable or improved. Her exceptional influence in the development of epidemiology as well as quality improvement is seen in early 20th century England's embracing similar methods led by Emory W. Groves (1908), a physician who championed outcome measurement. Dr. Grove's (1908) early work demonstrated variability in surgical mortality, fostering interest in understanding what should be considered "acceptable" rates of death, alongside standardization of medical approaches to diseases so that like comparisons could be made between providers and hospitals.

Interestingly, at the time of Dr. Grove's (1908) work in England, practitioners in the United States held a rather fatalistic view toward poor medical outcomes, with beliefs that poor outcomes were not linked to system structure, processes of care, or practitioner abilities, but instead were due to factors beyond human control. Massive social reform dominated the late 19th and early 20th centuries in the United States, with significant public administrative growth along with required performance auditing. Deficits in medical education were made public during this time with the publication of the Flexnor Report of 1910 which cited poor medical school educational standards and ultimately led to a retooling of American medical education (Fee, 1982). Nurse licensure formalized requirements for nursing education mandating preliminary education, professional training in nursing, licensing examinations, and formal state registration (Wyatt, 2019). While these measures acted to improve structural healthcare quality, it wasn't until 1914 that outcome evaluation formally emerged in the United States, when physician Ernest Codman publicly recommended 12-month postoperative patient follow-ups as a measure of surgical success (Codman, 1914). In 1917, Dr. Codman articulated this concept as the *End-Result Idea*, advocating for measurement and public reporting of results (outcomes), in an effort for hospitals to improve the medical care delivered at their facilities (Codman, 1917). Sadly, Dr. Codman's End-Result Idea was viewed as heretical and dangerous, stifling work on the science of outcome measurement and limiting health quality improvement to primarily structural and process description, until the work of Donabedian.

Donabedian

In 1966, Avedis Donabedian detailed descriptions of structure, process, and outcome measures and took up the torch for development of criteria to evaluate outcomes. In 1980, he described *structure* as stable attributes within the care setting, for example personnel manpower and available equipment; *processes* were described as interventions used by healthcare professionals, including how skillfully these interventions were executed; and, *outcomes* were defined as the resultant change in health status that is directly in-line with care structure and process (Donabedian, 1980). Donabedian (1980) identified that outcomes must be assessed in relation to both structure and process variables to provide a thorough understanding of *how* and *why* the outcome occurred. Figure 18.1 illustrates Donabedian's (1980) concepts showing the inter-relatedness of structure, process and outcome, with outcomes the result of the process and structural interactions. A shortcoming to the Donabedian (1980) model is the exclusion of individual patient factors or characteristics which may alter expected results, for example inherent susceptibility for different outcomes due to significant comorbidities, or health disparities affecting access to services. Although Donabedian's (1980) work defined the important relationship among structure, process, and outcome, practitioners rarely embraced outcome measurement in routine clinical practice until the 1990s when it became an expectation.

Ellwood's Outcomes Management

In 1988, Dr. Paul Ellwood published his definition of *Outcomes Management* (OM), describing it as ". . . a technology of patient experience designed to help patients, payers, and providers make rational medical care-related choices based on better insight into the effect of these choices on patient life" (p. 1549). The suggestion that knowledge of healthcare outcomes could drive patient, payer, and provider healthcare choices revolutionized contemporary medicine and nursing care at a time in the United States when hospital payment had become capitated with the emergence of *Diagnostic Related Groups* (DRGs). Ellwood's (1988) landmark paper prophetically predicted a dramatic shift in healthcare stakeholder engagement well before launch of consumer internet access, including requirements such as public reporting and standardized healthcare quality *core measures* that could be tied to reimbursement in association with the results produced.

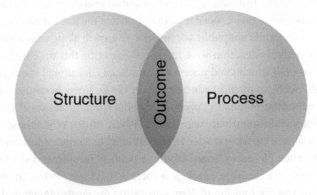

FIGURE 18.1 The Inter-relatedness of Donabedian's Structure and Process Concepts in the Production of Outcomes.

Ellwood (1988) suggested four essential principles for inclusion in an OM program:

1. An emphasis on standards that providers can use to select appropriate interventions;
2. The measurement of patient functional status and well-being, along with disease-specific outcomes;
3. A pooling of outcome data on a massive scale; and
4. The analysis and dissemination of the database to appropriate decision makers.

Today, Ellwood's (1988) principles support a number of initiatives that are now standard requirements for health systems, including:

- Use of evidence-based guidelines developed by scientific and professional practice agencies to support delivery of optimal healthcare;

- Use of valid and reliable tools to capture such factors as disease severity, disability, functional status, health consumer perceptions of service quality or satisfaction, and quality of life, with many of these developed to validly capture patient outcomes within a discrete population or diagnosis of interest;

- Use of large national registries to capture standardized payer-required core measures for pooling and analyses; and,

- Benchmarking of provider and/or institutional performance, along with publicly reported data.

Following publication of Ellwood's (1988) paper, the *Outcomes Management Model* (Figure 18.2) emerged, demonstrating four key steps in the measurement of outcomes using an effectiveness research approach (Wojner, 2001). The first of these steps centered on identification of outcome targets, along with other important variables that were theoretically in-line with the outcome, including those that could confound outcome attainment; this process lent itself to construction of an *outcome measurement repository* or database. The second step included review of the evidence supporting current and new or evolving practice processes, with collaborative agreement reached across all providers/stakeholders on an evidence-supported standardized approach to patient management. This effort resulted in the development of structured care methods consisting of care maps/pathways, order sets, decision-support algorithms, policies, and procedures to assist with provider compliance with the new agreed upon approach to patient management. The third step involved implementing the new care methods, with time provided to ensure the stability of care processes; once stability of the new practices was reached, data collection would then begin to capture structure, process, and outcome data. The last phase involved data analysis with interdisciplinary review of findings. This phase led to agreed upon next steps/changes to further outcome improvement, often recycling back to phase two where new approaches or further refinement of existing processes could be agreed upon and standardized for a subsequent phase of testing and evaluation (Wojner, 2001).

Models for Outcome Evaluation

When beginning an outcome measurement project, APRNs must start by considering the model that will best frame their efforts. Numerous methods to support outcome evaluation have emerged over time, but interestingly each contains similar approaches to the measurement of outcomes, although the Outcomes Management Model depicts the process as *effectiveness research* (Wojner, 2001). Most other models adhere to a *quality model* structure although elements are similar. For example, the *Plan-Do-Study-Act* (PDSA) model starts with identification of the quality (outcome)

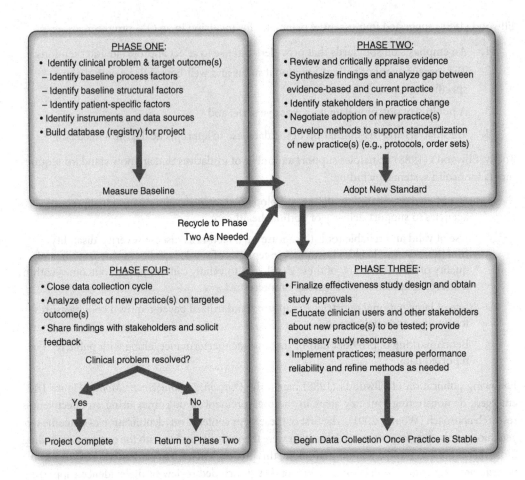

FIGURE 18.2 Wojner's outcomes management model.

Source: Reprinted with permission from the Health Outcomes Institute, LLC-P, Fountain Hills, Arizona.

target and planning, moving to standardization of an approach to care, followed by collecting performance data, and last, examining the results; findings often require a recycling through the process again as methods are refined and further improved upon, until the targeted outcome is achieved. PDSA is a popular quality model to guide the work of outcome evaluation under the authority of local quality improvement initiatives and extends from the work of Deming (1986) who first developed it as the Plan-Do-Check-Act (PDCA) framework. Six Sigma is another performance improvement model that is supported by similar elements and a cyclic methodology: Define-Measure-Analyze-Improve and Control (Council for Six Sigma Certification, 2018).

Selection of a model to support the work of outcome evaluation is largely dependent on the purpose. If the APRN intends to disseminate findings as effectiveness research in a publication or presentation, the Outcomes Management Model may provide the most appropriate framework for the project, including the attainment of local Ethics or Institutional Review Board approval (Alexandrov et al., 2019; Wojner, 2001). Conversely, if the project is only intended for internal quality improvement without external dissemination, selection of a quality model may be the best option. Table 18.1 provides elements that the APRN should consider in determining whether the project should be classified as effectiveness research or quality improvement.

TABLE 18.1 Effectiveness Research Versus Quality Improvement

CONSIDERATIONS	QUALITY IMPROVEMENT	RESEARCH
Project purpose	• Focuses on a specific local performance gap compared to the existing standard of care • Focus is to improve a specific aspect of health or healthcare delivery that is not consistently and appropriately being implemented	• Identifies a specific deficit in scientific knowledge in the literature and practice • Proposes to address specific research questions or test hypotheses to develop new knowledge or advance existing knowledge
Intended methods	• Focuses on the implementation of only scientifically acceptable evidence-based practice changes • Implementation methods may be staged and sequential over time based on feedback received, with the intent of tailoring the process to local resource availability • Intended analyses focus on structural and process changes alongside outcome measurement	• Focuses on the implementation of either a new/novel untested intervention, or testing of effectiveness in an intervention shown to be efficacious in another sample • Protocol defines the intervention and its implementation in detail, along with a case report form that enables collection of patient characteristics and demographics, process fidelity, structural standardization, and outcome data using valid and reliable methods and instruments • Analytical strategies allow comparison between groups using experimental or mixed methods in relation to the intervention(s) being tested
Risk–benefit analysis	• The provider–patient relationship is not altered • Benefit to patients and other stakeholders is well established scientifically • Institutional benefit is specified (i.e., improved efficiency or cost per case) • Participant risk is associated with no participation	• Requires Ethics or Institutional Review Board approval • Use of personal health information extends to beyond the usual provider–patient relationship • Benefit to participants or the institution may be unknown • Risks to participants may occur and must be disclosed • Written informed consent may be required
Generalizability	• Generalizability to other settings is unlikely and is not the main intent	• Results may be generalizable depending on the sample, methods, and limitations cited
Dissemination	• Intended for internal process and structural improvement • Unlikely to be accepted or allowable for presentation or publication without Ethics or Institutional Review Board project approval	• Requires Ethics or Institutional Review Board approval, therefore making dissemination outside the organization possible according to the approvals received

Source: Adapted from the work of Stausmire, J. M. (2014). Quality improvement or research – deciding which road to take. *Critical Care Nurse, 34*(6), 58–63. https://doi.org/10.4037/ccn2014177

Selecting an Outcome Target

Determining the need to evaluate outcomes should be inherent to the role of the APRN. As the "attending nurse" for the service, the APRN should know where quality healthcare exists, as well as where there are significant performance issues that reduce healthcare quality (Alexandrov et al., 2019). Therefore, the choice to undertake an outcome evaluation project should extend not from intuition, but from a baseline empirical examination of actual service outcomes within a discrete patient population.

The rationale for selection of a specific or discrete patient cohort is tied to current knowledge and trends in what's been referred to as *personalized medicine*. Failed clinical trials across numerous healthcare specialties are now being criticized for failure to enroll homogeneous groups of patients with little to no baseline examination of a potential response, nor an understanding of what outcomes were valid, and how and when to measure these outcomes. Today, healthcare providers must carefully define potential responders to a therapeutic intervention and then craft processes that will support achievement of the targeted outcome; when the outcome is not achieved a critical analysis of "why" this happened should occur, followed by a reappraisal of structure and process methods, refinement, and improvement, and subsequent retesting of the intervention.

Examples of the need for a more homogeneous patient cohort during the conduct of health outcomes research include the failed mechanical thrombectomy trials in acute large vessel occlusion (LVO) stroke published in 2013 which showed no difference in 3-month outcome between medical management alone and interventional management (Broderick et al., 2013; Ciccone et al., 2013; Kidwell et al., 2013) as well as the failed HeadPoST study which claimed that it didn't matter if ischemic stroke or intracerebral hemorrhage patients were managed with the head of bed at 0- or 30-degrees (Anderson et al., 2017). Had the scientific community accepted these failures instead of analyzing what went wrong and how structure and process could be improved, management of acute stroke patients would never have evolved. Instead, 2015 saw the publication of results from five new mechanical thrombectomy trials demonstrating efficacy at 3-months compared to medical management alone (Berkhemer et al., 2015; Campbell et al., 2015; Goyal et al., 2015; Jovin et al., 2015; Saver et al., 2015), and the ongoing ZODIAC study led by an APRN clinical trialist sponsored by the National Institutes of Health's National Institute for Nursing Research is using evidence-based methods to understand the contribution of head positioning to patient stability in hyperacute LVO stroke (U.S. National Library of Medicine, 2020).

Outcome measures fall into several different categories, and depending on the source, many different classification systems can be used to group them together. For example, the National Quality Forum (NQF, 2020) categorizes interventions tied to outcomes as patient-centered, nurse-sensitive, and systems-sensitive, with only one intervention identified as nurse-sensitive, namely provision of smoking cessation counseling. The rationale for limiting the number of nurse-sensitive interventions in the NQF portfolio is that numerous other aspects of care contribute to the production of an outcome, not solely nursing care. To illustrate this point, consider pressure ulcer development, a National Database of Nursing Quality Indicators (NDNQI) measure (American Nurses Association, 2020); if the physician of record doesn't prescribe the appropriate diet and hydration for a frail patient, skin breakdown may ensue even with provision of an excellent nursing turning and mobility regimen. This example provides sound rationale for moving away from nurses accepting total responsibility for outcomes, to one of interdisciplinary teams accepting responsibility. Few nurses work strictly in isolation from other healthcare providers, and for those who do perhaps they may be positioned to assume a position of total responsibility for results seen in their patients. But for most, the evaluation of outcomes should be considered a "team sport," in that what is measured as the final result of care processes most likely reflects how the team as a whole, in concert with available system structural resources, manages the patient cohort. Because of this major shift in thinking, this chapter provides a broad classification of outcomes into general categories (Table 18.2).

The physiologic category contains outcomes which will vary significantly based on the population or discrete cohort under study. The outcomes listed here include such metrics as disease severity (which may be evaluated using disease-specific instruments), disease-related disability, complications which are common within the population of interest or of concern based on treatment methods used, as well as mortality.

Mortality is a measure that is frequently reported in benchmarked data that allow users, including the general public, to evaluate rates of death at different institutions. However, without careful, responsible risk adjustment, mortality data may be misinterpreted. For example, if a

TABLE 18.2 Outcome Measures

CATEGORY	EXAMPLES
Physiologic indicators	Time to targeted blood pressure Symptomatic intracerebral hemorrhage following reperfusion treatment in ischemic stroke Disability severity Nosocomial pneumonia Venous thromboembolism Mortality
National Database of Nursing Quality Indicators (NDQI)	Nosocomial pressure ulcers Failure to rescue Catheter-associated urinary tract infection rate Central line–associated bloodstream infection rate Ventilator-associated pneumonia rate Falls and fall-injuries
Functional status	Modified Rankin Scale Barthel Index Return to work or previous lifestyle
Quality of life	Disease-specific measures Short Form 36 (SF-36) taken as a whole, with subscales in the following domains: Physical functioning Role functioning Bodily pain General health Vitality Social functioning Role-emotional Mental health
Health consumer satisfaction	Hospital Consumer Assessment of Healthcare Providers and Systems (HCAHPS)© STROKE Perception Report©
Health economic indicators	Length of hospital stay Hospital readmission within 30-days of discharge Cost per case Patient annual health spending

small rural hospital transports complex patients with a specific diagnosis to higher level tertiary hospitals, we would expect the small rural hospital to hold a much lower mortality rate than the tertiary care hospital. This example illustrates what is referred to as *sample referral bias*, with hospitals accepting the most complex patients disadvantaged on mortality reports compared to those hospitals that only handle patients with minor problems (Hulley et al., 2013).

When selecting a physiologic outcome target, APRNs should choose those that can be tied clearly to processes and structures that are within their ability to impact. An example would be venous thromboembolism: The APRN can examine the use of anticoagulation and mobility measures, implement a new standard of practice within the cohort, and evaluate improvement in the outcome. Another example is time to target blood pressure in an outpatient hypertension cohort: The APRN can examine how patients are routinely followed and managed, implement a new approach that might include telemedicine, along with a new evidence-based medication management algorithm, and then reevaluate the outcome to see if time to targeted blood pressure decreases. Physiologic outcomes are often an important starting place for APRN evaluation and intervention, and they are ripe for use of additional outcome measures alongside implementation of new or novel approaches to care. For example, if new methods to reduce time to targeted blood pressure attainment are implemented, the APRN can also tack on measurement of patient satisfaction with this process. Similarly, if new methods to prevent venous thromboembolism are implemented, the APRN can also tack on measures for quality of life, resource utilization, health economic indicators, and functional status.

Functional status is another important outcome measure as it considers the ability of the patient to participate in activities of daily living (ADLs), with numerous valid and reliable measures available for use. Selection of measures that are considered the gold standard for a specific population is important to enable comparisons between groups. Setting specific measures should also be considered; for example, functional status measurement within a hospital setting will not be well served by a measure created for use within an inpatient rehabilitation or long-term care setting. Whenever possible, measurement of baseline ADL or functional limitations is recommended so that the APRN can statistically adjust findings in functional outcomes measured later in the care period.

Quality of life (QoL) is an important measure that allows providers to understand the patient experience of living with a number of different disease processes or psychosocial circumstances. As the number of people with chronic illnesses grow, use of QoL tools will continue to gain importance so that providers can better understand how to approach such problems as pain management, dyspnea, and other aspects of chronicity that limit return to a full, healthy life. A number of tools are available to measure QoL and many are disease, age, and/or condition specific. Use of a tool that has been found to be valid and reliable is essential, so the APRN is advised to search the literature for the best candidate instruments. The Short Form 36 (SF-36) is often categorized as a QoL instrument, although it consists of domains that cover a wide variety of content ranging from functional status to mental health; however, taken collectively, these content areas may provide a reasonable understanding of QoL. Beyond specific disease conditions, considerations when selecting a tool should also include the preferred-language of the patient, as well as patient culture.

Perceptions of satisfaction with healthcare services is another important area for measurement. Some key principles to consider when evaluating patient satisfaction tools include examination of reliability and validity, the specific concepts the tool is measuring, and the setting and sample on which it was tested. Keep in mind that the instrument's reliability and validity are only applicable to the setting in which the tool was tested. A tool highly valid and reliable in the acute care setting may not be valid and reliable in a home care setting (Polit & Beck, 2017). Additionally, some tools may be more focused on what has been referred to a *hospitality measures*, or measures associated with such things as room comfort and the quality of food served. Careful examination of the concepts targeted by the tool will allow the APRN to better understand its fit with the purpose of the study.

One of the drawbacks to using patient satisfaction as an outcome is the difficulty in determining what care delivery process is affecting the patient's response, as well as knowing whether the patient's disease outcome itself is the major factor impacting overall perceived health system quality. For example, when a patient states they were "not satisfied," it is often impossible to know whether the dissatisfaction was related to the nursing care received, the physician's care, or with the lack of cleanliness of the room. Additionally, if the patient's medical outcome is viewed by the patient/family as suboptimal, this may result in selection of a poor overall level of satisfaction with the services provided even though the services may have been fully evidence based. For this reason, use of disease and setting-specific satisfaction perception instruments is best as this may allow for severity adjustment of responses (Alexandrov, Brewer, Moore, et al., 2019). Despite potential shortcomings, measurement of patient experience and perceptions of care are becoming increasingly important. The Medicare value-based purchasing program provides incentives to hospitals that achieve higher levels of patient satisfaction (Centers for Medicare & Medicaid Services [CMS], 2020a), and the Magnet Recognition Program® also requires hospitals to demonstrate how they are outperforming their peer groups in patient satisfaction measures that are relevant to nursing care (American Nurses Credentialing Center [ANCC], 2020).

Practice Standardization and Fidelity Measurement

At the heart of outcome evaluation is the need for standardization of practice methods along with knowledge of the fidelity of these methods in relation to the outcome that is being measured. No other issue has been more polarizing to organized medicine internationally than the call for practice standardization around what's often been referred to as *best* or *evidence-based practice*. The most tumultuous period in medicine associated with practice standardization occurred in the mid-1990s through to the middle of the first decade of the 2000s, with calls for abandonment of "cookbook medicine" and an allowance of individual practitioner approaches to care, often resulting in highly heterogeneous practice methods associated with a wide variety of patient outcomes. But without structural and process standardization and measurement of adherence fidelity, end results or outcomes cannot validly be connected to the structures and processes used. Today, standardization is widely accepted due to the evolution of payer- and health consumer-inspired core measures which are now tied to pay-for-performance incentives. However, some degree of practice variation continues to exist, making clear the necessity to understand process fidelity alongside the measurement of outcomes. APRNs should consider existing evidence-based professional and scientific guidelines and other publications demonstrating efficacy or effectiveness in their selection of project methods and interventions.

Once the intervention has been clearly defined and adequately supported by evidence to ensure ethical project conduct, the APRN must consider methods to ensure fidelity of the intervention's implementation. Methods used will likely consist of a variety of strategies where education is provided to all stakeholders along with provision of process procedures, algorithms, and flow diagrams.

Additional supporting data elements will need to be considered and included in the development of a case report form to capture the outcome target, along with structural and process methods for fidelity evaluation, and patient factors such as demographics, co-morbidities, and disease-specific findings that may be important in risk adjustment, using valid and reliable tools (Polit & Beck, 2017). Caution should be used in defining the variables to be collected and should be largely driven by the intended analyses that will be performed. For example, if patient "obesity" is to be collected, should the APRN define this as "yes or no" based on a definition of body mass index (BMI) greater than 26, or should the actual BMI be recorded? Determining the correct level of data for variables that can be defined in numerous ways is essential. A good rule is to always collect interval or ratio level continuous data when they are available (e.g., actual age in years, weight, hemoglobin A1c levels); these can be recoded if necessary into categories later depending on the intended analyses.

Analyses should be pre-specified, in terms of both the statistical methods used as well as the point in time when they will occur (e.g., after enrollment of the first 30 subjects, quarterly), with fidelity measurement occurring at the time of outcome measurement so that results can be clearly understood (Piantadosi, 2017). The timing of analyses should be theoretically sound. For example, a patient with a disabling diagnosis such as stroke often requires several months of progressive rehabilitation before functional status improves. By reviewing leading research studies published in the field of acute stroke, the standard time for measurement of functional status is at 3-months from stroke onset. In designing a study testing an intervention that aims to improve functional status in acute stroke patients, investigators would be foolish to pursue a different time frame given the large body of work supporting this time period. While research studies may select both longitudinal and proximal measurement times, in the case of quality studies the APRN should consider a theoretically sound time frame that is conducive to measurement of the outcome while the patient is within the controlled setting, unless a system can be put in place to follow the patient over time and across different healthcare settings.

Fidelity measurement of standardization consists of the following key areas:

- Context:
  - Has overall standard of care changed to influence adherence or methods specified?
  - Have changes occurred that affect organizational capacity for the standard's performance?
  - Have users been exposed to biased messaging that may influence recruitment to the new standard and ultimately protocol adherence?
- Reach and recruitment:
  - To what extent is the new practice reaching intended patients?
  - Are unintended patients enrolled?
- Implementation:
  - To what extent is the practice implemented?
  - Dose delivered:
    - How much of the practice is being administered?
    - What, if anything, is omitted or performed inconsistently?
  - Dose received:
    - What is the average dose of the practice that is received?
- Overall fidelity:
  - How well does the practice execution maintain fidelity of the original design?

- Aggregate structural compliance
- Aggregate process compliance (Piantadosi, 2017)

The work of Anderson et al. (2013) provides a prime example of the importance of fidelity measurement to understand results. These investigators postulated that aggressive blood pressure lowering in patients with acute intracerebral hemorrhage would reduce hematoma expansion and improve 3-month outcome. Patients were randomized to one of two arms: The control arm allowed blood pressure to be elevated to as high as 180/105 mmHg per the standard of care, whereas in the experimental arm blood pressure was to be lowered to beneath 140/90 mmHg. Findings from the study showed that there was no difference in hematoma expansion between groups, but that the group in the experimental arm showed a trend toward improved 3-month functional outcome ($p = 0.06$; Anderson et al., 2013). Publication of the results of this study resulted in several scientific organizations immediately changing their guidelines to a recommended blood pressure of less than 140/90 mmHg. However, a later publication examined protocol fidelity in the Anderson et al. (2013) study, demonstrating that only 33% of patients in the experimental group actually achieved aggressive blood pressure lowering with maintenance to a blood pressure less than 140/90 mmHg as the study had proposed (Qureshi et al., 2016). Additionally, the starting blood pressures in the subjects in the experimental group were not extremely high, leaving it unknown how safe it would be to aggressively lower blood pressure in patients with extreme hypertension with acute intracerebral hemorrhage (Anderson et al., 2013). In short, without fidelity testing, the reader was left to assume that the trend in improved 3-month outcome was due solely to aggressive blood pressure lowering when this was not the case.

The importance of understanding protocol fidelity cannot be underestimated, since being able to attribute outcomes to the methods used is essential. In fact, this requirement now extends to the conduct of most interventional research studies funded by the United States federal agencies with an expectation of the reporting of protocol fidelity alongside experimental results so that readers can better understand the efficacy or effectiveness of new practice interventions (Piantadosi, 2017).

One of the most common methods to support measurement of process fidelity is development of *control charts*. Control charts were first developed in the business world by Walter Shewhart as a method to determine whether processes in manufacturing were in control (History-Biography, 2020). There are two types of control charts that can be constructed, *individual control charts* and *proportional control charts* (Wojner, 2001). *Individual control charts* are used for non-proportional data, such as minutes from emergency department arrival time to performance of first electrocardiogram (door to EKG time). *Proportional control charts* are used to capture proportional data, such as rates of patients receiving a newly proposed APRN consult or other intervention. Upper and lower control limits are calculated, and then actual performance is plotted against these limits; when practice becomes more stable over time, recalculation of upper and lower control limits may be necessary to ensure accurate capture of performance. Control charts are an excellent way to illustrate stability of process performance over time, but they can also be constructed to measure outcomes within quality projects; for example, length of stay can be monitored using an individual control chart, whereas complication rates such as pneumonia can be monitored using a proportional control chart.

Dissemination

The APRN has a responsibility to disseminate findings from outcome evaluation in a number of ways. First, those involved directly with the outcome evaluation effort should be intimately aware of what they have produced in comparison to baseline measures. Administrative authorities should also be made aware, as this is an important step in gaining APRN recognition for healthcare performance improvement leadership. When Ethics or Institutional Review Board approvals have been obtained, the APRN has a professional obligation to share their work with not only the advanced practice peer group, but also other interdisciplinary providers who may be interested in replicating the methods used. This can and should be accomplished through oral or poster presentation at scientific or clinical conferences, and always followed with publication of the project methods and results in a professional journal, because conference abstracts are not easily found and typically not recognized as evidence of significant role scholarship.

STAKEHOLDER SUPPORT FOR OUTCOME EVALUATION

The Seven Ps of Stakeholdership

A number of stakeholders have an interest in outcome evaluation, including:

- Patients
- Practitioners and Provider Programs
- Purchasers or Payers
- Product Producers
- Policymakers (Wojner, 2001)

That patients would have a stake in healthcare outcomes is hardly a surprise; in fact, patients should be viewed as active partners in the care they are provided. With availability of health information at their fingertips, patients can access information on a number of disease conditions, medications, available treatments, and service availability. Public reporting has made available an ability to compare the performance of physicians, as well as hospitals or clinics against their competitors so that patients are able to select the service provider and setting they believe will best meet their needs. Practitioners and the provider programs that hire them clearly have a stake in understanding the outcomes they produce. Not only will this knowledge help to improve processes used in care, including remediation of suboptimal practitioner skill, but it also can be used to understand important structural needs such as bed-demand, or the need to add new evolving services not previously available; in turn, when used to improve overall performance capabilities this knowledge betters market share. Purchasers' and payers' knowledge of key outcomes plays an important role in contracting health plans and also pay-for-performance, with suboptimal providers penalized for failure to perform up to par. Product producers use outcome evaluation to drive improvement in devices or development of new technology. Lastly, policymakers are using outcome evaluation to drive changes in reimbursement schedules, standardize approaches to care delivery, enlarge scope of practice for APRNs, and determine critical access needs where additional health service funding must be set aside.

Agencies Impacting Healthcare Outcomes and Quality

Briefly, a number of agencies are focused on outcome improvement in healthcare. The American Nurses Credentialing Center (ANCC, 2020) offers Magnet® recognition for hospitals that draw and retain nurses. This work began in the early 1980s when the American Academy of Nursing's (AAN) Task Force on Nursing Practice in Hospitals conducted a survey of approximately 160 hospitals in the United States and identified 41 hospitals where the environment attracted and retained nurses. In the early 1990s, the first U.S. hospital was given Magnet recognition and today Magnet is an international recognition that is available in both acute care hospitals and long-term care facilities (ANCC, 2020). Magnet recognition identifies care institutions where the quality of nursing care is exceptional and is based on 14 forces of Magnetism or standards of excellence that have five major themes or components: transformational leadership; structural empowerment; exemplary professional practice; new knowledge, innovations, and improvements; and empirical outcomes. Under the empirical outcomes model component, institutions must provide examples of the structures, processes, and outcomes they use for ongoing quality improvement efforts and the practitioners involved, with an emphasis on nurses. In addition, institutions must show that they are outperforming their peer group on outcome measures such as pressure ulcers, falls, catheter-associated urinary tract infections (UTIs), ventilator-associated events, central line–associated bloodstream infections, use of restraints, and pediatric intravenous (IV) infiltrations (ANCC, 2020).

Another influential agency is the AHRQ. The AHRQ is a part of the U.S. Department of Health and Human Services (DHHS) and not only funds health services research but is also very active in disseminating research results and evidence-based practices, which greatly influence health outcomes (AHRQ, 2020).

The NQF (2020) is a nonprofit organization developed in 1999 to address the need for valid and reliable healthcare performance indicators, with members that include a wide variety of public and private entities in roles such as healthcare consumer, healthcare provider (physicians, nurses, therapists, etc.), purchaser, and administrator. The NQF works as the endorsing agency for the CMS core measures that move on to pay-for-performance. Within this role, the NQF has endorsed hundreds of measures, most of which are process indicators. Efforts are taken to understand the necessity of process indicators over time, so that when high thresholds of adherence are identified, measures are retired from the core measure set. Presently, the primary interest of both the NQF and the CMS is development of valid and reliable outcome indicators as core measures.

The CMS is a federal agency that is charged with the administration of the Medicare and Medicaid programs within the United States (CMS, 2020b). Due to the high number of people and expenditures covered by Medicare and Medicaid, the CMS is one of the single biggest influencers of healthcare quality in the United States. The decisions of the CMS not only impact patients covered by Medicare and Medicaid but also those covered by private insurance as many private insurance companies adopt policies for reimbursement that are in alignment with CMS policies. The CMS's *value-based purchasing* program provides financial incentives for hospitals using their performance on process and outcome measures approved by the NQF, along with patients' experience of care measured by Hospital Consumer Assessment of Healthcare Providers and System (HCAHPS; CMS, 2020a). The CMS also posts the Hospital Compare website for consumer access to performance benchmarking (U.S. Department of Health and Human Services, 2020; www.medicare.gov/hospitalcompare/search.html).

Lastly, the Patient-Centered Outcomes Research Institute (PCORI, 2020) is an independent nonprofit, nongovernmental organization located in Washington, DC, that focuses on improving the quality of healthcare through the conduct of comparative effectiveness research that is wholly centered on outcomes of importance to patients and their families. The aim of PCORI is to provide evidence of alternative methods for healthcare delivery so that they may make informed decisions about how, where, and when to receive interventions that aim to improve health and well-being.

■ SUMMARY

Outcome evaluation ensures the development and delivery of quality healthcare services for numerous stakeholders. Advanced practice nurses must embrace outcome evaluation and become masterful in its methods. By measuring outcomes, APRNs are able to understand opportunities for improvement, develop and implement novel new approaches to care, and showcase the value of their contribution to patients and health institutions. Certainly, no other responsibility is more important in nursing than to improve the health of those the profession serves, and outcomes evaluation provides powerful guidance for how to do just that.

SUGGESTED LEARNING ACTIVITIES

1. Explore the CMS Hospital Compare website (www.medicare.gov/hospitalcompare/search.html) and compare two hospitals in your area.

    a. Based on the information presented, do you believe the findings to be accurate, or are their likely other intervening considerations?

    b. Develop a conceptual model that explains part, or all, of one of the reported outcomes. What structures and processes could be measured to explain differences in the outcome?

2. Develop a new outcome measure for the NQF that is important to a discrete group of patients. Support the importance of the measure using evidence that demonstrates value to at least three of the *seven P-stakeholders* cited in this chapter. Develop a valid evidence-supported definition for the measure that would support accurate and reliable data collection/documentation; determine its *measurement feasibility* (Are the data routinely available in the current medical record system?), as well as its usability in practice (How useful will the measure be to demonstrate practice quality?). What would need to change in how medical and nursing care are routinely performed and documented to help capture the outcome measure in a valid and reliable manner across numerous settings?

REFERENCES

Agency for Healthcare Research and Quality. (2020). *National Quality Indicators*. http://www.ahrq.gov

Alexandrov, A. W., Brewer, T. & Brewer, B. B. (2019). The role of outcomes and evidence-based practice quality improvement in enhancing and evaluating practice changes. In B. Melnyk & E. Finout-Overholt (Eds.), *Evidence-based practice in nursing and healthcare: A guide to best practice* (4th ed., pp. 293–312). Wolters Kluwer, Lippincott Williams & Wilkins.

Alexandrov, A. W., Brewer, B. B., Moore, K., Crau, C., Beenstock, D. J., Cudlip, R., Murphy, D. A., Klassman, L., Korsnack, A. M., Johnson, B., Parliament, C. F., Lane, P. C., . . . Alexandrov, A. V. (2019). Measurement ofpPatients' perceptions of the quality of acute stroke services: Development and validation of the STROKE Perception Report©. *Journal of Neuroscience Nursing, 51*(5), 208–216. https://doi.org/10.1097/JNN.0000000000000471

American Nurses Association. (2020). *The National Database of Nursing Quality Indicators*. http://ojin.nursingworld.org/MainMenuCategories/ANAMarketplace/ANAPeriodicals/OJIN/TableofContents/Volume122007/No3Sept07/NursingQualityIndicators.html

American Nurses Credentialing Center. (2020). *ANCC Magnet recognition program*. https://www.nursingworld.org/organizational-programs/magnet

Anderson, C. S., Heeley, E., Huang, Y., Wang, J., Stapf, C., Delcourt, C., Lindley, R., Robinson, T., Lavados, P., Neal, B., Hata, J., Arima, H., . . . INTERACT2 Investigators. (2013). Rapid blood-pressure lowering in patients with acute intracerebral hemorrhage. *New England Journal of Medicine, 368*(25), 2355–2365. https://doi.org/10.1056/NEJMoa1214609

Anderson, C. S., Arima, H., Lavados, P., Billot, L., Hackett, M. L., Olavarría, V. V., Muñoz, P. M., Brunser, A., Peng, B., Cui, L., Song, L., Rogers, K., . . . HeadPoST Investigators and Coordinators. (2017). Cluster-randomized, crossover trial of head pPositioning in acute stroke. *New England Journal of Medicine, 376*(25), 2437–2447. https://doi.org/10.1056/NEJMoa1615715

Berkhemer, O. A., Fransen, P. S., Beumer, D., van den Berg, L. A., Lingsma, H. F., Yoo, A. J., Schonewille, W. J., Vos, J. A., Nederkoorn, P. J., Wermer, M. J., van Walderveen, M. A., Staals, J., . . . MR CLEAN Investigators. (2015). A randomized trial of intraarterial treatment for acute ischemic stroke. *New England Journal of Medicine, 372*, 11–20.

Broderick, J. P., Palesch, Y. Y., Demchuk, A. M., Yeatts, S. D., Khatri, P., Hill, M. D., Jauch, E. C., Jovin, T. G., Yan, B., Silver, F. L., von Kummer, R., Molina, C. A., . . . Interventional Management of Stroke (IMS) III Investigators. (2013). Endovascular therapy after intravenous t-PA versus t-PA alone for stroke. *New England Journal of Medicine, 368*(10), 893–903. https://doi.org/10.1056/NEJMoa1214300

Campbell, B. C., Mitchell, P. J., Kleinig, T. J., Dewey, H. M., Churiloy, L., Yassi, N., Yan, B., Dowling, R. J., Parsons, M. W., Oxley, T. J., Wu, T. Y., Brooks, M., . . . EXTEND-IA Investigators. (2015). Endovascular therapy for ischemic stroke with perfusion-imaging selection. *New England Journal of Medicine, 372*, 1009–1018. https://doi.org/10.1056/NEJMoa1414792

Centers for Medicare & Medicaid Services. (2020a). *HCAHPS Hospital Consumer Assessment of Healthcare Providers and Systems.* www.hcahpsonline.org

Centers for Medicare & Medicaid Services. (2020b). *Centers for Medicare & Medicaid Services.* www.cms.gov

Ciccone, A., Valvassori, L., Nichelatti, M., Sgoifo, A., Ponzio, M., Sterzi, R., Boccardi, E., & SYNTHESIS Expansion Investigators. (2013). Endovascular treatment for acute ischemic stroke. *New England Journal of Medicine, 368*(10), 904–913. https://doi.org/10.1056/NEJMoa1213701

Codman, E. (1914). The product of a hospital. *Surgical Gynecology and Obstetrics, 18*, 491–494.

Codman, E. (1917). The value of case records in hospitals. *Modern Hospitals, 9*, 426–428.

Council for Six Sigma Certification. (2018). *Six Sigma: A Complete Step-by-Step Guide: A Complete Training & Reference Guide for White Belts, Yellow Belts, Green Belts, and Black Belts.* Council for Sigma Certification.

Deming, W. E. (1986). *Out of control.* Massachusetts Institute of Technology.

Donabedian, A. (1966). Evaluating the quality of medical care. *Milbank Memorial Fund Quarterly, 44*, 194–196. https://doi.org/10.2307/3348969

Donabedian, A. (1980). *The definition of quality and approaches to its assessment. Volume 1. An exploration in quality assessment and monitoring.* Health Administration Press.

Duncan, I. (2018). *Healthcare risk adjustment and predictive modeling* (2nd ed.). ACTEX Learning.

Ellwood, P. M. (1988). Outcomes management: A technology of patient experience. *New England Journal of Medicine, 318*, 1549–1556. https://doi.org/10.1056/NEJM198806093182329

Fee, E. (1982). A historical perspective on quality assurance and cost containment. In J. Williamson & Associates (Eds.), *Teaching quality assurance and cost containment in health care* (pp. 286–287). Jossey-Bass.

History-Biography. (2020). *Walter A. Shewhart.* https://history-biography.com/walter-a-shewhart

Goyal, M., Demchuk, A. M., Menon, B. K., Eesa, M., Rempel, J. L., Thornton, J., Roy, D., Jovin, T. G., Willinsky, R. A., Sapkota, B. L., Dowlatshahi, D., Frei, D. F., . . . ESCAPE Trial Investigators. (2015). Randomized assessment of rapid endovascular treatment of ischemic stroke. *New England Journal of Medicine, 372*, 1019–1030. https://doi.org/10.1056/NEJMoa1414905

Groves, E. (1908). A plea for uniform registration of operation results. *British Journal of Medicine, 2*, 1008–1009.

Hulley, S. B., Cummings, S. R., Browner, W. S., Grady, D. G., & Newman, T. B. (2013). *Designing clinical research* (4th ed.). Wolters Kluwer Health, Lippincott Williams & Wilkins.

Jovin, T. G., Chamorro, A., Cobo, E., de Miquel, M. A., Molina, C. A., Rovira, A., San Román, L., Serena, J., Abilleira, S., Ribó, M., Millán, M., Urra, X., . . . REVASCAT Trial Investigators. (2015). Thrombectomy within 8 hours after symptom onset in ischemic stroke. *New England Journal of Medicine, 372*, 2296–2306. https://doi.org/10.1056/NEJMoa1503780

Kidwell, C. S., Jahan, R., Gornbein, J., Alger, J. R., Nenov, V., Ajani, Z., Feng, L., Meyer, B. C., Olson, S., Schwamm, L. H., Yoo, A. J., Marshall, R. S., . . . MR RESCUE Investigators. (2013). A trial of imaging selection and endovascular treatment for ischemic stroke. *New England Journal of Medicine, 368*(10), 914–923. https://doi.org/10.1056/NEJMoa1212793

National Quality Forum. (2020). *Guidelines and measures.* https://www.qualitymeasures.ahrq.gov/browse/nqf-endorsed.aspx

Nightingale, F. (Ed.). (1863). *Notes on hospitals* (3rd ed.). Longman, Green, Longman, Roberts, and Green.

Patient-Centered Outcomes Research Institute. (2020). *Patient-Centered Outcomes Research Institute.* http://www.pcori.org

Piantadosi, S. (2017). *Clinical trials: A methodologic perspective* (3rd ed.). John Wiley & Sons.

Polit, D. F., & Beck, C. T. (2017). *Nursing research: Generating and assessing evidence for nursing practice.* Wolters Kluwer.

Qureshi, A. I., Palesch, Y. Y., Barsan, W. G., Hanley, D. F., Hsu, C. Y., Martin, R. L., Moy, C. S., Silbergleit, R., Steiner, T., Suarez, J. I., Toyoda, K., Wang, Y., . . . ATACH-2 Trial Investigators and the Neurological Emergency Treatment Trials Network. (2016). Intensive blood-pressure lowering in patients with acute cerebral hemorrhage. *New England Journal of Medicine, 375*(11), 1033–1043.

Saver, J. L., Goyal, M., Bonafe, A., Diener, H. C., Levy, E. I., Pereira, V. M., Albers, G. W., Cognard, C., Cohen, D. J., Hacke, W., Jansen, O., Jovin, T. G., . . . SWIFT PRIME Investigators. (2015). Stent-retriever thrombectomy after intravenous t-PA vs. t-PA alone in stroke. *New England Journal of Medicine, 372,* 2285–2295. https://doi.org/10.1056/NEJMoa1415061

Stausmire, J. M. (2014). Quality improvement or research – deciding which road to take. *Critical Care Nurse, 34*(6), 58–63. https://doi.org/10.4037/ccn2014177

U.S. Department of Health and Human Services. (2020). *Hospital compare.* http://www.medicare.gov/hospitalcompare/search.html

U.S. Food and Drug Administration. (2020). *Step 3. Clinical Research.* https://www.fda.gov/patients/drug-development-process/step-3-clinical-research

U.S. National Library of Medicine. (2020). *Clinical Trials.gov.* https://www.clinicaltrials.gov/ct2/show/NCT03728738?term=Alexandrov&cond=Stroke%2C+Ischemic&draw=2&rank=1

Wojner, A. W. (2001). *Outcomes management: Application to clinical practice.* Mosby.

Wyatt, L. (2019). *A History of Nursing.* Amberley.

ETHICAL ASPECTS OF PRACTICE SCHOLARSHIP

MARCIA PHILLIPS AND MARY HEITSCHMIDT

INTRODUCTION

The conduct of any research project requires consideration of ethical issues. The most important of these concerns includes obtaining informed consent of the participants, protecting participants from harm, and protection of participant privacy. Ethical principles are derived from various national and international statements of principles for the conduct of healthcare–related research, legal requirements primarily at the federal level, as well as regulations at the institutional, governmental, and professional levels. The foundations of the regulatory structure are processes for reviewing, approving, and monitoring research at the institutional level, with accountability to governmental, funding, and professional authorities. The primary responsibility for compliance rests with the individuals conducting the research, specifically the principal investigator and the institutions at which the research is conducted. If conducting international research the regulatory processes are different.

The process of obtaining approval to conduct a research study varies among clinical settings. Many organizations have a *nursing research committee* (Pintz et al., 2018) that promotes the integration and acculturation of evidence-based practice (EBP) generating nursing research. The research proposals are then submitted to the institutional review board (IRB) or the hospital nursing research committee to examine issues related to the protection of participants from the risks of participating in research. At institutions without a nursing research committee, research proposals may go to the director of nursing research or the institution's nurse scientist, if there is one, but generally go directly to the IRB for review with all of the other research protocols.

REVIEW COMMITTEES

Whether a nursing research committee review in addition to IRB approval is needed, the research investigator must also consider the following:

- *Frequency of the committee meetings.* Some organizations schedule meetings on an as-needed basis if the volume of clinical studies is small. If both a nursing research committee and an IRB exist, the institution's policies state whether a proposal for review can be submitted to both simultaneously or whether one must approve the proposal before it can be submitted to the other for review. It is important to know the structure and timeline of your institution's review process so that the investigator can factor this into the timeline of the study.

■ *Composition of the review committees.* It cannot be assumed that all review committees include a member who is familiar with nursing research. Therefore, it is important to write the proposal in lay terms for readers who may not have expertise in that particular content area and may not be familiar with nursing research. Advanced practice registered nurses (APRNs) are valuable members of research review committees. Active participation in these meetings provides APRNs a service scholarship opportunity.

■ *The presence of site-specific idiosyncrasies.* Some institutions require that an employee or physician be listed as principal investigator (PI) in a submission. This may require that the researcher set up collaborations in advance. IRBs require the PI and other research team members to complete initial training in research ethics before a protocol can be submitted. The Collaborative Institutional Training Initiative (CITI) provides online training for participating institutions and may be transferable; however, keep in mind that research training requirements are not the same at all institutions. Although these issues may seem trivial, such things can delay the process of approval while the committees seek additional information. By dealing directly and proactively with these issues, the investigator establishes credibility and demonstrates professionalism. Contact the site IRB to find out what research training requirements are needed to conduct the study.

Nursing Research Committees

Nursing research committees were initiated for the review of (a) scientific merit of a proposal for which an investigator is seeking support from nursing services, and (b) the nature and magnitude of the resources required of nursing services to implement the proposed research (Albert, 2016).

The nature and magnitude of resource consumption can range from minimal (e.g., a request merely to access participants for the study) to significant (e.g., an expectation that nursing staff will both implement various elements of an intervention and collect data regarding the feasibility and efficacy of the intervention).

Nursing research committees should be composed of members who have sufficient education and training in research to be able to examine the scientific merit of the study. Many institutions have PhD-prepared nurses lead these committees. APRNs leading or collaborating research teams, who are expert clinicians, are often valuable committee members. Committee membership may include those with a spectrum of experience from novice to expert (Albert, 2016). A goal of these committees would be to advance nursing science and, where possible, provide the research team with feedback that will improve the study (Parkosewich, 2013).

Institutional Review Boards

IRBs, also called human subject review committees, exist to provide fair and impartial review of research proposals and are responsible for the critical oversight of the research conducted on human subjects to protect them from any unnecessary risks associated with participation in research. In the United States, the Food and Drug Administration (FDA) and the Department of Health and Human Services (DHHS), specifically the Office for Human Research Protections (OHRP), regulations have empowered federally funded IRBs to approve, modify planned research prior to approval, or disapprove research. Institutions may not have a formal review structure if they do not receive federal funding, are small, or produce a limited volume of research. However, they can negotiate an agreement with a larger institution or external review committee to provide the required oversight.

In organizations in which a large volume of research is conducted, there may be more than one IRB committee (e.g., biomedical, social-behavioral, and/or biobehavioral). In the absence of federal funding and a formal review structure, the review may be done informally by an administrator of the institution. However, in this instance, the investigator should obtain a review from an external human subjects committee to document that the researcher has adhered to federal guidelines concerning the protection of human subjects from risk. Several independent IRBs can be found on the internet. Having approval from some type of IRB may be a journal or organizational requirement for dissemination and publication of the results. Also, IRB approved research studies are required for Magnet® recognition.

Guidelines for Review

IRBs usually have a set of guidelines or principles that govern their procedures and reviews. Institutions that receive federal funding must follow the 45 CFR 46. This section of the Code of Federal Regulations, the Common Rule, was recently revised and became effective in January 2019 and can be obtained at www.hhs.gov/ohrp/regulations-and-policy/regulations/finalized-revisions-common-rule/index.html.

Some small IRBs may use the principles set forth in the Belmont Report, which can be accessed at www.hhs.gov/ohrp/regulations-and-policy/belmont-report/index.html. The Belmont Report, published in 1979, was commissioned by the federal government to develop a set of principles that would offer guidance for the conduct of biomedical research and forms the basis for regulations and requirements imposed on IRBs. International review committees tend to use principles from the World Medical Association codified in the Declaration of Helsinki, found at www.wma.net/policies-post/wma-declaration-of-helsinki-ethical-principles-for-medical-research-involving-human-subjects. It is important to have an understanding of the principles in the Declaration of Helsinki for any research conducted, in whole or in part, outside the United States.

The Code of Federal Regulations stipulates the composition of the IRB (OHRP, DHHS, 2019a, 45 CFR 46.107). An IRB must consist of a minimum of five members with varying backgrounds to ensure a complete and adequate review of the research activities commonly conducted by the institution. Furthermore, by regulation, an IRB may not consist entirely of members of one profession, gender, or racial group. Collectively, the IRB must be sufficiently qualified through the experience and expertise of its membership to have knowledge of and sensitivity to prevailing attitudes. If the particular IRB routinely reviews research involving vulnerable participants, then the composition of the board must include one or more individuals knowledgeable about and experienced in working with these vulnerable populations. Also, the IRB must include at least one member whose primary concerns are in nonscientific areas and one who is not otherwise affiliated with the institution. One of the members should be able to discuss issues emanating from the perspective of the community and its values. No IRB member shall participate in the review if that person has a conflict of interest affiliated with the project. Lastly, an IRB may invite additional individuals with special areas of expertise to participate in the review and discussion of research proposals to enable the IRB to fulfill its purpose. Please see the regulations at 45 CFR 46.107 for complete information on all of the required qualifications to properly compose an IRB.

Jurisdiction of an IRB

The jurisdiction of an IRB is determined by answering two fundamental questions: "Is the activity research?" and "Does the activity involve human subjects?" For healthcare professionals, the first question may not be so easily answered because the distinction between research and therapy is not always readily apparent. Federal policy defines research as a "systematic investigation, including research development, testing and evaluation designed to develop or contribute to generalized knowledge" (OHRP, DHHS, 2019a, 45 CFR 46.102). Furthermore, research itself is not inherently therapeutic in that the therapeutic benefits of experimental interventions are unknown or may prove to be ineffective. If the focus of the proposed activity is currently accepted as standardized methods of care or if the research addresses institutional or patient-specific case issues, then the activity is generally not considered research and consequently may not require IRB reporting and review. However, if there is any uncertainty as to whether the activity is research, the activity should be treated as research and reported to the IRB. An activity is research if the answers to the following two questions are "yes": "Does the activity employ a systematic approach involving predetermined methods for studying a specific topic, answering a specific question, testing a specific hypothesis, or developing a theory?" and "Is the activity intended to contribute to generalizable knowledge by extending the results (e.g., publication of presentation) beyond a single individual or internal unit?" (OHRP, DHHS, 2019a, 45 CFR 46.102). It is ultimately up the IRB to determine if an activity is research.

There is one caveat. If the activity is to be disseminated (i.e., reported in a publication or presentation), the general practice has been to report it to the IRB for review. An activity that causes great confusion as to whether or not it constitutes research is continuous quality improvement (QI). QI is considered an essential component of responsible professional healthcare and a means for improving the processes, efficiencies, safety, and quality of care while preventing substandard care (Ogrinc et al., 2013). However, QI activities frequently consist of methods traditionally associated with randomized clinical trials, blurring the distinction between QI activities and research (Whicher et al., 2015). Some suggest that all activities should be reviewed by the IRB to ensure that the activity, research, or QI does not compromise patient autonomy or safety (Szanton et al., 2013). Those who advocate the review of all activities contend that once the activity receives IRB approval, it is sanctioned, thereby ensuring that the activity complies with commonly accepted ethical practices and involves a minimal level of risk for all participating parties, the human subjects, investigators, and the institution. However, many in the healthcare community believe that review of all activities would stall the research enterprise. According Ogrinc et al. (2013), if any of the following applies to the activity, it should be considered research and submitted to the IRB for review:

- Results are to be disseminated
- Results contribute to generalized knowledge
- Conditions are systematically assigned to patients
- Conditions are other than a standard of care
- Risks are explained in informed consent and may be minimal
- Information collected goes beyond routine patient care
- Risks to privacy and confidentiality exist

There is no consensus about universal criteria for making such a distinction between projects requiring IRB approval and those that are exempt (Whicher et al., 2015). However, the results of QI projects are often of interest to audiences outside the particular institution and dissemination of the results would be expected, and would not necessarily indicate that the QI project is research requiring IRB review (Gregory, 2015). Oermann et al. (2014) provide guidelines for writing QI and research manuscripts. To meet publication criteria, some institutions have separate processes in place that acknowledging the project as QI (Stausmire, 2014).

To determine if a project is a QI initiative that does not generally require IRB review, it is useful to contrast the aims and methods of research with those of QI projects. The federal regulation governing IRBs defines research as "a systematic investigation, including research development, testing and evaluation, designed to develop or contribute to generalizable knowledge" (OHRP, DHHS, 2019a, 45 CFR 46.102). In contrast, "the goal of QI is to analyze data to improve systems related to processes and outcomes (i.e., cost, productivity, quality)" (Gregory, 2015, p. 101). Several useful tools have been developed to assist researchers in differentiating research from QI and helping them determine if IRB review is required (Ogrinc et al., 2013; Stausmire, 2014).

Once the activity has been deemed research, the investigator should ask whether the research activity involves human subjects. A human subject is a living individual about whom an investigator obtains data or biospecimens through intervention or interaction with the individual or obtains identifiable private information (OHRP, DHHS, 2019a, 45 CFR 46.102). For example, an investigator whose research activities involve accessing health records of only patients who have died is not conducting research with human subjects.

■ LEVELS OF REVIEW

Once it has been established that the activity falls within the jurisdiction of the IRB, the level of IRB reporting and review must be identified. There are three levels of review, determined on the basis of the degree of risks inherent in the proposed research. Risk is the likelihood of harm or injury, whether it is physical or psychological, that occurs as a result of participation in research and can range from minimal to significant. The three levels of review are exempt, expedited, and full. It is important to determine which level of review is required because the extent of information required, the forms to be completed, and the time necessary for the review are determined by the type of review. For any questions about the level of review or the submission process you should consult your IRB.

The 2019 Common Rule revisions impacted all constituencies involved in human research protection programs. The intention was to reduce administrative burden and better protect the human subjects by making the informed consents more meaningful and focusing IRBs on higher risk research.

Exempt From Review

Research activities that are *exempt* from review by the IRB are those that pose minimal risks to participants, have no means by which a participant can be identified, and use human subjects who are capable of freely consenting to participate (OHRP, DHHS, 2019a, 45 CFR 46.104). Even though a research activity falls into the exempt category, it still must be submitted to the IRB for affirmation. Examples of activities that are exempt from review are listed in Exhibit 19.1.

Copies of surveys, interview guides, or questionnaires and the exact introductory remarks and consent forms to be used must be submitted to the IRB when requesting exempt status. If advertisements for participants are used, copies of the text for the planned advertisement must also be submitted. Although these materials may or may not be formally reviewed in the committee, a member of the IRB will assess the materials to verify that the activity meets the stipulations for exemption. The investigator will receive a document from the IRB indicating the exact criteria used

EXHIBIT 19.1

RESEARCH ACTIVITIES EXEMPT FROM 45 CFR 46

A. Research conducted in established or commonly accepted educational settings, involving normal educational practices, such as:

1. research on regular and special education instructional strategies, or

2. research on the effectiveness of or the comparison among instructional techniques, curricula, or classroom management methods.

B. Research involving the use of educational tests (cognitive, diagnostic, aptitude, achievement), survey procedures, interview procedures, or observation of public behavior, unless:

1. information obtained is recorded in such a manner that human subjects can be identified, directly or through identifiers linked to the subjects; and

2. any disclosure of the human subjects' responses outside the research could reasonably place the subjects at risk of criminal or civil liability or be damaging to the subjects' financial standing, employability, or reputation.

C. Research involving the collection or study of existing data, documents, records, pathological specimens, or diagnostic specimens, if these sources are publicly available or if the information is recorded in such a manner that subjects cannot be identified, directly or through identifiers linked to the subjects.

D. Research and demonstration projects that are conducted by or subject to the approval of department or agency heads, and that are designed to study, evaluate, or otherwise examine:

1. public benefit or service programs;

2. procedures for obtaining benefits or services under those programs;

3. possible changes in or alternatives to those programs or procedures; or

4. possible changes in methods or levels of payment for benefits or services under those programs.

E. Taste and food-quality evaluation and consumer acceptance studies:

1. if wholesome food without additives is consumed; or

2. if food is consumed that contains an ingredient at or below the level and for a use found to be safe, or agricultural chemical or environmental contaminant at or below the level found to be safe, by the Food and Drug Administration or approved by the Environmental Protection Agency or the Food Safety and Inspection Service of the U.S. Department of Agriculture.

Source: Adapted from Office for Human Research Protections, U.S. Department of Health and Human Services. (2019a). *Electronic Code of Regulations.* 45 CFR 46.104. https://ecfr.gov/cgi-bin/retrieveECFR?gp=1&SID=6eb266ca122b5ee13ee144cd3e74abe9&ty=HTML&h=L&mc=true&n=pt45.1.46&r=PART

to judge whether the activity does or does not meet the requirements for an exemption. If the IRB assessment determines that the activity does not fulfill the requirements for exemption, the investigator may be asked to submit additional justification or appropriate materials for IRB review.

Expedited Review

Activities that are considered within the exempt category but provide a means by which the individual participants can be identified must be reviewed at the expedited level because of the potential risk resulting from loss of anonymity and confidentiality. Materials required for an expedited review generally consist of the research protocol that presents the objectives, methods, participant selections, criteria, theoretical or potential risks and benefits, precautions and safeguards, and a sample of the informed consent. The application may be reviewed by a single member of the IRB.

There are two types of activities that receive an expedited review:

1. Activities that pose no more than a minimal risk to subjects for participation in the activity. Minimal risk is defined as "the probability and magnitude of harm or discomfort anticipated in the research are not greater in and of themselves than those ordinarily encountered in daily life or during the performance of routine physical or psychological examinations or tests" (OHRP, DHHS, 2019a, 45 CFR 46.102). If the risks are greater than minimal and if precautions, safeguards, or alternatives cannot be incorporated into the research activity to minimize the risks to such a level, then a full review is required.

2. Activities requiring minor changes in previously approved research, during the period for which approval is authorized (OHRP, DHHS, 2019a, 45 CFR 46.110).

As with all levels of review, the investigator receives a document from the IRB, indicating the exact criteria used to determine that the activity fulfills the requirements for an expedited review. If the initial assessment determines that the activity does not fulfill the requirements for expedited review, the investigator may be asked for justification or to submit the appropriate materials for a full review. Federal policy requires that all members of the IRB be advised of all proposals that have been approved under the expedited review process (OHRP, DHHS, 2019a, 45 CFR 46.110).

Full Review

A full review of any proposed research activity involving human subjects must occur in all other situations, such as those in which participation in the activity poses greater than minimal risk, those for which the participant cannot freely consent, and those involving vulnerable populations. Materials required for a full review are identical to those required for an expedited review. It is the IRB review process that differs. A full review varies in amount of time from the submission of materials to the notification of the disposition of the proposal. The proposal is reviewed by at least five members of the IRB. A member cannot participate in the discussion and determination of disposition of a project in which the member is an investigator. In such cases, where a conflict of interest is determined, the investigator member must be absent from the discussion and this absence must be reflected in the minutes of the meeting.

The criteria for IRB approval and review of the proposed research activity, which are listed in Exhibits 19.2 and 19.3, must occur at a convened meeting at which the majority of the members of the IRB are present. The review conducted by the IRB typically focuses on the mechanisms within the proposed research by which the participants are safeguarded or protected from any undue risks of participation, and the process and content of informed consent, that is, the ethics of the research. However, scrutiny of the research methodology also falls within the purview of the IRB because research that is poorly designed could identify and expose the participants, the investigator, and the institution to unnecessary risks. Although a proposal may be deemed ethically sound,

---

EXHIBIT 19.2

CRITERIA FOR INSTITUTIONAL REVIEW BOARD APPROVAL OF RESEARCH

All of the following requirements must be satisfied for approval of research:

1. Risks to participants are minimized;
2. Risks to participants are reasonable in relation to anticipated benefits;
3. Selection of participants is equitable;
4. Informed consent is sought for each prospective participant or the subject's legally authorized representative to the extent required;
5. Informed consent is documented or waived appropriately;
6. There is adequate provision for monitoring the data collected to ensure the safety of participants;
7. There are adequate provisions to protect the privacy of participants and to maintain the confidentiality of data; and
8. If any participant is vulnerable to coercion or undue influence, for example, pregnant women, human fetuses, neonates, prisoners, children, mentally disabled persons, or economically or educationally disadvantaged persons, additional safeguards have been included in the study to protect the rights and welfare of these participants.

Source: Adapted from Office for Human Research Protections, U.S. Department of Health and Human Services. (2019a). *Electronic Code of Regulations.* 45 CFR 46.111. https://ecfr.gov/cgi-bin/retrieveECFR?gp=1&SID=6eb266ca122b5ee13ee144cd3e74abe9&ty=HTML&h=L&mc=true&n=pt45.1.46&r=PART

EXHIBIT 19.3

BASIC INSTITUTIONAL REVIEW BOARD REVIEW

In the review of research proposals, the members of the IRB must follow the guidelines listed in the following:

1. Identify the risks associated with participation in the research;
2. Determine that the risks will be minimized to the extent possible;
3. Identify the possible benefits to be derived from the research;
4. Determine the risks are reasonable in relation to the benefits to the participants and the importance of the knowledge to be gained;
5. Determine the adequacy of the provisions to protect privacy and maintain confidentiality of the data; and
6. In the case of vulnerable population, determine that appropriate additional safeguards are in place to protect their rights and welfare.

Source: Adapted from Office for Human Research Protections, U.S. Department of Health and Human Services. (2019a). *Electronic Code of Regulations.* 45 CFR 46.111. https://ecfr.gov/cgi-bin/retrieveECFR?gp=1&SID=6eb266ca122b5ee13ee144cd3e74abe9&ty=HTML&h=L&mc=true&n=pt45.1.46&r=PART

if it is methodologically unsound, the IRB must disapprove the application. For proposed research to be approved, it must meet the criteria set forth by the IRB and other governing bodies (OHRP, DHHS, 2019a, 45 CFR 46.102).

A research proposal must receive approval from the IRB before the collection of data can be initiated. Once permission has been granted by the IRB, the researcher is obligated to conduct the study as proposed. The institution may have additional requirements before the research can commence which must be complied with, in addition to IRB approval. Any changes or alterations to the IRB-approved research must be reviewed and approved by the IRB before proceeding with the changes. For example, if the investigator wants to enroll more participants than originally requested, this step needs to be approved in advance before enrolling additional participants. The IRB defines a participant as anyone who has consented even if the individual did not participate in research activities. Any changes in the method of recruitment or changes in questionnaires must also receive IRB approval before the changes are implemented. Investigators are required to provide an annual IRB progress report unless:

- The application received exempt or expedited review at initial IRB submission
- The research includes only data analysis or standard of care clinical data review

The most common elements triggering periodic reviews are outlined in Exhibit 19.4. The IRB may require more frequent progress reports for high-risk protocols. Also, any increased risks or

EXHIBIT 19.4

ELEMENTS OF A PERIODIC REVIEW

Periodic reviews of research should include:

1. Any amendment to the currently approved research (e.g., the addition of research personnel, or a change in funding, research protocol, consent documents, Health Insurance Portability and Accountability Act [HIPAA] authorization, or any other change to the research);
2. Preliminary results, especially those that might suggest one intervention is better or worse than the other with respect to risks, benefits, alternatives, or willingness to participate;
3. Participant enrollment;
4. Information about any participant complaints, refusals, or withdrawals from participation, and safety;
5. Reportable events (e.g., study-related adverse events) and protocol violations;
6. Review by other IRBs;
7. Suspension of research activity;
8. Presentations and publications; and
9. Conflicts of interest.

Source: Adapted from Office for Human Research Protections, U.S. Department of Health and Human Services (2019a). Electronic Code of Regulations. 45 CFR 46.109. https://ecfr.gov/cgi-bin/retrieveECFR?gp=1&SID=6eb266ca122b5ee13ee144cd3e74abe9&ty=HTML&h=L&mc=true&n=pt45.1.46&r=PART

unforeseen problems should be reported to the IRB immediately. The individual study participants' data should not be identifiable.

Informed Consent

Informed consent is one of the primary ethical requirements related to research with humans. It reflects the basic principle of *respect for persons*. Informed consent ensures that prospective human participants have a clear understanding of the nature of the research and can knowledgably and *voluntarily* decide whether to participate in the research being proposed. "Voluntary" is defined as acting of one's own free will. The process of providing informed consent is not a distinct moment in time at which the participant simply signs a form. It is an ongoing educational process between the investigator and the participant. Consequently, informed, voluntary participation should be verified at every interaction between the investigator or a representative of the research team and the participant. Because of the nature and complexity of some studies (e.g., longitudinal, multiphase studies), informed consent may be required for various phases of the study.

Although some IRBs require the use of a standardized format for consent procedures, modifications are usually permitted as long as the process provides for full disclosure, adequate comprehension, and voluntary choice—elements easy to enumerate but not so easy to achieve (see Exhibit 19.5). Usually any element may be omitted that is not relevant to the study. However, a statement that the participant understands what will occur as a result of their participation in the study and

---

EXHIBIT 19.5

GENERAL REQUIREMENTS FOR INFORMED CONSENT

In seeking informed consent the initial process must include key information that assists the perspective subject's understanding why one may or may not want to participate in the research. The following information shall be provided to each participant:

1. A statement that the study involves research, including an explanation of the purposes, expected duration and procedures, especially if they are experimental

2. A description of any reasonably foreseeable risks or discomforts to the participant

3. A description of any benefits to the participant or to others that may reasonably be expected from the research

4. Disclosure of appropriate alternative procedures or course of treatment that might be advantageous to the participant

5. A description of how confidentiality of records will be maintained

6. If research is greater than minimal risk, a description of compensation for participation and what is to occur with injury from participation

7. An explanation with contact information for persons who can provide additional information regarding questions about the research and research participants' rights, and research-related injury

(continued)

8. A statement that participation is voluntary and that refusal has no consequent penalties or loss of benefits to which the participant is otherwise entitled

9. Additional elements when appropriate:

   a. Acknowledgment if the procedure may involve currently unforeseeable risks to the participant, or to the embryo or fetus, *if* the participant is or may become pregnant

   b. Circumstances under which the participant's participation may be terminated by the investigator without regard to the participant's consent

   c. Additional costs to the participant from participation in the research

   d. Consequences of withdrawal and procedures for orderly termination of participation

   e. Provision of new information that may influence the participant's willingness to continue to participate

   f. The approximate number of participants involved in the research

Source: Adapted from Office for Human Research Protections, U.S. Department of Health and Human Services. (2019a). *Electronic Code of Regulations.* 45 CFR 46.111. https://ecfr.gov/cgi-bin/retrieveECFR?gp=1&SID=6eb266ca122b5ee13ee144cd3e74abe9&ty=HTML&h=L&mc=true&n=pt45.1.46&r=PART

affirming that the participant freely agrees to participate must be included at the end of the form. There are two to three places for signatures and date at the end of the consent form:

1. The participant's;

2. The person obtaining consent and witnessing the participant's signature; and

3. If needed, the person only witnessing the participant's signature.

(See Exhibit 19.6 for an example of informed consent key elements.) When a parent or guardian signs for a participant, the participant's name should be clearly identified, as should the signatory's relationship to the participant. If the research is complex or poses a significant risk, the IRB may encourage the investigator to develop a "patient information sheet" that presents the information from the formal consent form in simple, unambiguous language that is devoid of all "legalese." Copies of the consent and information sheets are given to the participant, and the investigator should retain the originals for at least 2 years after the study is completed; however, depending on the type of study, a longer period of time may be necessary. Your IRB can provide guidance on study record retention. Consent length varies depending on the risk, nature of the research study, and the entire consent process to ensure subjects are fully informed. Guidelines for developing a consent form as well as institution specific template consents can usually be obtained from the IRB.

When the research involves a vulnerable population, there is a greater challenge for consenting. Vulnerable populations are those that may lack knowledge or understanding (i.e., children, pregnant women, fetuses, mentally impaired or seriously ill persons, and economically or educationally disadvantaged individuals). These populations may require special protection and abide by different guidelines. It is important that investigators working with these populations become familiar with subparts B, C, and D of 45 CFR 46 (OHRP, DHHS, 2019a, 45 CFR 46.201Sub B, C & D). Protected health information is listed in Exhibit 19.7. Passage of Genetic Information Nondiscrimination Act (GINA) in 2013 also includes that genetic information is protected by the Privacy Rule (National Human Genome Research Institute, 2019).

EXHIBIT 19.6

SAMPLE OF INFORMED CONSENT: LOW RISK STUDY

Key Information: You are invited to participate in a research study. The consent will give you information about the study. Taking part in this research is voluntary. The purpose of the research is to study the effects of hospitalization in elderly adults.

Your participation may last your entire hospital stay.

During this study we will collect data about your hospital care.

You are being asked to be a participant in research under the direction of Dr. _____, a professor in the College of Nursing at the University of _____. You are being told about this research and may be able to take part because of your current illness and hospitalization. Before you agree to be in this research, please read this form. Your participation is completely voluntary. Your decision will not affect your relations with the university, your physicians, the hospital staff, or your care. If you decide to participate, you are free to quit at any time.

The purpose of the research is to study the effects of hospitalization of older patients. Approximately 720 patients may take part in this research. We are interested in looking at the care you receive, such as bathing and eating; the use of healthcare services; and the severity, length, and outcome of your hospitalization.

If you agree to take part, I, or another member of the research team, will visit you daily while you are in the hospital to ask you questions about your thinking and your ability to perform daily activities. The first interview will last about 20 minutes. All other daily visits will last about 10 minutes. These visits will be scheduled at a time that is convenient for you and your caregiver. Each day, we would like to review your hospital record to obtain information about your care, medications, and any tests and their results. We would also like your permission to talk with a relative, friend, or caregiver about your recent illness. The risks of being in this research include possible inconvenience of interviews and possible breach of privacy and confidentiality.

There is no direct benefit to you. This research will not help in your current care or treatment. We hope that what we learn from this research will help to improve the care to patients like you in the future.

If you decide to take part, we will be careful to keep all information about you strictly confidential. Only members of the research team will have access to this information. All information about you will be kept under lock and key in the research office of Dr. _____. When results are published or discussed, no information will reveal your identity.

You have the option not to participate in this study.

There is no payment for your participation.

You may ask questions now. If you have questions later, you may contact Dr. _____ _____ at XXX.XXX.XXXX or by email at _____

If you have questions about your rights as a research participant, you can call the Office for Protection of Research Subjects at the _____ at XXX.XXX.XXXX.

Your participation in this research is entirely voluntary. Your decision will not affect your care. You can refuse to answer any question or stop answering altogether. You can stop participating in the research

(continued)

at any time without consequences of any kind. You will be given a copy of this form for your information and to keep for your records.

I have read the above information. I have been given a chance to ask questions, and my questions have been answered to my satisfaction. I have been given a copy of this form.

Signature of the Participant: _____ Date of signature: _____

Signature of Individual Obtaining Consent: _____ Date of signature: _____

Signature of Witness (if needed): _____ Date of signature: _____

EXHIBIT 19.7

PROTECTED HEALTH INFORMATION

1. Names
2. Any geographic subdivision smaller than a state (including street names, city, county, precinct, ZIP code)
3. Any element of dates directly related to an individual (e.g., birth date, admission date, date of death)
4. Telephone numbers
5. Facsimile numbers
6. Electronic mail addresses
7. Social Security numbers
8. Medical record numbers
9. Health plan beneficiary numbers
10. Account numbers
11. Certificate/license numbers
12. Vehicle identifiers
13. Device identifiers
14. Web universal resource locators (URLs)
15. Internet protocol (IP) address numbers
16. Biometric identifiers (e.g., fingerprints and voiceprints)
17. Full-face photographic images
18. Any other unique identifying number, characteristic, or code

Source: U.S. Department of Health and Human Services. (2003). (NIH publication number 03-5388). *Protecting personal health information in research: Understanding the HIPAA privacy rule.* https://privacyruleandresearch .nih.gov/pdf/hipaa_privacy_rule_booklet.pdf

Few circumstances allow for the waiver of consent. Situations in which waivers may be approved include the following: (a) the research involves no more than minimal risks to subjects; (b) the waiver or alteration will not adversely affect the rights and welfare of the subjects; (c) the research cannot practically be carried out without the waiver or alteration; and (d) whenever appropriate, the subjects will be provided with additional pertinent information after they have participated (OHRP, DHHS, 2019a, 45 CFR 46.116e) An example of a situation in which a waiver of consent is granted is a study that uses only data that have been previously collected for non-research purposes, such as the medical health record. The investigator must demonstrate that it would not be practicable to go back and obtain consent from the individuals whose records are to be used. It may be the case that a large number of individuals cannot be reached because their contact information has changed, because the patients are no longer affiliated with the medical center, or because they are deceased.

For individuals experiencing health emergencies, there is a provision by the FDA and the DHHS that allows emergency research to proceed without voluntary prospective informed consent by the patient (OHRP, DHHS, 2019b, 21 CFR 50.24). However, these health emergencies must render the patient incapable of providing informed consent. Examples of such health emergencies include patients who are experiencing life-threatening illnesses or trauma and those requiring resuscitation in which research is clearly necessary to identify safe and effective therapies (Baker & Merz, 2018). These health emergencies may occur out of the hospital or in the emergency department or intensive care unit. According to 21 CFR 50.24, exception from informed consent requirements for emergency research requires that the potential participant must be in a life-threatening situation and current treatments must be either unproven or unsatisfactory (OHRP, DHHS, 2019b, 21 CFR 50.24). In addition, it is required that obtaining informed consent is not feasible because the participant is unable to consent as a result of the health emergency, a surrogate is not readily available, and there is a limited window of opportunity to intervene. Another requirement is that participation may provide direct benefit to the participant, and the project must have been prospectively reviewed and approved with waiver of consent by an IRB. Additional protections of the rights and welfare of the participants also must be ensured; either the patient or their surrogate must provide informed consent as soon as practicable. However, it is important to understand that research in which participation does not hold the potential for "therapeutic benefit" continues to require informed consent of either the patient or a legal surrogate (Chen et al., 2008).

■ RESEARCH MISCONDUCT

Research misconduct occurs when a researcher fabricates or falsifies data and/or the results, or plagiarizes information within a research report (OHRP, DHHS, 2019c, 42 CFR 93). The misconduct must be committed intentionally, knowingly, or recklessly and the allegation must be proven with sufficient evidence. Research misconduct does not include honest error or differences of opinion. All institutions that receive Public Health Service (PHS) funding are required to have written policies and procedures for addressing any allegations of the misconduct. Research misconduct involving National Institutes of Health (NIH) awards ultimately falls under the authority of the Office of Research Integrity (ORI), which has specific procedures to handle allegations of misconduct.

An individual found guilty of misconduct can lose federal funding, be restricted to supervised research, or even lose their job. One may also be required to submit a correction or retraction of published articles. Thorough investigation of an allegation is extremely important considering the serious penalty that can be inflicted.

An excellent resource for further reading on research conduct is available at https://ori.hhs.gov/ori-intro.

CONFLICTS OF INTEREST

Conflicts of interest in research are an area of concern for all research activities. Potential conflicts can be financial or they may be personal (i.e., institutional, relationships). A conflict of interest is understood to describe situations in which financial or other considerations have the potential to compromise or bias professional judgment and objectivity. Financial conflicts of interest have received the most attention and are particularly of concern when research is funded by commercial entities that may have an interest in the outcomes of the research (Dunn et al., 2016). Other types of conflicts of interest include institutional or professional affiliations, or other relationships that may indicate the potential for bias. Conflicts of interest are not inherently improper, but consideration of how the conflict might impact the objectivity of the research is required to be considered by the IRB, and requires disclosure by the researcher at all stages of dissemination.

IRBs are required to consider any factors that may impact the risks and benefits of the proposed research, the potential for coercion, and selection of participants, including how conflicts of interest (financial or personal) may affect the rights and welfare of participants. It is important to disclose any potential conflicts of interest at the time of IRB review, and when the results of the research are disseminated (by publication or otherwise). IRBs and/or institutional specific conflict of interest committees are charged with determining any conditions required to mitigate the potential that a conflict will impact the integrity of the research project.

SUMMARY

The IRB process is a critical and essential step in ensuring the conduct of appropriate and ethical research. It can consume large amounts of time and increase the complexity of the research project. It is important to consider these requirements in developing a timeline for any research project. The recommendations offered are intended to facilitate development of a partnership among the IRB, the researcher, and the research participants in pursuing knowledge that results in a positive research experience for all, as well as the successful completion of the research.

SUGGESTED LEARNING ACTIVITIES

Persons who sustain a mild traumatic brain injury (mTBI) have been reported to experience difficulties with memory. It has been reported in the literature that using a smartphone with an appropriate app might help persons with mTBI with their memory. On the basis of your review of the literature, you decide to recruit participants for a study. Participants will be randomly assigned to times when they are scheduled to call a researcher's voicemail. A 2-week predetermined call schedule will be assigned to each participant. Half of the participants will use the smartphone app as a reminder, and half will not.

Before conducting the study, you are required to obtain IRB approval.

1. Acquire and complete the information the IRB at your institution requires.

2. Prepare a written informed consent for potential participants to read and sign.

3. Create an oral script that will be used when recruiting participants.

REFERENCES

Albert, N. M. (Ed.). (2016). *Building and sustaining a hospital-based nursing research program*. Springer Publishing Company.

Baker, F. X., & Merz, J. F. (2018). What gives them the right? Legal privilege and waivers of consent for research. *Clinical Trials (London, England), 15*(6), 579–586. https://doi.org/10.1177/1740774518803122

Chen, D. T., Meschia, J. F., Brott, T. G., Brown, R. D., & Worrall, B. B. (2008). Stroke genetic research and adults with impaired decision-making capacity: A survey of IRB and investigator practices. *Stroke, 39*(10), 2732–2735. https://doi.org/10.1161/STROKEAHA.108.515130

Dunn, A., Coiera, E., Mandl, K., & Bourgeois, F. (2016).Conflict of interest disclosure in biomedical research: a review of current practices, biases, and the role of public registries in improving transparency. *Research Integrity and Peer Review, 1*(1), 1–8. https://doi.org/10.1186/s41073-016-0006-7

Gregory, K. E. (2015). Differentiating between research and quality improvement. *The Journal of Perinatal & Neonatal Nursing, 29*(2), 100–102. https://doi.org/10.1097/JPN.0000000000000107

National Human Genome Research Institute. (2019). *Privacy in Genomics*. https://www.genome.gov/about-genomics/policy-issues/Privacy

Oermann, M. H., Turner, K., & Carman, M. (2014). Preparing quality improvement, research, and evidence-based practice manuscripts. *Journal of the Association of Occupational Health Professionals in Healthcare, 34*(3), 31–36.

Office for Human Research Protections, U.S. Department of Health and Human Services. (2019a). *Electronic Code of Regulations*. 45 CFR 46 Protection of Human Subjects. https://ecfr.gov/cgi-bin/retrieveECFR?gp=1&SID=6eb266ca122b5ee13ee144cd3e74abe9&ty=HTML&h=L&mc=true&n=pt45.1.46&r=PART

Office for Human Research Protections, U.S. Department of Health and Human Services. (2019b). *Electronic Code of Regulations*. 21 CFR 50.24 Exceptions of Informed Consents requirements for emergency research. https://ecfr.gov/cgi-bin/retrieveECFR?gp=1&SID=f8e5c60f6e28b0c2be5dd9442e4259f7&ty=HTML&h=L&mc=true&n=pt21.1.50&r=PART#se21.1.50_124

Office for Human Research Protections, U.S. Department of Health and Human Services. (2019c). *Electronic Code of Regulations*. 42 CFR 93 Public Health Service Policies on Research Misconduct. https://ecfr.gov/cgi-bin/retrieveECFR?gp=2&SID=3954d64b8d8a1d5032c337accdba75fe&ty=HTML&h=L&mc=true&r=PART&n=pt42.1.93

Ogrinc, G., Nelson, W. A., Adams, S. M., & O'Hara, A. E. (2013). An instrument to differentiate between clinical research and quality improvement. *Irb, 35*(5), 1–8.

Parkosewich, J. A. (2013). An infrastructure to advance the scholarly work of staff nurses. *The Yale Journal of Biology and Medicine, 86*(1), 63–77.

Pintz, C., Zhou, Q. P., McLaughlin, M. K., Kelly, K. P., & Guzzetta, C. E. (2018). National study of nursing research characteristics at Magnet®-designated hospitals. *Journal of Nursing Administration, 48*(5), 247–258. https://doi.org/10.1097/NNA.0000000000000609

Stausmire, J. M. (2014). Quality improvement or research--deciding which road to take. *Critical Care Nurse, 34*(6), 58–63. https://doi.org/10.4037/ccn2014177

Szanton, S. L., Taylor, H. A., & Terhaar, M. (2013). Development of an institutional review board preapproval process for doctor of nursing practice students: Process and outcome. *Journal of Nursing Education, 52*(1), 51–55. https://doi.org/10.3928/01484834-20121212-01

Whicher, D., Kass, N., Saghai, Y., Faden, R., Tunis, S., & Pronovost, P. (2015). The views of quality improvement professionals and comparative effectiveness researchers on ethics, IRBs, and oversight. *Journal of Empirical Research on Human Research Ethics: JERHRE, 10*(2), 132–144. https://doi.org/10.1177/1556264615571558

WEB RESOURCES

General Resources

Office for Human Research Protections (OHRP): http://www.hhs.gov/ohrp

U.S. Department of Veterans Affairs, Office of Research Oversight: http://www.va.gov/ORO/index.asp

U.S. Food and Drug Administration, Guidance, Compliance and Regulatory Information: http://www.fda.gov/drugs/guidancecomplianceregulatoryinformation/default.htm

For Information About the Registration of Clinical Trials

Clinical trial registration: http://www.icmje.org/recommendations/browse/publishing-and-editorial-issues
FDAAA 801 and the Final Rule: http://www.clinicaltrials.gov/ct2/manage-recs/fdaaa
Guidance on public law 110–85 enacted to expand the scope of clinicaltrials.gov registration: http://grants
.nih.gov/grants/guide/notice-files/not-od-08-014.html
Home-ClinicalTrials.gov: http://www.clinicaltrials.gov

For Online Ethics Training

Collaborative Institutional Training Initiative (CITI): https://www.citiprogram.org

COMMUNICATING PRACTICE SCHOLARSHIP THROUGH ORAL PRESENTATION

LISA A. RAUCH

▨ INTRODUCTION

Communicating research through oral presentations in the 21st century may look different from what you have experienced in the past. The rapid surge of technology keeps us on a constant learning curve as to best practices for delivering content and engaging audiences, whether in a classroom, conference, or workplace setting. Knowledge translation of research findings is a key step in reducing the research–practice gap (Curtis et al., 2016). Clearly and concisely communicating information about a completed study or a study in progress is vital to the growth of the profession's body of evidence. As the profession continues to increase the numbers of doctorally prepared nurses (American Association of Colleges of Nursing [AACN], 2017), it will be imperative for advanced practice registered nurses (APRNs) to disseminate research findings to transform patient care. Numerous opportunities to share research exist, including oral presentations in the academic, clinical, and community settings. Common venues include events sponsored by an organization, poster or podium session at conferences, webinars, podcasts, and traditional media. The growing availability of technology such as webcasting, broadcasting, and podcasting has led to the expedited dissemination of information, thereby reaching a larger and varied audience quickly.

▨ PREPARING THE PRESENTATION

Initial Planning

Ideally, dissemination of a study's findings is considered during the planning phase of the study. The Agency for Healthcare Research and Quality (AHRQ) provides a guideline for the planning of the dissemination of research results (www.ahrq.gov/patient-safety/resources/advances/vol4/planning.html). This guideline may assist researchers to think through their dissemination plans and suggests appropriate modes and venues for sharing findings early in the research process. An initial step is to identify opportunities to present at research, clinical, or educational conferences. Additional opportunities may arise in your work setting to present study findings with a focus on quality improvement and informing best practices. These presentations are typically brief, concise, and directed toward policy changes within an institution. Conference sponsors solicit presenters by announcing a call for papers or call for abstracts. Reviewing the conference focus to determine whether your study fits the focus of the conference is crucial. An abstract topic that is timely, congruent with conference objectives, and aligned with the interests of the anticipated target audience will have a greater likelihood of being accepted for presentation. After determining that your study is a good fit, carefully review the detailed requirements for submitting an abstract as outlined in the conference brochure or online.

Abstracts

Abstracts of completed research usually are considered for oral or poster presentations. Research in-progress is considered only for a poster session. The abstract, typically 150 to 300 words in length, is used by reviewers to determine the worthiness of a study. Thus, it is imperative that submission guidelines are followed precisely. Most guidelines for research abstracts require the inclusion of these major components of the study (Grove et al., 2015):

1. Titles—Should include key variables, participants, and setting

2. Purpose of the study

3. Brief description of sample—Number of subjects and distinct characteristics such as diagnosis, age range, and gender

4. Methods—Design, setting, data collection procedures, instruments including reliability and validity information

5. Findings—Summary of data and statistically significant results, level of significance

6. Conclusions—Summary of the results in relation to the purpose of the study and meaning of the data

In addition, an organization may require a brief author biography.

Criteria for Evaluating Abstracts

Criteria used to evaluate abstracts may include originality, scientific merit, clinical relevance, soundness of findings, overall quality, relevance to conference theme and objectives, and clarity. It is important to keep the organization's evaluative criteria in mind when writing the abstract.

Acceptance of the Abstract and Preparing for Oral or Poster Presentations

Acceptance of an abstract for either oral or poster presentation triggers the need to start preparing for a successful event. The letter of acceptance usually includes presentation guidelines. Although organizations' guidelines vary, most paper presentations are scheduled for 20 minutes with 15 minutes for content delivery and 5 minutes for questions. Poster presentations may occur over several days with designated times when presenters need to be at the poster to interact with conference participants.

Identifying the Content

Develop a detailed outline to serve as a roadmap when you write your script to practice the presentation. Include the key aspects of the study that were included in the abstract you submitted. Remember your time frame. It is important to "get to the punch line" (findings and implications for practice) and not spend too much time on the literature review. A sentence or two to set up the problem and purpose of the study is sufficient for most audiences.

Developing Visual Aids

An important aspect of your preparation is determining the audiovisual aids you will use to convey your information. Most conference presentations call for the use of slides that often are made available to participants before your presentation either online, on a USB drive, or through a conference mobile app. Less commonly, presenters may opt to distribute hard copies of their slides as a handout at the beginning of the presentation.

The Purpose of Slides

Slides enhance the presentation with a visual of your content. As you develop your presentation, determine the types and number of slides that will be used—word, pictorial, or a combination. There are numerous computer software programs (e.g., Harvard Graphics, PowerPoint, Prezi, or Keynote) that can be used for making slides. The most commonly used software at conferences is PowerPoint. Users of iPads are advised to check with the venue to see whether alternate presentation software such as Keynote will be supported.

Use of Color

Color combinations can be previewed before producing the slide. Whether to use a dark background with light type or a light background with dark type is debated (Blome et al., 2017). Nonetheless, color choice is vital for readability. For example, light pink text on a light-blue background is difficult to read. Combinations with higher contrast improve readability. According to Tomita (2017), color can have a powerful influence on the perception and atmosphere of a poster. Generally, analogous colors (those found next to each other on a color wheel) result in a warm, calm and harmonious appearance while complementary colors appear bold, striking, and sharp. Whatever colors you choose, a simple color scheme will be more appealing according to Berg and Hicks (2017).

Considerations for Developing Slides on a Computer

Developing slides on a computer allows easy preview and reordering of the slides. According to Wellstead et al. (2017), psychological analysis of PowerPoint presentations has demonstrated that people can only hold four concepts or topics of information at any one time. Therefore, limiting the detail on slides is important. One option is to limit the words to five or fewer in the title, on each line and in the number of lines per slide. There is debate about exactly which size font is best, but up to 32 points and no less than 24 points are commonly recommended according to Blome et al. (2017). In general, use a simple template, and select an easy to read font type such as Arial or Times consistently.

Many presenters are now creating multimedia presentations that include animation, audio, and video within slides to capture the audience's attention or to emphasize a point within the slide. If you are new to PowerPoint, or are having difficulty creating slides, there are many step-by-step guides available online.

Tools for Developing Charts and Graphics

There are numerous software tools that can help the presenter translate their data and make it into easy to understand and attractive charts, maps, graphs and other visualizations. Excel and Google Charts are perhaps the most commonly used chart and graphing softwares. If you are seeking to create more advanced graphics you can look to other software tools. The following software tools may be helpful in developing charts and graphs: D3. j. from Data-Driven Documents is available at d3js.org; Fusion Charts at fusioncharts.com, and Tableau at tableau.com (Chen, 2017).

Saving the Presentation

Slide presentations can be saved on a USB flash drive and easily transported. Experienced presenters recommend saving more than one copy of the file to be safe. Sending the presentation file to yourself via email or uploading it to a file hosting service such as Dropbox are other means of retrieving a file if the unexpected happens.

■ HOW TO DEVELOP PUBLIC SPEAKING SKILLS

Despite the anxiety some people feel when speaking publicly, the experience can be rewarding and exciting. Public speaking, like any skill, requires preparation. One suggestion is to conduct a practice run by presenting to colleagues and responding to their questions (Wellstead et al., 2017). This is a good time to remind yourself that your overarching goal is to deliver valuable and useful information to your audience. According to Maxey and O'Connor (2013), your audience will value your presentation more if they are able to link your content to their practice. There are several websites that provide a good overview of presentation skills. Examples of both good public speaking skills and, frankly, terrible public speaking skills abound on YouTube (www.youtube .com). A tutorial to aid in the development of presentation skills is available at cmsw.mit.edu/ writing-and-communication-center/resources/speakers.

Variance

Varying the presentation will make it much more memorable and interesting according to Kaltenbach and Soetikno (2016); this can be achieved by varying type of evidence (quantitative and qualitative), types of visuals, as well as the presenter's gestures and voice, volume, and tone. Furthermore, they recommend using varying types of evidence—qualitative information to develop a story line and quantitative information to back it up.

Relevance, Relatability, and the Power of Emotion

Kaltenbach and Soetikno (2016) also describe how to make data more impactful by making it more relevant and relatable to viewer's experience. They give the example "that stating 1 in 20 U.S. adults will develop colorectal cancer" is more relatable than stating "the lifetime risk of developing colorectal cancer is 6%" (p. 1059). They also note the importance of not simply reciting or reading slides which dulls the material and the audience. The best presenters speak naturally with expression, using the slides to reinforce the story rather than carry the story. Showing "enthusiasm, excitement or energy" is recommended by many presentation experts (Blome et al., 2017). Sometimes an interesting or humorous anecdote related to the conference location or your content serves to relax both you and the audience.

Storytelling

According to Lawrence and Paige (2016), storytelling is an ancient and powerful method for communicating and teaching. Storytelling is a powerful tool to engage your audience by letting them relate personal experiences to the information you are disseminating. Timbral (2017), in a discussion of student learning, explains how storytelling can help those without a specific or comparable experience to "imagine themselves applying the knowledge and skills they learn in a class." Urstad et al. (2018) describe how storytelling in a clinical classroom triggered student engagement and a deeper understanding of the material.

Managing Audience Engagement

We are accustomed to the rapid pace of information we receive daily via electronic means. Audience participants can easily become inattentive or distracted while listening to an oral presentation. Managing audience engagement is a useful skill when presenting to both large and small audiences. Using audience response systems such as Poll Everywhere during a PowerPoint presentation is one way to engage audience members. Participants are able to respond to questions in real time utilizing their mobile phones (iPhone or Android). This simple technology allows a presenter to assess the audience's interest, knowledge, biases, and specific areas of curiosity. Participants can respond individually or the presenter can request that participants work in pairs or groups to respond to queries. Audience responses are reflected in graphs or charts within your presentation and feedback can be shared with participants almost immediately. One advantage to using polling software is that they allow anonymous answering which may encourage participation. Poll questions require prior planning and setup. The template for inserting polling questions into a presentation is easy to use and fairly intuitive. More information can be found at www.polleverywhere.com.

Tips for Last Minute Preparations Before the Presentation

Review your notes on the day of your presentation. Arrive early to the room where you are scheduled to present so that you can meet the moderator and any fellow speakers. This gives you time to acquaint yourself with the podium and audiovisual setup and to practice advancing and backing up slides. As you begin your presentation, take time to briefly introduce yourself to the audience. This helps establish your credibility with the participants. Linking your presentation or findings to the conference theme or to a key concept presented at an earlier session promotes continuity and relatability while establishing context for the participants. When presenting after lunch, late in the afternoon or evening, or at the end of a conference be aware of the audience's energy level. Beginning your presentation with an entertaining opening, humor, picture, or other strategies such as group activities could help to maintain the audience's attention. A systematic review of expert opinion articles by Blome et al. (2017) identified the five most frequent recommendations for what makes an effective presentation:

- Keep slides simple;
- Adjust the talk to the audience;
- Rehearse;
- Do not read the talk from slides or manuscript;
- Make eye contact.

Exhibit 20.1 provides a summary of advice on strategies for presenting an engaging presentation.

▪ POSTER PRESENTATIONS

Poster presentations have distinct advantages over oral presentations or publications when disseminating research. By conducting a poster presentation, research findings are communicated to participants in an informal way. The informal exchange of ideas between the author and the participant promotes immediate feedback to the author, which may be useful in future presentations, preparation of manuscripts, clarification of unclear or confusing aspects of the study, and networking. Editors of nursing journals often solicit manuscripts after viewing posters and talking to the presenter.

EXHIBIT 20.1

STRATEGIES FOR PRESENTING AN ENGAGING PRESENTATION

- Know your audience. Speak their language and present your material in a way that is meaningful to them.
- Organize your thoughts.
- Use audiovisual aids.
- Use charts and graphs—most often, research findings can best be displayed with the use of tables, charts, graphs, figures, and so on. These tools help to better organize the findings for the audience.
- Speak to the audience and maintain eye contact.
- Watch your pace; nervousness increases speech rate.
- Remember to breathe.
- Rehearse your presentation and know the time it takes so that you can fit the schedule.
- Dress appropriately—if you are doing a presentation during working hours on-site at your organization, everyday work clothes may be appropriate. In other instances, when presenting off-site, business clothing is the appropriate attire.
- Elicit audience participation by asking questions or presenting a concept, idea, or finding, and then ask: "What does this mean to you?" or "What do you think about this study result?"
- Vary your tone of voice.
- Allow time for questions. The nature of research stimulates inquiry, so people will likely have questions.
- Always repeat the question so that everyone can hear it.
- Use tact in responding to criticism to your research and keep an open mind.
- Recognize people who have made significant contributions to the research.
- Thank the audience and let them know where you may be reached by email or phone. Provide your business card for those who wish to follow up with you.

Congruent with an oral presentation, the poster presents the major categories included in the abstract in a visually engaging manner without wordiness and busyness (Berg & Hicks, 2017).

Types of Posters

Determining the poster size depends on the presenting environment. Conference sponsors often have specific guidelines for preparing the poster; size, type of display (freestanding or wall), and how to sequence content (left to right horizontally vs. a vertical flow) are often stipulated. Poster displays are usually between 3 to 4 feet x 4 feet for easels or free standing. For a mounted bulletin board or wall presentation, 4 feet by 6 feet poster may be required. When a table is provided, use a stand-alone table-top display. A stand-alone display can be constructed by using a foam board or a portable commercial stand in which Velcro fasteners can be used to mount segments of the poster. A table top presentation also allows a spot for paper abstracts, business cards or other materials to be housed for participants. All formats require a method for mounting the poster such as pushpins or clips. This is a helpful online tutorial demonstrating poster presentation preparation: www.kumc.edu/SAH/OTEd/jradel/effective.html.

Font Choices

The American College of Physicians (ACP) recommends using no more than three font sizes for the title, section heads, and body type. Using both upper and lowercase letters is easier to read than all capital letters. The smallest type—usually 24 point—should be easily read from 3 to 5 feet (ACP, 2016). Berg and Hicks (2017) state that "sans serif fonts, such as Helvetica or Univers, are said to be good for titles, whereas Times Roman, Garamond, Palatino, or Century Schoolbook are suited for the body text" (p. 463).

Layout

At most poster presentations, there will be a large number of other posters lined up in many rows competing for attention. An attractive and easy to read layout will help draw viewers. Tomita (2017) states that columns are one of the most important visual design elements, suggesting that design focus around the use of three or four columns. There are many ways to organize the content in your poster. One strategy is to place your core message in the center with details on the sides. Others divide the poster into a grid, and there are other approaches. Whatever approach you choose, it is important to ensure the poster appears balanced.

Compelling and Understandable Graphics

Strong visuals and graphics may increase communication effectiveness. Labels should be detailed enough to communicate your message. Chen (2017) recommends "removing chart junk," which is anything that is "unnecessary for the viewer to understand the major points. Examples of chart junk include heavy or dark grid lines, superfluous text, and inappropriately ornate fonts." In other words, strip out anything that does not contribute to your points.

Constructing the Poster

Self-assembly involves using your personal computer to lay out the poster (using PowerPoint or other software) and a printer to print text in it. Make use of any in-house audiovisual department resources. Many hospitals and universities have the capability to produce posters and print. Check with the marketing, education, or media services department in your institution. Office supply stores (e.g., Staples and FedEx Office) can help produce your poster for a fee.

Portability

Consider the use of poster boards in separate pieces for portability as a hand-carry. If traveling by air, check with the airline ahead of time to determine whether a poster tube can be carried on the plane or if it must be checked. Be forewarned that an additional baggage charge may be levied if you are required to check the poster tube. Consider sending a poster "overnight" via FedEx or another carrier to the hotel or conference site. Be sure to call ahead to determine whether this is a viable option and inquire as to how to address the package (e.g., "future hotel guest").

Handouts

Have copies of the abstract, which includes authors, affiliations, address, email, and telephone number available. If you were given a proof copy of your poster prior to printing, consider making color copies available to those interested in your study. Another option is to condense your findings into a concise written document that is easy to read and saves paper (Wellstead et al., 2017).

Presenting Yourself and Your Poster

A poster presentation is an excellent way to meet others, share your work, and network. Many professional relationships have begun by meeting at a poster presentation (Berg & Hicks, 2017). With this in mind, use your body language to indicate your interest in sharing your research and answering questions. Furthermore, the authors suggest maintaining an open stance, eye contact, and a welcoming smile. Wear professional attire so that your poster can be the focus rather than your appearance.

Remain next to your poster and interact with the participants. This can be difficult when participants are approaching while you are engaged in a conversation. As multiple viewers approach, signal with body language that you recognize they are there and will turn your attention to them soon. Speak to your most important points, concepts, or contributions to current practice and acknowledge participants as they approach individually. Introduce yourself and ask attendees their research interests. Answer questions and accept constructive criticism gracefully. Do not become defensive if challenged about "Why didn't you do xyz?" Provide your rationale or respond with "That's a good suggestion for future research in this area." Be ready with business cards or handouts to provide the means of contacting each other later. Jot a note on any cards given to you to remind you of the person's interest or request.

Exhibit 20.2 summarizes common steps in preparing a poster preparation.

Posters are excellent vehicles for disseminating research findings to the community as well as to the profession. They can easily be used at community health fairs, at local professional meetings, and seminars, and can be developed for display in shopping malls, physicians' offices, and community and social service agencies. When the plan is to use a poster for different types of audiences, it is helpful if the entire poster is not developed as a whole piece. Develop separate

---

EXHIBIT 20.2

STEPS IN PREPARING AND GIVING A POSTER PRESENTATION

1. Conference Information
   - Conference date and location.
   - Length of time for poster session and requirement for being present at poster.
   - Type of display.
2. Poster information
   - Title: A short catchy, easily understood title that encourages people to read more (Berg & Hicks, 2017).

(continued)

- Author names, credentials and affiliations.
- Problem and a brief background.
- Method—Design, sample, setting, and data collection process.
- Data analysis.
- Results and implications.
- Acknowledgment—Sources of funds.

3. Poster assembly
   - Layout of poster—Consider the sequence of ideas, and use headings, arrows, or broken lines to guide the reader.
   - Use of color—Pictures, self-explanatory tables and graphs will attract viewers.
   - Available resources.
   - Portability.

4. Other considerations
   - Plan handouts.
   - Use of display items such as data collection tools: mark these as "for display only" and put them in a plastic sleeve or have them laminated.

5. Poster session
   - Dress professionally and wear comfortable shoes.
   - Set up the poster and take it down at designated times.
   - Be at the poster and interact with participants, note requests for information and offer your business card to attendees.
   - Observe other posters and seek permission from authors to take a picture of posters you find attractive.
   - Ask a colleague or another poster presenter to take a picture of you with your poster. These "photo ops" can be used in the future for agency newsletters, and so on.

6. Evaluation
   - Immediately following the presentation, jot down things you would do differently—format, colors, written content, type, and number of handouts.

segments for sections such as the research methods and conclusions so that these sections can be adapted for each audience.

DISSEMINATING RESEARCH FINDINGS THROUGH ELECTRONIC MEDIA

The media, including television, radio, and the internet, are powerful vehicles for disseminating nursing research.

Web-Based Presentations and Webinars

Although most presentations are delivered to a live audience in the same location, you may be offered the opportunity to present via a satellite teleconference or web-based platform. Virtual conferences are being offered with increasing frequency. Webinars may consist of the audience viewing slides and listening to the audio portion of the presentation or they may use an interactive format with video and audience participation. Conducting face-to-face oral presentations gives you the opportunity to see your audience, interact with them, and receive verbal and nonverbal feedback during the presentation. On the other hand, you only reach a small number of people. Web-based presentations may be viewed by large numbers of people but limit your ability to read your audience and interact with them. Regardless of the medium used, strategies for preparing the presentation are the same. Presenting via a teleconference or web-based format requires extra attention to fielding questions, and dealing with technical issues.

If cameras are available during your webinar the videographer may move between you and your slides. Less movement while speaking is better, so practice your presentation in a mirror prior to the actual event to identify any distracting mannerisms such as nervous hand gestures, wiping hair out of your eyes, and so on.

How to Handle Questions and Answers in Webinars

Discuss how the audience will be able to ask questions prior to your presentation. If they can call in, you may want to ask that questions be held until the end. If attendees can email or instant message questions, a facilitator is often available to collect these questions, group them by theme, and pose the questions to you at pre-planned times during the webinar. Be sure to provide your email, telephone, or other contact information for follow-up. Webinars may be available asynchronously, so it is important that people viewing your presentation at a later time will be able to contact you.

Coordinate With Technical Support

Technical assistance is a must. We have all witnessed a web conference that experienced technical difficulties. Technical support is needed initially to load your presentation, ensure that your microphone is working, and that you and your slides appear centered in the screen shots. Technical assistance also may be needed to troubleshoot issues arising from the attendees' end of the computer. Audio issues and visual issues may require adjustments from the technical support person. As you begin your presentation, ask the audience to email or phone the technical support line if they have difficulty accessing your presentation. A resource for additional tips and guidelines in developing a webinar presentation may be found at info.workcast.com/webinar-best-practices?utm_campaign=Bing%20eBooks&utm_source=pp.

Digital Posters

Computer poster sessions and digital poster sessions are two additional means of presenting research. A computerized poster may be presented during a standard poster viewing session. The poster typically is designed to be viewed on a laptop or tablet. Formats include a PowerPoint slide show, video clips, or other multimedia. Key elements remain the same as for a static poster. Digital poster sessions are web based and usually asynchronous. They may be accessed by many people over time. Digital poster sessions may incorporate PowerPoint slides, slide narration, video clips, audio clips, or other media. Digital presentations should adhere to the principles of universal design to meet accessibility standards. References and contact information must be included.

Television and Radio and News Media

Before considering the media as an outlet for disseminating information, check with your employer about existing policies and/or restrictions. There may be a staff member who is charged with assisting those who wish to communicate research findings to the media. Some organizations submit press releases—a written overview of events that are occurring. If this is being done, find out how you could submit your research findings.

Professional organizations often invite reporters from local television stations to conferences so that research of interest to the public can be identified. Because of this possibility, many organizations will ask you to sign a document indicating your willingness to share the study with the media.

Television, radio, and newspaper reporters often search the internet for evidence-based research reports on topics of current interest. If you have disseminated research in any way, always do an internet search on your topic and see if you find mention of yourself and your work. If you do, be prepared for the possibility of being contacted by a reporter. Develop key talking points related to your topic to manage the interview and make sure your message is heard. Always know and be ready to talk about the implications of your topic to the public. Many institutions have their own guidelines for how and when employees may interact with members of the press. Keep in mind that your main goal is to keep the focus on your research and "manage the message." Press releases from the National Institute for Nursing Research (www.ninr.nih.gov) serve as examples for sharing scientific information in a concise format. Television remains a powerful medium for disseminating research.

Reaching Out Proactively to the Media

Nurses can be proactive and contact local television stations to arrange a meeting with producers. Local stations often have a health segment that may be an appropriate fit with your research. Before contacting the local station, ensure that your institution is supportive. Have a clear idea of the type of local show that might broadcast your findings, know the type of people who watch particular shows, determine the fit between your topic and the show, and maintain confidentiality of study participants. If an interview is granted, inquire whether the interview will be live or taped and if you are the only person being interviewed or if there are other participants. If there are other participants, find out the background of each participant. Start preparing by creating an outline, scripting, and practicing with a colleague or by videotaping your presentation and reviewing the tape. Follow the guidelines for preparing an oral presentation and public speaking strategies presented in this chapter.

Preparing for an Interview

Carefully preparing for an interview with the media is important. Preparing for an interview with the media includes familiarity with the mechanics that will be used (i.e., face to face, by telephone, and video/audio taping for television or radio). There are several strategies for preparing for the various stages (prior to, during, and after the interview), which are highlighted in the following:

1. Be clear on ground rules related to topics you will and will not address and the opportunity to review and correct misstatements.
2. Identify possible questions that support and do not support your study and formulate a 10- to 30-second response.
3. Respond directly to a question, use citations, and do not predict when hypothetical situations are presented and an answer is being sought.

4. Determine the key points of your interview and emphasize the points each time you have the opportunity.

5. Look at the interviewer during the taping or when you are not being interviewed. See www.bottomlinemediacoaching.com/5-mistakes-to-avoid-during-a-tv-interview for more tips, including knowing the pronunciation of the interviewer's name.

6. Use terms that lay people will understand.

7. Limit your movements during the interview.

8. Immediately correct the interviewer when something that is said is incorrect.

9. Communicate enthusiasm and smile.

10. Wear a solid-color outfit.

11. Write a thank-you note to the host and the producer.

(Condensed from The Society for Neuroscience Tip Sheet accessible at: www.sfn.org/~/media/SfN/Documents/Public%20Outreach/baw_General_Techniques_for_Media_Interviews.ashx)

A local news channel is likely to be open to allowing a short segment presentation when the topic is one that is of great interest to its viewers. Consider a national channel if your research findings have major implications for the health of society. Reading newspapers and magazines that the public reads will give you an idea of topics that are relevant and interesting to the public as well as how this information is presented.

Radio

Radio also is a powerful medium for research dissemination. Most people invest some amount of time listening to the radio on a daily basis. The radio audience potential is vast. Many local stations host special interest shows and talk shows and invite people to participate. It would be wise to invest time in searching out these opportunities.

There are advantages and disadvantages for the use of the media in disseminating research findings. Distinct advantages are that this type of medium has a greater potential for reaching a larger audience and influencing the public's perception of nurses' contributions to their health. On the other hand, the short time allotment for the presentation increases the possibility of misinterpretation of your message. Thus, researchers must provide a comprehensive presentation of the research methodology, findings, and implications in an understandable and concise manner. To help counter the simplicity and brevity of this type of research presentation, provide your name and a work email, phone number, or address where you can be reached so that community members may contact you to learn more about your study. Do not give out home or personal contact information.

Videotaping

Most laptops and computer monitors now include web camera (webcam) capability. In addition to allowing individuals to participate interactively in web-based conferences or seminars, a webcam can be used to record video and audio. Software programs, such as Blender and Lightworks for the PC and iMovie for Apple, can be downloaded/purchased via the internet. When planning any video recording, consider the target audience, desired outcomes, and content. Identify the most effective ways to communicate your message and use visual aids that support the script or photography. Writing a script is important to ensure that the message is succinct and will be delivered within the allotted time. During the recording, it is helpful to consider the camera as the audience and to pretend that you are in your living room speaking to guests. After recording yourself discussing your research or presenting your poster, you may save it as a media file for viewing as a podcast, or post it on YouTube.com or another appropriate website. Podcasts may be an audio file only, audio with video clips, or even a pdf file (Digitalpodcast.com). Researchers may choose to audiotape their presentation and disseminate it via a podcast. This mobile learning strategy may be appreciated by those with an auditory learning style.

Summary of Electronic Media

As noted at the beginning of this chapter, technology plays a major role in providing opportunities for the dissemination of nursing research. The internet offers a fast and convenient means to not only obtain information but to effectively share new research findings. Web-based venues are transforming how we transfer knowledge and influence global healthcare. As an example, YouTube.com is a video-sharing website where users can upload, view, and share video clips. A quick search of YouTube with the keywords "nursing research" provides many ideas for disseminating your research findings to the world. Many journal websites are technology enabled, which allows authors of articles to post supplemental content, such as a video clip discussing research.

Social media and professional networking sites such as LinkedIn, blogs, Twitter, and listservs are more informal ways of sharing ideas, obtaining feedback from others, and identifying potential colleagues with whom to collaborate. Posting your research interests and a brief summary of research completed on appropriate sites may lead to further opportunities to share your findings. In order to keep postings very concise (Twitter has a 140-character limit) yet meaningful, judicious editing is needed.

A cautionary note is warranted. Postings to electronic media are in the public domain, even if the site is password protected or accessible by subscription only. Nurses are advised to reacquaint themselves with the Healthcare Insurance Portability and Accountability Act (HIPAA) regarding patient privacy and confidentiality rights. Likewise, state boards of nursing (National Council of State Boards of Registered Nursing [NCSBN], 2018) and the American Nurses Association (ANA, 2011) have developed guidelines to assist nurses in determining what content can be shared electronically. Nurses whose web postings (on blogs, Facebook, LinkedIn, etc.) violate HIPAA standards face professional and legal sanctions.

■ SUMMARY

In conclusion, the mode of disseminating research findings is varied. The goal is effective communication with the target audience. Oral and poster presenters must conform to the guidelines set forth by the sponsoring organization to contribute to the success of the event. Taking the time to reflect on and evaluate your poster or oral presentation is essential to further developing your professional presentation skills.

SUGGESTED LEARNING ACTIVITIES

1. After reviewing your research findings and the National Communication Association's media tips (www.natcom.org/advocacy-public-engagement/develop-your-media-strategy) complete these steps in preparation for a mock interview by a member of the press:

      b.   What is new or unique about your findings?

      c.   Why are your findings important? In what way will they contribute to safe, quality nursing care?

      d.   Who or what benefits as a result of your findings?

2.   Edit your presentation, poster, or written research to clearly answer the questions in question 1.

3.   Based on the context of your oral presentation content and your desire to maintain audience attention:

      a.   Develop an analogy that will help the audience understand the content you are presenting.

      b.   Identify a few key points in your talk that might be illustrated with humor (an anecdote, a cartoon, or a poem).

      c.   Develop several questions or polls to increase audience engagement and input during your presentation.

      d.   Integrate at least one of these methods into your presentation, poster, or written research.

ACKNOWLEDGMENTS

The author would like to acknowledge the work done by this chapter's original authors Dr. S. Smith, Dr. M. Mateo, and Dr. Stuenkel.

REFERENCES

American Association of Colleges of Nursing. (2017). *Fact sheet: The doctor of nursing practice (revised June 2017)*. http://www.aacn.nche.edu/media-relations/fact-sheets/dnp

American College of Physicians. (2016). *Preparing a poster presentation*. https://www.acponline.org/membership/residents/competitions-awards/acp-national-abstract-competitions/guide-to-preparing-for-the-abstract-competition/preparing-a-poster-presentation

American Nurses Association. (2011). *Principles for social networking and the nurse*. Author. https://www.nursingworld.org/~4af4f2/globalassets/docs/ana/ethics/social-networking.pdf

Berg, J., & Hicks, R., (2017). Successful design and delivery of a professional poster. *Journal of the American Association of Nurse Practitioners, 29*(8), 461–469. https://doi.org/10.1002/2327-6924.12478

Blome, C., Sondermann, H., & Augustin, M. (2017). Accepted standards on how to give a medical research presentation: A systematic review of expert opinion papers, *GMS Journal for Medical Education, 34*(1), 1–7.

Chen, H. (2017). *Design and conquer create compelling graphics*. Americanlibrariesmagazine.org (May, p. 55). https://americanlibrariesmagazine.org/2017/05/01/information-design-and-conquer

Curtis, K., Fry, M., Shaban, R. Z., & Considine, J. (2016). Translating research findings to clinical nursing practice. *Journal of Clinical Nursing, 26*, 862–872. https://doi.org/10.1111/jocn.13586

Grove, S. K., Gray, J. R., & Burns, N. (2015). *Understanding nursing research: Building an evidence-based practice* (6th ed., pp. 40–41). Elsevier.

Kaltenbach, H., & Soetikno, R. (2016). How to create and deliver an effective presentation. *Gastroenterology, 151*, 1058–1060. https://doi.org/10.1053/j.gastro.2016.10.009

Lawrence, R. L., & Paige, D. S. (2016). What our ancestors knew: Teaching and learning through storytelling. *New Directions for Adult and Continuing Education, 149*, 63–72. https://doi.org/10.1002/ace.20177

Maxey, C., & O'Connor, K. E. (2013). *Fearless facilitation: The ultimate field guide to engaging your audience* (pp. 8–17). Pfeifer.

National Council of State Boards of Registered Nursing. (2018). *A nurse's guide to the use of social media.* Author. https://www.ncsbn.org/NCSBN_SocialMedia.pdf

Timbral, J. (2017). Instructional storytelling: Application of the clinical judgement model in nursing. *Journal of Nursing Education, 56*(5), 305–308. https://doi.org/10.3928/01484834-20170421-10

Tomita, H. (2017). Visual design tips to develop an inviting poster for poster presentations. *Association for Educational Communication & Technology, 61*, 313–315. https://doi.org/10.1007/s11528-017-0197-x

Urstad, K., Ulfsby, K., Brandeggen, T., Bodsberg, K., Jensen, L., & Tjoflat, I. (2018). Digital storytelling in clinical replacement studies: Nursing students' experiences. *Nurse Education Today, 71*, 91–96. https://doi.org/10.1016/j.nedt.2018.09.016

Wellstead, G., Whitehurst, K., Gundogan, B., & Agha, R. (2017). How to deliver an oral presentation. *International Journal of Surgery Oncology, 2*(6), e25 https://doi.org/10.1097/IJ9.0000000000000025

21

REPORTING RESULTS THROUGH PUBLICATIONS

TRACY KLEIN AND PATRICIA F. PEARCE

▥ INTRODUCTION

The purpose of this chapter is to provide information regarding the opportunities for successfully publishing scholarly work. The focus will be on many options available for publishing and how they can be leveraged to secure successful publication. Further emphasis will be placed on the processes, planning, and strategies to adequately develop high-quality, professional publications as well as maneuvering challenges such as authorship, copyright, and attribution. Key questions an author should explore before submitting a manuscript for consideration will be provided, including discussion of peer-reviewed and non-peer-reviewed opportunities. Ethical parameters will be detailed, and helpful hints provided.

In order to change practice and improve patient outcomes, both researchers and advanced practice registered nurses (APRNs) need to disseminate findings from their scholarly and clinical work. APRNs can be educated through master's or doctoral level programs (DNP or PhD). Historically APRNs were educated at the master's level, which continues today. Education at the DNP level was added in the early 2000s. Notably, a number of APRNs completed doctoral work in PhD, EdD, or other doctoral programs. Many APRNs start their practice with or return to school to complete a doctor of nursing practice (DNP) or doctor of philosophy (PhD). Regardless of degrees completed, scholarship in the form of disseminating through publication is an integral part of the discipline. For the APRN who is a DNP or PhD student, the scholarly process and the plan for communicating findings is best developed at the time a scholarly project or dissertation is begun. Higher degree completion is accompanied by a parallel increase in expectations for publication and other forms of dissemination of scholarly work. In doctoral education there is an expectation that scholarly work completed in the program should be communicated and shared outside of the program. For those in clinical practice, whether or not enrolled in an additional advanced degree program, scholarly publication supports the foundation and continuance of moving patient care, systems of care, and research forward and further enhances the skills of the practitioner for scholarly work. Sharing scholarly work is a responsibility for all nurses (Kennedy, 2018).

A DNP project typically encompasses quality assurance, practice improvement, evidence-based practice, or policy recommendations (see Exhibit 21.1), while a PhD program includes dissertation research and analysis in qualitative, quantitative, or mixed method design. Both the DNP project and PhD dissertation entail scholarly work, but their focus and scope differ. Projects, theses, and dissertations are forms of scholarship, and practice itself is a form of scholarship, however audience and appropriate methods for dissemination vary considerably. Although the traditional approach to publishing scholarship is through professional journals, other publication options are available, including professional society newsletters, media from institutes or agencies such

---

EXHIBIT 21.1

SELECTED EXAMPLES OF SCHOLARLY PROJECTS

Health Promotion and Community Health

- Compare strategies for health promotion/disease prevention.
- Identify trends in patient visits, outreach programs.
- Evaluate screening protocols.

Policy-Related Scholarly Projects

- Implement new policy collaboratively with health department (e.g., HPV vaccine awareness).
- Evaluate or compare nursing home policies for treating chronic pain.
- Evaluate employer policies regarding health and the potential cost savings of new policies.

Integration of Technology in Care and Informatics-Related Projects

- Create a database for monitoring injuries in urgent care and evaluate its impact.
- Use technology to improve health (telehealth consultation, interactive "home" visits, etc.) and evaluate results.
- Evaluate technology's impact on care (information transfer to point of care, etc.).

Source: Adapted from National Organization of Nurse Practitioner Faculties. (2007). *NONPF recommended criteria for NP scholarly projects in the practice doctorate program.* https://cdn.ymaws.com/www.nonpf.org/resource/resmgr/imported/ScholarlyProjectCriteria.pdf

---

as the Centers for Disease Control and Prevention, the Pew Foundation, conference proceedings, electronic posters, and other media.

■ STARTING THE PROCESS OF PUBLICATION

The main categories for publishing forms include print or electronic, or simultaneously print and electronic. Electronic venues for publication comprise a number of options, including personal and organizational websites, and commercial ventures such as YouTube. Open access publications and web-based publications, such as videos, make up accessible means for nurses to watch and share original information that can be accessed through websites, mobile devices, blogs, and email. Further, surveys can be deployed, and results announced and promoted through social media platforms such as Twitter. Although open and web or mobile access methods greatly enhance the speed and scope of dissemination, there are tradeoffs to consider in selecting these options. It can be difficult to maintain both the integrity and the focus of research dissemination when expanded access occurs. Institutions, particularly for those in tenure-eligible positions, often have constraints or criteria related to publication completion which determine both how dissemination occurs and how it counts toward employment-related requirements. The expansion of options over the last decade also prompts discussion of ethical and scholarly considerations in developing a dissemination plan. A too-broad dissemination plan can also decrease the impact of results and potentially increases the risk for insecure sharing or plagiarism.

The multiple decision points, steps, and procedures necessary to ensure successful publication are highlighted in Figure 21.1, with a short annotation on each step. Step one is selecting a journal, triggering next steps included in the diagram. Each of the facets will be explained in detail, with recommendations for completing the process.

■ SELECTION OF PUBLICATION VENUE

Journals

According to the Cumulative Index to Nursing and Allied Health Literature (CINAHL) website (www.cinahl.com), there are over 4,000 journals indexed in the CINAHL repository; only a small

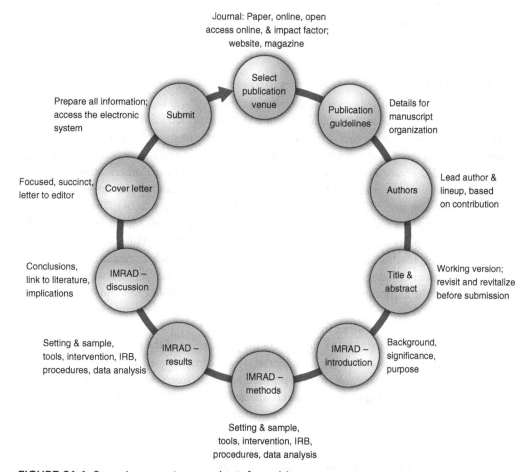

FIGURE 21.1 Steps in preparing to submit for publication.

Note: IMRAD is acronym representing a technique for organizing and presenting information in an abstract, highlighting the critical components: Introduction, Methods, Results, and Discussion

Source: From Nakayama, T., Hirai, N., Yamazaki, S., & Naito, M. (2005). Adoption of structured abstracts by general medical journals and format for a structured abstract. *Journal of the Medical Library Association, 93*(2), 237–242; Sollaci, L. B., & Pereira, M. G. (2004). The introduction, methods, results, and discussion (IMRAD) structure: A fifty-year survey. *Journal of the Medical Library Association, 92*, 364–372.

percentage are exclusively research journals. In PubMed, which includes MEDLINE and PubMed Central (PMC), there are 30,000 journal records indexed (www.nlm.nih.gov/bsd/serfile_added-info.html). There is some overlap between PubMed and CINAHL, but using both when searching for journals or published information will provide comprehensive information regarding what is already published in your field of interest, and where gaps can be explored.

Publishing in journals with a less strenuous research emphasis but a heavier emphasis on clinical application allows nurse clinicians and practitioners to report on evidence-based practices that improve health outcomes, but in work that does not necessarily meet the data-based and more highly controlled research methods requirements. Clinical articles often include problem-solving skills, clinical decision making, and discussion and debate regarding professional issues in nursing, all that are critical for nursing knowledge. Such articles focus on a variety of practice topics that improve nursing practice, including examining clinical guidelines in practice, brief reports, innovative clinical practice, case studies, healthcare outcome evaluations, and policy-based implementation strategies. Broome et al. (2013) found in a broad assessment of published DNP projects from 2005–2012 that the percentage published in peer reviewed journals has increased over time and that original clinical investigations were the most frequent, followed in frequency by practice-focused patient and provider studies.

Peer-Review

Peer-review (also called *juried review*) is the process through which scholarly work is assessed by others who have expertise on the topical content and methods used for the work being reported. Peer review can be an open process (authors and reviewers names are known to each other), a single blind review (reviewer is aware of author identify, but reviewers are unknown to authors), or double-blinded review (authors and reviewers are unaware of each other's identity) (Baker, 2012). Peer review is one method of assuring heightened accountability and integrity in publication, both linking to credibility of the work published (Dougherty, 2006). The credibility of publishing in a professional journal is based on the peer-review process intended to evaluate the quality of work by peers who are experts in the field (Dougherty, 2006). While peer review process can vary, clear explanation of how peer review occurs and under what criteria is important to assure the author of the integrity of a journal (Edie & Conklin, 2019). Peer review process should be explained in the author guidelines for the journal or site of publication and should include a description of the process, degree of confidentiality of review, and discussion of conflicts of interest, as well as how reviewers can be suggested if needed (Broga et al., 2014; Marusic, 2018; Marusic et al., 2019; Vervaart, 2014). Editors are the gatekeepers of the peer review process and assume the responsibility of selecting reviewers who have demonstrated advanced knowledge or practice in a particular nursing role, such as practice, administrator, researcher, educator, systems focus (e.g., informatics) or specific patient care specialty. Manuscripts are ideally reviewed by at least two reviewers, and often three or more. Reviewers screen the manuscripts for content and process quality, accuracy, timeliness, relevance, and appropriateness prior to the editor's consideration of the article for publication. Despite its potential weaknesses, peer review is the most appropriate means for selecting manuscripts for publication. Peer review gives readers assurance that the journal's content meets acceptable standards of scholarship, conferring validity and credibility on an author's work. Lack of rigorous peer review has also been implicated in the proliferation of predatory journal publications in nursing (Oermann et al., 2018).

Because of promotion and tenure criteria, faculty in institutions of higher education place weight on number and quality of publications, particularly for research intensive positions

(Oermann & Hays, 2018). Publication metrics can be used to determine the impact of a journal and is also considered in the criteria for some institutions (Carpenter et al., 2014). Although the quality of material published in a non-peer- reviewed journal may not be any different from that in a peer-reviewed journal, choice of a journal should be made in light of current job requirements as well as your planned career track, and always considering the audience intended to reach.

Non-Peer-Reviewed Publications

Non-peer-reviewed publications include many internet sites that report news or healthcare information, magazines, and newspapers as well as some journals (Wood & Ludwig, 2012). However, for journals that do not include peer review, an editor may still review manuscripts and decide which manuscripts will be published, using similar criteria to those used by peer-reviewed journals. A journal editor reviewing a manuscript submitted for publication does not qualify for peer-review status. Although the articles in such journals may be excellent, the lack of peer review other than an editor lessens their credibility. Journals that are peer reviewed will include a statement such as "peer-reviewed journal" somewhere within the journal information provided in each issue and typically on the journal website. If there is a lack of information about peer-review for a journal, or questions about the process, clarification should be done by contacting the editorial office, before completing a submission to the journal. Authors must be patient, because the peer review process takes time, but authors must also be aware that an acceptance for publication within a few days of submission can indicate need to investigate peer review process of the journal. Authors should also receive commentary provided by the peer reviewers, typically labeled for each reviewer (e.g., reviewer one, reviewer two), and the reviewers' comments.

The major limitation to publishing on websites or online is the lack of peer review which diminishes the credibility of the publication. For online publications not linked with a peer-reviewed journal or process, or from a well-known agency, such as the Centers for Disease Control or National Institutes of Health, control of quality potentially diminishes. Publishing a scholarly project abstract in a repository, which may be maintained by an individual university (Heselden et al., 2019) or a professional association such as Sigma Theta Tau's Virginia Henderson repository (www.sigmarepository.org) heightens accessibility, but does not include peer review necessarily. Innovation in interactivity is increasing also for repository work (Hodge et al., 2016). Authors must also be aware that works published electronically are used often by others without the author's knowledge or permissions. Additionally, the work posted is difficult to remove once posted, thus has potential to exist indefinitely. Authors must always be cautious in publication in any venue – once published, works are typically available for a lengthy period of time.

Paper-Print Journals

Publishers provide paper-print journals, but increasingly material in print is also available electronically, and some journals are transitioning to only digital, online access. Electronic access increases entrée to an author's work via internet searching, but journals provide differing access to publication content. Titles, author listing, abstract, keywords, and other identifying information is routinely available through internet searches. When submitting a manuscript for publication, publishers use web-based systems (i.e., Manuscript Central, Scholar One, etc.) to acquire, review, edit, and produce the journal's content. The manuscript is submitted electronically to an editor, forwarded by the editor to reviewers electronically, and revised and published electronically.

Electronic Journals and Open Access

There can be advantages to online publications. Once accepted for publication and processed, articles are often placed in an online database of the journal until it is assigned to an issue of the journal, named in some way for early access, like Online First (tcn.sagepub.com/content/early/recent) or directly into the journal online site. Manuscripts published in early print, or early online print, are considered published articles with an assigned *digital object identifier*, or DOI number, if the journal subscribed to the DOI system of identification. This reduces the time from generating knowledge to communicating the information to others. Another advantage of electronic systems is that resources are conserved—reducing paper use in generating and photocopying, as well as postage for shipping to publishers. In addition, further content can also easily be updated with new information and hypertext links to other related sites Additionally, readers can enter into a dialogue with the author and the editor through electronic mail or direct website linkage, which can be appended to the electronic article.

Online publishing is an increasing trend, but definitions, processes, parameters, and value are debated. There are journals that were begun as online journals specifically, and there are journals that have transitioned from in-print to online format. An additional model includes journals that are available in hard copy print as well as online, digital access. A fully open access journal is defined as a journal that provides open access to all readers at no charge to readers, and includes that the reader can download, share, distribute, and link the articles (Albert, 2006; Baker et al., 2019; Hua et al., 2017). For these journals, the funding model is typically through author payment directly to the publisher. Advertising and other activities provide additional financial base in this model. Open access journals are different from journals that have the option of in-print or online publications. Although some journals provide an option to authors to enable online access for their publication, the journal might not be completely open access, or it might be accessible only by members of a restricted group, such as a professional association like the Journal of the American Association of Nurse Practitioners (JAANP). JAANP is an example of a journal which has been in-print since its start, and only recently transitioned to online, digitally available content only. Members of AANP have full online access to all journal content, but some editorials and articles are made available online to non-members. There is an option for fully-online availability choice for authors, with monetary payment, or open access for those reports that are required to be made available by funding parameters.

Open access publication can be considered scholarly, and online journals may or may not be affiliated with a publisher, professional organization, or association. Open access journals depend on author payment for their publication funding. Baker et al. (2019) describe common categories of cost coverage – the gold model, green model, platinum, and hybrid model. There is an open access association to which open access journals belong, and within this association guidelines and ethical parameters are set (Albert, 2006; Baker et al., 2019; Hua et al., 2017). Open access journals might or might not include peer review. Most often there is a cost of approximately $500 to $5,000 to the author to submit a manuscript. Upon acceptance of the manuscript and payment if required, the article is published online and readily available for public viewing, thereby decreasing the time it takes for publication. In terms of audience, there is no cost for the reader to view the article or to purchase the article through online publishing companies as this fee is paid by the author to the publisher. There are groups that identify high-quality, peer-reviewed open access research journals and periodicals like the Directory of Open Access Journals (DOAJ) (doaj.org) which provides an ongoing listing of open access journals. The DOAJ is maintained as a non-profit organization, through member funding, and the list changes as updated are made.

Members are drawn from individuals and groups, including organizations such as libraries, publishers, and government organizations. Removal of a journal from the DOAJ which was previously listed may indicate that is has been identified as a "predatory journal."

Predatory Journals

Increasing availability of predatory journals is a major concern in publishing, and a concern to most disciplines, including nursing (INANE Predatory Publishing Practices Collaborative, 2014; International Academy of Nursing Editors Predatory Publishing Practices, 2015; Kearney & INANE Predatory Publishing Practices Collaborative, 2015). Research completed in the area of predatory journals indicate an increasing problem in nursing and other disciplines (Baker et al., 2019; Mercier et al., 2018; Oermann et al., 2016; Wahyudi, 2017). A predatory journal is one that charges fees for publishing and for editorial services, but without providing those services expected, resulting in a substantial lack of rigor (Baker et al., 2019; Beall, 2012; Beall, 2016; Strinzel et al., 2019; Wahyudi, 2017). Typically, predatory journals are online and open access, and prey upon naïve authors, or authors seeking a quick publication. Predatory journals are often fleeting and locating a home address for the journal is difficult. These online journals exploit authors by using an open access publishing model that involves illegitimate journals, journals that actually do not exist, or a journal created specifically to exploit unsuspecting authors. Invitation to publish from predatory journals, or to participate in their editorial board, appear in seemingly random emails or spam from a predatory journal may seem quite legitimate at first. Mercier et al. (2018) demonstrated predatory journals targeting new, novice professionals with promises of publication, conference presentations, and editorial board positions. Many professionals feel honored to have been asked to serve on editorial boards and often agree, unaware that their name is being used to support an illegitimate journal (Wahyudi, 2017).

Although there is discussion about the use of the term *predatory* in publishing, with concern that fledgling journals or smaller publishers are at risk of being mislabeled with this negative term, there is a general consensus that authors must be aware of exploitative practices in publishing, most notably with journals that provide little attention to rigor, questionable business practices, and poor service overall to science (Baker et al., 2019; Memon, 2019; Mercier et al., 2018; Oermann et al., 2016). Lack of focus by a journal on a particular clinical area or content focus has been identified as a common characteristic of predatory journals (Baker et al., 2019; Oermann et al., 2016). There is evidence of heightened plagiarism in predatory journals. Plagiarized content was identified in a descriptive comparative study of three nursing journals that represented authors from 26 countries (Owens & Nicoll, 2019).

Determining the status of a journal as predatory is challenging. Beall's List of Predatory Journals, formerly developed by Beall, is now a compilation online that is periodically updated by an anonymous source (beallslist.weebly.com/contact.html) after the original list was described by Beall (2016). Strinzel et al. (2019) reported a descriptive mixed method study of journals, and demonstrated 72 journals from 42 publishers were included in predatory and non-predatory journal lists. Peer review, editorial services, policies, and business practices were some of the factors explored by Strinzel et al. (2019). Oermann et al. (2016) investigated predatory journals in nursing, identifying in descriptive research a total of 140 predatory journals involving 75 publishers. Noted by the Oermann team (2016) was a pattern of journals publishing only a few issues and then stopping, as well as relative youth of 1 to 2 years of age for the journals. Commentary by Baker et al. (2019), and research reported by Cobey et al. (2019) and Wahyudi (2017) provide lists of items that should raise question regarding the status of a journal as predatory. The initiative

---

EXHIBIT 21.2

EXAMPLES OF THE MOST COMMON SIGNS THAT A JOURNAL MIGHT BE PREDATORY

CHARACTERISTIC		EXPLANATION
Publisher solicited	→	Publisher solicitation is often overly solicitous, flattering, and includes promises of quick publication and far-ranging dissemination.
Author payment requested ahead-of-acceptance to publish	→	Many models of open access publishing have author fees involved. Predatory journals often request fees ahead of acceptance, versus after peer-review and official notification of acceptance.
Fast publication turnaround time	→	Very fast turnaround time to publication promised, with a range of only several weeks to a month or so.
Plagiarism	→	Obvious plagiarism in existing published articles in journal.

Think. Check. Submit (thinkchecksubmit.org) provides guidance for those seeking to submit to a legitimate journal, and offers checklists and helpful questions to ask when evaluating potential options for publication. Exhibit 21.2 includes several of the most frequently acknowledged characteristics of predatory journals found in research of predatory journals (Baker et al., 2019; Mercier et al., 2018; Oermann et al., 2016, 2019; Wahyudi, 2017).

■ SUCCESSFUL PUBLISHING

Journal publication is the most frequent method for scholarly dissemination because many nurses and others can be reached by one effort—publishing a high-quality, focused manuscript that will remain accessible by others on a long-term, stable basis. To increase the chance of having your manuscript accepted for publication (Happell, 2005, 2012; Oermann, 2018; Oermann & Hays, 2018; Price, 2010; Yancey, 2016), following critical factors for successful publishing is vital (Exhibit 21.3). Several of these factors are discussed in more detail in the upcoming sections.

■ JOURNAL SELECTION

Audience

Knowing the audience reading the journal is an important first step in selecting a journal for publication, and then selecting a journal based on that audience is critical. Additionally, determining who would most readily benefit from gaining the information being published is the basis for

---

EXHIBIT 21.3

CRITICAL FACTORS FOR SUCCESSFUL PUBLISHING

- Identify the appropriate audience.
- Select the appropriate journal, based on audience desired, topic, and methods.
- Conform to submission guidelines.
- Adhere to copyright laws.
- Include implications for practice.
- Use recent and seminal references which are appropriately integrated.
- Organize manuscript based strictly on author guidelines and style requirements.
- Use tables and graphs creatively, logically, and rationally.
- Determine authorship attribution.
- Acknowledge appropriately.
- Conform to ethical practices.

---

determining an appropriate audience. Editors know their journal audience and will reject outright an article that is inappropriate for the journal audience.

Identifying the audience clearly in the introduction will help to draw in the editor, the audience later, and will keep the author on point while generating the manuscript. For example, if findings suggested a cost-effective way to deliver nursing care, practitioners and administrators would be interested in the topic. However, it is likely that practitioners would be more interested in the clinical implications, whereas administrators might be more interested in the management aspects—targeting the work to the audience is an exceedingly important step in securing publication.

Funding Requirements for Publication

One factor that can influence dissemination of findings from a scholarly project includes requirements of the funding agency and organization that supported the project. The author is responsible for meeting funding agency guidelines. Some funding agencies and organizations require a review of results before findings are disseminated and expect to be listed in the acknowledgments. Most journals delineate that funding or sponsored projects related to the work being reported must include indicator of the funding organization, as this is a component of assuring transparency in funding, heightening scientific integrity, and reduction of potential bias. Funders may also require review or approval of submission of the manuscript before it is submitted. Because funding agency requirements can potentially delay the dissemination process, it is important to be familiar with requirements of funding or supporting agencies, including employers in the circumstance of a research endeavor or project done in an institution of employment. Intellectual property considerations of academic institutions vary between institutions and might allow, as an example, for collaboration and review but not approval by funding agencies who may attempt to influence findings and outcomes.

Evaluating Impact Factor

Choosing a high-quality journal to publish a manuscript is important. There is a variety of publication metrics to measure the productivity of the journal. The first and most common is the impact factor (IF), produced by the Institute for Information Science, held by Thompson-Reuters. The IF is an objective indicator of the relative importance of a journal, thus is linked to the article published in the rated journal. The higher the IF, the greater the importance of the journal in its field. The IF reports are available at the Institute of Scientific Information (ISI), owned by Thompson-Reuters. An author can find out how many times a paper was cited and in which journals. Nursing is challenged with strengthening citation of publications, thus also with strengthening IFs for nursing journals. The criteria remain debatable in the publishing world (Carpenter et al., 2014). Meeting with a medical librarian can assist in evaluation of a prospective journal, including the impact of its authors and its publications. Medical libraries, such as that found at Cornell University, have a wealth of resources on their websites to evaluate and better understand the IF (guides.library.cornell.edu/impact). There are also tools such as JANE (Journal Author Name Estimator; jane.biosemantics.org/) which pull from PubMed to identify journals for good fit based on input of the abstract or proposed subject, using an article influence calculation indicator measuring how often articles in the journal are cited after their first five years of publication.

■ AUTHORSHIP

Identifying authors and contribution for the manuscript is a critical step in developing a manuscript for publication. Authorship implies significant involvement in writing an article and in the work that led to that writing. The reality is that authorship is often given to (or insisted on by) people with minimal involvement in the writing project—perhaps a supervisor, a data collector, or a statistician. The International Committee of Medical Journal Editors (ICMJE, 2019) authorship guidelines recommend that authorship be based on the following four criteria: (a) substantial contributions to the conception or design of the work, or the acquisition, analysis, or interpretation of data for the work; (b) drafting the work or revising it critically for important intellectual content; (c) final approval of the version to be published; and (d) agreement to be accountable for all aspects of the work in ensuring that questions related to the accuracy or integrity of any part of the work are appropriately investigated and resolved (ICMJE, 2019). Brand and colleagues (2015) detail specific information about contribution, collaboration, and credit allocation that is helpful for determining authorship as well. Ascertaining steps in the project or research endeavor, along with steps in the dissemination process, and delineating responsibilities early on in the work will facilitate decision-making regarding dissemination.

In large, multi-site research projects, it is becoming common to list the research group as the author, with individuals mentioned in a footnote. When this is the case, all members of the group still must meet the stringent requirements for authorship. There is no specific rule for order of authorship (Bosch et al., 2012; Brand et al., 2015; Cleary et al., 2012; ICMJE, 2019), but authorship must be related to contribution to the work being published. Ideally, the order of authorship should be discussed before beginning the writing process, which helps to expedite the writing process overall and diminishes conflicts later in the writing process. The joint decision of the co-authors, after analysis of each author's contribution to the work, can further determine whether adjustments should be made. Order of authorship in nursing journals often indicates greatest to smallest contribution, paralleling first to last author. This order might be based on the amount of time given or on the importance of the contribution. In other journals, authorship may be alphabetically ordered, but alphabetical listing does not align with recommendations for appropriate attribution (Brand et al., 2015; ICMJE, 2019). An additional model includes the practice of listing the senior investigator as the last author. Most journals request identification of the corresponding author, which is typically the first author who has primary responsibility for managing all activities related to the publication, ensuring all parameters are met, guidelines followed, and timelines achieved. Although timing of authorship decisions is often begun with planning of the manuscript, the process can be changed through the point of submission, and should be changed if there is shifting contribution (Brand et al., 2015; ICMJE, 2016).

Acknowledge Appropriately

If not everyone who contributed to a research endeavor is entitled to authorship, then certainly each person who contributed substantially should be acknowledged (Bosch et al., 2012; Brand et al., 2015; Cleary et al., 2012; ICMJE, 2019). There is almost as much controversy about who is entitled to acknowledgment as there is to authorship entitlement. As a rule of thumb, acknowledgments are reserved for those who have made a substantial contribution to the project being reported in an article, including editorial and writing assistance (ICMJE, 2016, 2019). Those who might be acknowledged are data collectors, a project director, an editorial assistant, or a faculty advisor. The primary author must also ensure that acknowledgments are acceptable to those who will be acknowledged, because not everyone wishes to be acknowledged publicly. Obtaining written permission ahead of manuscript submission from those named in an acknowledgment is best practice to ensure approval of the acknowledgment, and that the acknowledgment will be included in often widely disseminated materials.

■ CONSTRUCTING AND SUBMITTING THE MANUSCRIPT

Title

A well-written title is a product of both science and art, as well as patience. Crafting the perfect title starts with a working title and ends with finalizing at completion of the manuscript. A clearly written title will draw the searcher or reviewer into the work and stimulate interest, while a poorly written title will not. Recommendation for the appropriate number of words for a title is equivocal, with general guidelines recommending between 10 to 15 primary terms (i.e., American Psychological Association [APA] guidelines), relevant concepts and variables of interest, and terms related to design and sample (Alexandrov & Hennerici, 2007; Langford & Pearce, 2019). Research is indeterminant regarding influence of sub-titles, semi-colons, dashes, but these can be easily used if appropriate for the work being published.

Formatting and Abstract Development

Every journal will provide parameters for formatting citations and the reference list, as well as for general writing of the article. In nursing, citations and the manuscript body typically, but not always, follow the APA format. However, even when the format is clearly a published format such as APA, each journal will have specific and often nuanced items the journal requires that are different than published formats like APA. The specific guidance regarding journal expectations for format and structure is typically located in author guidelines included on the journal website or located in a print journal issue.

The abstract is one of the most important aspects of the manuscript because it is one of the related items seen in electronic searches, and provides the information a searcher will use to make a decision regarding locating and reading the related article (Alexandrov & Hennerici, 2007; Pearce & Ferguson, 2017; Pierson, 2016). An abstract is required with submission of any manuscript. Since the recommendation to use a standardized reporting structure for scientific abstracts in the 1940s, many journals use some variation of the IMRAD (Introduction, Methods, Results, Discussion) format for abstracts and publications (Nakayama et al., 2005; Sollaci & Pereira, 2004). Components of IMRAD are detailed in Exhibit 21.4. The introduction includes a brief background of the topic and the study purpose(s). Methods comprise the design, setting, sample description, intervention, measurement tools, and outcome measures. Results include the primary findings. Finally, the discussion is the section in which conclusions and implications for practice and research are presented.

Specific journal format for the abstract should be detailed in the author guidelines for the particular journal, and can require a word count of approximately 100 to 750 words that provides key

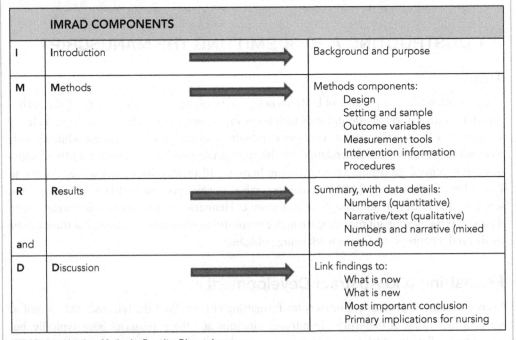

EXHIBIT 21.4

INTRODUCTION, METHODS, RESULTS, DISCUSSION COMPONENTS AND INCLUSION INFORMATION

IMRAD COMPONENTS		
I	Introduction	Background and purpose
M	Methods	Methods components: Design Setting and sample Outcome variables Measurement tools Intervention information Procedures
R and	Results	Summary, with data details: Numbers (quantitative) Narrative/text (qualitative) Numbers and narrative (mixed method)
D	Discussion	Link findings to: What is now What is new Most important conclusion Primary implications for nursing

IMRAD, Introduction, Methods, Results, Discussion.

information about the work being reported, and serves to invite the reader to read the manuscript (Alexandrov & Hennerici, 2007; Pearce & Ferguson, 2017). Abstract format can range from an unstructured paragraph to a structured paragraph, but to ensure all information is placed properly, using the headers found in a structured abstract is helpful, with removal of those headers if the journal requires an unstructured abstract (Alexandrov & Hennerici, 2007; Pearce & Ferguson, 2017). The abstract is an exceedingly important aspect of publication because it is often the first thing a reader will assess, and will serve as the basis for the reader's decision to further pursue information housed in the article; a poorly written abstract does not invite the reader to pursue more information on the topic, and ends up being rejected by a reader (Alexandrov & Hennerici, 2007; Pearce & Ferguson, 2017; Pierson, 2016).

Moving beyond the abstract into the manuscript, a more exact process to standardize reports of scholarly endeavors is the format Consolidated Standards of Reporting Trials (CONSORT), which was developed to decrease inadequate reporting of randomized controlled trials (RCTs) and develop consistency among articles to improve evidence-based practice (Altman et al., 2012; Moher et al., 2012). The CONSORT statement is used to report the minimum set of recommendations for reporting clinical trials. This standardization of publication allows facilitation of complete and transparent reporting with critical appraisal and interpretation. A checklist and diagram are provided to assist the authors to organize the text of the manuscript. Although the CONSORT statement is used for clinical trials, use of the CONSORT format has been integrated for other than clinical trials, simply because of the user-friendliness and practical orientation of the graphical modeling for authors and readers. Journal editors are critically aware of the need to have a data-driven practice base and are eagerly seeking research-based information or clinically relevant projects that hold the potential for transforming nursing practice. Editors are receptive to working with authors to ensure the best and most relevant product possible.

Query Letters

Editors are professionals and experts in writing for publication. Editors know the types of manuscripts they would like to obtain for publication. A query letter must include details about the research that will be reported, and plans for publication, such as timing (Table 21.1). The editor will consider the material provided and might suggest alternate plans to increase the chance of

TABLE 21.1 Components of a Query Letter

COMPONENT	RATIONALE AND INSTRUCTION

Letterhead	• Use professional letterhead—formal from institution or create a letter head with contact information.
	• Streamline to relevant information, with no additional pictures, graphics, or other decoration.
	• Include:
	  • Name, credentials
	  • Street address
	  • City, state ZIP
	  • Contract phone, email

(continued)

TABLE 21.1 Components of a Query Letter (*continued*)

COMPONENT	RATIONALE AND INSTRUCTION
Date	• If formal letter is being used, include date. • If email, the date will be obvious in email.
Dear Formal Editor Name Journal Name	• Include salutation with name. Helpful information, whether formal letter or email, because it makes it clear you are writing to the editor and not the editorial staff. Editorial staff might be the receiving individual, so is really helpful to address to the editor.
Body of the Letter Example of the Body of a Letter: I wish to submit a manuscript to *journal name*. I will be reporting research that included examination of processes of change used in smoking cessation by 190 smokers and former smokers selected through random-digit dialing. An 84% response rate was demonstrated with mailed cross-sectional survey. Multivariate analysis of variance of ten processes of change across five stages of smoking cessation (precontemplation, contemplation, relapse, recent, and long-term quitting) was significant, $F (40,590)$ = 5.02, p = .0001. Post hoc analysis revealed statistically significant differences on seven of the ten processes of change ($p < .05$). The information will be applicable by the readers of *journal name here* to help clients complete smoking cessation. (Optional to add content outline here if above paragraph is not self-explanatory as to approach.) The manuscript will be ready for submission within 6 weeks of receiving your positive reply. I look forward to hearing from you.	• Intent must be stipulated (to submit manuscript for consideration for publication). • Topic, processes, and outcomes should be identified—use salient information, writing precisely, and providing sufficient information such that the editor is intrigued to know more. Do not report entire study completed. • Interest for reader should be stated. • Outcomes application is useful to include.
Optional brief paragraph here indicating qualifications (self and/or team) for writing on a topic if that is not obvious in ending signature information.	• Clear linkage regarding author (and/or team) indicating qualifications for writing on the topic is particularly useful for the editor.
The manuscript will be ready for submission within *[time estimate]* of receiving your positive reply.	• It is useful to provide a generic, estimated timeline for completion of the manuscript, making sure the timeline is not overly zealous, but within reason for authors (team) to complete the writing. The editor might suggest an alternate time frame. For example, if the editor is preparing a special edition that happens to be on the topic of the research, an invitation to submit for consideration for a special issue might be made.
Sincerely,	• A closing term is in good form for professional correspondence.
Corresponding author	• Inclusion of the corresponding author (typically the primary, lead author, is critical to include, so the editor and staff have full information for contact.

acceptance. However, the editor might also indicate a lack of interest in the manuscript. Often the rationale for indicating lack of interest is provided, but not always. Frequent reasons include similarity to already published or soon-to-be published material in the journal, mismatch with readership interest, or other issues. Regardless of the information provided in response, the substance can be helpful in moving to the next step—the information provided should expedite move to submission or change to another journal.

Implications for Practice

Often a manuscript is rejected for publication because the author does not discuss the implications of the findings for the journal's readership. In the case of nursing focused work, the term *nurse* or variation should be apparent in the work. As the topic expert, readers expect a discussion of the utility of findings to practice, typically addressing one or more areas of practice, education, advocacy, research, administration, or leadership. The length of the implications section will vary depending on the journal's purpose as well as the information and emphasis provided in the manuscript. The implications section in a research journal is often short compared to a clinical journal's focus on application. When discussing implications for the study, findings are presented in relation to similar studies. Highlighting how findings support and differ from those of others of similar studies have been reported. If no similar work has been reported, note that lack of information. Finally, suggesting directions for next steps, future investigations, and projections of additional questions are expected.

Conforming to the Submission Requirements

All journals have requirements for formatting and submitting manuscripts. Although these requirements are not always printed in the journal issues, they can usually be found on the journal's website. Journal editors have a bias toward manuscripts that are formatted as precisely as possible to the journal guidelines. An incorrectly formatted manuscript can be a minor "red flag" to an extreme of being considered a fatal flaw, with rejection outright (Kennedy, 2018). Often, editors assume that if the author of an article was serious about publication in the journal, the author would have made an effort to send the document properly formatted to meet journal guidelines. A lingering thought in the editor's mind might be, "If the author did not pay attention to simple formatting requirements, what attention has been paid to ensure the integrity of the research and the manuscript?" as well as "How difficult will be to work with the author(s) if the author(s) cannot seem to follow basic instructions?"

Developing Manuscript References

References should be formatted in whatever format is delineated by the specific journal. References should be as current as possible but can also include older, more dated references if those are relevant, gold standard, or seminal sources, sources of reference for methods, or, in the case of replicating a study, the original study cited appropriately. References should also be highly relevant to the topic of the work, reflecting a solid background for the work being published. Specific guidelines for a journal should be included in the author guidelines. Using current references conveys to the editor and readers that the information included in the manuscript positions the work in appropriate and contemporary context and will contribute to development of knowledge.

Modeling Appropriate Tables and Figures

Graphical displays, including tables and figures, are highly useful in most publications, if they are well designed. *Infographics* is an umbrella term to represent graphical displays, with special attention to heightening usability of information (Nicol & Pexman, 2010). Graphical displays convey a level of sophistication editors embrace and readers are drawn to. Well-designed graphical displays help to organize even complex information succinctly, and to convey complex concepts and processes in a user-friendly manner for readers. Florence Nightingale created a legacy in nursing that involved a substantial amount of evidence, epidemiologic principles, and creative and talented use of graphical displays, detailed by hand and without computer generation. Highlights from Nightingale's work specifically with data and graphical display of data are reported in Thompson (2016).

Considering which concepts lend themselves to data display is critical in the process of generating a manuscript. Attending to journal guidelines for the number of graphical displays allowed, as well as formatting requirements, is also important. Titling, describing, and placing graphical displays depends heavily on journal guidelines. While generating the manuscript, placing a graphic in the body of the manuscript, as being written, is acceptable; when completing submission, author guidelines for the journal will provide guidance for submission. When discussing table or graph information in text, do not restate every piece of information. Highlight one or two key points and refer the reader to the table or graph. Highly useful guidelines such as Nicol and Pexman (2010) for graphical display will aid best use. Examples of tables and figures can be found in almost every published article and every research textbook and mostly are useful as models to emulate, as they have been through peer review.

Tables are graphical displays that include rows and columns of information; figures are generally more pictorial. A table is used for presentation of variables and related results. A figure is generally a more pictorial display, such as a Venn diagram, flow, timeline, or process diagram. Tables and figures are especially useful for conveying a large amount of information in a concise manner that help readers to grasp the information quickly and effectively. Tables and figures are highly recommended for use in effective writing (Alexandrov & Hennerici, 2007; Oermann & Hays, 2018; Pearce & Ferguson, 2017; Tornquist, 1999) and detailed instructions are included in publication guideline manuals (e.g., American Medical Association [AMA], 2007; APA, 2009) and textbooks (e.g., Polit & Beck, 2017). Graphical displays can be used to depict theoretical foundation, process, timelines, and a wide variety of other items in writing. Examples from a training manual (Figure 21.2), from generation within Microsoft Word (Figure 21.3), of a grant proposal timeline (Figure 21.4), and of a Venn diagram demonstrating integrated components (Figure 21.5) are demonstrated.

Timelines are especially useful if reporting processes, or with need to demonstrate time investment. An example of a timeline projection used in a successful grant proposal (Pearce & Reel, 2019, unpublished data) for Spanish translation for a questionnaire is shown in Figure 21.4.

Although graphical displays are used throughout publications, with research studies, tables and figures are most consistently seen with reporting results. Results can always be summarized in the narrative of a manuscript, but integration of tables and figures helps to convey sufficient detail that the reader is well informed regarding the information being reported. Writing results is a challenging activity that requires author precision and creativity, as well as thoughtfulness in considering the reader. Tables and figures are generally required for presenting anything more than a single item result. Clear, concise, precise, and well-organized information will help to walk the reader through the information, and make the results readily visible and available.

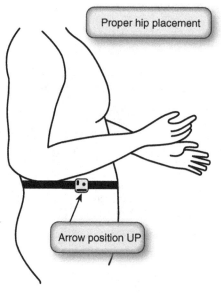

FIGURE 21.2 Graphical example from appropriate hip placement for Actical® motion monitor.
Source: Training Manual, Pearce & Reel, 2019, unpublished data.

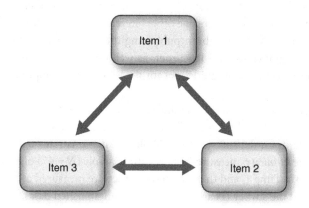

FIGURE 21.3 Three-item flow diagram.
Source: Generation in Microsoft Word Tools.

Approximately 4 months total time span.

| 20 hrs total/ over 4 weeks | 4 hrs total/ over 1 week | 20 hrs total/ over 4 weeks | 20 hrs total/ over 4 weeks | 60 hrs total/over 6 weeks Programming and Evaluation |

| Develop: Activity list, METs Categories | Verification | Translation → Spanish | Back translation → English Verification | Programming Verification | Evaluation Algorithm reliability Readability |

FIGURE 21.4 Example of a timeline.

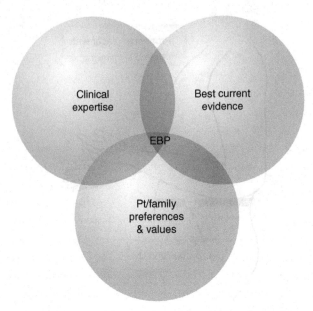

FIGURE 21.5 Venn diagram representing evidence-based practice cornerstones.

Every journal will provide instructions regarding the maximum number of tables and figures, as well as formatting, for any manuscript submitted. Investing time and effort in designing well-crafted tables and figures will help to engage others in reading the manuscript, including editors and reviewers, who make decisions about publishing the manuscript. Assuring that statistical tests, precise results, significance and level met, as well as any other relevant information are presented clearly, and meet relevant guidelines for the journal, will support chance of successful publication.

Complexity of tables and figures will parallel the complexity of the study being reported. The following examples are gathered from small studies with relatively straightforward information and provide helpful hints for data presentation. Table 21.2 demonstrates self-reported data for the demographic variable *Ethnicity*, measured twice, with a sample ($N = 47$) of middle school adolescents in a sport camp at Time 1, and then again when they are measured at Time 2, when only 31 adolescents completed the survey (Pearce & Reel, 2019, unpublished data). Note the information follows recommendation of highest to lowest frequency count for Time 1, and subsequent change for Time 2, as well as alignment of the digits, per recommendations (AMA, 2007; APA, 2009; Nicol & Pexman, 2010). There is no specific rule for presentation order (e.g., highest to lowest counts, or lowest to highest, alphabetical), but the consistent recommendation is to present in a logical fashion to heighten understanding by the reader. A traditional highest to lowest, or lowest to highest pattern is a common pattern among researchers reporting numeric data. Also note that the numbers included in Table 21.3 reflect a total of 100%; ensuring that the numbers are precise, reflect the actual data from the research, and are presented in a clean, clear, and precise manner are exceedingly important in writing. If numbers do not logically sum to 100% of reporting material, a notation of rationale should be provided (see APA manual). The statistical calculation (e.g., mean, *t*-test) and the significance level used ($p = .05$) must be indicated clearly in the table. Labeling the table can be done clearly using the content of the columns and rows, such as variable name (e.g., Ethnicity) and points of measurement (Time 1 and Time 2).

TABLE 21.2 Participant Ethnicity by Time 1 and Time 2

ETHNICITY	TIME1		TIME 2	
	N (%)			
Hispanic	30	(.638)	23	(.742)
Caucasian	3	(.064)	1	(.032)
African American	3	(.064)	3	(.097)
American Indian	2	(.043)	1	(.032)
Asian	1	(.021)	1	(.032)
Pacific Islander	1	(.021)	1	(.032)
"I'm not sure"	7	(.149)	1	(.032)
Total	47	(1.00)	31	(1.00)

TABLE 21.3 Mean Activities, Minutes, and Metabolic Equivalents (MET) Minutes by Time 1 and Time 2 Measurement

ITEM	TIME 1	TIME 2	t-TEST
Reported Number Activities	5.38	5.27	$t = 0.29$
Minutes in Activity	240	263	$t = .129$
Calculated MET minutes	954	958	$t = .3$
No significant differences Time 1 and Time 2 ($p > .05$)			

■ THE ETHICS OF DISSEMINATION

Adhere to Copyright Laws

Once a manuscript is accepted for publication, authors are required by the publisher to sign an agreement that either transfers copyright of the author's material to the publisher or delineates exact procedures for handling the copyrighted material if the copyright is not officially transferred. Copyright and intellectual property laws are complex and challenging to understand, but authors must understand the agreements being signed for copyright (Adeney, 2015; Anfray et al., 2012; Carroll, 2015; Dames, 2012; Murphy et al., 2015). The author must work within the parameters of details explicated in the copyright document. Author(s) have responsibility to know the agreed upon copyright parameters. Violation of copyright is a serious legal issue. When in doubt about using copyrighted work, call and/or write the copyright holder (Adeney, 2015; Anfray et al., 2012; Carroll, 2015; Dames, 2012; Murphy et al., 2015).

Conform to Ethical Practices

Adhering to ethical practices when publishing is vital; unethical practices can ruin chances for future publication. Two easily avoided unethical practices are submitting the same manuscript to different journals at the same time and plagiarism.

It is considered unethical to submit a manuscript to more than one journal at the same time. Every journal's *Information for Authors* guidelines has a statement to the effect that the author warrants that he or she is submitting original, unpublished material, under consideration by no other publisher. So, although it is acceptable to query as many editors as desired about interest in your manuscript, it can only be submitted to one journal at a time. If a manuscript is rejected, it is then permissible to submit to another journal.

Plagiarism is defined as claiming someone's ideas and work, published or unpublished, as your own (American Psychological Association, 2009). The four common types of plagiarism are (a) verbatim lifting of passages, (b) rewording ideas from an original source as an author's own, (c) paraphrasing an original work without attribution, and (d) noting the original source of only some of what is borrowed (AMA, 2007; APA , 2009). Authors must be acutely aware of their own writing, with attention to appropriate attribution to the original source for any point at which the writing reflects the ideas of others. Integrating a significant amount of material (copyright law does not define "significant") through paraphrasing or direct quotation, requires formal correspondence with the copyright holder, which is usually the publishing company, to obtain written permission. Likewise, any published item, no matter how large or small that is complete unto itself, such as a table, figure, chart, graph, art work, poem, or picture, requires permission from the copyright holder to reproduce the item.

There is a variety of plagiarism detection programs available for use in considering originality of the manuscript. Examples include: TurnItIn (www.turnitin.com), iThenticate (www.ithenticate.com), Plagiarism Checker by Grammarly (www.grammarly.com/plagiarism-checker), and QueText (www.quetext.com). Plagiarism detection software is used by editors in the publication processes. It is a helpful step for authors to utilize the plagiarism detector prior to submitting for publication. This step provides an opportunity to remedy any problems with plagiarism that might have inadvertently occurred in the writing process. Further discussion of the intricacies of copyright in order to avoid plagiarism or copyright law violation, can be found in publications and information sponsored by www.copyright.gov.

Many are surprised to find out that it is possible to plagiarize their own work ("self-plagiarism"). Roig (2015) published a guide to avoiding plagiarism which defines self-plagiarism as: "several distinct practices in which some or all elements of a previous publication (e.g., text, data, and images) are reused in a new publication with ambiguous acknowledgement or no acknowledgement at all as to their prior dissemination" (p. 16). Many journals now require disclosure before a submission is accepted of any prior publications that include similar data or concepts, in addition to a prohibition of duplicate submission or publication.

Managing Rejection and Planning for New Submission

If a manuscript is not accepted for publication know there is another journal that will provide an appropriate space for publication. Many published authors have had their works rejected for publication. The art of writing requires practice and study. Receiving feedback about a manuscript's strengths and weaknesses from reviewers and editors helps authors focus on developing the manuscript further, and in the process honing publication skills. There is a great deal of feedback for improvement that arises out of a rejection process. If a manuscript is rejected, there are options for follow through. One involves an email to the editor personally, clarifying any instructions regarding whether to revise and resubmit. A good editor will be honest about the quality of a manuscript and may recommend other journals that may be more appropriate for the work.

The second option is to revise and submit the manuscript to another journal. This process requires backstepping to revise the manuscript according to the newly selected journal's readership, guidelines, and focus. Many excellent manuscripts are needlessly rejected because the author did not target content for a journal's readership or conform to its style. Re-evaluation and engagement in the revision process can be exhilarating and positive. The helpful hints and tools discussed in this chapter can be used to re-evaluate and re-engage in the appropriately fitting topic, method, or findings to the new journal.

Other opportunities might be to also ask respected peers to complete an evaluative read before resubmission. Presentation of work in a poster or podium presentation can provide an additional source of feedback before revision and resubmission.

■ SUMMARY

Scholarly work, whether related to academic program activities such as a master's thesis, DNP scholarly project, PhD dissertation, or work beyond academic programming, contributes positively to the healthcare delivery system. As more nurses are prepared with expanded expertise through graduate levels of education and analytics, the impact of nursing practice and outcomes are being disseminated in clinical, administrative, and education settings. Nurses who conduct scientific investigations have a professional obligation to share their findings, thus providing the foundation for the profession's growth and maturation. Although the focus of this chapter has been on dissemination through publications, it is important for nurses to consider the many opportunities to share their findings with those inside and outside of the profession. Too often it is observed that the public does not always understand what nurses do and how they impact healthcare. Efforts in demonstrating the work of nurses via publication can change practice, encourage peers, and help demonstrate to the public the importance of nursing in the promotion of optimal health and well-being.

SUGGESTED LEARNING ACTIVITIES

Identify a topic of interest through the development of a question of inquiry and a brief literature review. Test your question with a few trusted peers. Then follow the steps below to perform and build a plan for your topic development.

The OWL (Online Writing Lab) at Purdue (owl.purdue.edu/owl/purdue_owl.html) is an excellent site at which to hone your writing and research skills.

1. Go to owl.purdue.edu/owl/subject_specific_writing/professional_technical_writing/audience_analysis/index.html and complete an "Audience Analysis."

2. Go to owl.purdue.edu/owl/general_writing/the_writing_process/writers_block/more_writers_block_strategies.html and identify your blocks to writing and try two of the suggested intervention strategies.

3. Go to owl.purdue.edu/owl/research_and_citation/conducting_research/evaluating_
    sources_of_information/index.html and evaluate the value of the next three sources of
    information you plan to use in your research.

REFERENCES

Adeney, E. (2015). Medical and scientific authorship: A conflict between discipline rules and the law. *Journal of Law and Medicine, 23*(2), 413–426. https://doi.org/10.2139/ssrn.2853171

Albert, K. M. (2006). Open access: Implications for scholarly publishing and medical libraries. *Journal of the Medical Library Association, 94*(3), 253–262.

Alexandrov, A. V., & Hennerici, M. G. (2007). Writing good abstracts. *Cerebrovascular Diseases, 23*(4), 256–259. https://doi.org/10.1159/000098324

Altman, D. G., Moher, D., & Schulz, K. F. (2012). Improving the reporting of randomised trials: the CONSORT Statement and beyond. *Statistics in Medicine, 31*(25), 2985–2997. https://doi.org/10.1002/sim.5402

American Medical Association. (2007). *AMA manual of style* (10th ed.). University Press.

American Psychological Association. (2009). *Publication manual of the American Psychological Association* (6th ed.). Author.

Anfray, C., Emery, M. P., Conway, K., & Acquadro, C. (2012). Questions of copyright. *Health and Quality of Life Outcomes, 10*, 16. https://doi.org/10.1186/1477-7525-10-16

Baker, J. D. (2012). The quid pro quo of peer review. *AORN Journal, 96*(4), 356–360. https://doi.org/10.1016/j.aorn.2012.08.013

Baker, E. F., Iserson, K. V., Aswegan, A. L., Larkin, G. L., Derse, A. R., & Kraus, C. K. (2019). Open access medical journals: Promise, perils, and pitfalls. *Academic Medicine, 94*(5), 634–639. https://doi.org/10.1097/ACM.0000000000002563

Beall, J. (2012). Predatory publishers are corrupting open access. *Nature, 489*(7415), 179. https://doi.org/10.1038/489179a

Beall, J. (2016). Essential information about predatory publishers and journals. *International Higher Education, 86*, 2–3. https://doi.org/10.6017/ihe.2016.86.9358

Bosch, X., Pericas, J. M., Hernandez, C., & Torrents, A. (2012). A comparison of authorship policies at top-ranked peer-reviewed biomedical journals. *Archives of Internal Medicine, 172*(1), 70–72. https://doi.org/10.1001/archinternmed.2011.600

Brand, A., Allen, L., Altman, M., Hlava, M., & Scott, J. (2015). Beyond authorship: Attribution, contribution, collaboration, and credit. *Learned Publishing, 28*, 151–155. https://doi.org/10.1087/20150211

Broga, M., Mijaljica, G., Waligora, M., Keis, A., & Marusic, A. (2014). Publication ethics in biomedical journals from countries in Central and Eastern Europe. *Science and Engineering Ethics, 20*(1), 99–109. https://doi.org/10.1007/s11948-013-9431-x

Broome, M. E., Riner, M. E., & Allam, E. S. (2013). Scholarly publication practices of Doctor of Nursing Practice-prepared nurses. *Journal of Nursing Education, 52*(8), 429–434. https://doi.org/10.3928/01484834-20130718-02

Carpenter, C. R., Cone, D. C., & Sarli, C. C. (2014). Using publication metrics to highlight academic productivity and research impact. *Academic Emergency Medicine, 21*(10), 1160–1172. https://doi.org/10.1111/acem.12482

Carroll, M. W. (2015). Sharing research data and intellectual property law: A primer. *PLoS Biology, 13*(8), e1002235. https://doi.org/10.1371/journal.pbio.1002235

Cleary, M., Jackson, D., Walter, G., Watson, R., & Hunt, G. E. (2012). Editorial: Location, location, location—the position of authors in scholarly publishing. *Journal of Clinical Nursing, 21*(5–6), 809–811. https://doi.org/10.1111/j.1365-2702.2011.04062.x

Cobey, K. D., Grudniewicz, A., Lalu, M. M., Rice, D. B., Raffoul, H., & Moher, D. (2019). Knowledge and motivations of researchers publishing in presumed predatory journals: A survey. *BMJ Open, 9*(3), e026516. https://doi.org/10.1136/bmjopen-2018-026516

Dames, K. (2012). The coming copyright clash in higher education. *Information Today, 297*(7), 24–25.

Dougherty, M. C. (2006). The value of peer review. *Nursing Research, 55*(2), 73–74. https://doi.org/10.1097/00006199-200603000-00001

Edie, A. H., & Conklin, J. L. (2019). Avoiding predatory journals: Quick peer review processes too good to be true. *Nursing Forum, 54*(3), 336–339. https://doi.org/10.1111/nuf.12333

Happell, B. (2005). Disseminating nursing knowledge—A guide to writing for publication. *International Journal of Psychiatric Nursing Research, 10*(3), 1147–1155.

Happell, B. (2012). Writing and publishing clinical articles: A practical guide. *Emergency Nurse, 20*(1), 33–37. https://doi.org/10.7748/en2012.04.20.1.33.c9042

Heselden, M., Malliarakis, K. D., Lunsford, B., Linton, A., Sullo, E., Cardenas, D., Ingram, C., Smith, L., & Austin, J. (2019). Establishing an open access repository for doctor of nursing practice projects. *Journal of Professional Nursing, 35*(6), 467–472. https://doi.org/10.1016/j.profnurs.2019.06.001

Hodge, V., Jessop, M., Fletcher, M., Weeks, M., Turner, A., Jackson, T., Ingram, C., Smith, L., & Austin, J. (2016). A digital repository and execution platform for interactive scholarly publications in neuroscience. *Neuroinformatics, 14*(1), 23–40. https://doi.org/10.1007/s12021-015-9276-3

Hua, F., Shen, C., Walsh, T., Glenny, A. M., & Worthington, H. (2017). Open Access: Concepts, findings, and recommendations for stakeholders in dentistry. *Journal of Dentistry, 64*, 13–22. https://doi.org/10.1016/j.jdent.2017.06.012

INANE Predatory Publishing Practices Collaborative. (2014). Predatory publishing. *Journal of Midwfery & Women's Health, 59*(6), 569–571. https://doi.org/10.1111/jmwh.12273

International Academy of Nursing Editors Predatory Publishing Practices Collaborative. (2015). Predatory publishers: What the nursing community needs to know. *Journal of Perianesthesia Nursing, 30*(2), 87–90. https://doi.org/10.1016/j.jopan.2015.02.002

International Committee of Medical Journal Editors. (2016). *Defining the role of authors and contributors* (pp. 1–3). Author.

International Committee of Medical Journal Editors. (2019). *Recommendations for the conduct, reporting, editing, and publication of scholarly work in medical journals* (pp. 1–19). Author.

Kearney, M. H., & INANE Predatory Publishing Practices Collaborative. (2015). Predatory publishing: What authors need to know. *Research in Nursing and Health, 38*(1), 1–3. https://doi.org/10.1002/nur.21640

Kennedy, M. S. (2018). Journal publishing: A review of the basics. *Seminars in Oncology Nursing, 34*(4), 361–371. https://doi.org/10.1016/j.soncn.2018.09.004

Langford, C. A., & Pearce, P. F. (2019). Increasing visibility for your work: The importance of a well-written title. *Journal of the American Association of Nurse Practitioners, 31*(4), 217–218. https://doi.org/10.1097/JXX.0000000000000212

Marusic, A. (2018). The role of the peer review process. In F. O. Wells & M. J. G. Farthing (Eds.), *Fraud and misconduct in biomedical research (e-book version)* (4th ed., pp. 135–160). CRC Press.

Marusic, A., Rudan, I., & Campbell, H. (2019). Declarations of conflicts of interest from the editors of the *Journal of Global Health* - 2019. *Journal of Global Health, 9*(1), 010102. https://doi.org/10.7189/jogh.09.010102

Memon, A. R. (2019). Revisiting the term predatory open access publishing. *Journal of Korean Medical Science, 34*(13), e99. https://doi.org/10.3346/jkms.2019.34.e99

Mercier, E., Tardif, P. A., Moore, L., Le Sage, N., & Cameron, P. A. (2018). Invitations received from potential predatory publishers and fraudulent conferences: A 12-month early-career researcher experience. *Postgraduate Medical Journal, 94*(1108), 104–108. https://doi.org/10.1136/postgradmedj-2017-135097

Moher, D., Hopewell, S., Schulz, K. F., Montori, V., Gotzsche, P. C., Devereaux, P. J., Elbourne, D., & Egger, M. (2012). CONSORT 2010 explanation and elaboration: Updated guidelines for reporting parallel group randomised trials. *International Journal of Surgery (London, England), 10*(1), 28–55. https://doi.org/10.1016/j.ijsu.2011.10.001

Murphy, A., Stramiello, M., Lewis, S., & Irving, T. (2015). Introduction to intellectual property: A U.S. perspective. *Cold Spring Harbor Perspectives in Medicine, 5*(8), a020776. https://doi.org/10.1101/cshperspect.a020776

Nakayama, T., Hirai, N., Yamazaki, S., & Naito, M. (2005). Adoption of structured abstracts by general medical journals and format for a structured abstract. *Journal of the Medical Library Association, 93*(2), 237–242.

Nicol, A. A. M., & Pexman, P. M. (2010). *Displaying your findings: A practical guide for creating figures, posters, and presentations* (6th ed.). American Psychological Association.

Oermann, M. H. (2018). Writing publishable review, research, quality improvement, and evidence-based practice manuscripts. *Nursing Economics, 36*(6), 268–275.

Oermann, M. H., Conklin, J. L., Nicoll, L. H., Chinn, P. L., Ashton, K. S., Edie, A. H., Amarasekara, S., & Budinger, S. C. (2016). Study of predatory open access nursing journals. *Journal of Nursing Scholarship, 48*(6), 624–632. https://doi.org/10.1111/jnu.12248

Oermann, M. H., & Hays, J. C. (2018). *Writing for publication in nursing* (4th ed., pp. 1–357). Springer Publishing Company.

Oermann, M. H., Nicoll, L. H., Carter-Templeton, H., Woodward, A., Kidayi, P. L., Neal, L. B., Edie, A. H., Ashton, K. S., Chinn, P. L., & Amarasekara, S. (2019). Citations of articles in predatory nursing journals. *Nursing Outlook, 67*(6), 664–670. https://doi.org/10.1016/j.outlook.2019.05.001

Oermann, M. H., Nicoll, L. H., Chinn, P. L., Ashton, K. S., Conklin, J. L., Edie, A. H., Amarasekara, S., & Williams, B. L. (2018). Quality of articles published in predatory nursing journals. *Nursing Outlook, 66*(1), 4–10. https://doi.org/10.1016/j.outlook.2017.05.005

Owens, J. K., & Nicoll, L. H. (2019). Plagiarism in predatory publications: A comparative study of three nursing journals. *Journal of Nursing Scholarship, 51*(3), 356–363. https://doi.org/10.1111/jnu.12475

Pearce, P. F., & Ferguson, L. A. (2017). How to write abstracts for manuscripts, presentations, and grants: Maximizing information in a 30-s sound bite world. *Journal of the American Association of Nurse Practitioners, 29*(8), 452–460. https://doi.org/10.1002/2327-6924.12486

Pierson, C. A. (2016). Structured abstracts improve clarity and reach your intended audience. *Journal of the American Association of Nurse Practitioners, 28*(7), 346. https://doi.org/10.1002/2327-6924.12392

Polit, D. F., & Beck, C. T. (2017). *Nursing research: Generating and assessing evidence for nursing practice* (10th ed.). Wolters Kluwer Health.

Price, B. (2010). Disseminating best practice through publication in journals. *Nursing Standard, 24*(26), 35–41. https://doi.org/10.7748/ns2010.03.24.26.35.c7568

Roig, M. (2015). *Avoiding plagarism, self-plagarism, and other questionable writing practices: A guide to ethical writing.* https://ori.hhs.gov/sites/default/files/plagiarism.pdf

Sollaci, L. B., & Pereira, M. G. (2004). The introduction, methods, results, and discussion (IMRAD) structure: A fifty-year survey. *Journal of the Medical Library Association, 92*, 364–372.

Strinzel, M., Severin, A., Milzow, K., & Egger, M. (2019). Blacklists and whitelists to tackle predatory publishing: A cross-sectional comparison and thematic analysis. *MBio, 10*(3), e00411–e00419. https://doi.org/10.1128/mBio.00411-19

Thompson, C. (2016). How data won the west. *Smithsonian Magazine,* pp. 23–27.

Tornquist, E. M. (1999). *From proposal to publication: An informal guide to writing about nursing research* (pp. 1–215). Addison-Wesley.

Vervaart, P. (2014). Ethics in online publications. *Electronic Journal of the International Federation of Clinical Chemistry and Laboratory Medicine, 25*(3), 244–251.

Wahyudi, R. (2017). The generic structure of the call for papers of predatory journals: A social semiotic perspective. In P. Mickan & E. Lopez (Eds.), *Text-based research and teaching* (pp. 117–136). Palgrace Macmillan.

Wood, B. D., & Ludwig, R. L. (2012). The difference between peer review and nonpeer review. *Radiologic Technology, 84*(1), 90–92.

Yancey, N. R. (2016). The challenge of writing for publication: Implications for teaching-learning nursing. *Nursing Science Quarterly, 29*(4), 277–282. https://doi.org/10.1177/0894318416662931

EXEMPLARS OF APRN-LED INITIATIVES

BETH A. STAFFILENO, MARCIA PENCAK MURPHY, LINDSEY GRADONE, IZABELA KAZANA, CLAIRE CUNNINGHAM, AND JESSICA MAULEON

■ INTRODUCTION

The pervasive problems of the nation's healthcare system call for increasing numbers of advanced practice registered nurses (APRNs) prepared as highly proficient, competent providers and equipped with evidence-based knowledge and skills to improve the health of the population (Trautman et al., 2018). APRNs are prepared to improve the health and outcomes of patient populations and/or delivery systems. APRNs improve outcomes through systems leadership, quality improvement processes and by translating evidence into practice settings and are well situated to identify clinical problems that require collaborative partnerships and problem-solving skills, using evidence-based resources to improve outcomes and transform systems of care.

The American Association of Colleges of Nursing (AACN) Task Force Report (2015) on the Implementation of the Doctor of Nursing Practice (DNP) defined scholarship as "the mechanism that provides knowledge development within a discipline" and highlighted that nurses with a practice-focused doctorate "are prepared to generate new knowledge through practice innovation" (p. 2). APRNs are prepared to contribute to the scholarly output in the discipline, particularly in the area of clinical practice. APRNs translate knowledge into practice by working with interdisciplinary teams, using translational research methods, and disseminating practice-focused scholarly products.

This chapter describes four APRN-led initiatives implemented across diverse settings including acute care, long-term care, assisted living, and home care. These exemplars highlight how APRNs serve as change agents to improve processes and healthcare outcomes. Key strategies to promote successful change are evident across these exemplars including identifying the problem with data, using evidence-based approaches, collaborating with key stakeholders, and identifying evidence-based methods that were feasible within the specific setting. Moreover, these exemplars show that using collaborative teams promote high value care and positive outcomes for the populations served.

■ EXEMPLAR 1: INTEGRATION OF EVIDENCE-BASED PRACTICE AT AN ACADEMIC MEDICAL CENTER

Background

Evidence-based practice (EBP) is a systematic problem-solving strategy that integrates high quality, current evidence in conjunction with clinicians' expertise and patients' preferences for determining patient care (Stannard, 2019). EBP improves the safety, efficiency, and quality of healthcare when used to direct clinical decision-making (Dols et al., 2019; Melnyk & Fineout-Overholt, 2019). Research has demonstrated EBP is better than care based on tradition (Melnyk & Fineout-Overholt, 2019). Melnyk and Fineout-Overholt (2019) reported implementation of EBP contributes to improved quality of care and patient outcomes as well as decreased costs.

Identifying the Problem

Although nurses value EBP, barriers to implementation remain and many nurses do not consistently use evidence in their daily practice (Jun et al., 2016; Melnyk et al., 2016, 2018). Individual barriers to using EBP include perceived lack of time, lack of EBP knowledge and skills, and lack of authority to change practice (McKinney et al., 2019). The most frequently cited and impactful organizational barriers are a lack of administrative and cultural support (e.g., resistance from colleagues, leadership, and other professions) as well as insufficient resources (Duncombe, 2017; Jun et al., 2016). Therefore, the purpose of this project was to increase registered nurses' (RNs) knowledge of EBP processes and organizational resources available to support practice changes.

Methods to Address the Problem

This project was conducted at a large, academic medical center in Chicago, Illinois. It used a pre-post design involving RNs on six adult inpatient units from the medical, surgical, and psychiatric service lines. The pre-survey was exploratory, designed to identify any gaps in RNs' understanding and use of EBP so that the intervention could be tailored to the desired outcome.

A 20-item survey was developed to assess RNs' understanding of how EBP is operationalized, the degree to which they use it in their daily practice, and their ability to make practice changes. The survey was developed based on validated surveys (Melnyk et al., 2008; Pravikoff et al., 2005), then expanded and tailored to the practices and resources at the project site. The survey was developed in collaboration with key stakeholders and found to have face validity by those stakeholders.

Surveys were formatted electronically. A link to the surveys was sent to RNs' work email addresses. Emails also described the purpose of the survey, indicating participation was voluntary and responses were confidential. A pre-survey was sent June 2016 and a post-survey was sent in July 2017. Returned survey data were compiled automatically then exported to Excel for analysis. Survey responses were anonymous as no unique identifiers were collected.

The pre-survey was sent to 308 RNs with 106 respondents (34.4%). Surveyed RNs reported lacking knowledge of how to change a clinical practice. Specifically, 57.4% ($n = 58$) did not know how to change clinical practice on their unit if it was not evidence based, and 53.5% ($n = 54$) did not know how to change an operational standard (policy, procedure, or care plan) if it no longer reflected the best evidence.

A flowchart was developed based on the pre-survey results to provide guidance to RNs on EBP processes and how to change a clinical practice if it is no longer evidence based. It directs RNs to first check institutional policies, procedures and protocols when they have a clinical question, but also to consult evidence-based resources to verify that they reflect current best practice before implementation. If the institutional resources are no longer evidence based, the flowchart directs RNs to the appropriate shared governance committees for changing practice. Supplementary EBP resources are also highlighted as a quick reference.

Additionally, the RNs received a 10-minute unit-based education session covering (a) the pre-survey findings, (b) a review of EBP concepts, and (c) an overview of the flowchart. Educational sessions were offered for 2 days on each unit at each day/night shift change to reach as many RNs as possible. Printed copies of the presentation and flowchart were displayed in prominent locations throughout the unit as visual reminders. The flowchart was also uploaded to the nursing intranet for long-term availability.

Evaluation

Descriptive statistics were used to assess demographic characteristics and categorical survey items. Percentage change was calculated to determine the impact of pre-post EBP unit-based education. Survey items with Likert scales were collapsed into dichotomous categories, then Chi-square analysis was used to compare changes before and after implementation. Items with Likert scales for agreement were collapsed into categories of either agreement (strongly agree and agree) or disagreement (strongly disagree and disagree). Five-point scales of frequency were collapsed into categories of minimal occurrence (never and rarely) and more frequent occurrence (sometimes, frequently, and always). Statistical significance was determined using a p-value <0.05 for these data.

Results

Most respondents were BSN-prepared and had more than 5 years of nursing experience. More than half of the RNs were from critical care units with fewer RNs reporting from general medical-surgical units or psychiatry. Some RNs did not respond to all questions. A significant ($p < 0.05$) increase was found in RNs' awareness of organizational resources for EBP projects at the project site. Although there was no significant change in RNs' self-reported knowledge of how to access online resources or ability to access resources in a time-efficient way, there was strong agreement at baseline as well as respective 2.2% and 8.8% increases in agreement on the post-survey. Similarly, there was a 6.9% increase in respondents' agreement concerning the need to stay up to date with nursing practice by reading research publications. A significant increase was found in RNs' self-reported confidence to change clinical practice on their units, as well as organizational policies and procedures if they were not evidence-based ($p < 0.001$).

Discussion

This project aimed to increase RNs' knowledge of EBP processes and organizational resources available to support practice changes. As reported in Gradone and Staffileno (2019) the most significant changes were in RNs' self-reported confidence to change clinical practice. This reflected the intended impact of the flowchart and unit-based education sessions, which were to direct RNs through the EBP process and the process of making a practice change if needed. This was consistent with research findings that suggested providing educational courses in a clinical setting can improve RNs' attitudes and perception of skills related to EBP (Connor et al., 2016; Sim et al., 2016).

This outcome also reflected the importance of organizational support as a facilitator of EBP, which is consistent with other reports in the literature (Lavenberg et al., 2019; Wu et al., 2018). Brockhopp et al. (2016) reported use of their model also highlighted the importance of contacting appropriate administrative groups with the ability to enact change. This is similar to the flowchart for this current project, which directs RNs to the proper shared governance committees with the power to make organizational changes at the medical center.

Conclusion

Results of this quality improvement project indicated a significant increase in RNs' self-reported confidence to make EBP changes on their units and at an organizational level. This was consistent with research findings that provision of educational courses in a clinical setting can improve RNs' attitudes and perception of skills related to EBP (Connor et al., 2016; Sim et al., 2016).

Recommendations for Clinical Practice

APRNs have the requisite knowledge and skills to integrate evidence-based changes into daily practice. Moreover, APRNs are in a key position to guide direct care RNs with responding to clinical questions using the best available evidence to improve patient outcomes.

Summary

This first exemplar highlights key components addressed in Chapter 5, Establishing and Sustaining an Evidence-Based Practice Environment. Essential to the success of this APRN-led project was key stakeholder buy-in, especially organizational support from nursing leadership. Importantly, this project provided unit-based education and access to resources for RNs.

▧ EXEMPLAR 2: ENGAGING LONG-TERM CARE RESIDENTS IN WALKING ACTIVITY: A QUALITY IMPROVEMENT PROJECT

Background

Physical activity is recommended for all Americans, including older adults and individuals with chronic conditions (Centers for Disease Control and Prevention, 2019; U.S. Department of Health and Human Services [DHHS], 2018). The health risks related to sedentary lifestyle and potential health benefits routine walking are well known (DHHS, 2018). International experts in geriatrics and physical therapy recommended "reducing sedentary behaviors for all Long-Term Care (LTC) residents" (de Souto Barreto et al., 2016).

Identifying the Problem

Physical inactivity in LTC facilities is prevalent as residents spend almost all of their time sitting or lying (den Ouden et al., 2015; Parry et al., 2019). There is a concern that wheelchair overuse in LTC may contribute to physical inactivity. While the majority of LTC residents have multiple chronic conditions (Moore et al., 2014), physical inactivity may further exacerbate declining health (Patterson et al., 2018), cognitive abilities (Ku et al., 2017; Tan et al., 2017), and bone mass (Rodriguez-Gómez et al., 2018). There are several studies and clinical guidelines suggesting that moderate levels of physical activity may have significant positive impacts on body systems, regardless of gender or age (Frändin et al., 2016; HHS, 2018; Schnelle et al., 2003; Soares-Miranda et al., 2016) and mortality reduction (Esteban-Cornejo et al., 2019; DHHS, 2018). One LTC inner-city facility had a *Walk-to-Dine* program, but it was offered to residents inconsistently. Therefore, the purpose of this project was to engage eligible LTC residents into participating in daily self-paced walking to promote physical activity.

Methods to Address the Problem

The Model for Improvement with its Plan-Do-Study-Act method (Langley et al., 2009), recommended by the Institute for Healthcare Improvement (n.d.), was used as a framework to guide this project. The APRN-project lead identified key stakeholders and obtained a letter of support from senior LTC facility leadership. A literature review helped identify an evidence-based walking program for LTC residents (MacRae et al., 1996; Schnelle et al., 2002; Schnelle et al., 1995). Additional interventions were selected to support the implementation of a consistent walking program including (a) an environment and policy assessment, (b) identifying a champion, (c) staff training, and (d) mentoring and motivating (Galik et al., 2014; Taylor et al., 2015). The LTC facility's leadership commitment and support allowed securing the resources essential for the project implementation. A critical step in the planning phase was the assessment of all residents for eligibility and enrollment in a walking program that was provided 5 days a week. The APRN-project lead, with input from the facility's staff, designed the tools to collect data and manually completed data collection. The first assessment was completed based on a mobility screening questionnaire used in previous research studies (Schnelle et al., 1995). Then, the final eligibility of residents for a walking program was assessed during walking trials. The project was implemented on one floor of the LTC facility over 20 weeks. It was monitored closely by the APRN-project lead and a facility champion-restorative nurse.

Evaluation

The process evaluation was ongoing and focused on three sections of the Logic Model-inputs, activities, and outputs (W. K. Kellogg Foundation, 2017). The evaluation included questions and measures to describe how the walking program was working and why. The main measures were designed to describe the impact of walking activity on residents enrolled in the program.

Results

All staff participated and completed education about the walking program and its potential benefits. Among the 78 residents screened, 17% ($n = 13$) were eligible and enrolled in the walking program whereas severe functional decline and/or physical disability were the primary reasons for exclusion. Of all enrolled residents, 77% were identified with severe or moderate cognitive impairment with the Brief Interview for Mental Status assessment score between 6 and 12, the majority were African American (70%), female (62%), and 70 years of age (ranging from 42–91). The residents' length of stay at the LTC facility was between 6 months to 6 years. As reported by Kazana and Pencak Murphy (2018), after 20 weeks, 69% ($n = 9$) of residents continued their participation in the walking program. None of the residents experienced a fall or any acute symptoms during walking activity. None of the residents stopped participation in the walking activity due to dissatisfaction with the program. With respect to walking, 77% of the residents were provided the activity at least 60% of the time, 23% of the residents only one to two times per week, and no residents received the activity 100% (or five times a week) as intended.

Discussion

The project results supported feasibility of a walking program implementation for LTC residents and demonstrated that residents tolerated walking well without any adverse events during activity. Our observations were consistent with Danilovich et al. (2017) who claimed that even frail older adults tolerated high-intensity walking activity well. In addition, Fien et al. (2019) reported that LTC residents in their 80s, cognitively impaired, using a walker or a cane tolerated a structured exercise program and increased their gait speed. One of our unanswered questions was why 23% of the residents were provided activity only one to two times a week. Kuk et al. (2018) suggested that gaps in communication and lack of accountability within teams had strong negative effect on promoting functional activity in LTC, possibly more than short staffing. Thus, multiple changes in management and senior leadership in our LTC facility during the project planning and implementation might have been a contributing factor.

Conclusion

While challenges to implement a sustainable walking program for LTC residents may arise from multiple organizational factors (Douma et al., 2017), they can be mitigated with leadership support and staff engagement (Slaughter et al., 2018). Often, the residents with chronic pain, dementia, or physical frailty can do more than they or healthcare providers think they can do. While walking activity has a potential for maintaining or even improving residents' functional status (Frändin et al., 2016; DHHS, 2018; Schnelle et al., 2003), acute decline in walking distance or in gait speed might be an early signal of change in a resident's health (Danilovich et al., 2017). Usually restorative nurses oversee physical activity of LTC residents, and nurse assistants play an instrumental role in daily care provided to the residents. However, implementation of a sustainable and effective walking program requires commitment and ongoing support from LTC providers, including nurse practitioners, and LTC leadership (Kagwa et al., 2018).

Recommendations for Clinical Practice

APRNs can play a critical role in engaging LTC residents in walking activity. First, APRNs working in LTC can recommend or even prescribe physical activity when it is appropriate. Also, many APRNs, especially those doctorally prepared, can lead transformation efforts and become quality improvement (QI) project leaders. In addition, by implementing resident-centered components with measuring the distance (Kazana & Pencak Murphy, 2018) or the time residents walk could enhance understanding of those residents' well-being overall (Middleton et al., 2015).

Summary

This exemplar highlights content from Chapter 4, Continuous Quality Improvement. A key component for any practice change is to evaluate its impact on patient outcomes and processes. This APRN-led project incorporated a continuous QI model to guide the Plan, Do, Study, Act phases as described.

▓ EXEMPLAR 3: FALL PREVENTION PROGRAM IN AN ASSISTED LIVING FACILITY

Background

Among adults 65 and older, falls are the seventh highest cause of death and the leader in fatal and non-fatal injuries (Bergen et al., 2016; Burns & Kakara, 2018). When compared to community-dwelling older adults, assisted living facility (ALF) residents are at a greater risk of falling due to a higher level of care needs and functional dependence (Kistler et al., 2016; Matthews et al., 2016;

Towne et al., 2017). Subsequently, ALF average fall rates range from 3 to 13 falls per 1,000 resident bed days of care (Francis-Coad et al., 2018).

Identifying the Problem

At one non-profit religiously affiliated ALF in suburban Chicago, the resident fall rate was 14.5 falls per 1,000 resident bed days of care, over 11.5% higher than the average ALF fall rate. Consequently, the facility's fall-related minor injury rate per 1,000 resident bed days was 3.57. Therefore, the purpose of this project was to (a) decrease the rate of falls and fall-related minor injuries, and (b) increase staff knowledge about falls among older adults in the pilot ALF through the development of a multicomponent evidence-based fall prevention program.

Methods to Address the Problem

Care complexity and functional impairment of ALF residents closely resembles that of nursing home (NH) patients (Kistler et al., 2016; Matthews et al., 2016). Therefore, the Agency for Healthcare Research and Quality's (AHRQs) Falls Management Program for NHs served as the foundation of the pilot ALF's fall prevention program. The AHRQs Falls Management Program components used in the program included (a) formation of an interdisciplinary fall committee, (b) delivery of the general fall education and the new protocol training, (c) completion of the multifactorial fall risk assessments, and (d) establishment of individualized fall prevention care plans using evidence-based interventions (Taylor et al., 2005).

Lewin's Change Theory was used to engage key stakeholders and promote positive behavior change. Lewin's change stages and project activities aligned in the following manner: (a) *unfreezing*: identification of key stakeholders (director of nursing, residents, physical therapist, pharmacist, RNs, and certified nurse assistants) and creating motivation for change by providing evidence of the problem and education about the significant of falls; (b) *moving*: formation of the fall committee with stakeholders, development of fall program, preparation of staff through training sessions, and implementation of new protocol; (c) *refreezing*: maintenance of behavior and system change with monthly booster sessions, project evaluation, communication of result to stakeholders, and transition of project leader role to director of nursing (Tetef, 2017; Wojciechowski et al., 2016).

Evaluation Plan

This quality improvement project used a pre-post approach to evaluate staff knowledge, fall rates, and fall-related minor injury rates. Descriptive statistics were used to assess pre- and post-intervention measures. Changes in continuous variables were examined using t-tests or one-way analysis of variance and categorical variables were examined using Chi-square analysis.

Results

The fall prevention program spanned 3 months followed by a 3-month post evaluation. The sample included 29 residents with 79% being female and 21% male. Average resident age was 89.7 years. Staff consisted of eight full-time equivalent (FTE) RNs and 36 FTE certified nursing assistants. Of the RNs, all were female and held associate nursing degrees. Of the certified nursing assistants, 8% were male and 92% female.

Both RN and certified nursing assistant average post-education test scores increased, indicating a change in knowledge of falls (+6.7%, $p = .022$; +6.7%, $p = .007$, respectively). Although resident fall-related minor injury rates reduced in months 1 and 3 of the program and at the 3-month post-evaluation (33%, 28%, and 11%, respectively), no statistically significant changes were noted. Fall rates reduced in months 1 and 3 of the program and 3-months post-evaluation (33% and 73%, respectively), with significance reductions noted at the 3-month evaluation (44%, −10.44 falls per 1,000 resident bed days, $p = .01$). Month 2 of the program showed a rise in both fall-related minor injury and fall rates by 72% and 12%, respectively. One resident accounted for 40% of falls and injuries in this month, which impacted the overall increase in injury and fall rates as reported in Cunningham et al. (2018).

Discussion

Both the American Geriatrics Society (AGS; Kenny et al., 2011) and the National Institute for Health and Care Excellence (2017) guidelines support the use of a multifactorial intervention, in which a multifactorial fall risk assessment is completed followed by tailored fall interventions. This APRN-led project integrated similar evidence-based recommendations for the 3-month fall prevention program. Similarly, Vlaeyen et al. (2015) also used multifactorial interventions which resulted in both decreased falls and recurrent falls. However, a recent Cochrane Review reported that a multifactorial intervention has uncertain or minimal impact on reducing fall rates or risk (Cameron et al., 2018). These varying outcomes among project results presented in the literature poses challenges for standardizing fall prevention protocol for ALFs.

Currently, there is no standardized fall prevention program to reduce or prevent falls in ALFs. However, this project serves as a useful model for developing and implementing a fall prevention program in an ALF. Key stakeholders were engaged in project strategies which may have positively influenced positive outcomes. At the staff level, direct care staff provide 80% of the resident's care (Gray et al., 2016); therefore, significantly improving the staff's baseline fall knowledge and utilizing both the RNs and certified nursing assistants as the main personnel to deliver the new protocol may have contributed to the program's success (Walker et al., 2016; Wilson et al., 2016).

Conclusion

These program results support that a multifactorial fall program using AHRQs FMP components can effectively improve staff knowledge of falls and reduce the rate of falls and fall-related minor injuries among ALF residents. Outcomes support that an APRN-led quality improvement project can positively impact resident outcomes and successfully create a system change in the assisted living setting.

Recommendations for Practice

APRNs will play an important role in the care of older adults across a variety of practice settings. Moreover, DNP-prepared APRNs are instrumental in integrating evidence-based research into clinical practice, which can ultimately translate into delivery of higher quality care outcomes (Trautman et al., 2018). The strategies used in this fall prevention program can be used by APRNs to reduce falls and falls with injuries in ALFs.

Summary

This exemplar highlights content from Chapter 16, Implementing Evidence-Based Practice. The use of a change theory was the framework for the implementation plan.

Essential for the success of this APRN-led project was establishing a team, ongoing effective communication, and planning for sustainability.

■ EXEMPLAR 4: INTEGRATION OF AN ADVANCE CARE PLANNING MODEL IN HOME HEALTH

Background

Chronically ill individuals often fail to recognize the significance of a life-limiting prognosis and continue to seek aggressive medical care largely due to poor communication with their healthcare team (Lewis et al., 2016). Evidence demonstrates that lack of advance care planning (ACP) and documented advance directives (ADs) is directly correlated to higher hospital readmission rates and a lower hospice length of stay at the end-of-life.

Identifying the Problem

Only 2.3% of patients at a Midwest home health (HH) agency had documented ADs, compared to 28% nationally. Of concern, this HH agency lacked standardized procedures for ACP leading to inadequate staff knowledge regarding end-of-life, avoidable hospital readmissions, and delayed transitions into hospice care. The purpose of this initiative was to develop evidence-based procedures using the Respecting Choices® ACP model to: (a) educate staff, (b) increase ACP conversations offered and completed among high-risk patients, (c) increase Practitioner Orders for Life-Sustaining Treatment (POLST) rates, (d) reduce 60-day hospital readmissions, and (e) support hospice care admissions.

Methods to Address the Problem

Staff trained for this ACP initiative included licensed clinical social workers (LCSWs), RNs, physical therapists (PTs), occupational therapists (OTs), and speech therapists (STs). Stakeholder support was obtained early on as the identified problem aligned with the organization's mission to provide patient-centered care. This initiative used a pre-post design. The Respecting Choices® model was adapted for an evidence-based approach to ACP conversations and AD completion. Three intervention phases were delineated including: (a) system redesign, (b) staff education, and (c) dissemination. Inclusion criteria for the ACP initiative consisted of HH patients identified as: (a) high-risk for hospital readmission and/or (b) high-risk for needing a hospice referral. Identification of high-risk patients was accomplished through Outcome and Assessment Information Set M1033, a 10-item Medicare Electronic Medical Record (EMR) tool, which was completed on all patient admissions to this HH agency (Centers for Medicare & Medicaid Services, 2018).

Standard procedures were developed for high-risk HH patients to be identified and approached regarding ACP conversations. During *system redesign,* a multidisciplinary process was created to outline each staff member's role and responsibilities. Two ACP tools were developed and integrated into the EMR system for staff to document: ACP goals, code status, healthcare power of attorney, and completed POLST forms (Hammes & Briggs, 2011). For *staff education* the Knowledge-Attitudinal-Experiential Survey on Advance Directives (KAESAD) was used to assess staff pre-intervention knowledge, confidence, and experiences surrounding ACP/ADs. Staff received a 2-hour mandatory educational session on the new ACP initiative and the last education sessional session was filmed for those unable to attend a live-course. The KAESAD was administered after this educational session as a post-test. Moreover, three LCSWs achieved Respecting Choices® First Steps facilitator certification and also attended a 2-hour educational session regarding Respecting Choices® Last Steps ACP. Lastly, during the *dissemination* phase, an interdisciplinary ACP steering committee was assembled to serve as champions and routinely assess the initiative's progress.

Evaluation

Staff knowledge, confidence, and experiences within this HH agency were measured pre- and post-education using the KAESAD instrument. Additionally, standardized EMR tools that were created for this initiative were used to track ACP conversations, POLST rates, 60-day hospital readmissions and hospice admissions. Paired *t*-test and Chi square analyses compared changes pre- and post-implementation.

Results

The KAESAD survey was analyzed for 75 staff (100% response rate) and demonstrated improvement in ACP/AD knowledge, confidence, and experiences, as reported by Mauleon and Staffileno (2019). Among the 50 pre and 179 post patient charts reviewed there were increases in ACP offered 6% to 80% ($p < 0.001$); ACP conversations completed 4% to 31% ($p < .001$); POLST rates 26% to 43.6%, ($p = .059$); decreased 60-day hospital readmissions 40% to 20% ($p = .025$); while hospice care admissions was not impacted 10% to 5.5% ($p = .381$).

Discussion

The purpose of the initiative was to develop an evidence-based ACP procedure to improve ACP conversations and POLST rates, reduce 60-day hospital readmissions, and support hospice care admissions. Several notable findings were observed. First, significant improvement occurred in both the rate of ACP conversations offered and ACP conversations completed by trained LCSW Respecting Choices® ACP facilitators. The results of this project were congruent with a recent Cochrane Review that examined outcomes of the Respecting Choices® model and derivative ACP models conducted in inpatient and outpatient settings (MacKenzie et al., 2018). The review validates that using the Respecting Choices® ACP model increases ACP conversations and enhances patient/surrogate congruency surrounding treatment (MacKenzie et al., 2018). A second finding was a substantial increase in POLST rates documented in the EMR. Studies specifically involving Respecting Choices® Last Steps, ACP, and POLST facilitation found that ACP conversations increase the likelihood of a completed POLST form in a patient's chart (Hickman et al., 2016; Torke et al., 2018). Third, there was a notable reduction in 60-day hospital readmissions, but no difference in hospice admission rates. Fewer studies have examined the correlation between implementation of the Respecting Choices® ACP model and healthcare utilization at the end-of-life and weaker correlations with a high-risk of bias exist (MacKenzie et al., 2018; Rocque et al., 2017).

This initiative was distinctive, as it was conducted in an agency with patients receiving traditional HH services. Comparably, ACP programs in recent literature have been piloted in hospitals, ambulatory settings, assisted livings, skilled nursing facilities, and home-based palliative care programs.

Conclusion

Chronically ill patients are inconsistently approached regarding end-of-life decision-making and often seek out continued aggressive treatment largely due to poor communication with their healthcare team. HH agencies care for individuals as they near the end of life and therefore have an unprecedented opportunity to engage patients and families in ACP discussions and assist them with ADs to ensure life-sustaining treatments are consistent with their personal goals and values (Hammes & Briggs, 2011).

Recommendation for Clinical Practice

This ARPN-led initiative validates that implementing evidence-based ACP procedures within a HH agency significantly improves ACP conversations, increased POLST rate completion, and reduces 60-day hospital readmissions. Hospice care admissions were not impacted in this particular HH population and future well-designed studies are needed to determine the long-term impact of ACP initiatives within other HH settings. Moreover, APRNs are well positioned to lead healthcare system changes surrounding ACP and AD completion and help to advocate for patients at the end of life.

Summary

This exemplar highlights content from Chapter 7, Identifying a Focus of Practice Inquiry. This APRN-led project focused on a timely and significant problem that was supported with data from the practice site. The knowledge gained from this project can be used by APRNs and transferred to similar practice settings.

▬ SUMMARY

This book teaches APRNs prepared at the masters and doctoral levels how to (a) find relevant and current evidence, (b) appraise the evidence, and (c) translate evidence into practice to improve patient care and outcomes. The exemplars presented in this chapter showcase APRNs using this knowledge and skill in real-world settings to address important clinical problems. As described in each exemplar, key strategies for addressing clinical problems include engaging key stakeholders, using an evidence-based approach, and using collaborative communication and skills to lead teams. Skills required to lead effective change initiatives evident across the exemplars include searching for evidence, critical appraisal of evidence, identifying a theoretical or implementation framework, developing a rigorous evaluation plan, and disseminating results. As practice scholars, APRNs generate new knowledge through practice innovation. Furthermore, this new knowledge and lessons learned can be of value when implementing to other practice settings to improve patient outcomes.

REFERENCES

Bergen, G., Stevens, M. R., & Burns, E. R. (2016). Falls and fall injuries among adults aged ≥65 years: United States 2014. *Morbidity and Mortality Weekly Report, 65*(37), 993–998. https://doi.org/10.15585/mmwr.mm6537a2

Brockhopp, D., Hill, K., Moe, K., & Wright, L. (2016). Transforming practice through publication: A community hospital approach to the creation of a research- intensive environment. *The Journal of Nursing Administration, 46*(1), 38–42. https://doi.org/10.1097/NNA.0000000000000294

Burns, E., & Kakara, R. (2018) Deaths from falls among persons aged ≥65 years: United States, 2007-2016. *Morbidity and Mortality Weekly Report, 67*(18), 509–514. https://doi.org/10.15585/mmwr.mm6718a1

Cameron, I. D., Dyer, S. M., Panagoda, C. E., Murray G. R., Hill, K. D., Cumming, R. G., & Kerse, N. (2018). Interventions for preventing falls in older people in care facilities and hospitals. *The Cochrane Database of Systematic Reviews 2018, 9,* CD005465. https://doi.org/10.1002/14651858.CD005465.pub4

Centers for Disease Prevention and Prevention. (2019). *Physical activity. Walking.* https://www.cdc.gov/physicalactivity/walking/index.htm

Centers for Medicare & Medicaid Services. (2018). *Outcome and assessment information set (OASIS) quality measure development and maintenance project.* https://www.cms.gov/Medicare/Quality-Initiatives-Patient-Assessment-Instruments/HomeHealthQualityInits/Downloads/OASIS-Field-Test-Summary-Report_02-2018.pdf

Connor, L., Dwyer, P., & Oliveira, J. (2016). Nurses' use of evidence-based practice in clinical practice after attending a formal evidence-based practice course. *Journal for Nurses in Professional Development, 32*(1), E1–E7. https://doi.org/10.1097/NND.0000000000000229

Cunningham, C., Murphy, M. P., Lamb, K. V., & Fogg, L. (2018). *Reduction of Falls in an Assisted Living Facility.* Poster presentation at Gerontological Advanced Practice Nursing Association annual conference, Washington, DC.

Danilovich, M. K., Conroy, D. E., & Hornby, T. G. (2017). Feasibility and impact of high-intensity walking training in frail older adults. *Journal of Aging & Physical Activity, 25*(4), 533–538. https://doi.org/10.1123/japa.2016-0305

de Souto Barreto, P., Morley, J. E., Chodzko-Zajko, W., Pitkala, K. H., Weening-Djiksterhuis, E., Rodriguez-Manas, L., Barbagallo, M., Rosendahl, E., Sinclair, A., Landi, F., Izquierdo, M., Vellas, B., & Rolland, Y. (2016). International Association of Gerontology and Geriatrics-Global Aging Research Network (IAGG-GARN) and the IAGG European Region Clinical Section. Recommendations on physical activity and exercise for older adults living in long-term care facilities: A taskforce report. *Journal of the American Medical Directors Association, 17*(5), 381–392. https://doi.org/10.1016/j.jamda.2016.01.021

den Ouden, M., Bleijlevens, M. H., Meijers, J. M., Zwakhalen, S. M., Braun, S. M., Tan, F. E., & Hamers, J. P. (2015). Daily (in)activities of nursing home residents in their wards: An observational study. *Journal of American Medical Directors Association, 16*(11), 963–968. https://doi.org/10.1016/j.jamda.2015.05.016

Dols, J. D., Hoke, M. M., & Allen, D. (2019). Building a practice-focused academic-practice partnership. *The Journal of Nursing Administration, 49*(7/8), 377–383. https://doi.org/10.1097/NNA.0000000000000771

Douma, J. G., Volkers, K. M., Engels, G., Sonnevald, M. H., Goossens, R. H. M., & Schreder, E. J. A. (2017). Setting-related influences on physical inactivity of older adults in residential care settings: A review. *BMC Geriatrics, 17,* 97. https://doi.org/10.1186/s12877-017-0487-3

Duncombe, D. C. (2017). A multi-institutional study of the perceived barriers and facilitators to implementing evidence-based practice. *Journal of Clinical Nursing, 27*(1), 1216–1226. https://doi.org/10.1111/jocn.14168

Esteban-Cornejo, I., Cabanas-Sánchez, V., Higueras-Fresnillo, S., Ortega, F. B., Kramer, A. F., Rodriguez-Artalejo, F., & Martinez-Gomez, D. (2019). Cognitive frailty and mortality in a national cohort of older adults: The role of physical activity. *Mayo Clinic Proceedings, 94*(7), 1180–1189. https://doi.org/10.1016/j.mayocp.2018.10.027

Fien, S., Henwood, T., Climstein, M., Rathbone, E., & Keogh, J. (2019). Exploring the feasibility, sustainability and the benefits of the GrACE + GAIT exercise programme in the residential aged care setting. *PeerJ-the Journal of Life and Environmental Sciences, 7,* e6973. https://doi.org/10.7717/peerj.6973

Francis-Coad, J., Etherton-Beer, C., Burton, E., Naseri, C., & Hill, A. M. (2018). Effectiveness of complex falls prevention interventions in residential aged care settings: A systematic review. *JBI Database of Systematic Reviews and Implementation Reports, 16*(4), 973–1002. https://doi.org/10.11124/JBISRIR-2017-003485

Frändin, K., Grönstedt, H., Helbostad, J. L., Bergland, A., Andresen, M., Puggaard, L., Harms-Ringdahl, K., Granbo, R., & Hellström, K. (2016). Long-term effects of individually tailored physical training and activity on physical function, well-being and cognition in Scandinavian nursing home residents: A randomized controlled trial. *Gerontology, 62,* 571–580. https://doi.org/10.1159/000443611

Galik, E., Resnick, B., Hammersla, M., & Brightwater, J. (2014). Optimizing function and physical activity among nursing home residents with dementia: Testing the impact of function-focused care. *The Gerontologist, 54*(6), 930–943. https://doi.org/10.1093/geront/gnt108

Gradone, L. D., & Staffileno, B. A. (2019). Integration of evidence-based practice at an academic medical center. *Medical Surgical Nursing, 28*(1), 53–58.

Gray, M., Shadden, B., Henry, J., Brezzo, R. D., Ferguson, A., & Fort, I. (2016) Meaning making in long-term care: What do certified nursing assistants think? *Nursing Inquiry, 23*(3), 244–252. https://doi.org/10.1111/nin.12137

Hammes, B. J., & Briggs, L. (2011). *Building a systems approach to advance care planning.* Bereavement and Advance Care Planning Services, Gundersen Lutheran Medical Foundation, Incorporated.

Hickman, S. E., Unroe, K. T., Ersek, M. T., Buente, B., Nazir, A., & Sachs, G. A. (2016). An interim analysis of an advance care planning intervention in the nursing home setting. *Journal of the American Geriatrics Society, 64*(11), 2385–2392. https://doi.org/10.1111/jgs.14463

Institute for Healthcare Improvement. (n.d.). *Resources. How to improve.* http://www.ihi.org/resources/Pages/HowtoImprove/default.aspx

Jun, J., Kovner, C. T., & Stimpfel, A. W. (2016). Barriers and facilitators of nurses' use of clinical practice guidelines: An integrative review. *International Journal of Nursing Studies, 60*, 54–68. https://doi.org/10.1016/j.ijnurstu.2016.03.006

Kagwa, S. A., Boström, A. M., Ickert, C., & Slaughter, S. E. (2018). Optimising mobility through the sit-to-stand activity for older people living in residential care facilities: A qualitative interview study of healthcare aide experiences. *International Journal of Older People Nursing, 13*, e12169. https://doi.org/10.1111/opn.12169

Kazana, I., & Pencak Murphy, M. (2018). Implementing a patient-centered walking program for residents in long-term care: A quality improvement project. *Journal of American Association of Nurse Practitioners, 30*(7), 383–391. https://doi.org/10.1097/JXX.0000000000000037

Kenny, R. A., Rubenstein, L. Z., Tinetti, M. E., Brewer, K., Cameron, K. A., Capezuti, E. A., John, D. P., Lamb, S., Martin, F., Rockey, P. H., Suther, M., Peterson, E., . . . Panel on Prevention of Falls in Older Persons, American Geriatrics Society and British Geriatrics Society. (2011). Summary of the updated American Geriatrics Society/British Geriatrics Society clinical practice guideline for prevention of falls in older persons. *Journal of American Geriatric Society, 59*(1), 148–157. https://doi.org/10.1111/j.1532-5415.2010.03234.x

Kistler, C. E., Zimmerman, S., Ward, K. T., Reed, D., Golin, C., & Lewis, C. L. (2016). Health of older adults in assisted living and implications for preventive care. *The Gerontologist, 57*(5), 949–954. https://doi.org/10.1093/geront/gnw053

Ku, P. W., Liu, Y. T., Lo, M. K., Chen, L. J., & Stubbs, B. (2017). Higher levels of objectively measured sedentary behavior is associated with worse cognitive ability: Two-year follow-up study in community-dwelling older adults. *Experimental Gerontology, 99*, 110–114. https://doi.org/10.1016/j.exger.2017.09.014

Kuk, N. O., Zijlstra, G. A. R., Bours, G. J. J. W., Hamers, J. P. H., Tan, F. E. S., & Kempen, G. I. J. M. (2018). Promoting functional activity among nursing home residents: A cross-sectional study on barriers experienced by nursing staff. *Journal of Aging and Health, 30*(4), 605–623. https://doi.org/10.1177/0898264316687407

Langley, G. L., Moen, R., Nolan, K. M., Nolan, T. W., Norman, C. L., & Provost, L. P. (2009). Chapter Five. Using the Model for Improvement. In G. L. Langley, R. Moen, K. M. Nolan, T. Nolan, C. L. Norman, & L. P. Provost, *The improvement guide: A practical approach to enhancing organizational performance* (2nd ed., pp. 89–107). Jossey-Bass Publishers.

Lavenberg, J. G., Cacchione, P. Z., Jayakumar, K. L., Leas, B. F., Mitchell, M. D., Mull, N. K., & Umscheid, C.A. (2019). Impact of a hospital evidence-based practice center (EPC) on nursing policy and practice. *Worldviews on Evidence-Based Nursing, 16*(1), 4–11. https://doi.org/10.1111/wvn.12346

Lewis, E., Cardona-Morrell, M., Ong, K. Y., Trankle, S. A., & Hillman, K. (2016). Evidence still insufficient that advance care documentation leads to engagement of health care professionals in end-of-life discussions: A systematic review. *Palliative Medicine, 30*(9), 807–824. https://doi.org/10.1177/0269216316637239

MacKenzie, M. A., Smith-Howell, E., Bomba, P. A., & Meghani, S. H. (2018). Respecting choices and related models of advance care planning: A systematic review of published evidence. *The American Journal of Hospice & Palliative Care, 35*(6), 897–907. https://doi.org/10.1177/1049909117745789

Matthews, F. E., Bennett, H., Wittenberg, R., Jagger, C., Dening, T., & Brayne, C. (2016). Who lives where and does it matter? Changes in the health profiles of older people living in long term care and the community over two decades in a high-income country. *PLOS ONE, 11*(9), e0161705. https://doi.org/10.1371/journal.pone.0161705

Mauleon, J., & Staffileno, B. A. (2019). Integration of an advance care planning model in home health: Favorable outcomes in end-of-life discussions, POLST rates, and 60-day hospital readmissions. *Home Healthcare Now, 37*(6), 337–344. https://doi.org/10.1097/NHH.0000000000000797

MacRae, P. G., Asplund L. A., Schnelle J. F., Ouslander J. G., Abrahamse A., & Morris C. (1996). A walking program for nursing home residents: Effects on walk endurance, physical activity, mobility, and quality of life. *Journal of American Geriatric Society, 44*, 175–180. https://doi.org/10.1111/j.1532-5415.1996.tb02435.x

McKinney, I., DellowStritto, R. A., & Branham, S. (2019). Nurses' use of evidence-based practice at point of care: A literature review. *Critical Care Nursing Quarterly, 42*(3), 256–264. https://doi.org/10.1097/CNQ.0000000000000266

Melnyk, B. M., & Fineout-Overholt, E. (2019). Making the case for evidence-based practice and cultivating a spirit of inquiry. In B. M. Melnyk & E. Fineout-Overholt (Eds.), *Evidence-based practice in nursing & healthcare* (pp. 7–32). Wolters Kluwer.

Melnyk, B. M., Fineoult-Overholt, E., & Mays, M. Z. (2008). The evidence-based practice beliefs and implementation scales: Psychometric properties of two new instruments. *Worldviews on Evidence-Based Nursing, 5*(4), 208–216. https://doi.org/10.1111/j.1741-6787.2008.00126.x

Melnyk, B. M., Gallagher-Ford, L., Thomas, B. K., Troseth, M., & Szalacha, L. (2016). A study of chief nurse executives indicates low prioritization of evidence-based practice and shortcomings in hospital performance metrics across the United States. *Worldviews on Evidence-Based Nursing, 13*(1), 6–14. https://doi.org/10.1111/wvn.12133

Melnyk, B. M., Gallagher-Ford, L., Zellefrow, C., Tucker, S., Thomas, B., Sinnott, L. T., & Tan, A. (2018). The first U.S. study on nurses' evidence-based practice competencies indicates major deficits that threaten healthcare quality, safety, and patient outcomes. *Worldviews on Evidence-Based Nursing, 15*(1), 16–25. https://doi.org/10.1111/wvn.12269

Middleton, A., Fritz, S. L., & Lusardi, M. (2015). Walking speed: The functional vital sign. *Journal of Aging & Physical Activity, 23*(2), 314–322. https://doi.org/10.1123/japa.23.2.314

Moore, K. L., Boscardin, W. J., Steinman, M. A., & Schwartz, J. B. (2014). Patterns of chronic co-morbid medical conditions in older residents of U.S. nursing homes: Differences between the sexes and across the age span. *The Journal of Nutrition, Health & Aging, 18*(4), 429–436. https://doi.org/10.1007/s12603-014-0001-y

National Institute for Health and Care Excellence. (2017). *Falls in older people*. https://www.nice.org.uk/guidance/qs86/resources/falls-in-older-people-pdf-2098911933637

Parry, S., Chow, M., Batchelor, F., & Fary, R. E. (2019). Physical activity and sedentary behavior in a residential aged care facility. *Australasian Journal on Ageing, 38*(1), E12–E18. https://doi.org/10.1111/ajag.12589

Patterson, R., McNamara, E., Tainio, M., de Sá, T. H., Smith, A. D., Sharp, S. J., Edwards, P., Woodcock, J., Brage, S., & Wijndaele, K. (2018). Sedentary behaviour and risk of all-cause, cardiovascular and cancer mortality, and incident type 2 diabetes: A systematic review and dose response meta-analysis. *European Journal of Epidemiology, 33*(9), 811–829. https://doi.org/10.1007/s10654-018-0380-1

Pravikoff, D. S., Tanner, A. B., & Pierce, S. T. (2005). Readiness of U.S. nurses for evidence-based practice. *The American Journal of Nursing, 105*(9), 40–51. https://doi.org/10.1097/00000446-200509000-00025

Rocque, G. B., Dionne-Odom, J. N., Huang, C. H. S., Niranjan, S. J., Williams, C. P., Jackson, B. E., Halilova, K. I., Kenzik, K. M., Bevis, K. S., Wallace, A. S., Lisovicz, N., . . . Taylor, R. A. (2017). Implementation and impact of patient lay navigator-led advance care planning conversations. *Journal of Pain and Symptom Management, 53*(4), 682–692. https://doi.org/10.1016/j.jpainsymman.2016.11.012

Rodríguez-Gómez, I., Mañas, A., Losa-Reyna, J., Rodríguez-Mañas, L., Chastin, S., Alegre, L. M., García-García, F. J., & Ara, I. (2018). Associations between sedentary time, physical activity and bone health among older people using compositional data analysis. *PloS One, 13*(10), e0206013. https://doi.org/10.1371/journal.pone.0206013

Schnelle, J. F., Alessi, C. A., Simmons, S. F., Al-Samarrai, N. R., Beck, J. C., & Ouslander, J. G. (2002). Translating clinical research into practice: A Randomized Controlled Trial of exercise and Incontinence Care with Nursing Home Residents. *Journal of the American Geriatrics Society, 50*, 1476–1483. https://doi.org/10.1046/j.1532-5415.2002.50401.x

Schnelle, J. F., Kapur, K., Alessi, C., Osterweil, D., Beck, J. G., Al-Samarrai, N. R., & Ouslander, J. G. (2003). Does an exercise and incontinence intervention save healthcare costs in a nursing home population? *Journal of the American Geriatrics Society, 51*(2), 161–168. https://doi.org/10.1046/j.1532-5415.2003.51053.x

Schnelle, J. F., MacRae, P. G., Ouslander, J. G., Simmons, S. F., & Nitta, M. (1995). Functional incidental training, mobility performance, and incontinence care with nursing home residents. *Journal of the American Geriatrics Society, 43*(12), 1356–1362. https://doi.org/10.1111/j.1532-5415.1995.tb06614.x

Sim, J. Y., Jang, K. S., & Kim, N. M. (2016). Effects of education programs on evidence-based practice implementation for clinical nurses. *Journal of Continuing Education in Nursing, 47*(8), 363–371. https://doi.org/10.3928/00220124-20160715-08

Slaughter, S. E., Bampton, E., Erin, D. F., Ickert, C., Wagg, A., Jones, C. A., Schalm, C., & Eastabrooks, C. (2018). Knowledge translation interventions to sustain direct care provider behaviour change in long-term care: A process evaluation. *Journal of Evaluation in Clinical Practice, 24*(1), 159–165. https://doi.org/10.1111/jep.12784

Soares-Miranda, L., Siscovick, D. S., Psaty, B. M., Longstreth, W.T. Jr., & Mozaffarian, D. (2016). Physical activity and risk of coronary heart disease and stroke in older adults: The cardiovascular health study, *Circulation, 133*(2), 147–155. https://doi.org/10.1161/CIRCULATIONAHA.115.018323

Stannard, D. (2019). A practical definition of evidence-based practice for nursing. *Journal of PeriAnesthesia Nursing, 34*(5), 1080–1084. https://doi.org/10.1016/j.jopan.2019.07.002

Taylor, J., Barker, A., Hill, H., & Haines, T. (2015). Improving person-centered mobility   care in nursing homes: A feasibility study. *Geriatric Nursing, 36*(2), 98–105. https://doi.org/10.1016/j.gerinurse.2014.11.002

Taylor, J. A., Parmelee, P., Brown, H., & Ouslander, J. (2005). *The falls management program: A quality improvement initiative for nursing facilities.* Agency for Healthcare Research and Qaulity. https://www.ahrq.gov/sites/default/files/publications/files/fallspxmanual.pdf

Tan, Z. S., Spartano, N. L., Beiser, A. S., DeCarli, C., Auerbach, S. H., Vasan, R. S., & Seshadri, S. (2017). Physical activity, brain volume, and dementia risk: The Framingham Study. *Journals of Gerontology. Series A, Biological Sciences and Medical Sciences, 72*(6), 789–795. https://doi.org/10.1093/gerona/glw130

Tetef, S. (2017). Successful implementation of new technology using an interdepartmental collaborative approach. *Journal of PeriAnestehsia Nurses, 32*(3), 225–230. https://doi.org/10.1016/j.jopan.2015.05.118

Torke, A., Hickman, S., Hammes, B., Counsell, S., Inger, L., Slaven, J., & Butler, D. (2018). POLST facilitation in complex care management: A feasibility study. *American Journal of Hospice & Palliative Medicine, 36,* 5–12. https://doi.org/10.1177/1049909118797077

Towne, S. D., Cho, J., Smith, M. L., & Ory, M. G. (2017). Factors associated with injurious falls in residential care facilities. *Journal of Aging and Health, 29*(4), 669–687. https://doi.org/10.1177/0898264316641083

Trautman, D. E., Idzik, S., Hammersla, M., & Rosseter, R. (2018). Advancing scholarship through translational research: The role of PhD and DNP prepared nurses. *The Online Journal of Issues in Nursing, 23*(2). https://doi.org/10.3912/OJIN.Vol23No02Man02

U.S. Department of Health and Human Services (HHS), The 2018 Physical Activity Guidelines Advisory Committee. (2018). *Physical Activity Guidelines for Americans* (2nd ed.). https://health.gov/paguidelines/second-edition/committee

Vlaeyen, E., Coussement, J., Leysens, G., Van der Elst, E., Delbaere, K., Cambier, D., Denhaerynck, K., Goemaere, S., Wertelaers, A., Dobbels, F., Dejaeger, E., Milisen, K., & the Center of Expertise for Fall and Fracture Prevention Flanders. (2015). Characteristics and effectiveness of fall prevention programs in nursing homes: A systematic review and meta-analysis of randomized controlled trials. *Journal of the American Geriatrics Society, 63,* 211–221. https://doi.org/10.1111/jgs.13254

Walker, G. M., Armstrong, S., Gordon, A. L., Gladman, J., Robertson, K., Ward, M., Conroy, S., Arnold, G., Darby, J., Frowd, N., Williams, W., Knowles, S., & Logan, P. A. (2016). The falls in care home study: A feasibility randomized controlled trial of the use of a risk assessment and decision to support tool to prevent falls in care homes. *Clinical Rehabilitation, 30*(10), 972–983. https://doi.org/10.1177/0269215515604672

Wilson, D. S., Montie, M., Conlon, P., Reynolds, M., Ripley, R., & Titler, M. G. (2016). Nurses' perceptions of implementing fall prevention interventions to mitigate patient-specific fall risk factors. *Western Journal of Nursing Research, 38*(8), 1012–1034. https://doi.org/10.1177/0193945916644995

W. K. Kellogg Foundation. (2017, November). *W. K. Kellogg Foundation step-by-step guide to evaluation: How to become savvy evaluation consumers.* https://www.wkkf.org/resource-directory/resources/2017/11/the-step-by-step-guide-to-evaluation--how-to-become-savvy-evaluation-consumers

Wojciechowski, E., Pearsall, T., Murphy, P., & French, E. (2016). A case review: Integrating Lewin's theory with the Lean's system approach for changes. *The Journal of Issues in Nursing, 21*(2), 4. https://doi.org/10.3912/OJIN.Vol21No02Man04

Wu, Y., Brettle, A., Zhou, C., Ou, J., Wang, Y., & Wang, S. (2018). Do educational interventions aimed at nurses to support the implementation of evidence-based practice improve patient outcomes? A systematic review. *Nurse Education Today, 70,* 109–114. https://doi.org/10.1016/j.nedt.2018.08.026

INDEX

Printed in the United States
by Baker & Taylor Publisher Services